HEMOSTASIS LABORATORY YEARBOOK

VOLUME 1

HEMOSTASIS LABORATORY YEARBOOK

Additional books in this series can be found on Nova's website under the Series tab.

Additional E-books in this series can be found on Nova's website under the E-book tab.

HEMOSTASIS LABORATORY YEARBOOK

VOLUME 1

THOMAS W. STIEF
EDITOR

Nova Science Publishers, Inc.
New York

For permission to use material from this book please contact us:
Telephone 631-231-7269; Fax 631-231-8175
Web Site: http://www.novapublishers.com

Library of Congress Cataloging-in-Publication Data

ISSN: 2159-8746

ISBN: 978-1-60741-089-8

Published by Nova Science Publishers, Inc. + New York

CONTENTS

PREFACE

Hemostasis (coagulation and fibrinolysis) is of importance in a broad range of medical disciplines. A high-quality hemostasis diagnosis enables a good therapy, which can be rather complicated without laboratory help. This new yearbook gathers important contributions in this field and presents them in a coherent and logical format.

Article 1 –Hemostasis is classified in Analytical Hemostasis and Clinical Hemostasis. Hemostasis Laboratory focuses on Analytical Hemostasis = the laboratory aspects of hemostasis. Detailed test information allows a better understanding of the hemostasis state of the individual patient.

The topic of this issue is Hemostasis and Infection/Inflammation. Hemostasis, Infection, and Inflammation are complex biologic systems with many important cross reactions. Hemostasis is classified in primary, secondary, and tertiary hemostasis. Primary hemostasis is the medicine (physiology, biochemistry, pathophysiology, pathobiochemistry) of the thrombocytes and their interaction with cells of the blood stream and the vessel wall. Secondary hemostasis is the medicine of plasmatic coagulation. The central enzyme of plasmatic coagulation is thrombin (IIa). Blood contact with unphysiologic, polynegative surfaces generates via kallikrein-genesis the intrinsic tenase. Tissue factor (TF) generates the extrinsic tenase. The generation and the inactivation of the factors Xa or IIa are of clinical importance. Tertiary hemostasis is the medicine of cellular and plasmatic fibrinolysis. Polymorphonuclear neutrophil granulocytes (PMN) are the main cells of cellular fibrinolysis. The central enzyme of fibrinolysis is plasmin. Urokinase and tissue-plasminogen activator (t-PA) are the human activators of plasminogen, plasmin is inhibited by plasmin-inhibitor.

Article 2 – The rapid laboratory diagnosis of the pre-phase of pathologic disseminated intravascular coagulation (PDIC phase 0) is a major clinical challenge. PDIC means multiple micro-thrombi that obstruct vital organ areas, and that can cause multi-organ failure. There is clinical need for reliable hemostasis parameters to diagnose the pre-phase of PDIC to start the adequate treatment in time. The routine hemostasis tests such as prothrombin time and activated partial thromboplastin time are too blunted to diagnose the early phases of PDIC; furthermore, thrombocytes might be dysfunctional, cell fragments might be counted as platelets, platelets-count or fibrinogen concentration are acute phase parameters that might increase instead of decrease, and antithrombin activity might change only slightly or it might be altered in an artificially diluted test matrix.

In the present review new routine parameters for diagnosis of the early phases of PDIC are presented: basal chromogenic thrombin activity (IIa-Test), thrombin (IIa) generation after plasma recalcification (RECA), IIa generation after intrinsic activation of plasma (INCA), or

IIa generation after extrinsic activation of plasma (EXCA), fibrinogen function+antigen+ratio, undiluted antithrombin activity, and active endotoxin (here clinically understood as active lipopolysaccharide or active ß-glucan). A combination of these new assays allows to diagnose the pre-phase of PDIC within minutes. Especially the functional ultra-specific IIa-Test (normal range 100±20%; 100%=5.5 mIU/ml) or the therefrom derived standardized RECA helps to distinguish the normal systemic intravascular coagulation from the dynamic PDIC phase 0 (120-150% of normal basal IIa) or from the PDIC phase 1 (> 150% of normal basal IIa). All these simple photometric assays do not require special hemostasis machines to test the dynamic coagulation state of each individual patient.

Article 3 – Usual drugs against human immuno deficiency virus (HIV) have complex heterocyclic or homocyclic structures; the cytochrome P-450 system (CYP450) hydroxylates such organic ring structures and can transform them into generators of reactive oxygen species (H2O2, ·OH, 1ΔO2) that might be a main therapeutic way to destroy HIV. The lipid membrane of HIV is stabilized by only about 14 protein spikes (gp160 trimers) per virion and contains more molecules of oxidizable unsaturated fatty acids or cholesterol per nm^2 than the human cell membrane, and is thus more susceptible to 1ΔO2 than human cells. Nonradical generators of 1ΔO2 (e.g. the physiological taurine-chloramine) could be new therapeutics against AIDS. Chloramines at blood concentrations of about 1 mM are still tolerable to hemostasis of human blood: the 50 % inhibitory concentration (IC50) of 1ΔO2 sensible thrombocytes, fibrinogen, factor VIII, factor V, factor X, antithrombin, and plasmin-inhibitor is > 1 mM chloramine. Thrombin generation in the ultra-specific, ultra-sensitive recalcified coagulation activity assay (RECA) does not increase in 1 mM chloramine–oxidized whole citrated blood with hemolysis being < 0.1 g/l free hemoglobin. HIV or other lipid enveloped viruses in blood might be eliminated by slow infusion of about 1 mM chloramine, a pro-drug of 1ΔO2.

Article 4 – There is clinical need for a simple rapid assay that detects active endotoxin (here clinically understood as active lipopolysaccharide (LPS) or active ß-glucan) in blood of patients. Hitherto Limulus-based endotoxin tests cannot be used for plasma testing due to the presence of strong plasmatic serine protease inhibitors of the Limulus clotting system. It was the aim of the present study to destroy these inhibitors without affecting the true content of active endotoxin in plasma.

10 µl citrated or EDTA plasma were oxidized with 10 µl 60 mM chloramine-T® for 10 min (37°C). 10 µl 230 mM methionine without or with 0.63 mg/ml of the LPS inhibitor polymyxin B were added. Then 30 µl Limulus reagent, that contained the factors C,B,G,A and the chromogenic substrate for activated factor A (FAa) Ile-Glu-Gly-Arg-pNA, were added and the increase in absorbance with time was measured.

The normal range is 0.8±0.2 ng/ml LPS reactivity (MV±1SD) and < 0.1 µg/ml ß-glucan reactivity. This method allows to quantify plasmatic LPS reactivities from 0.1 to 1000 ng/ml (about 10-100000 % of normal) and ß-glucan reactivities from 0.1 to 100 µg/ml; e.g. an extreme LPS reactivity of 100 ng/ml means that this plasma behaves in the Limulus assay as if pooled normal plasma with 0.8 ng/ml LPS would have been supplemented with 99.2 ng purified LPS/ml plasma. Only about 1 % of added purified LPS or about 10 % of added purified ß-glucan is free=unbound=active. These new assays will help to diagnose the very early phase of gram-negative or fungal sepsis.

Article 5 – Background: Early diagnosis and rapid treatment are important for survival in patients with severe sepsis. However, conventional microbiological techniques are time consuming. Therefore, new plasma methods have been developed to accelerate diagnosis and to permit rapid evaluation of the antibiotic treatment. Active endotoxin (here clinically understood as free lipopolysaccharide (LPS) or free ß-glucan) is proposed to indicate the diagnosis and severity of sepsis syndrome and the patient´s risk to develop infection-associated severe complications such as pathologic disseminated intravascular coagulation (PDIC).

Material and Methods: Active plasmatic endotoxin is measured via a modified Limulus test: 10 µl EDTA-plasma of 63 patients with severe sepsis at their first day in intensive care unit and of 48 healthy donors and plasmatic reactivity standards supplemented with 0-1000 ng/ml purified LPS or with 0-100 µg/ml purified Zymosan A (a ß-glucan) were incubated with 5 µl 106 mM sodium citrate, pH 7.4, and with 10 µl 60 mM chloramine-T® for 10 min (37°C). 10 µl 230 mM methionine without (testing for active LPS + active ß-glucan) or with 0.63 mg/ml polymyxin B (testing only for active ß-glucan) were added. Then 30 µl Limulus factors / Ile-Glu-Gly-Arg-pNA reagent were added and the increase in absorbance with time was measured. An exemplary LPS reactivity of 20.8 ng/ml means that this plasma is as active as pooled normal plasma (with 0.8 ng/ml LPS reactivity) that had been supplemented with additional 20 ng/ml purified LPS.

Results: The patients with severe sepsis had ≥ 3 ng/ml LPS reactivity or ≥ 0.5 µg/ml ß-glucan reactivity, or both. 81 % of the patients had a LPS reactivity ≥ 3 ng/ml: these had 25.3±19.1 ng/ml, range 3.9-98 ng/ml (normal range: 0.8±0.2 ng/ml). Thus, LPS reactivity increases up to about 100fold in patients with severe sepsis. 75 % of the patients had a ß-glucan reactivity ≥ 0.5 µg/ml: these had 6.3±7.5 µg/ml, range 0.5-36.2 µg/ml (normal range: < 0.1 µg/ml). Dividing the ß-glucan reactivity [ng/ml] by 300 and adding the LPS reactivity [ng/ml] gives the total endotoxin reactivity of plasma [ng/ml]. The sepsis-associated organ failure assessment (SOFA) score displayed significantly positive correlations with active LPS ($p = 0.03$), active ß-glucan ($p = 0.035$), and active total endotoxin ($p = 0.0004$).

Discussion: Plasmatic LPS reactivities of about 2-3 ng/ml or plasmatic ß-glucan reactivities of about 0.5 µg/ml are considered as threshold concentrations to cause severe hemostasis complications such as PDIC. These new plasma assays for active LPS or active ß-glucan could help to diagnose the very early phase of gram-negative or fungal sepsis.

Article 6 – The aim of this laboratory study was to test new assays that focus on fibrinolysis alterations in septic patients, aberrance of the results from normal values, and correlation to coagulation markers.

For the present work, samples of potassium-ethylene-diamine-tetraacetic acid (K3-EDTA)-plasma and citrated plasma were collected from n=48 intensive care patients with a clinical diagnosis of sepsis. Additionally, a subset of K3-EDTA-plasma was stabilized 1+1 with 2.5 M arginine, pH 8.6, to conserve the real state of fibrinolysis activation in unstable plasma samples as e.g. from critically ill patients.

At admission to the intensive care unit the patients had 127±118% (mean value ± 1 standard deviation) (normal range (N)=100±20%) amidolytic plasmatic plasmin activity, 43±18% (N=100±20%) plasminogen function, 130±53% (N=100±20%) antiplasmin activity, 12.5±7.9 (N=1.1±0.7) anti-urokinase units/ml PAI-1, 3.05±2.52 (N=0.049±0.025) µg/ml D-dimer, 371±142% (N=100±30%) plasmin-antiplasmin complex, 20±14% (N=100±15%)

fibrinolysis parameters assay (FIPA) activity, 1.06±0.28 (N=1.0±0.1) fibrinogen function/fibrinogen antigen ratio, and 0.58±0.59 (N=0.44±0.14) nmol/l prothrombin fragment F1+2. The intra-assay coefficients of variation of all functional or antigenic tests were < 5% or < 10%, respectively. Most patients showed a significantly decreased plasmatic fibrinolytic state, when compared with healthy individuals; amidolytic plasmin activity in EDTA-1.25 M arginine-stabilized plasma presented large aberrations in some septic patients. The FIPA mean values approximately doubled within about 1 week in the intensive care unit. The results will be the basis of further clinical studies.

Article 7 – Polymorphonuclear granulocytes (PMN = neutrophils) lyse thrombi. To study this important cellular part of fibrinolysis, 50 µl plasma-clots (without and with 0.5 µmoles chloramine) were incubated with the possible PMN modulator and with 50 µl PMN-rich citrated plasma. The turbidity decrease was measured at 405 nm and the approximate effective doses were determined (microtiter plate clot lysis assay with PMN-rich plasma = PMN-CLA).

G-CSF had an approximate 50% stimulatory concentration (SC50) of 1.5 µg/ml, 50 % thrombolysis occured within 1d. The prooxidative SC50 of G-CSF was 0.5 µg/ml. Singlet oxygen (1ΔO2) generator chloramine stimulated thrombolysis of unoxidized or oxidized clots (SC50 = 5 mM or 2 mM). 1.4 mM vancomycin was the SC50 against oxidized clots. The approximate inhibitory concentrations 50% (IC50) for unoxidized clots were: 12 mM glucose, 51 µg/ml vitamin K1 (phytomenadione=2-methyl-3-phytyl-1,4-naphtoquinone), 2 µg/ml doxycyclin, 3.4 mg/ml hydrocortisone, 0.06 mg/ml dexamethasone, > 20 IU/ml heparin, 25 IU/ml dalteparin, 4 IU/ml certoparin, 56 µg/ml pentosanpolysulphate, 0.26 mM tranexamic acid, 1.2 mM epsilon-amino-caproid-acid, 9.3 KIU/ml aprotinin, 52 mM arginine. Vitamin K1 and dexamethasone also stimulated thrombolysis at 10-20fold higher concentrations. Plasmin in unoxidized clot supernatants increased from 2 mU/ml to 10 mU/ml within 4.5d. Plasmin in oxidized clot supernatants increased 5-10fold. After 18 h (37°C) maximally about 0.16 mM chloramine was generated by 245 PMN/µl that were stimulated by 3 µg/ml G-CSF. This means that about 10000 activated PMN/µl could generate 5-10 mM chloramine. PMN enhance fibrinolysis by activation of their 1ΔO2 generating respiratory burst.

It is suggested to diagnose the cellular fibrinolysis by means of the present PMN-CLA in each individual patient, and to treat a patient with with hypo- or hyper-reactive PMN with an adequate PMN modulator.

Article 8 – Knowledge of the composition and protein release pattern of human thrombi is of importance to understand hemostasis. 9 ml pooled normal human citrated plasma were recalcified. The generated clots (about 2x10cm) were incubated in duplicate with 41 ml 0.9% NaCl or H2O. After 0-4d (37°C) the clot supernatants and the unclotted plasma were analyzed for routine clinical-chemical analytes. Plasmin was determined by incubation of 50 µl sample with 100 µl 1.5 M arginine, pH 8.7, and 150 µl 0.93 mM HD-Val-Leu-Lys-pNA, 938 mM KCl. About 50-60 % of all plasma components are initially entrapped in a plasma clot with a large surface. After 1-6 h still about 30-40 % of plasmatic proteins or cholesterol, triglycerides are entrapped in the clot. After 24 h the entrapment is only about 20 %. Active plasmin in the supernatants was < 1 mIU/ml at 0-24h, plasmin activity in the supernatants after 4d was about 5 mIU/ml. The here demonstrated plasma entrapment in a clot within the first 3h (37°C) after clot generation facilitates the study of lysis of blood thrombi, e.g. by replacing radioactive markers by gamma-glutamyl transferase (GGT) or pseudocholine esterase.

Article 9 – Activated phagocytes are important cells in hemostasis and inflammation. Essential phagocyte mediators are urokinase (u-PA), singlet oxygen (1ΔO2), and cationic proteins/polypeptides (polycations). The aim of the present work was to study the interaction of u-PA, 1O2, and polycations with plasmatic fibrinolysis.

0-60 µg poly-L-lysine (PLL; MW=60 kDa) were incubated with 0.5 IU u-PA in 100 µl 100 mM Tris, 25 mM sodium citrate, 63 mM NaCl, 1 % polygelin, 0.1 % Triton X 100®, pH 7.7 (assay buffer) for 0-3 h (37°C). Then 25 µl plasminogen activator inhibitor (PAI)–1 depleted citrated plasma and pooled plasma with 5.7 U (u-PA inhibiting units)/ml PAI–1 or with 5.7 U/ml PAI-2 were added. After 10 min (37°C) the remaining u-PA activity was determined by addition of plasminogen, 1ΔO2 generating chloramine, and chromogenic plasmin substrate.

The activity of 0.5 IU u-PA preincubated for 3h (37°C) with 25 µg PLL in 100 µl assay buffer was about 40 % higher than that of untreated u-PA. Plasmatic PAI-1 lost function when it was incubated with u-PA/PLL: the approximate 50 % inhibitory concentration (IC50) was 0.2-0.3 mg/ml for PLL of 60 kDa and 3h (37°C) u-PA/PLL preincubation. Polycations neutralize the function of PAI-1 and enhance that of PAI-2 in plasma.

Activated phagocytes release large amounts of polycations (cationic proteins or defensins). Therefore, the interactions between polycations and u-PA and that between polycations and PAI modulate inflammation, enhancing (→PAI-1) or inhibiting (→PAI-2) plasmin generation in the microenvironment of activated phagocytes.

Article 10 – Tissue factor (TF) triggers extrinsic hemostasis. Monocytes/macrophages (MØ) contain high amounts of pre-TF or TF. Upon MØ activation these cells generate large concentrations of singlet oxygen (1ΔO2). The question arises, if TF is resistant against this important oxidant.

150 µl 2.3 ng/ml placental TF in 6 % human albumin, PBS was incubated at 37°C at final chloramineT®-concentrations of 0-20 mM for 10 min. Then 150 µl 258 mM methionine were added. After 15 min (23°C) 30 µl 2.75 M CaCl2 were added. 5 µl of this oxidized 1 ng/ml TF, 239 mM Ca++ were incubated with 50 µl unfrozen pooled normal citrated plasma and the extrinsic coagulation activity assay (EXCA) was performed. For control 1, plasmatic fibrinogen was oxidized similarly and the fibrinogen function turbidimetric assay (FIFTA) was performed. For control 2, the FIFTA-reagent (0.3 IU/ml thrombin in 6 % human albumin, PBS) was oxidized similarly and the FIFTA was performed with pooled normal citrated plasma.

1-2 mM chloramine enhance the TF activity by about 40 %. The approximate 50 % inhibitory concentration (IC50) of chloramine-T® against TF is 17 mM, which is comparable to that of thrombin that is resistant to oxidation (IC50=16 mM). Plasmatic fibrinogen is sensible to singlet oxygen: the approximate IC50 of its generator chloramine is 2 mM.

The TF-resistance against 1ΔO2 might be of importance in inflammatory areas, where MØ might generate both, TF and 1ΔO2. TF causes coagulation and 1ΔO2 prevents the generation of fibrin that would limitate the inflammatory focus.

Article 11 – Activated granulocytes respond to foci of inflammation or of fibrin with the generation of millimolar concentrations of chloramines that are generators of nonradical singlet oxygen (1ΔO2). Protein C and antithrombin are the main down-regulators of plasmatic thrombin activity. Here the interaction between chloramines and these important coagulation regulators was investigated.

Pooled normal human citrated plasma (pH 7.4) was oxidized with the nonradicalic oxidant chloramine-T® for 20 min at 37°C. Then the activities of protein C and antithrombin were chromogenically tested. For control, also plasmin inhibitor was functionally determined and the global plasmatic fibrinolysis parameters assay (FIPA) was performed. Oxidative inactivation of protein C at pH 7.4 by 1.5 mM chloramine-T® is quenched by 21 mM of the 1ΔO2 - inhibitor methionine and is not affected by 21 mM or 75 mM of the hydroxyl radical (·OH)- inhibitor mannitol. Chloramine-consumption in plasma was tested by supplementation of citrated plasma with chloramine-T®. Remaining chloramine was photometrically determined at 405 nm after addition of 200 µl 4 M KI in phosphate buffered saline (PBS) to 20 µl oxidized plasma.

The approximate inhibitory concentrations 50% (IC50) of chloramine-T® against protein C, antithrombin, or plasmin-inhibitor were 2 mM, 3 mM, or 1.5 mM, respectively; 1.5 mM chloramine enhanced FIPA by 50 %. Chloramines might inactivate 1ΔO2-susceptible hemostasis factors via oxidation of critical methionines or cysteines. About 1 mM chloramine had a plasma half life of less than 1 minute. 1ΔO2 generators down-regulate the inhibition of coagulation and of fibrinolysis and possibly facilitate inflammation.

Article 12 – The aim of the present study was to compare ultra low doses of heparin and of the low molecular weight heparin enoxaparin, when the anticoagulants were added to plasma directly out of the original siliconized glass vial to obtain the final plasma concentration without further plasma dilution steps. This imitates the continuous administration of these heparins. The recalcified coagulation activity assay (RECA) was performed with n=10 citrated plasmas of healthy donors and with n=32 citrated plasmas of patients without hemostasis alterations, 50 µl plasma being supplemented with 2 µl 0, 2.6, 26, or 260 mIU/ml heparin or enoxaparin, generating final concentrations of 0, 0.1, 1, or 10 mIU/ml. Venous blood had been collected in polypropylene tubes, recalcified thrombin generation with 40 min (37°C) coagulation reaction time was performed in polystyrol microwells with flat bottom.

0.1 mIU/ml enoxaparin decreased the thrombin generation by about 30-60 %, when compared with unsupplemented plasma; the thrombin generation in plasma with 0.1 mIU/ml heparin was nearly identical or even about 20 % higher than that in unsupplemented plasma. The data demonstrate that ultra low concentrations of heparin, as e.g. occurring in the end of heparin infusions, might be dangerous especially for some susceptible patients. It is suggested to replace heparin by enoxaparin or to "bridge" the end of a heparin infusion with administration of enoxaparin, and to monitor the correct dosage of enoxaparin in each individual patient by means of a specific thrombin generation assay.

Article 13 – Background: The activity of low-molecular-weight-heparin (LMWH) or unfractionated heparin towards individual plasmatic thrombin (IIa) generation is clinically important. Here the individual anticoagulant efficiency of heparins was determined, imitating their continuous administration.

Methods: To 50 µl citrated plasma of 51 healthy donors or of 213 patients (without anticoagulation therapy; with normal PT and APTT) in polystyrol microwells 2 µl of the anticoagulants in 0.9 % NaCl were added directly out of a siliconized glass vial, resulting in final plasma concentrations of 0-1 IU/ml of the heparins without further plasma dilutions. After 10 min (23°C) the extrinsic coagulation activity assay (EXCA) was performed. Pooled unfrozen normal plasma supplemented with these heparins was simultaneously analyzed for APTT and EXCA.

Results and Discussion: The approximate 50 % inhibitory concentration (IC50) of heparin in EXCA is 0.08 IU/ml, the approximate IC50 of enoxaparin is 0.14 IU/ml. 0.1 IU/ml heparin or enoxaparin in individual normal plasmas results in a thrombin generation of 43±16 % or 57±12 % of normal, respectively (MV±1SD) of the unsupplemented plasma control; 0.2 IU/ml enoxaparin results in a thrombin generation of 42±11 % of normal. Normal thrombin generation at 0.1 IU/ml heparin correlates only slightly to normal thrombin generation at 0.1 IU/ml enoxaparin (r= 0.334). 0.01 IU/ml heparin or enoxaparin reduce normal thrombin generation by about 10 % or 20 %, respectively. At 1 IU/ml enoxaparin there is still approximately 13 % of normal thrombin generation, whereas at 1 IU/ml heparin there is nearly no thrombin generation. Thus, heparin at concentrations in the range of 0.01 IU/ml might be too weak, at concentrations in the range of 1 IU/ml heparin might be too strong. About 5-10 % of samples are partially resistant to heparin or enoxaparin: a thrombin generation > MV+1SD of normal indicates plasmatic resistance against heparin or LMWH; a thrombin generation < MV–1SD of normal indicates plasmatic hyper-responsiveness to heparin or LMWH. The APTT in pooled normal plasma is 1.5fold or 2fold prolonged by 0.11 IU/ml of 0.15 IU/ml heparin, respectively, which corresponds to about 40 % or 20 % of normal thrombin generation in EXCA; the plasmatic LMWH concentration that is prophylactic (about 40 % of normal EXCA) or therapeutic (about 10-20 % of normal EXCA) is about 0.3 IU/ml enoxaparin or about 0.6–1 IU/ml enoxaparin, respectively. The LMWH dosage of each patient should be adjusted with an ultra-specific thrombin generation assay.

Article 14 – Heparins (unfractionated heparin UFH or low molecular weight heparin LMWH) are among the most important physiological anticoagulants. They gain anticoagulant function in blood not until complexation with antithrombin III. What is the necessary incubation time of heparins at low dose to obtain full anticoagulant activity in plasma?

50 µl unfrozen pooled normal plasma was supplemented with 2 µl 2.6 IU/ml UFH (0.1 IU/ml final concentration) or with 2 µl 2.6 IU/ml of the LMWH enoxaparin (0.1 IU/ml final concentration) in 0.9% NaCl out of siliconized glass vials. After 1-11 min (37°C or 23°C) the extrinsic coagulation activity assay (EXCA) was performed. The EXCA is a new ultra-specific and close-to-physiological thrombin generation assay.

The approximate 50% inhibitory time point (ITP50 = 50% of the complete anticoagulant activity) was a pre-incubation time of 1 min (37°C) for low dose UFH and of 3 min (37°C) for low dose enoxaparin prior to performing the EXCA. The respective ITP50 values at 23°C were about 1.5-fold prolonged. This work demonstrates the importance of the pre-incubation time of plasmatic heparins on thrombin generation assays that analyze the sensibility of individual plasmas to heparins: after plasma supplementation with heparins there should be a minimal pre-incubation time of at least 2-fold the ITP50 to obtain nearly full function of heparins. Furthermore, these data provide evidence for an anticoagulant lack phase of some minutes that might be required in clinical heparinization (especially in low dose heparinization) of individual patients.

Article 15 – When cells are fragmented, microparticles (MP) arise that are phospholipid vesicles with strange polynegative niches. MP may cause serious pro-thrombotic hemostasis problems. The ultra-specific, ultra-sensitive thrombin generation assay RECA (recalcified coagulation activity assay) detects subtle alterations of plasmatic coagulation. MP enhance thrombin generation in the RECA. The aim of the present work was to investigate a possible influence of MP without tissue factor (TF) on extrinsic coagulation.

The EXCA (extrinsic coagulation activity assay) was performed with 7 individual unfrozen normal citrated plasma samples that had been supplemented with 0-1.5 g/l hemoglobin/MP, derived from hypotonic lysis of erythrocytes of the respective subject. About 1 g/l free plasmatic hemoglobin is a clinically relevant hemoglobin concentration if a patient suffers from in vivo hemolysis.

Plasmatic MP modulated extrinsic thrombin generation: first, thrombin generation was inhibited with a 25% inhibitory concentration (IC25) of about 0.1 g/l Hb-MP; the IC50 was approximately 0.75 g/l HB-MP; plasmatic Hb-MP concentrations > 1 g/l might enhance extrinsic IIa generation, possibly by kallikrein-thrombin-mediated activation of factor V. Thus, TF-lacking microparticles are primarily an activator of the intrinsic (and not of the extrinsic) phase of blood coagulation.

Article 16 – Phospholipids are the main components of human cell membranes. With their negatively charged phosphatidyl-heads oriented towards inside or outside the cell they form polynegative bilayers. They differ with respect to the ligands at the phosphatidyl-group: there might be a choline (PC), a ethanolamine (PE), or a serine (PS). PS is slightly more negatively charged than PE or PC, which might have an effect on coagulation. The aim of the present work was to measure the thrombin generating capacity of different phospholipids in the ultra-specific, ultra-sensitive thrombin generation tests recalcified coagulation activity assay (RECA), intrinsic coagulation activity assay (INCA), and extrinsic coagulation activity assay (EXCA).

20 μl samples of individual and pooled unfrozen normal citrated plasma was supplemented with 20 μl PC, PE, or PS of different concentrations and were analyzed in the ultra-specific, ultra-sensitive thrombin generation assays RECA, INCA, and EXCA.

The approximate 200% stimulatory concentrations (SC200) for pooled normal plasma in RECA-20 were 0.5 mM PS, 1.3 mM PE, and 4.8 mM PC. When individual plasmas were tested, there were only slight differerences in the action of the PS, PE, or PC. The approximate 50% inhibitory concentrations (IC50) on the usual INCA-4 were 0.5 mM PE, 0.6 mM PS, or 1.1 mM PC. The phospholipids inhibited tissue factor - triggered thrombin generation in the EXCA at approximate IC50 values of 0.5 mM PS, PE, or PC.

It seems that the real cause of prothrombotic tendencies of some cell membranes is not the PS flop (PS translocation towards outside) but rather the membrane instability itself with generation of multiple polynegative niches within the altered membrane or within PL microparticles.

Article 17 – Severe hemorrhage or shock are clinical indications for replacement of volume. For volume replacement plasma expanders of the type of hydroxy-ethyl-starch (HES) or of the dextran type might be used or the volume is replaced by infusion of a crystalloid. Since such changes of the plasma matrix might influence normal hemostasis, the aim of this work was to measure thrombin generation in the ultra-specific, ultra-sensitive recalcified coagulation activity assay (RECA) upon recalcification of 20 μl pooled unfrozen normal citrated plasma that had been supplemented with HES of 200 kDa, HES of 70 kDa, dextran of 40 kDa, or 0.9% NaCl.

If increasing amounts of 0.9% NaCl were added to pooled normal plasma, the thrombin generation in RECA increased from < 50 mIU/ml IIa for 0-4 μl 0.9% NaCl added to 20 μl plasma to about 600 mIU/ml IIa for 6-14 μl NaCl added to 20 μl plasma, i.e. infusion of > 0.5-1 litre of volume per 3 litres of plasma can be prothrombotic. Using this volume of HES-200kDa or of HES-70kDa, the thrombin generation in RECA-30 increased about 5fold or about 8fold, respectively; with this volume of dextran the thrombin generation in RECA-30 increased about twice, when compared with the 0.9 % NaCl control.

Thus, HES may trigger the intrinsic phase of blood coagulation, especially at final plasma concentrations > 0.5%. The present data support the concept that for clinically mandatory volume replacement the plasma expanders of the HES or the dextran type might induce more hemostasis problems than just the replacement with NaCl-like solutions.

Article 18 – Human albumin is therapeutically used for a broad range of diseases. Commercial preparations may contain activators of the intrinsic phase of hemostasis. The ultra-specific, ultra-sensitive, and close to physiologic recalcified coagulation activity assay (RECA) detects subtle prothrombotic changes of any material that comes in contact with blood. Therefore, here 3 different commercial human albumins (Behring, Baxter, Talecris) were tested for contact phase activation in the RECA with 20 min coagulation reaction time in untreated polystyrol microwells (RECA-20) and for 50% inhibitory concentration (IC50) of aprotinin against amidolysis of a chromogenic substrate.

Pooled unfrozen normal human citrated plasma supplemented with 17-33 g/l Behring-albumin had a plasmatic thrombin generation in RECA-20 of about 0.1-0.2 IU/ml; the same concentration of added albumin from Baxter or Talecris induced a plasmatic thrombin generation of about 0.2-0.6 IU/ml. The 0.9% NaCl control generated less than 0.05 IU/ml thrombin in the present RECA-20 experiment.

The approximate IC50 of aprotinin against amidolysis was 1 KIU/ml, 4 KIU/ml, or 11 KIU/ml for 5% albumin from Behring, Talecris, or Baxter, respectively, when assayed in 1+1 dilution with phosphate buffered saline. The lowest amidolytic acitivity corresponded to the lowest RECA activity.

It is suggested to test all commercial lots of human albumin before releasing them to the market with the RECA. A given industrial product should be below certain still to be defined limits of RECA, e.g., an ideal albumin lot would be one that behaves similarly as the 0.9% NaCl control. Albumin lots with elevated RECA might trigger pathologic disseminated intravascular coagulation in the patient.

Article 19 – Free endotoxin in human blood can cause pathologic disseminated intravascular coagulation (PDIC). Its rapid functional determination is therefore of great clinical importance. The chromogenic Limulus test is sensitive to free lipopolysaccharide (LPS) in pg/ml quantities. Normally, the kinetic of the enzymes of the Limulus clotting system (factors C, B, G, A) is hyperbolic, as it is also typical for the human clotting system. The aim of the present study was to find out how this complicated hyperbolic kinetic can be transformed at an ideal time point into a linear kinetic.

Plasmatic LPS reactivity was determined after singlet oxygen – mediated destruction of plasmatic serine protease inhibitors. The chromogenic Limulus reagent was added in presence of different concentrations of arginine, a known competitive inhibitor of serine proteases.

The approximate 50% inhibitory concentration (IC50) of arginine against the Limulus clotting system was 50 mM. The approximate IC50 against the amidolytic activity of activated factor A was 150 mM. Since the normal range of LPS-reactivity in human plasma is 100±25% of normal (100% = about 0.8 ng/ml) and LPS-reactivities > 300% of normal may cause PDIC, the dangerous grey-zone of about 200% of normal LPS-reactivity must be determined precisely in patients at risk for PDIC. It is suggested to add 300-400 mM (final conc.) sterile arginine to a Limulus reaction, that detects pg/ml quantities of free LPS, e.g. at that reaction time point (37°C) when pooled normal plasma with about 0.8 ng/ml LPS reactivity generates an absorbance at 405 nm that is about 5-10 % of the maximal absorbance, i.e. when precise quantifications of plasmatic LPS reactivities in the critical 1-3 ng/ml range are possible.

Article 20 – Background: FEIBA (factor eight inhibitor bypassing activity) is an established drug to enhance plasmatic thrombin generation in patients at risk for bleeding due to inhibitors of the intrinsic pathway of coagulation. The aim of the present work was to determine the 200 % effective dose (ED200) of FEIBA on plasmatic thrombin generation.

Material and Methods: Pools of unfrozen citrated plasma (normal or from patients on coumarin, INR=1.8) were supplemented with 0-10 U/ml FEIBA (Immuno; S-TIM4) on polystyrol U-well microtiter plates (Brand®701300) at 23°C. Immediately thereafter the ultra-specific, ultra-sensitive thrombin generation assays RECA-10 (recalcified coagulation activity assay with 10 min coagulation reaction time (CRT) at 37°C), INCA-4 (intrinsic coagulation activity assay with 4 min CRT), and EXCA-1 (extrinsic coagulation activity assay with 1 min CRT) were performed with 20 µl or 50 µl plasma samples. Thrombin generation = thrombin activity after CRT minus basal thrombin activity in citrated plasma (without CRT).

Results: The approximate ED200 of FEIBA in pooled normal plasma was about 0.02 U/ml in RECA-10, about 0.04 U/ml in INCA-4, and about 0.05 U/ml in EXCA-1. The ED200 of FEIBA added to pooled plasma from patients on coumarin was about 0.03 U/ml FEIBA in RECA-10; about 0.06 U/ml FEIBA were necessary to obtain a RECA value that is 33 % of normal.

Discussion: The RECA is a new instrument to predict and to monitor the hemostatic power of FEIBA: in patients at risk for bleeding or already in bleeding the target RECA value might be about 33-50 % of the normal one: FEIBA therapy should be individually adjusted according to the RECA value.

Article 21 – Background: The generation of plasmatic thrombin is of major importance in hemostasis regulation. The purpose of the present work was to modulate thrombin generation by addition of low activities of thrombin to citrated plasma and to quantify the resulting thrombin generation after recalcification of these plasmas.

Material and Methods: Pools of unfrozen citrated plasma (normal or from patients on coumarin) were supplemented with 0-63 mIU/ml bovine or human thrombin on polystyrol U-well microtiter plates (Brand®701300) at 23°C. Immediately thereafter the ultra-specific, ultra-sensitive thrombin generation assays RECA-10 (recalcified coagulation activity assay with 10 min coagulation reaction time (CRT) at 37°C) and EXCA-1 (extrinsic coagulation activity assay with 1 min CRT) were performed with 20 µl or 50 µl plasma samples. Thrombin generation = thrombin activity after CRT minus basal thrombin activity in citrated plasma (without CRT).

Results: The approximate 200 % effective dose (ED200) of added bovine or human thrombin on thrombin generation of pooled normal plasma in the RECA-10 was about 2-4 mIU/ml. The respective approximate ED200 in the EXCA-1 was about 5 mIU/ml added thrombin. The ED200 of thrombin added to pooled plasma from patients on coumarin (international normalized ratio = 1.8) on thrombin generation in RECA-10 was about 8 mIU/ml. To obtain in pooled coumarin-plasma a thrombin generation that is about one third of the normal RECA value about 14 mIU/ml thrombin had to be added.

Discussion: Addition of only about 2-4 mIU/ml thrombin to pooled unfrozen normal citrated plasma approximately doubles the thrombin activity generated in RECA-10 which corresponds well to the about 3 mIU/ml thrombin in pooled normal plasma that is necessary for a normal hyperbolic rate phase in the intrinsic hemostasis assay RECA. The present findings may be of importance in diagnosis and therapy of individual dysgenerations of plasmatic thrombin.

Article 22 – Background: Tissue factor (TF) as one of the main triggers of hemostasis activates factor VII (F VII) to FVIIa, a possible prothrombinic drug against severe bleeding. The purpose of the present study was to quantifiy the 200 % effective dose (ED200) of TF on thrombin generation as assayed by the new ultra-specific, ultra-sensitive thrombin generation assay RECA.

Material and Methods: Pools of unfrozen citrated plasma (normal or from patients on coumarin, INR = 1.8) were supplemented with 0-25 pg/ml human placental TF on polystyrol U-well microtiter plates (Brand®701300) at 23°C. Immediately thereafter the ultra-specific, ultra-sensitive thrombin generation assays RECA-10 (recalcified coagulation activity assay) with 10 min coagulation reaction time at 37°C (CRT) and EXCA-1 (extrinsic coagulation activity assay with 1 min CRT) were performed with 20 μl or 50 μl plasma samples. Thrombin generation = thrombin activity after CRT minus basal thrombin activity in citrated plasma (without CRT).

Results: The approximate ED200 of TF in normal RECA-10 was about 1 pg/ml. The approximate ED200 in pooled plasma of patients on coumarin (INR=1.8) was about 2.5 pg/ml; here about 12 pg/ml TF are necessary to obtain a RECA-10 value that is one third of normal.

Discussion: The present work quantifies for the first time the amount of TF that is necessary to double normal recalcified thrombin generation. This ED200 of about 1 pg/ml for pooled normal plasma and about 3fold this amount for pooled plasma of INR=1.8 is of physiological and clinical interest, e.g. in the development of TF as prothrombinic economical drug against severe bleeding. The dosis of such a prothrombinic drug amount should be individually established for each individual patient by means of an ultra-specific, ultra-sensitive thrombin generation assay, such as the RECA.

Article 23 – Background: Factor VIIa (F VIIa) is the enzyme part of the extrinsic tenase that activates factor X. F VIIa is used since about a decade to prevent or treat severe hemorrhages. Until now there has been no simple physiologic assay that quantifies the prothrombinic capacity of F VIIa in patient plasma, allowing individual adjustments of the F VIIa dosage. Here this thrombin activity is quantified with new ultra-specific, ultra-sensitive thrombin generation assays.

Material and Methods: Pools of unfrozen citrated plasma (normal or from patients on coumarin, INR=1.8) were supplemented with 0-20 μg/ml recombinant F VIIa on polystyrol U-well microtiter plates (Brand®701300) at 23°C. Immediately thereafter the thrombin generation assays RECA-10 (recalcified coagulation activity assay) with 10 min coagulation reaction time at 37°C (CRT), INCA-4 (intrinsic coagulation activity assay with 4 min CRT), and EXCA-1 (extrinsic coagulation activity assay with 1 min CRT) were performed with 20 μl or 50 μl plasma samples. Thrombin generation = thrombin activity after CRT minus basal thrombin activity in citrated plasma (without CRT).

Results: The approximate 200 % effective dose (ED200) was about 0.3 μg/ml in RECA-10 or in INCA-4, in EXCA-1 no 200% of normal thrombin generation could be reached. The ED200 of FEIBA added to pooled plasma from patients on coumarin was about 1 μg/ml

FEIBA in RECA-10; about 3 μg/ml FEIBA were necessary to obtain a RECA value that is one third of normal.

Discussion: The RECA is a new instrument to predict and to monitor the hemostatic power of procoagulants, such as e.g. F VIIa: in severely bleeding patients or patients at risk for severe bleeding the target RECA value might be about 33-50 % of the normal one: therapy with prothrombinic drugs should be individually adjusted according to the RECA value.

Article 24 – Background: Finding the correct individual dosage of bypassing procoagulants in patients with inhibitors of factor VIII (F VIII) or IX (F IX) is a clinical challenge for every good hemostasis laboratory. The aim of the present work was to use the ultra-specific thrombin generation assay RECA (recalcified coagulation activity assay) to quantify activated thrombin generation in commercial hemophilia-like plasmas. What is the effective dose of a coagulation trigger to get a thrombin generation that is about 100 mIU/ml, which is in the range of thrombin generation in clotting normal plasma ?

Material and Methods: 20 μl plasmas completely deficient in F VIII or F IX, with 1 % F VIII or F IX, or with 10 % F VIII or F IX were supplemented in U-well plates (Brand®701300) with 0-33 mIU/ml thrombin, 0-852 mIU/ml F Xa, 0-10 U/ml FEIBA (factor eight inhibitor bypassing activity; STIM-4), 0-20 μg/ml recombinant F VII, or 0-25 pg/ml tissue factor (TF). Immediately thereafter the RECA was started with 2 μl RECA-trigger = 250 mM CaCl2.

Results: The effective doses of different coagulation triggers to obtain RECA values in the range of 100 mIU/ml thrombin in commercial plasma containing 10 % F VIII or 10 % F IX were about 30-40 mIU/ml thrombin, 25-40 mIU/ml F Xa, 2.5 U/ml FEIBA, 12 μg/ml F VIIa, or 5 pg/ml TF. For 1 % F VIII plasma or 1 % F IX plasma the respective doses of F Xa or of TF are about 3-4fold higher.

Discussion: The present work might contribute to characterize the biochemistry, physiology, and pharmacology of coagulation factors VIII and IX. The ideal RECA target value for patients with deficiencies of the intrinsic pathway of blood coagulation might be about 33-50 % (about one third to one half) of normal generation of thrombin, preventing hemorrhagic and thrombotic complications.

Article 25 – Background: Factor Xa (F Xa) generation and activity is important to maintain a physiologic hemostasis. F Xa is the enzyme part in the prothrombinase, that converts prothrombin into thrombin, the central enzyme of coagulation. The aim of the present work was to determine the 200 % effective dose (ED200) of F Xa on plasmatic thrombin generation.

Material and Methods: Pools of unfrozen citrated plasma (normal or from patients on coumarin, INR=1.8) were supplemented with 0-0.852 IU/ml bovine F Xa on polystyrol U-well microtiter plates (Brand®701300) at 23°C. Immediately thereafter the ultra-specific, ultra-sensitive thrombin generation assays RECA-10 (recalcified coagulation activity assay with 10 min coagulation reaction time (CRT) at 37°C) and EXCA-1 (extrinsic coagulation activity assay with 1 min CRT) were performed with 20 μl or 50 μl plasma samples. Thrombin generation = thrombin activity after CRT minus basal thrombin activity in citrated plasma (without CRT).

Results: The approximate ED200 of added F Xa on thrombin generation of pooled normal plasma in the RECA-10 was about 5 mIU/ml F Xa. The respective approximate ED200 of added F Xa in the EXCA-1 was about 80 mIU/ml F Xa. The approximate ED200 of added F Xa on thrombin generation in RECA-10 of pooled plasma of patients on coumarin (INR=1.8) was about 8 mIU/l added F Xa. To obtain in pooled coumarin-plasma a thrombin generation that is about one third of the normal RECA value about 28 mIU/ml factor Xa had to be added.

Discussion: Only about 5 mIU/ml F Xa added to pooled unfrozen normal citrated plasma approximately doubles the thrombin activity generated in RECA-10. These data may be of interest to develop new therapeutics, such as close-to-physiologic anti- F Xa anticoagulants.

Article 26 – Endotoxin (here clinically understood as lipopolysaccharide (LPS) or ß-glucan) that is not neutralized by plasma proteins is of toxicologic and of pathophysiologic importance. The aim of the present study was to find out the approximate proportion of free endotoxin in relation to the total amount of endotoxin when LPS or ß-glucan are supplemented to pooled normal citrated plasma.

5 % human albumin (HA) or pooled normal citrated plasma supplemented with additional 0-95 µg/ml zymosan A (ZyA) or additional 0-1000 ng/ml LPS were incubated for 10 min at 37°C. 10 µl 60 mM chloramine-T® in 50 mM sodium citrate, pH 7.8, were added to 10 µl endotoxin-sample in half area microwells and incubated for 10 min (37°C). Then 10 µl 230 mM methionine were added. After 3 min (23°C) 30 µl Limulus reagent Coamatic®Chromo-LAL were added. The specific increase in absorbance (ΔA) was determined as ΔA at 405 nm minus ΔA at 450 nm after 0-210 min incubation time (37°C).

If the oxidative Limulus assay is performed with plasma instead of human albumin, the LPS activity in plasma is far lower than its activity in 5 % human albumin: only about 0.1 % of added LPS is active, about 99.9 % of added LPS is inactive, presumably because LPS is bound to strong plasmatic LPS inhibitors such as immunoglobulins that neutralize LPS. The reactivity of ZyA in plasma is nearly identical to that of ZyA in 5 % HA. The reactivity of LPS that enters plasma at total concentrations between 1 and 10 ng/ml is of major clinical importance. Plasmatic LPS reactivities > 200 % of normal are the threshold for PDIC. Therefore, for the purpose of clinical endotoxin analysis of patient blood with singlet oxygen treated plasmas the Pyrochrome® reagent should be used that is at least 10fold more sensitive than the Coamatic® reagent.

Article 27 – This review focuses on the antithrombotic action of activated polymorphonuclear neutrophil granulocytes (PMN). PMN with about 4000 cells/µl are the main leukocyte type in normal human blood. They are the first line of defence against invading bacteria or fungi. About 50 % of all blood PMN are always slightly activated and express adhesion molecules (e.g. CD11b/CD18) that bind endothelial surface proteins (e.g. ICAM-1). PMN roll over the endothelium to patrol for the existence of any pathogen that may stick to the endothelium and that may threaten vessel patency. In this sense also fibrin might be considered as a special type of pathogen. CD11b/CD18 receptors of PMN bind to fibrin and activate the cell. Activated PMN via membrane assembly of NADPH-oxidase (Nox2) generate high concentrations of H2O2 that reacts via catalysis of released myeloperoxidase to HOCl. The hypochlorite reacts with amino groups to chloramines, an important biological source of the excited nonradical oxidant singlet molecular oxygen (1O2*). 1O2* is an inter- and intra- cellular communication signal and a destructive bullet. Light quants (hν, especially those at about 425 nm) may enhance PMN patrolling and may direct and recruit PMN to a pathologic focus, such as a pathologic thrombus. CD11b/CD18 binding induces H2O2 generation and viceversa.

1O2* is a selective oxidant. Due to its nonradical nature, 1O2* is relatively inoffensive to normal mammalian cells but highly destructive against pathogens. 1O2* inactivates important components of hemostasis, such as thrombocytes, fibrinogen, factors V, VIII, X, α2-antiplasmin, and PAI-1 with 50 % inhibitory concentrations of 1-2 mM in blood or plasma. It is suggested to imitate the physiologic PMN mediated thrombolysis by intravascular injection of blue photons or of sub-millimolar concentrations of chloramines.

Article 28 – Background: Plastic tubes or siliconized glass tubes are currently used for diagnostic blood sampling. In the present work thrombin generation of pooled normal plasma stored in different tubes was studied in the ultra-specific, ultra-sensitive thrombin generation assay RECA (recalcified coagulation activity assay).

Material and Methods: 600 μl unfrozen pooled normal citrated plasma was incubated for 30 min at 23°C in emptied polypropylene (PP) tubes from Sarstedt, or emptied polyethylene (PE) tubes, emptied siliconized glass tubes, unsiliconized glass tubes from Becton Dickinson. Then the recalcified coagulation activity assay (RECA) was performed with 50 μl pooled normal plasma in U-polystyrol-microwells (Brand®701300), 5 μl RECA-trigger (250 mM CaC12), 0-35 min coagulation reaction time at 37°C (CRT), 100 μl arginine-reagent (2.5 M arginine, pH 8.6, 0.16 % Triton X 100®), 3 min incubation, addition of 25 μl 1 mM chromogenic thrombin substrate HD-CHG-Ala-Arg-pNA in 1.25 M arginine, pH 8.7, and determination of ΔA at 405 nm.

Results: The plastic tubes (either made of PP or of PE) generated much less thrombin in RECA than glass tubes. PE tubes behaved very similarly as PP tubes: at 20 min CRT (=RECA-20) the plastic tubes generated 0.04-0.05 IU/ml thrombin. Siliconized glass tubes generated about 10fold more thrombin at RECA-20 and unsiliconized glass tubes generated about 10fold more thrombin than siliconized glass tubes, when analyzed at RECA-10 or RECA-15.

Discussion: Pre-analytic alteration of plasma should be minimized. For ultra-specific, ultra-sensitive thrombin generation assays there should be neither blood-collection-tube-induced increased thrombin generation nor blood-collection-tube-induced decreased thrombin generation of the recalcified plasma sample. For this purpose plastic tubes of the type of polypropylene or of polyethylene are preferable to procoagulant siliconized glass tubes.

Article 29 – Background: Enzyme reactions often are coupled with the generation of coloured substances. If the enzyme kinetic is still in its linear part, it is easy to convert the respective concentration of a coloured substance into the correct enzyme activity. The aim of the present work was to convert ΔA-values in the non-linear part of an enzyme kinetic into the true ones.

Material and Methods: As exemplary enzyme the hemostasis enzyme thrombin was used. As exemplary substrate HD-CHG-Ala-Arg-pNA at 0.14 mM final concentration, which here is approximately 0.5fold the Km value, was used. 50 μl 0-1 IU/ml bovine thrombin in 6.7 % human albumin were incubated in polystyrol U-well microtiter plates with 100 μl 2.5 M arginine, pH 8.6, 0.16 % Triton X 100®, 5 μl 0.9 % NaCl and 25 μl 1 mM chromogenic pNA-substrate in 1.25 M arginine, pH 8.7 were added and ΔA at

405 nm was determined after 40 min or after 105 min at 23°C.

Results and Discussion: The enzyme kinetic leaves the linear part of the curve at about 40 % of the maximal ΔA. ΔA-values in the non-linear part of the enzyme kinetic can be converted into true ΔA-values by usage of one of the following transformation formulas: y =

111.09e0.0033x or y = 0.0032x2 – 0.9853x + 331.81 with "x" being the ΔA value measured and "y" being the true ΔA-value. These conversion formulas may help to diagnose a pathological enzyme activity within short time periods, avoiding repetition of measurements.

Article 30 – Background: The bacterial enzyme asparaginase that attacks asparagines or glutamines is clinically used as part of the therapy of acute lymphoblastic leukaemia (ALL). Asparaginase is known to be pro-thrombotic in some patients. It was the aim of the present work to identify such problematic plasmas by means of in-vitro addition of asparaginase immediately followed by performance of a new ultra-specific and -sensitive thrombin generation assay: the recalcified coagulation activity assay (RECA).

Material and Methods: 50 μl samples of n=57 individual unfrozen citrated normal plasmas and of n=7 pools of 7±1 individual unfrozen citrated normal plasmas were supplemented by repetitive 1+1 dilution in polystyrol U-microwells (Brand®701300) with 0-100 U/ml Escherichia coli - asparaginase. Immediately thereafter the RECA was performed with coagulation reaction times (CRT) of 0-20 min (37°C). The approximate 200 % stimulatory concentrations (SC200) or the approximate 50 % inhibitory concentrations (IC50) of plasmatic asparaginase were determined using the respective most sensible CRT.

Results: For 29 plasma samples (51 %) there appeared only a SC200 (approx. SC200-mean = 10 U/ml asparaginase). 12 samples (21 %) had only an IC50 (approx. IC50-mean = 10 U/ml asparaginase). 14 samples (24.5 %) had both a SC200 and an IC50 (approx. SC200-mean = 40 U/ml and approx. IC50-mean = 4 U/ml asparaginase). 2 plasma samples (3.5 %) had neither a SC200 nor an IC50. Of the n=29 individual plasma samples with only a SC200 for asparaginase about one third (10/29) had a SC200 < 3 U/ml, about one third (10/29) had a SC200 of 3-20 U/ml, and about one third (9/29) had a SC200 > 20 U/ml.

Discussion: The present asparaginase preparation might pathologically activate or pathologically inactivate intrinsic coagulation. The present work demonstrates that the coagulation - altering capacity of any drug (e.g. asparaginase) in individual plasma samples can be measured prior to the administration of this drug to the patient. With the RECA, the patient's individual coagulation response to any drug can be pre-viewed, allowing individual dosage adjustments.

Versions of these chapters were also published in *Hemostasis Laboratory,* Volume 1, Numbers 1-4, edited by Thomas W. Stief, published by Nova Science Publishers, Inc. They were submitted for appropriate modifications in an effort to encourage wider dissemination of research.

In: Hemostasis Laboratory Yearbook, Volume 2
Editor: Thomas W. Stief, pp. 1-2
ISBN: 978-1-60741-089-8

HEMOSTASIS AND INFECTION/INFLAMMATION

Hemostasis is classified in Analytical Hemostasis and Clinical Hemostasis. *Hemostasis Laboratory* focuses on Analytical Hemostasis = the laboratory aspects of hemostasis. Detailed test information allows a better understanding of the hemostasis state of the individual patient.

The topic of this issue is Hemostasis and Infection/Inflammation. Hemostasis, Infection, and Inflammation are complex biologic systems with many important cross reactions. Hemostasis is classified in primary, secondary, and tertiary hemostasis. Primary hemostasis is the medicine (physiology, biochemistry, pathophysiology, pathobiochemistry) of the thrombocytes and their interaction with cells of the blood stream and the vessel wall. Secondary hemostasis is the medicine of plasmatic coagulation. The central enzyme of plasmatic coagulation is thrombin (IIa). Blood contact with unphysiologic, polynegative surfaces generates via kallikrein-genesis the intrinsic tenase. Tissue factor (TF) generates the extrinsic tenase. The generation and the inactivation of the factors Xa or IIa are of clinical importance. Tertiary hemostasis is the medicine of cellular and plasmatic fibrinolysis. Polymorphonuclear neutrophil granulocytes (PMN) are the main cells of cellular fibrinolysis. The central enzyme of fibrinolysis is plasmin. Urokinase and tissue-plasminogen activator (t-PA) are the human activators of plasminogen, plasmin is inhibited by plasmin-inhibitor.

Inflammation means tissue activation by whatever pathogen, e.g. by germs or fibrin. Blood might be considered as a liquid tissue. Inflammation can be physiologic (defensive) or pathologic (offensive=auto-aggressive). Activated phagocytes generate high concentrations of reactive oxygen species that mediate inflammation. The nonradicalic singlet oxygen ($^1\Delta O_2$) is more typical for physiologic inflammation, the hydroxyl radical (·OH) is more typical for pathologic inflammation. Two main phagocyte types participate in inflammation: the macrophages (activated monocytes (MØ) from blood or tissue) and the PMN. Especially activated PMN have important anti-pathogen functions: they destroy bacteria, fungi, and fibrin. In the blood stream about half of the PMN are rolling over the endothelium, patrolling for pathogenic material attached to the endothelium. The CD11b/18 receptors of activated PMN bind to intercellular adhesion molecule (ICAM)-1 of activated endothelial cells or to fibrin deposits on the endothelium. CD11b/18 binding activates the oxidative respiratory burst of PMN, activated PMN can produce microenvironments of $^1\Delta O_2$ generating chloramines, e.g. taurine–chloramine, in the range of 10 mM. So the pathogens in the surrounding of activated PMN are destroyed.

The article, *"Diagnosis of the pre-phase of pathologic disseminated intravascular coagulation"* of this issue is a review of the diagnosis of the pre-phase of pathologic disseminated intravascular coagulation (PDIC). PDIC is a feared complication in all clinical disciplines. Sepsis, tissue hypoxia, or major trauma are typical causes of PDIC. Up to now there have been no ultra-specific, ultra-sensitive markers to diagnose the very early activation of hemostasis. This article presents new laboratory developments that will help the clinician to therapy patients with PDIC, e.g. the chromogenic ultra-specific, ultra-sensitive IIa-Test determines basal IIa activity in 1.25 M arginine – stabilized plasma of EDTA-blood (normal range: 100 ± 20 % = 5.5 ± 1.1 mIU/ml; mean value ± 1 standard deviation) or the therefrom derived recalcified coagulation activity assay (RECA) measures the pro-thrombotic capacity of citrated plasma generated at standardized pre-analytic conditions.

The article *"Hemostasis tolerable singlet oxygen ($^1\Delta O_2$) as a perspective in AIDS therapy"* reviews the importance of $^1\Delta O_2$, which at low blood concentrations is a beneficial oxidant against thrombi and lipid-enveloped viruses, such as the human immunodeficiency virus that causes aquired immune deficiency syndrome (AIDS). The adequate blood concentration of chloramine (= $^1\Delta O_2$ generator = pro-drug of $^1\Delta O_2$) against lipid enveloped viruses as being about 1 mM in human blood has been found by cooperative research between laboratories of virology and hemostasis.

The human organism is especially susceptible to endotoxin (here clinically understood as lipopolysaccharide or ß-glucan). A technique is presented in article Nr. 3 *"Determination of active endotoxin in plasma"* that measures only the toxicologically relevant part of the endotoxin molecules in blood, i.e. only free = unbound = active endotoxin. Analytical data on active endotoxin in plasma are presented in article Nr. 4 *"Active endotoxin in sepsis"*. The hemostasis system is severely altered in endotoxin-sepsis. Article Nr. 5 *"Plasmatic fibrinolysis in sepsis"* focuses on plasmatic fibrinolysis in intensive care patients with severe sepsis.

The cellular part of fibrinolysis is investigated in article Nr. 6 *"Modulation of granulocyte mediated thrombolysis"*, using the microwell clot lysis assay (CLA) that detects decrease in turbidity upon PMN-mediated clot lysis. Article Nr. 7 *"Entrapment of plasma components in a clot"* describes the biochemical/chemical components of a plasma clot in dependence of spontaneous lysis at 37°C.

Inflammation is a complex interplay of different compounds, many of them stem from activated phagocytes. Article 8 *"Polycations neutralize plasmatic PAI-1"* describes the interaction between polycations, $^1\Delta O_2$, urokinase, which are inflammation mediators of activated PMN or MØ, and plasmatic plasminogen activator inhibitor (PAI) – 1. MØ generate TF and $^1\Delta O_2$; article Nr. 9 *"Tissue factor is resistant against singlet oxygen"* describes the resistance of TF to $^1\Delta O_2$. Plasmatic protein C, whose activated form down-regulates thrombin generation, is sensible to $^1\Delta O_2$, as described in article Nr. 10 *"Singlet oxygen inactivates plasmatic protein C"*.

Clinical hemostasis physicians are interested in physiologic drugs against IIa generation and in monitoring their individual action in analytical hemostasis. The low molecular weight heparins (LMWH) are such close-to-ideal drugs. Ultra-specific, ultra-sensitive chromogenic IIa generation assays, such as the RECA, the INCA (intrinsic coagulation activity assay), or the EXCA (extrinsic coagulation activity assay), diagnose the correct LMWH dose for each individual patient, as described in articles Nr. 11 *"Loss of anticoagulant action of ultra-low-dose heparin"* and Nr. 12 *"The sensibility of individual plasma to heparins"*.

Priv.-Doz. Dr. Med. Thomas W. Stief
Department of Clinical Chemistry,
University Hospital
D-35043 Marburg, Germany
Email: thstief@med.uni-marburg.de

In: Hemostasis Laboratory Yearbook, Volume 2
Editor: Thomas W. Stief, pp. 3-18
ISBN: 978-1-60741-089-8

THE LABORATORY DIAGNOSIS OF THE PRE-PHASE OF PATHOLOGIC DISSEMINATED INTRAVASCULAR COAGULATION

Thomas W. Stief*

Department of Clinical Chemistry, University Hospital, Giessen & Marburg, Germany

ABSTRACT

The rapid laboratory diagnosis of the pre-phase of pathologic disseminated intravascular coagulation (PDIC phase 0) is a major clinical challenge. PDIC means multiple micro-thrombi that obstruct vital organ areas, and that can cause multi-organ failure. There is clinical need for reliable hemostasis parameters to diagnose the pre-phase of PDIC to start the adequate treatment in time. The routine hemostasis tests such as prothrombin time and activated partial thromboplastin time are too blunted to diagnose the early phases of PDIC; furthermore, thrombocytes might be dysfunctional, cell fragments might be counted as platelets, platelets-count or fibrinogen concentration are acute phase parameters that might increase instead of decrease, and antithrombin activity might change only slightly or it might be altered in an artificially diluted test matrix.

In the present review new routine parameters for diagnosis of the early phases of PDIC are presented: basal chromogenic thrombin activity (IIa-Test), thrombin (IIa) generation after plasma recalcification (RECA), IIa generation after intrinsic activation of plasma (INCA), or IIa generation after extrinsic activation of plasma (EXCA), fibrinogen function+antigen+ratio, undiluted antithrombin activity, and active endotoxin (here clinically understood as active lipopolysaccharide or active ß-glucan). A combination of these new assays allows to diagnose the pre-phase of PDIC within minutes. Especially the functional ultra-specific IIa-Test (normal range 100±20%; 100%=5.5 mIU/ml) or the therefrom derived standardized RECA helps to distinguish the normal systemic intravascular coagulation from the dynamic PDIC phase 0 (120-150% of normal basal IIa) or from the PDIC phase 1 (> 150% of normal basal IIa). All these simple photometric assays do not require special hemostasis machines to test the dynamic coagulation state of each individual patient.

Key words: Pathologic disseminated intravascular coagulation (PDIC), pre-phase of PDIC, thrombin, endotoxin.

---

* Send correspondence to: PD Dr. med. T. Stief, Department of Clinical Chemistry, University Hospital, D-35043 Marburg, Germany; Email: thstief@med.uni-marburg.de; Tel.: +49-6421-58 64471; FAX: +49-6421-58 65594

INTRODUCTION

In normal human blood there is always a basal level of hemostasis activation, that leads to the generation of small amounts of thrombin. Systemic thrombin can be dangerous, because it converts fibrinogen into fibrin that might occlude blood vessels, the resulting micro-thrombi or thrombi cause ischemia/infarction of organs [1-3,42]. Thrombin is therefore physiologically neutralized by antithrombins: antithrombin III (= antithrombin = the main inhibitor of thrombin), heparin cofactor II, antithrombin I (= fibrinogen [4]), or α2-macroglobulin. Healthy normal plasma has 5.5±1.1 mIU/ml amidolytically active thrombin (IIa) that is mainly entrapped in α2-macroglobulin [5]. If hemostasis is pathologically activated by intrinsic or extrinsic triggers, pathologically elevated IIa activities arise [6]. Over-activation of intravascular coagulation is called pathologic disseminated intravascular coagulation (PDIC); the most common causes are trauma, surgery, tissue hypoxia, liver disease, or sepsis [7,8]. Intrinsic triggers are e.g. cell fragments such as membrane vesicles or DNA, the extrinsic trigger tissue factor (TF) is released upon damage of cells in TF-rich tissue, e.g. brain or placenta. Pathologic activities of systemic (non-local) thrombin generate multiple fibrin-thrombi in the blood circulation, which might cause multi-organ failure.

PDIC can be either acute or chronic; in acute PDIC a large amount of thrombin in a brief time period is generated, in chronic (compensated) PDIC small amounts of coagulation triggers lead to increased but still compensated levels of thrombin activity [9]. The PDIC phases are:

(0) hypercoagulable pre-phase, still without thrombotic complications
(1) hypercoagulable phase, leading to multiple micro-thrombi
(2) hypocoagulable phase, caused by consumption of clotting factors, leading to bleeding
(3) hyperfibrinolysis, leading to severe bleeding

Of major clinical importance are the phases (0) and (1), since many patients die in phase (1). PDIC is relatively easy to diagnose in phases (2) and (3) (overt PDIC with poor prognosis), when the patient is bleeding, as abnormalities can be detected in global coagulation tests [9-11]. The diagnosis of phase (1) of PDIC, and especially the diagnosis of phase (0) of PDIC (the pre-phase of PDIC) is difficult, because the usual laboratory parameters remain normal in very early PDIC, eventually with the exception of a decrease in circulating platelets [7,9]. The non-overt PDIC syndrome (chronic, compensated) remains often undetected [8]. There is clinical need for reliable hemostasis parameters that diagnose the pre-phase of PDIC (phase 0) to start the adequate treatment in time [7,12].

HITHERTO ROUTINE HEMOSTASIS TESTS FOR PDIC DIAGNOSIS

Prothrombin time (PT) and activated partial thromboplastin time (APTT) are blunted assays. They are of interest in hypo-coagulation, as it occurs e.g. in anticoagulant treatment either by coumarins or by unfractionated heparin, respectively. These tests do not detect spurious tendencies of hyper-coagulation, as it is typical for the very early phase of PDIC. For PDIC diagnosis, the traditional diagnostic trias of 1) decreasing platelet count, 2) decreasing antithrombin III activity, and 3) decreasing fibrinogen activity is better. However, 1) platelets might be dysfunctional, cell fragments (e.g. microparticles) might be counted as platelets, or the platelet number might increase in inflammation, 2) fibrinogen is an acute phase reactant that might increase in inflammation instead of decrease, and 3) antithrombin III activity changes only slightly or it might be altered in an artificially diluted test matrix. D-dimer concentrations depend on the activities of •thrombin, •factor XIIIa, and •plasmin, i.e. D-dimer assays do not distinguish between activation of coagulation as e.g. in PDIC and activation of fibrinolysis as e.g. in primary hyper-fibrinolysis. Besides, D-dimer may not increase in PDIC [13]. Furthermore, the usual diagnosis of hemostasis activation is performed in citrated plasma, which is rather unstable: critically ill patients have pathologic activities of proteases in their blood [14] that might artificially modulate parameter concentrations, such as D-dimer, in the pre-analytic time interval.

New Routine Hemostasis Tests for Diagnosis of Early PDIC

Basal chromogenic thrombin (IIa) activity and therefrom derived ultra-specific, ultra-sensitive IIa generation tests, fibrinogen function+antigen+ratio, undiluted antithrombin activity, and active endotoxin (here clinically understood as active lipopolysaccharide or active ß-glucan) are new simple rapid routine tests to diagnose the early phases of PDIC.

IIa -Test

Reliable data on *in vivo* thrombin generation in the blood of a critically ill patient are of great clinical interest to intervene in time in any pathologic disturbance of hemostasis. Previously, thrombin-antithrombin-complex (TAT) has been considered a marker for *in vivo* thrombin generation [15], however the TAT concentration depends also on the function of antithrombin III and on the function of the liver. A new marker for *in vivo* thrombin activity is the amidolytic thrombin activity in plasma: the thrombin trapped in the α2-macroglobulin molecule is chromogenically determined via cleavage of a tri-amino acids–paranitroanilide (pNA)- substrate [5]: EDTA blood of patients is centrifuged within 60 min (23°C), and the resulting plasma is immediately stabilized 1+1 with 2.5 M arginine, pH 8.6. In the IIa-Test one part (e.g 20 µl) of arginine-stabilized EDTA plasma is incubated with one part of 0.77 mM chromogenic thrombin substrate (e.g. HD-CHG-Ala-Arg-pNA; molecular weight= 624.6 Dalton; Pentapharm, Basel, Switzerland) in 1.25 M arginine, pH 8.7, preferably in half area microwells (e.g. Corning, costar® 3695, Schiphol-Rijk, The Netherlands), and the increase in absorbance at 405 nm with time (ΔA/t) at 37°C is determined by a microtitre plate reader with a 1 mA resolution (e.g. Milenia; DPC, Los Angeles, USA) (Table 1). The IIa-Test is standardized against pooled normal EDTA-plasma (100 % of normal), also stabilized 1+1 with 2.5 M arginine, pH 8.6. Arginine-stabilization of EDTA-plasma conserves the hemostasis activation state of plasma even against freezing/thawing [14]. With the IIa-Test, the basal coagulation activation in normal blood can be measured, which might be called normal intravascular coagulation (NIC). The normal range for basal IIa activity is 100±20 % (mean value (MV) ± 1 standard deviation (SD); 100 % is equivalent to 5.5 mIU/ml thrombin, which is 2.17 ng/ml active IIa; 1 mg IIa = 2525 IU IIa). In septic patients with prothrombotic changes of hemostasis the basal IIa activity increases to about 173±62 % of normal (MV±1SD) [14]. Therefore, the expression PDIC (pathologic DIC) might be better than just the abbreviation DIC. The IIa-Test is especially useful for phase (0) and phase (1) of PDIC. At phases (2) or (3) the basal IIa activity might paradoxically decrease due to destruction of the α2-macroglobulin cage by high activities of aggressive proteases in the blood of a severely ill patient. Therefore, in these, e.g., in Caucasians rather seldom late phases of PDIC (phases (2) and (3)) an abnormal PT or APTT might occasionally reflect better the extreme illness of the patient.

Table 1. IIa-Test.

20 µl EDTA-1.25 M arginine, pH 8.7 plasma 20 µl 0.77 mM HD-CHG-Ala-Arg-pNA in 1.25 M arginine, pH 8.7
ΔA_{405nm}/t (37°C)

Table 2a. FIFTA (fibrinogen function).

20 µl citrated plasma 40 µl 0.3 IU/ml thrombin, 0.4 mg/ml polybrene®, 6 % human albumin, PBS
ΔA_{405nm}/2 min (37°C)

Table 2b. FIATA (fibrinogen antigen).

10 µl plasma 20 µl PBS
A_{405nm}
20 µl 4.4 mM vancomycin in PBS
ΔA_{405nm}/2 min (23°C)

Table 3. Undiluted AT3 activity.

10 µl plasma 2 µl 58 IU/ml thrombin, 6 % human albumin, 54 IU/ml heparin, 1600 mM arginine, pH 7.4
30s (23°C)
50 µl 2.5 M arginine, pH 8.6, 0.124 % TritonX100® 20 µl 1 mM HD-CHG-Ala-Arg-pNA, 1.25 M arginine, pH 8.7
ΔA_{405nm}/t

Table 4a. Active endotoxin (here: active LPS + active ß-glucan).

10 µl plasma 10 µl 60 mM chloramine-T® in 50 mM sodium citrate, pH 7.8
10 min (37°C)
10 µl 230 mM methionine
1 min (37°C)
30 µl *Limulus*-reagent (*Limulus* factors + chromogenic substrate)
0, 10, 30, 60 min (37°C)
ΔA_{405nm}

Table 4b. Active ß-glucan.

10 µl plasma 10 µl 60 mM chloramine-T® in 50 mM sodium citrate, pH 7.8
10 min (37°C)
10 µl 230 mM methionine, 0.63 mg/ml (4957 IU/ml) polymyxin B
1 min (37°C)
30 µl *Limulus*-reagent (*Limulus* factors + chromogenic substrate)
0, 10, 30, 60 min (37°C)
ΔA_{405nm}

LPS reactivity [mA/t] = endotoxin reactivity [mA/t] minus ß-glucan reactivity [mA/t]

The IIa-Test is ultra-specific and ultra-sensitive for thrombin. Supra-molar concentrations of arginine completely inhibit kallikrein and depolymerize uncrosslinked fibrin. Blood of patients with severe pancreatitis might contain 100-1000 ng/ml active trypsin. In presence of supra-molar concentrations of arginine, 100 ng/ml active trypsin acts in the IIa-Test only like about 2 ng/ml active thrombin (= approximately 100 % of normal basal thrombin in plasma). Since trypsin activates the intrinsic phase of coagulation [16], a strongly positive result of the IIa-Test in severe pancreatitis really reflects a clinical prothrombotic state.

ULTRA-SPECIFIC IIA GENERATION TESTS

Derived from the above described IIa-Test, 3 ultra-specific, ultra-sensitive chromogenic tests of IIa generation have been developed:

1. RECA (recalcified coagulation activity assay [17])
2. INCA (intrinsic coagulation activity assay [18])
3. EXCA (extrinsic coagulation activity assay [19]).

In all these tests, 10 parts of fresh citrated plasma (e.g. 20 µl) are incubated with 1 part of coagulation trigger, which is 250 mM $CaCl_2$ in the RECA, SiO_2 + 250 mM $CaCl_2$ in the INCA, and 1 ng/ml tissue factor in 5 % human albumin + 250 mM $CaCl_2$ in the EXCA. In this coagulation reaction time (CRT; 37°C) thrombin is generated. The CRT for RECA is about 20 min (main value) and about 30 min (control value). For INCA the CRT is 4 min (main value) and 5 min (control value). For EXCA the CRT is 1 min (main value) and 2 min (control value). The assay results are only valid, if the ratio: (IIa in main value)/ (IIa in control value) < 1, i.e. if the thrombin generation curve is in its ascending part (thrombin is not significantly trapped within antithrombin I (= fibrin [4])). The test results can be calibrated against purified thrombin in 6.7 % human albumin, against pooled normal plasma, or against the mean value of unfrozen individual normal plasmas. The approximate normal ranges of these new thrombin generation tests are 100%±20-30% of normal; 100 % of normal = about 0.15 IU/ml IIa in the RECA, depending on the nature of the microwell, e.g. untreated polystyrol being best suitable (e.g. U-well 701300, Brand, Wertheim, Germany), 100 % of normal = about 0.5 IU/ml IIa in the INCA or in the EXCA. The RECA diagnoses the pro-thrombotic capacity of citrated plasma [6], if it is performed under well standardized pre-analytic conditions, i.e. immediate transport of citrated blood sample at 23±2°C to the central laboratory, e.g. by a suitable pneumatic delivery, immediate centrifugation at 2800 g for 5 min (23°C), and immediate analysis of plasma.

Fibrinogen Function+Antigen+Ratio

Normal fibrinogen activity is important for normal hemostasis function. Too much fibrinogen function (> 140 % of normal) might be pro-thrombotic, too few fibrinogen function (< 60 % of normal) might predispose to cerebral hemorrhage. Fibrinogen function is usually measured by addition of unphysiologically high activities of thrombin (> 10 IU/ml final assay concentration). Recently, two new fibrinogen tests have been described, the FIFTA (fibrinogen functional turbidimetric assay) (Table 2a) [20] and the FIATA (fibrinogen antigen turbidimetric assay) (Table 2b) [21]. In contrast to hitherto fibrinogen tests, the FIFTA works with a final physiologic thrombin activity of only 0.2 IU/ml, i.e. with the approximate thrombin activity in recalcified clotting normal plasma [17,22]. Many commercial functional fibrinogen tests depend on the plasma matrix: pathologically low albumin concentrations might alter the turbidimetric fibrin signal: this can result in a false fibrinogen concentration in patients with severe changes of the plasma matrix (plasmas of critically ill patients in intensive care units often have albumin concentrations of only 10-20 g/l (normal MV±1SD= 44±4g/l)). In the FIFTA, 1 part of citrated plasma (e.g. 20 µl) is incubated with 2 parts of FIFTA-reagent, containing 0.3 IU/ml thrombin, 0.4 mg/ml polybrene®, 6 % human albumin, phosphate buffered saline (PBS). The turbidity increase at 405 nm within 2 min (37°C) or within 5 min (23°C) is measured.

In the FIATA, fibrinogen and fibrinogen-like molecules are precipitated by the antibiotic vancomycin: 1 part of plasma (e.g. 10 µl) is incubated with 2 parts of PBS, the turbidity at 405 nm is determined, 2 parts of 4.4 mM vancomycin in PBS are added and the turbidity increase is measured after 2 min (23°C) or 40 s (37°C).

FIFTA and FIATA are standardized with pooled normal citrated plasma (=100 % of normal). The FIFTA/FIATA ratio (FI ratio) indicates the presence of normo-reactive (ratio=1.0±0.1), over-reactive (FI ratio > 1.1), or under-reactive (FI ratio < 0.9) fibrinogen. Over-reactive fibrinogen might occur in presence of enhancers of fibrin-polymerization such as soluble fibrin; under-reactive fibrinogen might occur in presence of dysfibrinogens or fibrinogen degradation products by plasmin.

The normal range for FIFTA is 100±20%, septic patients have 188±66% of normal, the normal range for FIATA is 100±20%, septic patients have 179±66% of normal, and the normal range of FIFTA/FIATA ratio is 1.0±0.1, septic patients have 1.12±0.32.

Undiluted Antithrombin III Activity (AT3)

AT3 is the most important physiological inhibitor of thrombin [23-25]. Decreased activity of AT3 results in increased thrombin generation. Therefore, AT3 activity must be determined routinely. Usual AT3 determinations work with a > 50fold dilution of plasma to overcome turbidity problems with in the assay nascending fibrin [26-28]. Recently, a new AT3 test has been developed, that works with nearly undiluted plasma [29]: in the thrombin reaction phase, 10 µl plasma or standards (100 % of normal pooled plasma and this plasma diluted with 0.9 % NaCl) are incubated with 2 µl thrombin reagent = 58 IU/ml (9.7 IU/ml final) thrombin, 6 % human albumin, 54 IU/ml (9 IU/ml final) unfractionated heparin, 1600 mM (267 mM final) arginine, pH 7.4, for 30s (23°C) in microwells with flat bottom (F-wells). 50 µl 2.5 M arginine, pH 8.6, 0.124 % Triton X 100® are added. After 3 min (23°C), the thrombin detection phase starts with addition of 20 µl 1 mM (0.24 mM final) chromogenic thrombin substrate HD-CHG-Ala-Arg-pNA in 1.25 M (1.87 M final) arginine, pH 8.7. ΔA/t at 405 nm is determined (Table 3). The normal range for this new AT3 test is 100±15% (MV±1SD), septic patients have 47±27% of normal active AT3. An improvement of AT3 activity might correlate with survival of the patient.

Active Endotoxin = Endotoxin Reactivity

Endotoxin is here clinically understood as lipopolysaccharide (LPS) from gram-negative bacteria or ß-glucan from fungi. The human organism is especially susceptible to active endotoxin [30]. Active (=free, unbound) endotoxin destroys susceptible cells in the blood stream (e.g. monocytes), which triggers intrinsic coagulation. Kallikrein and thrombin are formed and a PDIC may arise. Therefore, it is of great clinical importance to measure active endotoxin routinely to diagnose a possible pre-phase of sepsis and of PDIC as soon as possible to start the adequate treatment in time. Active endotoxin can be measured in plasma within minutes by coagulation factors of the *Limulus* cascade: 10 µl plasma (with EDTA or citrate) or plasma-standards (1, 10, 100, 1000 ng/ml LPS reactivity) are incubated for 10 min (37°C) with 60 mM chloramine-T® in 50 mM sodium citrate, pH 7.8. 10 µl 230 mM methionine are added. After 1 min (37°C) 30 µl *Limulus*-reagent (*Limulus* factors + chromogenic substrate Ile-Glu-Gly-Arg-pNA) are added and the increase in absorbance with time (ΔA/t) is measured (Table 4a).

If only active ß-glucan is to be quantified, the reaction conditions are the same as for active endotoxin, with the exception that the methionine reagent contains also 0.63 mg/ml of the LPS-inhibitor polymyxin B, which inhibits LPS reactivities of up to 1000 ng/ml LPS added to normal plasma (Table 4b).

Active LPS (LPS reactivity) is calculated with the formula:
LPS reactivity [mA/t] = endotoxin reactivity [mA/t] minus ß-glucan reactivity [mA/t]

Reactivity examples: 10 ng/ml LPS reactivity corresponds to the LPS reactivity of normal plasma containing 1 ng/ml LPS that had been supplemented with additional 9 ng/ml purified LPS. 10 μg/ml ß-glucan reactivity corresponds to the ß-glucan reactivity of normal plasma containing < 0.1 μg/ml ß-glucan that had been supplemented with 10 μg/ml purified ß-glucan.

The normal range of LPS reactivity is 100±25 % (100% = 0.8 ng/ml). Pre-septic patients have about 2 ng/ml (200-300 % of normal) LPS reactivity. The LPS reactivity in patients with severe sepsis can increase to a range of 100 ng/ml (mean value=20.5 ng/ml, standard deviation=19.6 ng/ml).

The fungal pathology should never be underestimated: massive fungal infection or a combined bacterial/fungal sepsis can cause PDIC [31,32]. Normal human plasma has < 0.1 μg/ml ß-glucan reactiviy. Pre-septic patients have about 0.5 μg/ml ß-glucan reactivity.The ß-glucan reactivity in patients with severe sepsis can increase to a range of 50 μg/ml (mean value = 4.7 μg/ml, standard deviation =7.0 μg/ml). Since free LPS is about 300fold as toxic as free ß-glucan [6,14], the load of active endotoxin of a patient can be calculated as: LPS [ng/ml] + ß-glucan [ng/ml]/300. Then patients with severe sepsis have 36.2±26.3 ng/ml active endotoxin [14]. In normal plasma, only about 1 % of the LPS molecules or about 10 % of the ß-glucan molecules are active=unbound=free.

Special Antigentic Parameters for PDIC Diagnosis

Intercellular adhesion molecule-1 (ICAM-1) is a parameter for endothelial damage (normal range: 0.19±0.04 μg/ml, septic patients: 2.56±2.48 μg/ml) [14]. Plasmin-antiplasmin-complex (PAP; normal range: 100±30%, septic patients: 313±307%) and D-dimer (normal range: 0.05±0.03 μg/ml, septic patients: 4.0±3.6 μg/ml) indicate fibrinolysis activation [14]. Since D-dimer is a final product of the combined action thrombin, factor XIIIa, and plasmin, D-dimer tests cannot distinguish between coagulation activation and fibrinolysis activation. To obtain reliable test results for unstable blood, these antigenic parameters should be measured in 1.25 M arginine - stabilized EDTA-plasma [14]. The inhibited plasmatic fibrinolysis in severe sepsis can be monitored by determination of plasminogen activator inhibitor-1 (PAI-1) activity or of the global assay FIPA (fibrinolysis parameters assay with 10 min reaction time) that measures the global plasmatic fibrinolytic state [33]: PAI-1 is about 10fold elevated and FIPA is about 5fold depressed in the begin of severe sepsis. An improvement of fibrinolysis seems to correlate with survival of the patient: the FIPA mean value approximately doubles within a stay of about 1 week in intensive care unit [34].

Conclusions

Acute PDIC is a terrible complication of many diseases; its high mortality is often caused by too late diagnosis and treatment [8]. Acute PDIC is comparable with a toxic snake bite [30,35] and very often results into severe pro-thrombotic hemostasis alterations with insufficient (frustrane) activation of cellular fibrinolysis [42].

The IIa-Test (normal range 100±20%; 100%= 5.5 mIU/ml basal IIa) or the standardized RECA helps to distinguish the normal intravascular coagulation (NIC; 100±20 % basal IIa; IIa generation in RECA = 100 % ± 30 % of normal) from a pre-phase of PDIC or from chronic PDIC [36] where the basal IIa activity is 120-150% or the basal IIa activity is dynamically increasing, or the RECA values are > 130 % of normal. The blood half life of α2-macroglobulin/protease complexes is only 15-60 min, especially cells of the reticuloenthelial system possess such receptors [37,38], which means that the α2-macroglobulin/thrombin concentration is not primarily dependent on the liver function.

The dynamic hemostasis state of each individual patient should be determined routinely, as indicated in exemplary figures 1-5 [14,30]. The low plasma volumes needed for these new tests allows the determination of a complete state of hemostasis activation also in pediatrics [25,39-41]. The above reviewed new hemostasis assays help to diagnose the very early phase of PDIC within minutes.

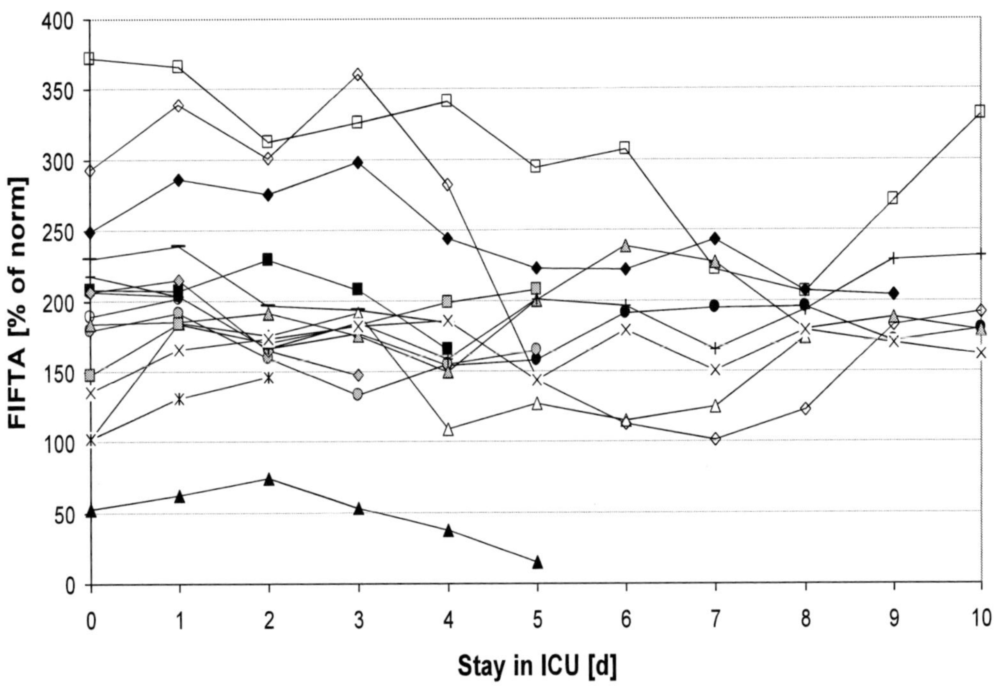

Figure 1. (Continued)

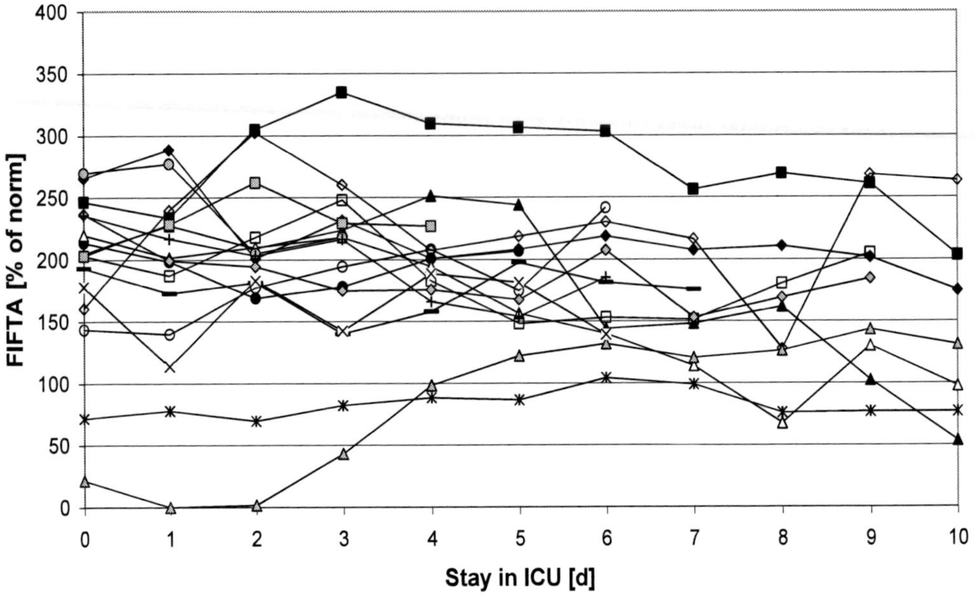

Figure 1. Fibrinogen function (FIFTA) in septic patients. Citrated plasma of 32 intensive care unit (ICU) patients with severe sepsis was analyzed for fibrinogen function with the FIFTA. Fig. 1a= patients 1-16, Fig. 1b= patients 17-32, each patient has his individual symbol. Patients with < 80 % FIFTA have pathologically decreased fibrinogen activities, e.g. by consumption of fibrinogen (PDIC phase (2)) or by destruction of fibrinogen by plasmin (PDIC phase (3)); patients with > 120 % FIFTA have pathologically increased fibrinogen activities, e.g. by hyper-fibrinogenemia or by enhancers of fibrin polymerization.

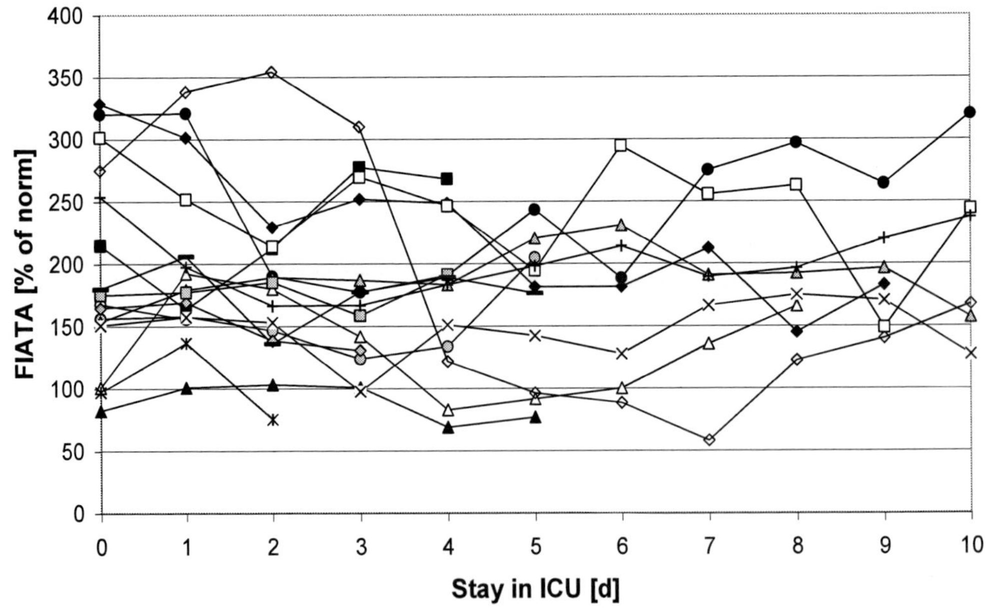

Figure 2. (Continued)

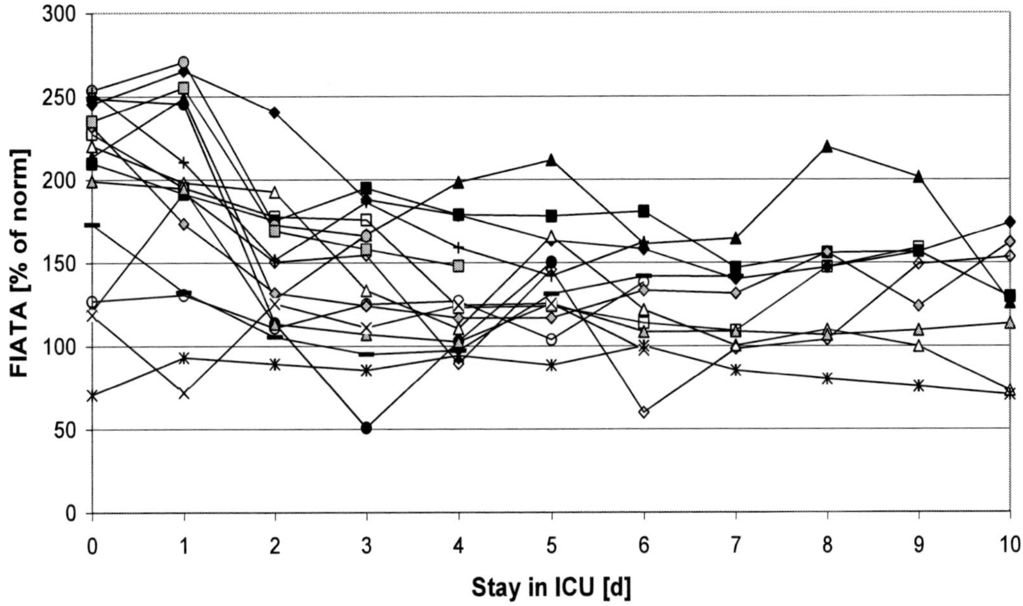

Figure 2. Fibrinogen antigen (FIATA) in septic patients. Citrated plasma of 32 intensive care patients with severe sepsis was analyzed for fibrinogen antigen by the FIFTA. Fig. 2a= patients 1-16, Fig. 2b= patients 17-32, each patient has his individual symbol.

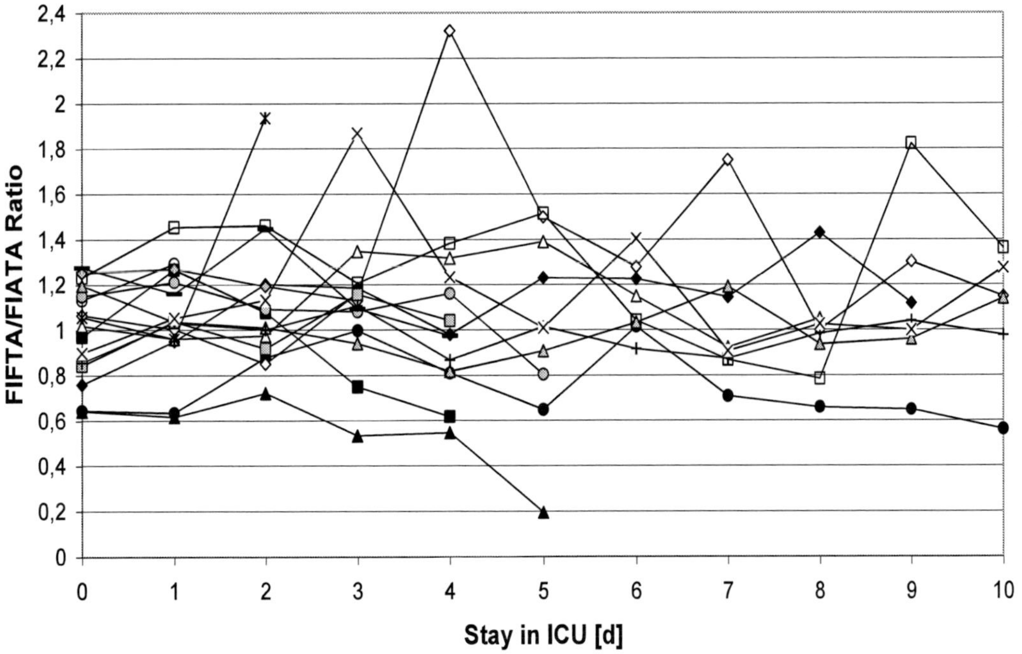

Figure 3. (Continued)

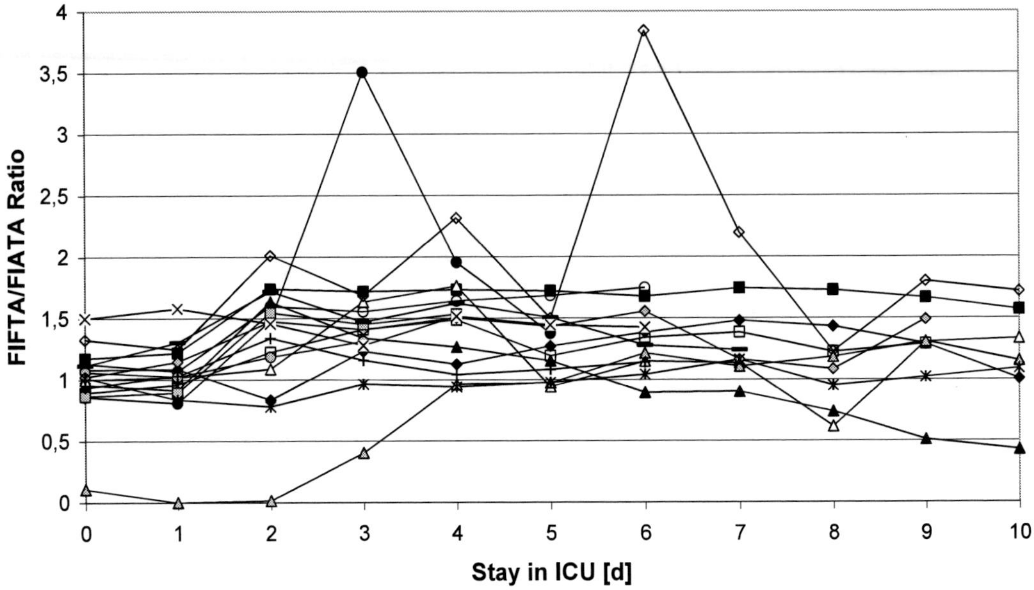

Figure 3. FIFTA/FIATA ratio in septic patients._The FIFTA/FIATA ratio (FI ratio) of the patient plasmas of Fig.1 and Fig. 2 was calculated. Fig. 3a= patients 1-16, Fig. 3b= patients 17-32, each patient has his individual symbol. Patients with a FIFTA/FIATA ratio < 0.9 have under-reactive fibrinogen, e.g. fibrinogen degradation products as occurring in PDIC phase (3) or dysfibrinogens; patients with a FI ratio > 1.1 have fibrinogen, whose function is over-reactive, e.g. due to enhancers of fibrin polymerization.

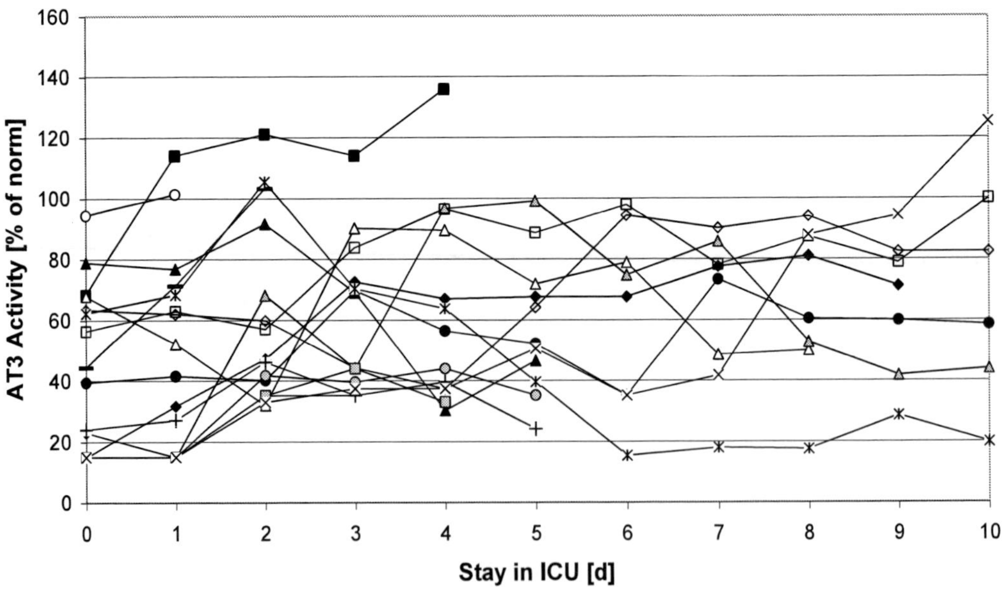

Figure 4. (Continued)

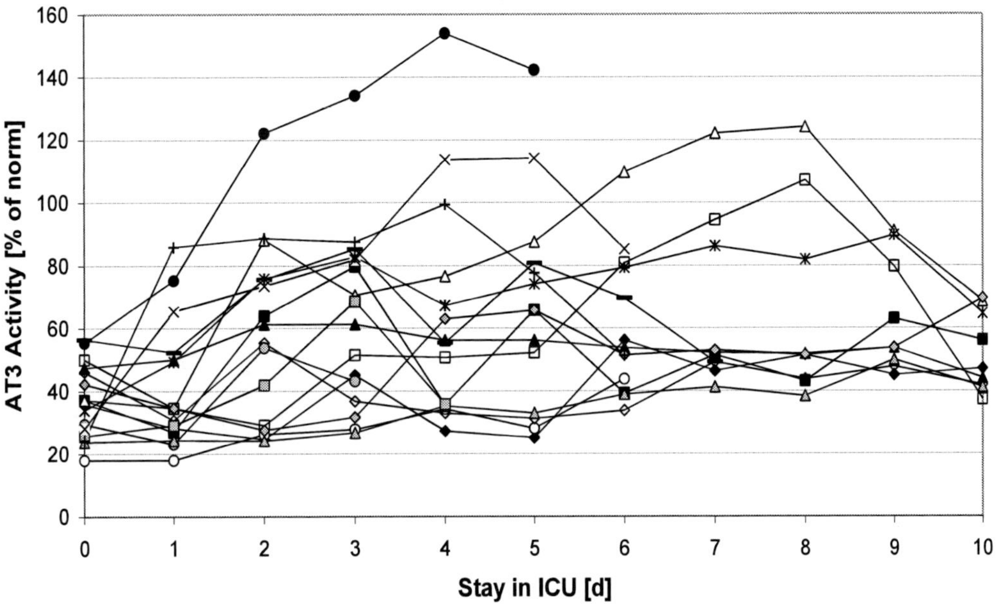

Figure 4. Undiluted antithrombin III function in septic patients. Citrated plasma of 32 intensive care patients with severe sepsis was analyzed for undiluted AT3 activity. Fig. 4a= patients 1-16, Fig. 4b= patients 17-32, each patient has his individual symbol. Normal range = 100 ±15 %.

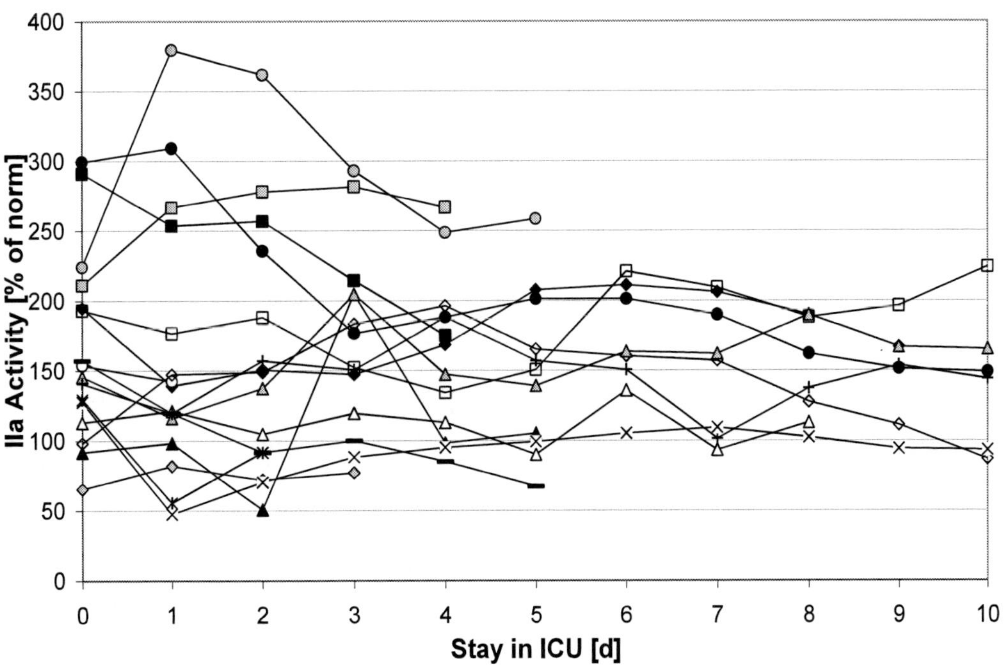

Figure 5. (Continued)

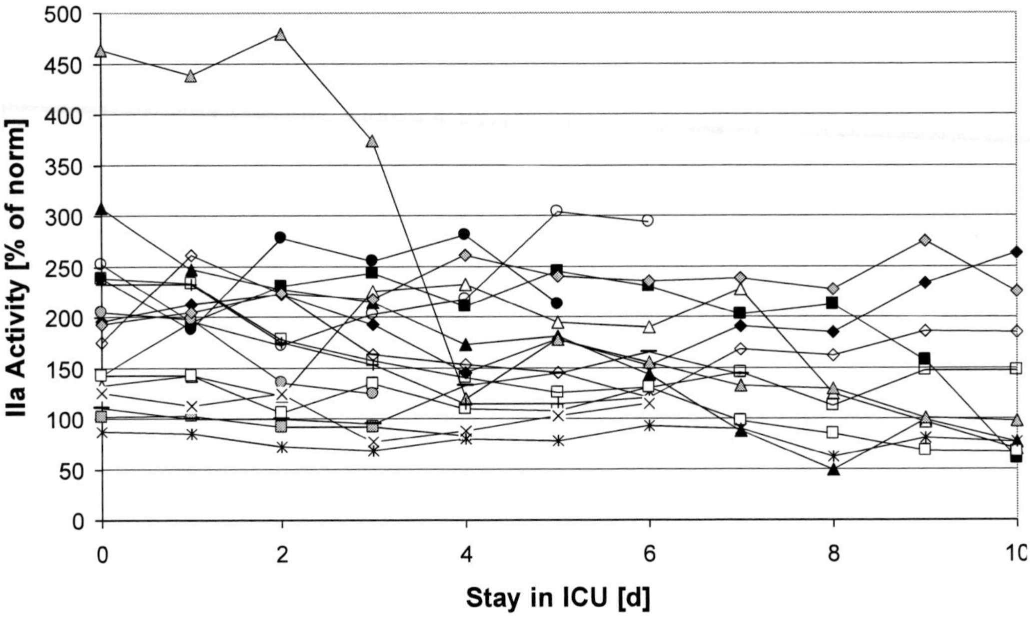

Figure 5. IIa-Test in septic patients. EDTA-1.25 M arginine plasma of 32 intensive care patients with severe sepsis was analyzed for basal thrombin (IIa) activity. Fig. 5a= patients 1-16, Fig. 5b= patients 17-32, each patient has his individual symbol. Patient 26 (greyΔ) had pancreatitis, his IIa activities in Fig. 5b (ICU days 0-3) have to be 2fold multiplied. IIa activities of 120-150% of norm and/or dynamically increasing IIa activities below 120 % of norm are characteristic for PDIC phase (0). IIa activities > 150 % of norm and/or dynamically increasing IIa activities in the range 120-150 % of norm are characteristic for PDIC phase (1).

References

[1] Bick RL. Disseminated intravascular coagulation current concepts of etiology, pathophysiology, diagnosis, and treatment. *Hematol Oncol Clin North Am* 2003; 17: 149-76.

[2] Pasternak JJ, Hertzfeldt DN, Stanger SR, Walter KR, Werts TD, Marienau ME, Lanier WL. Disseminated intravascular coagulation after craniotomy. *J Neurosurg Anesthesiol* 2008; 20: 15-20.

[3] Cotovio M, Monreal L, Navarro M, Segura D, Prada J, Alves A. Detection of fibrin deposits in horse tissues by immunohistochemistry. J Vet Intern Med 2007; 21: 1083-9.

[4] Mosesson MW. Fibrinogen and fibrin structure and functions. *J Thromb Haemost* 2005; 3: 1894-904.

[5] Stief TW. Specific determination of plasmatic thrombin activity. *Clin Appl Thromb Hemost* 2006; 12: 324-9.

[6] Stief TW. Thrombin generation by exposure of blood to endotoxin: a simple model to study disseminated intravascular coagulation. *Clin Appl Thromb Hemost* 2006; 12: 137-61.

[7] Bick RL. Disseminated intravascular coagulation. Objective laboratory diagnostic criteria and guidelines for management. *Clinics in Laboratory Medicine* 1994; 14: 729-69.

[8] Urge J, Strojil J. Early diagnosis of DIC development into the overt phase. *Biomed Pap Med Fac Univ Palacky Olomouc Czech Repub* 2006; 150: 267-9.

[9] Saba HI, Morelli GA. The pathogenesis and management of disseminated intravascular coagulation. *Clin Adv Hematol Oncol.* 2006; 4: 919-26.

[10] Gando S, Saitoh D, Ogura H, Mayumi T, Koseki K, Ikeda T, Ishikura H, Iba T, Ueyama M, Eguchi Y, Ohtomo Y, Okamoto K, Kushimoto S, Endo S, Shimazaki S; Japanese Association for Acute Medicine Disseminated Intravascular Coagulation (JAAM DIC) Study Group. Natural history of disseminated intravascular coagulation diagnosed based on the newly established diagnostic criteria for critically ill patients: Results of a multicenter, prospective survey. *Crit Care Med* 2008; 36: 145-50.

[11] Wada H, Hatada T. Pathophysiology and diagnostic criteria for disseminated intravascular coagulation associated with sepsis. *Crit Care Med* 2008; 36: 348-9.

[12] Levi M. Disseminated intravascular coagulation. *Crit Care Med* 2007; 35: 2191-5.

[13] Constantinescu AA, Berendes PB, Levin MD. Disseminated intravascular coagulation and a negative D-dimer test. *Neth J Med* 2007; 65: 398-400

[14] Stief TW, Ijagha O, Weiste B, Herzum I, Renz H, Max M. Analysis of hemostasis alterations in sepsis. *Blood Coagul Fibrinolysis* 2007; 18: 179-86.

[15] Bauer KA, Rosenberg RD. Thrombin generation in acute promyelocytic leukemia. *Blood* 1984; 64: 791-6.

[16] Stief TW. Quantification of thrombin generation by trypsin. *Medical and Biological Sciences* (Scientific Journals International) 2007; 1/ 2: 1-8.

[17] Stief TW. The Recalcified Coagulation Activity. *Clin Appl Thromb Hemost* 2007 Dec 26; [Epub ahead of print]

[18] Stief TW, Otto S, Renz H. The intrinsic coagulation activity assay. *Blood Coagul Fibrinolysis* 2006; 17: 369-78.

[19] Stief TW, Wieczerzak A, Renz H. The extrinsic coagulation activity assay. *Clin Appl Thromb Hemost* (in press)

[20] Stief TW. The fibrinogen functional turbidimetric assay. *Clin Appl Thromb Hemost* 2008; 14: 84-96.

[21] Stief TW. The fibrinogen antigen turbidimetric assay (FIATA): the $X^2\bar{x}$ test--the corrected chi-square comparison against the control-mean. *Clin Appl Thromb Hemost* 2007; 13: 73-100.

[22] Stief TW. Inhibition of thrombin generation in recalcified plasma. *Blood Coagul Fibrinolysis* 2007; 18: 751-60.

[23] Abildgaard U. Antithrombin--early prophecies and present challenges. *Thromb Haemost* 2007; 98: 97-104.

[24] Sorg H, Hoffmann JN, Rumbaut RE, Menger MD, Lindenblatt N, Vollmar B. Efficacy of antithrombin in the prevention of microvascular thrombosis during endotoxemia: An intravital microscopic study. *Thromb Res* 2007; 121: 241-8.

[25] St Peter SD, Little DC, Calkins CM, Holcomb GW 3rd, Snyder CL, Ostlie DJ. The initial experience of antithrombin III in the management of neonates with necrotizing enterocolitis. *J Pediatr Surg* 2007; 42: 704-8.

[26] Blomback M, Blomback B, Olsson P, Svendsen L. The assay of antithrombin using a synthetic chromogenic substrate for thrombin. *Thromb Res* 1974; 5: 621-32.

[27] Fareed J, Messmore HL, Walenga JM, Bermes EW, Bick RL. Laboratory evaluation of antithrombin III: a critical overview of currently available methods for antithrombin III measurements. *Semin Thromb Hemost* 1982; 8: 288-301.

[28] Gallimore MJ, Friberger P. Chromogenic peptide substrate assays and their clinical applications. *Blood Rev* 1991; 5: 117-27.

[29] Stief TW. Antithrombin III determination in nearly undiluted plasma. *Laboratory Medicine* 2008; 39: 46-8.

[30] Stief TW. Coagulation Activation by Lipopolysaccharides. *Clin Appl Thromb Hemost* 2007 Dec 26; [Epub ahead of print]

[31] Kalinski T, Jentsch-Ullrich K, Fill S, König B, Costa SD, Roessner A. Lethal candida sepsis associated with myeloperoxidase deficiency and pre-eclampsia. *APMIS* 2007; 115: 875-80.

[32] Lai CC, Liaw SJ, Lee LN, Hsiao CH, Yu CJ, Hsueh PR. Invasive pulmonary aspergillosis: high incidence of disseminated intravascular coagulation in fatal cases. *J Microbiol Immunol Infect* 2007; 40: 141-7.

[33] Stief TW, Fröhlich S, Renz H. Determination of the global fibrinolytic state. *Blood Coagul Fibrinolysis* 2007; 18: 479-87.

[34] Stief TW, Ulbricht K, Renz H, Max M. Plasmatic fibrinolysis in sepsis. (this issue)

[35] Paul V, Pudoor A, Earali J, John B, Anil Kumar CS, Anthony T. Trial of low molecular weight heparin in the treatment of viper bites. *J Assoc Physicians India* 2007; 55: 338-42.

[36] Iyoda M, Suzuki H, Ashikaga E, Nagai H, Kuroki A, Shibata T, Kitazawa K, Akizawa T. Elderly onset systemic lupus erythematosus (SLE) presenting with disseminated intravascular coagulation (DIC). *Clin Rheumatol* 2007 Dec 19; [Epub ahead of print]

[37] Ohlsson K. Elimination of 125-I-trypsin alpha-macroglobulin complexes from blood by reticuloendothelial cells in dogs. *Acta Physiol Scand* 1971; 81: 269-72.

[38] Borth W. Alpha 2-macroglobulin, a multifunctional binding protein with targeting characteristics. *FASEB J* 1992; 6: 3345-53.

[39] Goldenberg NA, Manco-Johnson MJ. Pediatric hemostasis and use of plasma components. *Best Pract Res Clin Haematol* 2006; 19: 143-55.

[40] Kowalik MM, Smiatacz T, Hlebowicz M, Pajuro R, Trocha H. Coagulation, coma, and outcome in bacterial meningitis--an observational study of 38 adult cases. *J Infect* 2007; 55: 141-8. Epub 2007 Apr 2.

[41] Moloney-Harmon PA. Pediatric sepsis: the infection unto death. *Crit Care Nurs Clin North Am* 2005; 17: 417-29.

[42] Langer F, Spath B, Haubold K, Holstein K, Marx G, Wierecky J, Brümmendorf TH, Dierlamm J, Bokemeyer C, Eifrig B. Tissue factor procoagulant activity of plasma microparticles in patients with cancer-associated disseminated intravascular coagulation. *Ann Hematol* 2008; 87: 451-7.

In: Hemostasis Laboratory Yearbook, Volume 2
Editor: Thomas W. Stief, pp. 19-38
ISBN: 978-1-60741-089-8

HEMOSTASIS TOLERABLE SINGLET OXYGEN ($^1\Delta O_2$) AS A PERSPECTIVE IN AIDS THERAPY

*Thomas W. Stief**
Department of Clinical Chemistry, University Hospital, Giessen & Marburg, Germany

ABSTRACT

Usual drugs against human immuno deficiency virus (HIV) have complex heterocyclic or homocyclic structures; the cytochrome P-450 system (CYP450) hydroxylates such organic ring structures and can transform them into generators of reactive oxygen species (H_2O_2, ·OH, $^1\Delta O_2$) that might be a main therapeutic way to destroy HIV. The lipid membrane of HIV is stabilized by only about 14 protein spikes (gp160 trimers) per virion and contains more molecules of oxidizable unsaturated fatty acids or cholesterol per nm^2 than the human cell membrane, and is thus more susceptible to $^1\Delta O_2$ than human cells. Nonradical generators of $^1\Delta O_2$ (e.g. the physiological taurine-chloramine) could be new therapeutics against AIDS. Chloramines at blood concentrations of about 1 mM are still tolerable to hemostasis of human blood: the 50 % inhibitory concentration (IC50) of $^1\Delta O_2$ sensible thrombocytes, fibrinogen, factor VIII, factor V, factor X, antithrombin, and plasmin-inhibitor is > 1 mM chloramine. Thrombin generation in the ultra-specific, ultra-sensitive recalcified coagulation activity assay (RECA) does not increase in 1 mM chloramine–oxidized whole citrated blood with hemolysis being < 0.1 g/l free hemoglobin. HIV or other lipid enveloped viruses in blood might be eliminated by slow infusion of about 1 mM chloramine, a pro-drug of $^1\Delta O_2$.

Keywords: Human immunodeficiency virus (HIV), cytochrome P-450 (CYP450), singlet oxygen ($^1\Delta O_2$), chloramines (R-NHCl), hemostasis

PATHOPHYSIOLOGY OF HIV

HIV-1 is a lentivirus belonging to the retrovirus family. The virus has a lipid bilayer membrane that contains two copies of a single RNA strand. The RNA encodes only 9 genes that are translated into about 15 proteins; among them are Gag, Pol, Env, Tat, Rev, Nef, Vif, Vpu, and Vpr, of which the first five are essential for virus replication [1,2]. Hitherto main

* Send correspondence to: T. Stief, MD, Priv.-Doz., Department of Clinical Chemistry, University Hospital, D-35043 Marburg, Germany; Email: thstief@med.uni-marburg.de; Tel.: 06421-5864471; Fax: 06421-5865594

targets in anti-HIV therapy are the enzymes reverse transcriptase and protease. HIV-1 primarily infects $CD4^+$ T-lymphocytes and monocytes/macrophages [2]. HIV attaches to surface CD4 receptors via the gp120Env protein, the modulated gp120 protein interacts with the HIV-coreceptors CCR5 or CXCR4, and the HIV-virus fuses with the host cell, a mechanism involving gp41Env, a protein located below gp120Env [3]. After fusion with the host cell the reverse transcriptase of the HIV-virus transcribes its RNA into DNA. This viral DNA together with the viral proteins integrase, matrix, Vpr, and some host proteins is the viral preintegration complex. The virus is either integrated as latent provirus into the host genome or it starts replicating itself. The transactivator of transcription protein (Tat) triggers the expression of all HIV genes. The Rev gene product is involved in the nuclear export of viral RNAs. Nef enhances the infectivity of virions and downregulates surface expression of CD4, possibly a mechanism of immune evasion. HIV virions are assembled by the viral protease that cleaves the HIV Pr55 Gag protein to produce the matrix, capsid, nucleocapsid and p6 proteins. HIV latency is a clinical problem [3-5]; the latent HIV reservoir are mainly the CD4 T-memory lymphocytes; patients require antiviral treatment for decades to eliminate these infected CD4 T-cells.

Targets of Usual Anti-HIV Drugs

Usual targets of anti-HIV drugs are:

1. CD4 as the primary human cell receptor for viral entry;
2. gp 120 as the viral glycoprotein attaching to the human cell;
3. CXCR4 (stromal derived factor (SDF) – 1) receptor on T-lymphocytes, CCR5, and MIP-1 (macrophage inflammatory protein - 1) receptor on macrophages as the coreceptors for viral entry;
4. gp 41 as the viral glycoprotein necessary for fusion of virus with human cell membrane;
5. reverse transcription of the viral RNA into proviral DNA;
6. viral integrase that integrates the proviral DNA into the host cell genome;
7. proviral DNA expression (Tat-dependent transactivation and HIV replication);
8. HIV-protease, an aspartyl-protease like renin and pepsin [6], that cleaves the gag and gag-pol precursor polyproteins to the structural proteins p17, p24, p7, p6, p2, p1 and the functional proteins protease p11, reverse transcriptase p66/p51, and integrase p32;
9. ubiquitin ligases as parts of the ubiquitin-proteasome system, regulating HIV assembly and budding.

Usual Anti-HIV Drugs

Examplary anti-HIV drugs with organic ring structures [7] (possible substrates for cytochrome P450) against these targets are:

ad 1: the cellular CD4 receptor antagonist cyclo-triaza-disulfonamide;

ad 2: plant lectins [8], 4-benzoyl-1-[4-methoxy-1*H*-pyrrolo[2,3-*b*]pyridine-3-yl)oxo acetyl]-w-(*R*)-methylpiperazine, or vancomycin, teicoplanin;

ad 3: Bicyclam AMD3100 (a bis-macrocyclic molecule), TAK-779 (an ammonium derivative with 3 benzole groups), 2,6-dimethyl-isonicotinamide, 2,6-dimethylpyrimidine-5-carboxamides;

ad 4: tri-phenyl-drivatives as fusion inhibitors;

ad 5a: the nucleoside analogue reverse transcriptase inhibitors (NRTI) that inhibit DNA synthesis by abnormal pyrimidines or purines; the thymidine analogues zidovudine (3′-azido-2′,3′-dideoxythymidine; AZT, retrovir®) and stavudine, the cytidine analogues zalcitabine, lamivudine, and emtricitabine ((2′,3′-dideoxy-3′-thia-5-fluorocytidine = FTC), the guanosine analogue abacavir, the inosine analogue didanosine (2′,3′-dideoxyinosine), and the purine analogue amdoxovir (diaminopurine dioxolane);

ad 5b: the nucleotide (adenosine 5′-monophosphate) analogue reverse transcriptase inhibitors (NtRTI) adefovir (phosphonyl-methoxyethyl-adenine) or tenofovir (phosphonyl-methoxypropyl-adenine;

ad 5c: the non-nucleoside analogue reverse transciptase inhibitors (NNRTI) nevirapine, delavirdine, the diarylpyrimidine (DAPY) R278474, the thiocarboxanilide UC-781 with a chlorinated phenyl-group, capravirine with a twofold chlorinated phenyl-group, tetrahydro-methylimidazo-benzodiazepin-one (TIBO), etravirine (R165335 TMC 125 [14]), efavirenz or DPC 083, the latter two with a trifluoro-methyl-group and a chlorinated phenyl-group; at an oral dose of 100 mg once daily DPC 083 effected a viral load reduction of 1.28 $\log_{10}$ after 8 weeks of treatment in patients with NNRTI-resistant HIV mutants;

ad 5d: Inhibitors of HIV ribonuclease H (RNase H), the enzyme that cleaves the RNA strand of the RNA/DNA heteroduplex (p15 domain of the p66 subunit of the p66/p51 reverse transcriptase heterodimer), are tipranavir, benzoylamino-dioxobutanoic acid, or hydroxyl-isoquinoline-1,3-dione;

ad 6: Naphthyridine (L-870,81), L-chicoric acid with 2 hydrochinone-like groups, pyranodipyrimide, or diketo acids (S-1360) [3,13];

ad 7: Aminoquinolone, neplanocin A, PKF 050-638, N-aminoimidazoles, 5fold-chlorinated pyridine oxides (JPL-32);

ad 8: Saquinavir, ritonavir, indinavir, nelfinavir, amprenavir, lopinavir, atazanavir, fosamprenavir [14], triterpenoid derivative of betulinic acid (PA-457) [3], or the coumarin-derivative tipranavir [15]; all drugs consist of several organic ring structures with a hydroxyethylene bond that replaces the normal peptidic bond;

ad 9: HIV-1 virions contain a small amount of mono-ubiquitinylated Gag proteins; two ubiquitin ligases conjugate ubiquitin to HIV-proteins, regulating virus budding. Therefore, ubiquitin analogues or Gag-inhibitors might act against HIV [16]. The virion infectivity factor (Vif) induces the poly-ubiquitin-binding and proteasome-mediated degradation of the anti-HIV enzyme APOBEC3G [17]. So, four main classes of actual antiretroviral drugs exist:

1. Nucleoside (or nucleotide) reverse transcriptase inhibitors (NRTI);
2. Non-Nucleoside reverse transcriptase inhibitors (NNRTI);

3. Protease inhibitors (PI);
4. Fusion inhibitors.

The main requirements for an ideal antiviral drug [1] are:

a) high antiviral activity against wild-type and mutant viruses
b) minimal adverse effects
c) easy to synthesize
d) cheap.

About 20 anti-HIV compounds have been approved in the USA in 2005: 7 NRTI, 1 NtRTI, 3 NNRTI, 8 PI, 1 fusion inhibitor [1]. The action of these drugs seems to involve inhibition of HIV-1 reverse transcriptase, protease, or virus entry. In 1996 the triple drug therapy was named highly active anti-retroviral therapy (HAART), typically a combination of 2 nucleoside analogues and a protease inhibitor (PI): zidovudine, lamivudine, and efavirenz or abacavir are typical initial HAART drugs [18]. HAART usually means cycles of 8 weeks of treatment and 8 weeks off treatment [19]. Unfortunately, HAART has massive side effects and complicated drug interactions [7]. Inspite of HAART there appears a long-term failure rate of up to 50 % [20].

Side Effects of Usual Anti-HIV Drugs

HIV infection and HAART are prothrombotic conditions: the incidence of venous thrombosis is increased severalfold in HIV-patients [21]; increased endothelial tissue factor expression, decreased antithrombin III function, and cell fragments (e.g. microparticles or DNA) are procoagulant. The lipodystrophy syndrome is a typical side effect of HIV-drugs; lipodystrophy is fat redistribution with accumulation of neck and abdominal fat, loss of facial, gluteal, or extremity fat with glucose intolerance and hyperlipidemia [6]. The side effects of HAART include drug interactions, especially with antituberculous drugs, mitochondrial toxicity [22-24], lactic acidosis, hepatotoxicity, pancreatitis, bone marrow-suppression [25], neuropathy, atherogenic dyslipidemia [26,27], and cardiomyopathy [28,29]. However, AIDS itself can cause cardiomyopathy, wasting syndrome, or nephropathy; therefore it may be difficult to judge, if the illness results from HAART or from HIV [30].

The exact route of metabolism of many anti-HIV drugs has yet not been fully clarified, but the cytochrome P-450 (CYP450) system seems to play a key role: drug metabolites may act as CYP450 modulators, thereby disrupting oxidative phosphorylation, resulting in accumulation of nonesterified fatty acids, dicarboxylic acids, and free radicals causing mitochondrial dysfunction.

Cytochrome P-450 as a Generator of Reactive Oxygen Species

The NADPH dependent cytochrome P-450 monooxygenase complex (CYP450) hydroxylates organic compounds, especially those with organic homocyclic or heterocyclic structures [31-33]: in Phase I drug metabolism (= hydroxylation and dealkylation) the compound is hydroxylated and becomes more hydrophilic. The CYP450 chain is located in the endoplasmatic reticulum and in the mitochondria and has important functions in cell activation and metabolism. Reducing cell enzymes (e.g. the CYP450 chain enzymes CYP450-reductase) or hypoxic environments can reduce xenobiotics and thereby can activate redox cyclers of the quinone or of the nitro-imidazole type [34]: a redox cycler is a compound, that undergoes repetitive reversible reduction/oxidation cycles with radical states and thereby generates reactive oxygen species (ROS = H_2O_2, ·OH, $^1\Delta O_2$). The redox cycler is activated by reduction of the molecule, e.g. by reaction with NADPH. A typical redox cycling reaction is quinone → hydroquinone → quinone. The thereby generated ROS ($H_2O_2 \rightarrow$ 2 ·OH or $H_2O_2 \rightarrow H_2 + {}^1\Delta O_2$) can modulate the CYP450 chain, the CYP450 electron transfer system is broken and becomes uncoupled. Examples for redox cyclers are chloroquin, adriamycin, tetracycline, 6-hydroxydopamine, clofibrate, dipyridamole, nitrofurantoin, metronidazole, many antiparasitic agents or their metabolites [35-37]. Strong ROS generators injure the mitochondria: quinones, antiparasitic drugs such as lapachone, nifurtimox, clioquinol, iod-chlor-hydroxychinoline, dinitrophenol, chloramphenicol, or carbonylcyanid-p-trifluoro-methoxy-phenylhydrazone [38]: they uncouple the CYP450 chain, the generated ROS destroy the proton gradient that is necessary for ATP synthesis and uncouple the oxidative phosphorylation.

The CYP450 chain interacts particularly with organic ring structures of phenolic or of planar aromatic nature (e.g. ß-naphthoflavone or 3-methylcholanthrene). Pro-oxidative compounds such as ethanol [39], paracetamol, or organic halogenated molecules favour the expression of certain CYP450 isoenzymes, preferably of the mitochondrial type [40]. The CYP450 chain can generate compounds that modulate the chain [41], by reaction of redox cyclers with NADPH or adrenodoxin, or by modulation of the catalytic centre of CYP450. These reactants destroy mitochondria [41-42]. CYP450- modulators are the by CYP450 generated metabolites of itraconazole, ketoconazole, diconazole, miconazole, clotrimazole, oxfendazole, 2-phenyl-imidazole, omeprazole, cimetidine, isoniazid, rifampicin, disulfiram, or alkylhydrazines. These metabolites bind strongly to CYP450 and are noncompetitive inhibitors or modulators of CYP450 [43]. Figure 1 demonstrates the action of a mechanism based inhibitor of CYP450: CYP450 converts the substrate into a reactive intermediate that binds irreversibly to CYP450, inactivates the specific hydroxylation activity of CYP450, and transforms CYP450 into a ROS generator [44], the imidazole of the azole drugs replaces a natural histidine residue. CYP450 is modified into an uncontrolled ROS generator. Generated ROS might react with other CYP450 enzymes, the heme stabilizing cysteinates (Fig. 1) of nearby CYP450 enzymes could be oxidized, converting also these enzymes into oxidases/ROS generators. A "chain reaction" could start, ROS are massively generated.

The ROS generated by CYP450 chain modulators attack susceptible membrane lipids. Ultraweak chemiluminescence, caused by $^1\Delta O_2$ [34], occurs when these lipid peroxides break down. Thus, the metabolizer CYP450 might become a ROS-generator/photons-emitter. A combination of a CYP450 modifyer (e.g. an azole) with a CYP450-inducer (e.g. a naphtoflavone) results into greatly enhanced ROS generation, that destructs membranes and the respiratory chain [41].

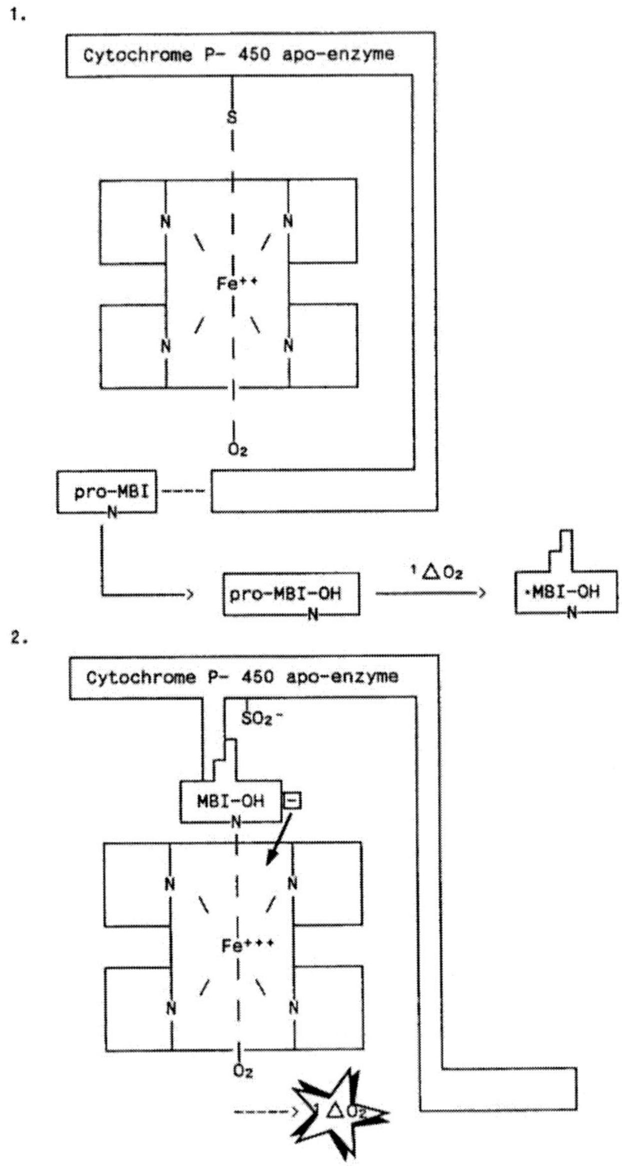

Figure 1. Mechanism based modulation of CP 450. CYP450 hydroxylates the potential mechanism based inhibitor (MBI) to pro-MBI-OH. If CYP450 is not occupied by excessive substrate, the CYP450 action or a redox reaction may convert pro-MBI-OH into MBI-OH. Reactive oxygen species (ROS: H_2O_2, $\cdot OH$, or $^1\Delta O_2$) favour the transition into the reactive radical intermediate ·MBI-OH, which may covalently bind nearby the reactive centre of CYP450, may oxidize the sulphur axial ligand of heme and may replace it by a N-Fe bond. This oxidation would induce a major conformational change in the apo-enzyme, redoxcycling MBI-OH may become a second prosthetic group, that may provide heme with electrons to generate ROS. The hydroxylase CYP450 might then behave as a singlet oxygen-generator/photons-emitter ($^1\Delta O_2/hv$).

Interestingly, the structures of CYP450 reductase and NO synthase are similar; NO synthase has recognition sites for NADPH, FAD, flavin mononucleotide, calmodulin and can be phosphorylated; both enzymes have a central role of CYP450 and NO synthase in cell activation [45]. CYP450 activity shows a day/night rhythm [46-48]. Since CYP450 cannot discriminate between physiological and pathophysiological substances, also harmless compounds can be hydroxylated into carcinogens or into ROS generators.

In conclusion, CYP450 often detoxifies xenobiotics, especially with organic ring structures, hydroxylating them. CYP450 interacts with substrates, inhibitors, or inducers of the enzyme. Cytochrome P-450 3A4 is the most abundant isoform and metabolizes approximately 60 % of the therapeutic drugs. Mechanism-based inactivation of CYP450 3A4 by drugs is often due to chemical modification of the heme. Examplary CYP-modifyers are the antibiotics erythromycin and isoniazid, the cytostatic tamoxifen, the antidepressant fluoxetine, the antihypertensives dihydralazine and verapamil, the herbal compounds bergamottin and glabridin, or the anti-HIV agents ritonavir and delavirdine [49].

CYP450 acts synergistically with P-glycoprotein, a 170 kDa phosphorylated and glycosylated plasma membrane transport protein [50]. P-glycoproteins "pump out" xenobiotics from cells. Most CYP450 3A4 inhibitors are also P-glycoprotein substrates/inhibitors [49,51]. Quinidine, for instance, is a P-glycoprotein inhibitor and consequently results into elevated concentrations of substrates for P-glycoprotein [6].

INTERACTION OF ANTI-HIV DRUGS WITH CYTOCHROME P-450

The anti-HIV protease inhibitors (PI) are metabolized by cytochrome P-450 enzymes (mainly 3A4 and 3A5) in liver and gut [52,53]. PI can induce or inhibit the CYP450 system, therefore the PI/CYP450 interaction is difficult to predict [54], e.g. fosamprenavir often acts as an inducer of CYP450 3A4 metabolism [55]. Many PI, such as amprenavir, DPC 681, L-734,394, nelfinavir, or ritonavir and also other anti HIV-drugs, such as the NNRTI delavirdine, act as mechanism based inhibitors of CYP450 [57]. Blood-level monitoring of tricyclic antidepressants is necessary, if a CYP450 inhibitor like ritonavir is given; a combination of PI and a statin (against lipodystrophy syndrome) may result into mitochondrial dysfunction and rhabdomyolysis, so simvastatin should not be combined with a PI [6]. Some CYP450 inhibitors are ciprofloxacin, clarithromycin, diltiazem, erythromycin, itraconazole, ketoconazole, or nefazodone. Typical inducers of CYP450 3A4 are the NNRTI efavirenz and nevirapine; general CYP450 inducers are rifampycin, carbamazepin, phenytoin, ethanol, and barbiturates [6]. The anti-HIV action of zidovudine is associated with myelosuppression and intense mitochondrial dysfunction [56].

Singlet oxygen generation of a drug seems to correlate with its anti-HIV power [57,58]. Examples for other prooxidative drugs that might improve the outcome of HIV-infection are antimalarials, e.g. atovaquone, clindamycin/primaquine, chloroquine or hydroxychloroquine [59].

Oxidative Inactivation of Viruses

Oxidants are virucid; the main targets are the lipids of the enveloped viruses [60]: the HIV membrane is rich in $^1\Delta O_2$ oxidizable unsaturated fatty acids or cholesterol, so-called lipid rafts. Photoillumination modulates the activation state of HIV [61-63].

Similarities between Anti-Parasite Drugs and Anti-HIV Drugs

Parasite infections are treated by drugs that increase the ROS concentration mostly by redox cycling mechanisms [64]. ROS generators (e.g. arising from CYP450 MBI) destroy HIV-1 infected cells similarly as they destroy parasites, e.g. trypanosomes. One pro-oxidative trypanocidal drug is suramin; suramin consists of a complicated organic ring structure: hexasodium-sym-bis(m-amino-benzoyl-m-amino-p-methylbenzoyl-1-naphthylamino-4,6,8-trisulfonate) carbamide. At higher concentrations suramin inhibits mitocondria and suppresses cells. Primarily, suramin was considered an anti-HIV drug because it inhibits in vitro the reverse transcriptase, the 50 % inhibitory concentration of suramin being similar to that of 3′-azido-3′deoxythymidine (AZT) [65]. However, suramin also inactivates the hepatitis delta virus (a virus without reverse transcriptase) by inhibition of virus uncoating and budding [66]. Unfortunately, suramin at > 10 μg/ml (the approximate plasma concentration of high dose suramin – treated AIDS patients), is toxic [65].

Trypanosomes can also be treated with the antifungal agent ketoconazole, which is a CYP450-MBI. The azoles might act as antiparasitic by mechanism based inhibition of CYP450, they cause mitochondrial swelling and alter plasma membrane [44,67,68]. Similarly to HIV-drugs in HAART, the anti-parasitic efficiency of a drug is potentiated, when it is combined with another type of anti-parasitic drug [69,70].

Biogenesis of Chloramines/$^1\Delta O_2$ and their Biologic Actions Against Lipid Membranes

Chloramines are physiological oxidants of activated phagocytes [71]: activated neutrophils (PMN) generate millimolar (in the 1-10 mM range) concentrations of chloramines by a combined action of NADPH-oxidase and myeloperoxidase (Fig. 2). $^1\mathbf{O_2}$ arises by the interaction of chloramines with hydrogen peroxide (Mallet-reaction); chloramines are nonradical oxidants, at physiologic pH and in physiologic concentrations they oxidize targets solely by singlet oxygen, and not by oxygen radicals [9,12,72].

Lipid enveloped viruses can be destroyed at blood concentrations of chloramines that are tolerable to the normal hemostasis system. Of particular interest would be the study of in-vitro destruction of HIV by chloramine. A harmless lipid enveloped virus was studied as a model virus: 10 μl vesicular stomatitis virus (VSV) concentrate was added to 80 μl heparinized venous blood (15 IU/ml) of a healthy donor. 10 μl chloramine-T® (sodium salt of N-chloro-toluene-sulfonamide; final blood concentration 0 - 8 mM) in PBS (with Ca^{2+},

Mg^{2+}) was added and after 30 min at 37°C 900 µl PBS (with Ca^{2+}, Mg^{2+}) was added, centrifuged, and the 10^{-2} titre of the supernatant was diluted 10^6 fold; 100 µl of this diluted supernatant were incubated with 1000 µl Vero-cells in culture medium for 3 days at 37°C. Then the vitality of the Vero-cells was checked by microscope: 1 mM chloramine in whole blood inactivated 90 %, 2 mM 99 % , and 4 mM 99.9 % of vesicular stomatitis virus added to normal blood, the singlet oxygen ($^1\Delta O_2$) generator chloramine was highly efficient against this lipid enveloped virus [72,135].

NADPH-Oxidase	
1.	$NADPH + H^+ + O_2 \rightarrow H_2O_2 + NADP^+$
Myeloperoxidase	
2.	$H_2O_2 + Cl^- \rightarrow HOCl + HO^-$
3.	$HOCl + R\text{-}NH_2 \rightarrow R\text{-}NHCl + H_2O$
4.	$R\text{-}NHCl + H_2O_2 \rightarrow {}^1\Delta O_2 + R\text{-}NH_2 + HCl$

Figure 2. Biogenesis of chloramines (R-NHCl) and a release reaction of singlet oxygen ($^1\Delta O_2$)

1 mM choramine decreases whole blood platelet aggregation by about 30 %, 2 mM completely inactivates aggregation; 1 mM chloramine in platelet rich plasma decreases platelet aggregation by 41 %, 2 mM completely inactivates aggregation, 1 mM or 2 mM chloramine decreases plasmatic fibrinogen activity by 33 % or 56 %, plasmatic factor V activity by 11 % or 42 %, plasmatic factor VIII activity by 26 %, or 61 %, and plasmatic factor X by 28 %, or 68 %, respectively; the global coagulation assays prothrombin time (PT) and activated partial thromboplastin time (APTT) increase < 1.5 fold by 1 mM chloramine-oxidation of plasma [12]. Thrombin generation in recalcified plasma of 1 mM chloramine-oxidized whole blood does not increase, it decreases by about 20 % [96]. Antithrombin III is the most important physiological inactivator of thrombin: its activity changes only by ≤ 10 % in ≤ 1 mM chloramine – oxidized blood or plasma. Oxidation of blood is similarly effective as oxidation of plasma, because the erythrocytes dispose of a reductive capacity, that compensates the about 2fold increase of plasmatic oxidant concentrations if the oxidant is added to whole blood.

In 22 individual samples of citrated blood (0.5 ml 106 mM sodium citrate + 4.5 ml blood) 0.75 mM chloramine increased free hemoglobin by 0.012 ± 0.018 g/l, 1.5 mM chloramine increased free hemoglobin by 0.026 ± 0.024 g/l, and 3 mM chloramines increased free hemoglobin by 0.14 ± 0.32 g/l. At 3 mM chloramine in blood, 2 of 22 samples had > 0.5 g/l free hemoglobin. None of the 22 blood samples oxidized at 1.5 mM chloramine, had > 0.1 g/l free hemoglobin (Fig. 3); the individual cell counts of granulocytes, lymphocytes, monocytes and of thrombocytes (MAXM; Beckman-Coulter, Krefeld, Germany) were constant up to final chloramine concentrations of 2 mM in whole citrated blood.

About 1 mM chloramine in plasma has a half life of less than 1 minute (37°C) (Fig. 4).

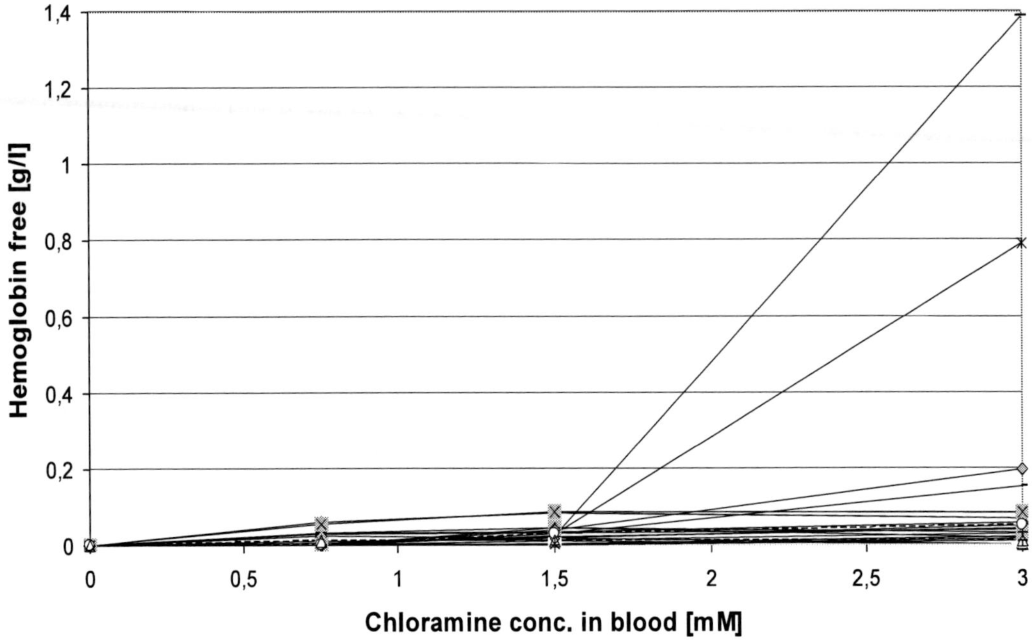

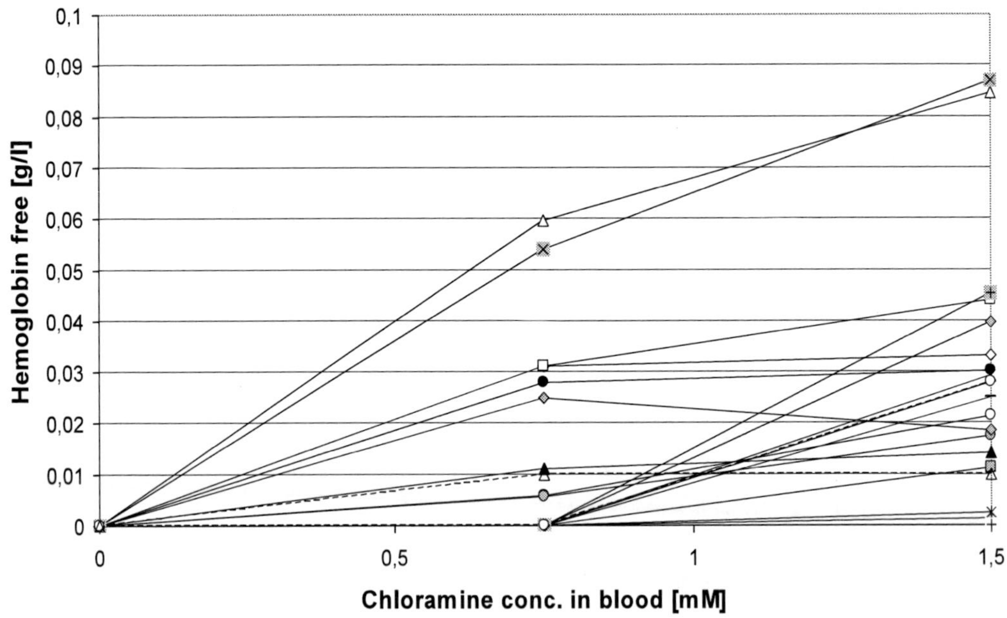

Figure 3. Hemolysis by chloramine. 500 µl of 22 individual citrated blood samples were incubated at 0, 0.75, 1.5, or 3 mM chloramine-T® for 10 min (37°C). After centrifugation for 10 min at 2500g 50 µl plasma was pipetted into V-wells polystyrol microtitre plates and the absorption at 405 nm was determined. The control absorption was that without addition of chloramine. 0.13 g/l hemoglobin (frozen/thawed diluted whole citrated blood) had an absorption of 209 mA. Each individual plasma sample has an individual symbol.

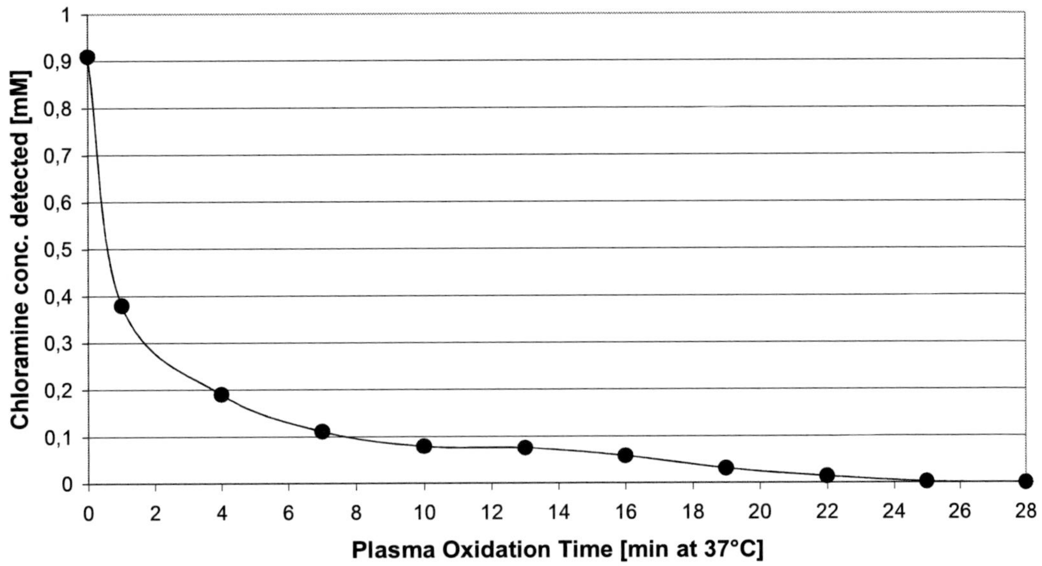

Figure 4: Half life of chloramine in human plasma. 20 µl pooled unfrozen pooled normal citrated plasma were supplemented in duplicate with 2 µl 10 mM (final conc. 0.91 mM) chloramine-T®. After 1-28 min at 37°C (0 min = replacing 20 µl plasma by 20 µl 0.9 % NaCl) 200 µl 4 M KI in PBS were added (23°C) and the increase in absorbance at 405 nm (23°C) was determined. 0.91 mM chloramine in 0.9 % NaCl - standard resulted in 453 mA. For matrix control, 20 µl pooled plasma were added to 200 µl 4 M KI in PBS that had been reacted with 2 µl 10 mM chloramine-T®. The generated absorbance was stable for chloramine in 0.9 % NaCl and decreased by about 1 % of the initial value per minute (23°C) for chloramine in plasma.

EVIDENCE AND PERSPECTIVES FOR ANTIVIRAL CHLORAMINES/SINGLET OXYGEN

Current drugs inhibit HIV-replication, they attenuate but cannot cure HIV infection. Many viruses are lipid-enveloped (e.g. herpes, influenza, HIV, or hepatitis viruses). The viral membrane has important functions for attachment of the virus to the outside of the human cell and budding of the nascent new virus inside the cell. The viral membrane consists of viral proteins and of host lipids. The lipids are not incorporated randomly and do not represent an average of the lipid composition of the human cell membrane. Specific lipid microdomains, so-called lipid rafts, are important in virus attachment, entry, uncoating, protein transport, and budding. Rafts concentrate viral proteins to the budding site and vice versa viral proteins organize rafts [73].

Blocking the first phase of HIV/cell interaction seems to be a very interesting approach in HIV therapy, i.e. the virus is eliminated before it enters the human cell [74]. Of major interest might be the destruction of the viral envelope. There is need for anti-HIV drugs with activity against HIV forms that are resistant to currently available agents [75] and for a HIV vaccine [76]. An ideal drug will be extremely effective against the primary target of the virus and against variations of this target. Hitherto drugs are designed upon the lock-and-key hypothesis [77]. Singlet oxygen generators, such as physiologic chloramines, might be a new type of anti-HIV drug that acts against all types of HIV or even against many other lipid enveloped viruses.

Nearly all the approved HIV-drugs have in common a complicate organic structure with benzole rings, heterocyclics, or halogenated C-atoms [78]. Many of these xenobiotics are substrates of CYP450: CYP450 might transform these molecules into redox-active agents that generate large amounts of singlet oxygen; the PI tipranavir for instance is of coumarinic nature [15]. Coumarins can act as redox cylcers of the quinone type, generating excited oxygen of the type of $^1\Delta O_2$ [79]. Singlet oxygen both destroys the viral envelope and activates dormant viruses incorporated into the host genome, the infected cells get unmasked and can be eliminated by the normal immune defense. The question arises, if the ROS generation in AIDS patients [80-82] belongs to the physiologic response. This altered redox status with serious energetic problems in the mitochondria [83,84] might be due to the viral infection [85,86] or due to the anti-viral drugs [87].

The pathophysiology of elevated ROS or nitric oxide in AIDS is still unclear [88,89]. The increased basal production of oxidants by phagocytes [90] might be physiological to combat HIV. Therefore, impaired PMN function might result in AIDS progression [91]. In contrast, prooxidative changes of the patient´s redox status correlate with therapeutic efficiency of HAART [92,93]. Therefore, ROS generators [94], particularly generators of singlet oxygen, may be a physiologic therapy [95,96]: *dosis sola venenum facit* (Paracelsus; it is only the dosage that makes an agent to a toxic one). Infusion of chloramines, e.g. the physiological taurine-chloramine, slowly (within 60 min) reaching a final blood concentration of 1 mM about twice a week might be tolerable to human hemostasis and might reduce the viral load by several $\log_{10}$ within 1 month. Chloramines have blood half-lifes of less than 1 minute and do not culminate like usual oral anti-HIV drugs. Chloramines at blood concentrations ≥ 3 mM might provoke harmful hemolysis. The so generated erythrocyte microparticles trigger the intrinsic phase of hemostasis: they activate pre-kallikrein to kallikrein and factor XII to factor XIIa. This potential pathologic action of chloramines should be tested in vitro before in vivo infusion, e.g. by the thrombin generation assay RECA (recalcified coagulation activity assay) [96]. At excessive blood concentrations of ≥ 3 mM the chloramines might act as anti- and as pro-coagulants, which would complicate the therapy.

HIV membranes are rather "naked", they have nearly no stabilizing membrane proteins (only about 14 spikes of trimers of gp160 (Env) per virion) [97] and thus seem to be especially vulnerable to oxidative attack against their membranes: HIV-1 is more vulnerable than e.g. VSV against $^1\Delta O_2$ [98]. Small amounts of pro-oxidative compounds bound to a purified substance might be truly responsible for the antiviral action of this substance [99]. Many *in vitro* anti-oxidative compounds such as flavonoids [100] become *in vivo* pro-oxidative [101-107], depending on the intra- and peri-cellular micro-milieau. CYP450 can transform antioxidants into redox cyclers [103,108,109] that could be activated to singlet oxygen generators via celluar reducing enzymes, e.g. flavonoids induce the expression of NAD(P)H-quinone oxidoreductase [103]. Singlet oxygen might then disorganize the viral membrane [110-112], which destroys the enveloped virus [113-120].

Thus, the diagnosis of the adequate dosis of $^1\Delta O_2$ generators could be important in therapy of thrombotic [72,103,121-126] or viral diseases [127-136]. Singlet oxygen might be superior to any of the known complicated therapy forms of lipid enveloped viruses, such as HIV [137-147].

REFERENCES

[1] Janssen PA, Lewi PJ, Arnold E, et al. In search of a novel anti-HIV drug: multidisciplinary coordination in the discovery of 4-[[4-[[4-[(1E)-2-cyanoethenyl]-2,6-dimethylphenyl]amino]-2-pyrimidinyl]amino]benzonitrile (R278474, rilpivirine). *J Med Chem.* 2005; 48: 1901-1909.

[2] Nielsen MH, Pedersen FS, Kjems J. Molecular strategies to inhibit HIV-I replication. *Retrovirology* 2005; 2: 10.

[3] Greene WC. The brightening future of HIV therapeutics. *Nat Immunol.* 2004; 5: 867-871.

[4] Simmons R, Siliciano RF. Can antiretroviral therapy ever be stopped ? An update. *AIDS Read.* 2004; 14: 435-8, 441-2.

[5] Blankson JN, Siliciano JD, Siliciano RF. The Effect of Early Treatment on the Latent Reservoir of HIV-1. *J Infect Dis.* 2005; 191: 1394-1396.

[6] Wynn GH, Zapor MJ, Smith BH, Wortmann G, Oesterheld JR, Armstrong SC, Cozza KL. Antiretrovirals, part 1: overview, history, and focus on protease inhibitors. *Psychosomatics.* 2005; 45: 262-270.

[7] De Clercq E. New approaches toward anti-HIV chemotherapy. *J Med Chem* 2005; 48: 1297-1313.

[8] Botos I, Wlodawer A. Proteins that bind high-mannose sugars of the HIV envelope. *Prog Biophys Mol Biol* 2005; 88: 233-282.

[9] Shechter Y, Burstein Y, Patchornik A. Selective oxidation of methionine residues in proteins. *Biochemistry* 1975; 14: 4497-503.

[10] Greenberg M, Cammack N, Salgo M, Smiley L. HIV fusion and its inhibition in antiretroviral therapy. *Rev Med Virol* 2004; 14: 321-337.

[11] De Corte BL. From 4,5,6,7-Tetrahydro-5-methylimidazo[4,5,1-jk](1,4)benzodiazepin-2(1H)-one (TIBO) to etravirine (TMC125): fifteen years of research on non-nucleoside inhibitors of HIV-1 reverse transcriptase. *J Med Chem* 2005; 48: 1689-1696.

[12] Stief TW, Kurz J, Doss MO, Fareed J. Singlet oxygen inactivates fibrinogen, factor V, factor VIII, factor X, and platelet aggregation of human blood. *Thromb Res* 2000; 97: 473-80.

[13] Pommier Y, Johnson AA, Marchand C. Integrase inhibitors to treat HIV/AIDS. *Nature Reviews Drug Discovery* 2005; 4: 236-248.

[14] Chapman TM, Plosker GL, Perry CM. Fosamprenavir: a review of its use in the management of antiretroviral therapy-naive patients with HIV infection. *Drugs* 2004; 64: 2101-2124.

[15] Kandula VR, Khanlou H, Farthing C. Tipranavir: a novel second-generation nonpeptidic protease inhibitor. *Expert Review of Anti-infective Therapy* 2005; 3: 9-21.

[16] Li F, Wild C. HIV-1 assembly and budding as targets for drug discovery. *Curr Opin Investig Drugs* 2005; 6: 148-154.

[17] Stopak K, Greene WC. Protecting APOBEC3G: a potential new target for HIV drug discovery. *Curr Opin Investig Drugs* 2005; 6: 141-147.

[18] Chang YC, Tyring SK. Therapy of HIV infection. *Dermatologic Therapy* 2004; 17: 449-464.

[19] Ananworanich J, Hirschel B. Interrupting highly active antiretroviral therapy in patients with HIV. *Expert Rev Anti Infect Ther*. 2005; 3: 51-60.

[20] Alberdi Leniz A, Tuset Creus M, Martin Conde M, del Cacho del Cacho E, Nigorra Caro M, Codina Jane C, Ribas I Sala J. Resistance to antiretroviral therapy. *Farm Hosp*. 2004; 28 (Suppl 1) : 55-71.

[21] Nolan D, Reiss P, Mallal S. Adverse effects of antiretroviral therapy for HIV infection: a review of selected topics. *Expert Opin Drug Saf* 2005; 4: 201-218.

[22] Schweinburg BC, Taylor MJ, Alhassoon OM, et al. Brain mitochondrial injury in human immunodeficiency virus-seropositive (HIV+) individuals taking nucleoside reverse transcriptase inhibitors. *J Neurovirol*. 2005; 11: 356-64.

[23] Moyle G. Mitochondrial toxicity: myths and facts. *HIV Ther* 2004; 9: 45-47.

[24] Setzer B, Schlesier M, Thomas AK, Walker UA. Mitochondrial toxicity of nucleoside analogues in primary human lymphocytes. *Antivir Ther*. 2005; 10: 327-334.

[25] Piscitelli SC, Polis MA. An update on drug interactions with zidovudine. *AIDS Patient Care STDS* 1998; 12: 687-690.

[26] Mehta N, Reilly M. Atherosclerotic cardiovascular disease risk in the HAART-treated HIV-1 population. *HIV Clin Trials* 2005; 6: 5-24.

[27] Fichtenbaum CJ. Coronary heart disease risk, dyslipidemia, and management in HIV-infected persons. *HIV Clin Trials* 2004; 5: 416-433.

[28] Hatherill M, Paed FC. Sepsis predisposition in children with human immunodeficiency virus. *Pediatr Crit Care Med* 2005; 6: S92-S98.

[29] Lazerow SK, Abdi MS, Lewis JH. Drug-induced liver disease 2004. *Curr Opin Gastroenterol* 2005; 21: 283-292.

[30] Torre D, Speranza F, Martegani R. Impact of highly active antiretroviral therapy on organ-specific manifestations of HIV-1 infection. *HIV Medicine* 2005; 6: 66-78.

[31] Bernhardt R. Cytochrome P450: structure, function, and generation of reactive oxygen species. *Rev Phyiol Biochem Pharmacol* 1995; 127: 137-221.

[32] Turrens JF, Giulivi C, Pinus C, Roldan E, Lavagno C, Boveris A. Low level chemiluminescence from isolated rat hepatocytes, intact lung and intestine in situ. *Basic Life Sci* 1988; 49: 239-242.

[33] Roy D. Cytochrome P-450 catalyzed redox cycling of orthophenyl-phenol. *Biochem Int* 1990; 22: 849-857.

[34] Cadenas E. Oxidative stress and formation of excited species. In: *Oxidative Stress*. Sies H (Ed.), Academic Press, London, UK, 1985; 311-326.

[35] Giulivi C, Turrens JF, Boveris A. Chemiluminescence enhancement by trypanocidal drugs and by inhibitors of antioxidant enzymes in Tripanosoma cruzi. *Mol Biochem Parasitol* 1988; 30: 243-251.

[36] Golenser J , Chevion M. Oxidant stress and malaria: host-parasite interrelationships in normal and abnormal erythrocytes. *Semin Hematol* 1989; 26: 313-325.

[37] Klotz LO, Kroncke KD, Sies H. Singlet oxygen-induced signaling effects in mammalian cells. *Photochem Photobiol Sci*. 2003; 2: 88-94.

[38] Terada H. Uncouplers of oxidative phosphorylation. *Environ Health Perspect* 1990; 87: 213-218.

[39] Tindberg N, Ingelman-Sundberg M. Cytochrome P-450 and oxygen toxicity. Oxygen-dependent induction of ethanol- and inducible cytochrome P-450 (IIE1) in rat liver and lung. *Biochemistry* 1989; 28: 4499-4504.

[40] Labbe G, Descatoire V, Beaune P, Letteron P, Larrey D, Pessayre D. Suicide inactivation of cytochrome P-450 by methoxsalen. Evidence for the covalent binding of a reactive intermediate to the protein moiety. *J Pharmacol Exp Ther* 1989; 250: 1034-1042.

[41] Salet C, Moreno G. Photosensitization of mitochondria. Molecular and cellular aspects. *J Photochem Photobiol* B 1990; 5: 133-150.

[42] Lazardi K, Urbina JA, de Souza W. Ultrastructural alterations induced by ICI 195,739, a bis-triazole derivative with strong antiproliferative action against Trypanosoma (Schizotrypanum) cruzi. *Antimicrob Agents Chemother* 1991; 35: 736-740.

[43] Zhang ZY, Wong YN. Enzyme kinetics for clinically relevant CYP inhibition. *Curr Drug Metab*. 2005; 6: 241-57.

[44] Rando RR Mechanism-based enzyme inactivators. *Pharmacol Rev*. 1984; 36: 111-142.

[45] Bredt DS, Hwang PM, Glatt CE, Lowenstein C, Reed RR, Snyder SH. Cloned and expressed nitric oxide synthase structurally resembles cytochrome P-450 reductase. *Nature* 1991; 351: 714-718.

[46] Gruler H, Müller-Enoch D. Slaving the cytochrome P-450 dependent monooxygenase system by periodically applied light pulses. *Eur Biophys* J 1991; 19: 217-219.

[47] Kobayashi Y, Motohashi Y, Miyazaki Y, Yatagai M, Takano T. Immunohistochemical study of temporal variations in cytochrome P-450 isoenzymes in rat testes and their modifications by the inductive effects of cadinenes. *Int J Biometerol* 1991; 35: 234-238.

[48] Belanger PM, Desgagne M, Bruguerolle B. Temporal variations in microsomal lipid peroxidation and in glutathione concentration of rat liver. *Drug Metab Dispos* 1991; 19: 241-244.

[49] Zhou S, Chan E, Lim LY, Boelsterli UA, Li SC, Wang J, Zhang Q, Huang M, Xu A. Therapeutic drugs that behave as mechanism-based inhibitors of cytochrome P450 3A4. *Curr Drug Metab* 2004; 5: 415-442.

[50] Ford J, Khoo SH, Back DJ. The intracellular pharmacology of antiretroviral protease inhibitors. *J Antimicrobioal Chemother* 2004; 54: 982-990.

[51] Martin AM, Nolan D, Gaudieri S, Phillips E, Mallal S. Pharmacogenetics of antiretroviral therapy: genetic variation of response and toxicity. *Pharmacogenomics* 2004; 5: 643-655.

[52] Inaba T, Fischer NE, Riddick DS, Stewart DJ, Hidaka T. HIV protease inhibitors, saquinavir, indinavir and ritonavir: inhibition of CYP3A4-mediated metabolism of testosterone and benzoxazinorifamycin, KRM-1648, in human liver microsomes. *Toxicol Lett.* 1997; 93: 215-219.

[53] Owen A, Khoo SH. Intracellular pharmacokinetics of antiretroviral agents. *J HIV Ther* 2004; 9: 97-101.

[54] Boffito M, Maitland D, Samarasinghe Y, Pozniak A. The pharmacokinetics of HIV protease inhibitor combinations. *Curr Opin Infect Dis* 2005; 18: 1-7.

[55] Huang L, Wring SA, Woolley JL, Brouwer KR, Serabjit-Singh C, Polli JW. Induction of P-glycoprotein and cytochrome P450 3A by HIV protease inhibitors. *Drug Metab Dispos* 2001; 29: 754-760.

[56] Lewis W, Gonzalez B, Chomyn A, Papoian T. Zidovudine induces molecular, biochemical, and ultrastructural changes in rat skeletal muscle mitochondria. *J Clin Invest* 1992; 89: 1354-1360.

[57] Kitagawa S, Yuo A, Souza LM, Saito M, Miura Y, Takaku F. Recombinant human granulocyte colony-stimulating factor enhances superoxide release in human granulocytes stimulated by the chemotactic peptide. *Biochem Biophys Res Commun.* 1987; 144: 1143-6.

[58] Aladdin H, Ullum H, Dam Nielsen S, et al. Granulocyte colony-stimulating factor increases CD4+ T cell counts of human immunodeficiency virus-infected patients receiving stable, highly active antiretroviral therapy: results from a randomized, placebo-controlled trial. *J Infect Dis.* 2000; 181: 1148-1152.

[59] Romanelli F, Smith KM, Hoven AD. Chloroquine and hydroxychloroquine as inhibitors of human immunodeficiency virus (HIV-1) activity. *Curr Pharm Des 2004*; 10: 2643-2648.

[60] Sieber F, O´Brien JM, Gaffney DK. Merocyanine- sensitized photoinactivation of enveloped viruses. *Blood Cells* 1992; 18: 117-127.

[61] Matthews JL, Skiles H, Newman JT, Chanh TC. Preliminary studies of photoinactivation of human immunodeficiency virus in blood. *Transfusion* 1991; 31: 636-641.

[62] Legrand-Poels S, Hoebeke M, Vaira D, Rentier B, Piette J. HIV-1 promoter activation following an oxidative stress mediated by singlet oxygen. *J Photochem Photobiol B.* 1993; 17: 229-237.

[63] Schuitemaker H, Kootstra NA, van Oers M, et al. Induction of monocyte proliferation and HIV expression by IL-3 does not interfere with anti-viral activity of zidovudine. *Blood* 1990; 76: 1490-1493.

[64] Bouteille B, Oukem O, Bisser S, Dumas M. Treatment perspectives for human African trypanosomiasis. *Fundam Clin Pharmacol.* 2003; 17: 171-181.

[65] Kaur M, Reed E, Sartor O, et al. Suramin's development: what did we learn? *Invest New Drugs.* 2002; 20: 209-219.

[66] Mitsuya H, Popovic M, Yarchoan R, et al. Suramin protection of T cells in vitro against infectivity and cytopathic effect of HTLV-III. *Science* 1984; 226: 172-174.

[67] Lazardi K, Urbina JA, de Souza W. Ultrastructural alterations induced by ICI 195,739, a bis-triazole derivative with strong antiproliferative action against Trypanosoma (Schizotrypanum) cruzi. *Antimicrob Agents Chemother* 1991; 35: 736-740.

[68] Dresser GK, Spence JD, Bailey DG. Pharmacokinetic-pharmacodynamic consequences and clinical relevance of cytochrome P450 3A4 inhibition. *Clin Pharmacokinet.* 2000; 38: 41-57.

[69] Resnick L, Markham PD, Veren K, et al. In vitro suppression of HTLV-III/LAV infectivity by a combination of acyclovir and suramin. *J Infect Dis* 1986; 154: 1027-1030.

[70] van Voornis WC. Therapy and prophylaxis of systemic protozoan infections. *Drugs* 1990; 40: 176-202.

[71] Weiss SJ. Tissue destruction by neutrophils. *N Engl J Med.* 1989; 320: 365-376.

[72] Stief TW. Regulation of hemostasis by singlet-oxygen ($^1\Delta O_2$*). *Curr Vasc Pharmacol* 2004; 2: 357-362.

[73] Nayak DP, Hui EK. The role of lipid microdomains in virus biology. *Subcell Biochem* 2004; 37: 443-491.

[74] Borkow G, Lapidot A. Multi-targeting the entrance door to block HIV-1. *Curr Drug Targets Infect Disord* 2005; 5: 3-15.

[75] Wainberg MA, Sawyer JP, Montaner JS, et al. Challenges for the clinical development of new nucleoside reverse transciptase inhibitors for HIV infection. *Antivir Ther* 2005; 10: 13-28.
[76] Tonini T, Barnett S, Donnelly J, Rappuoli R. Current approaches to developing a preventive HIV vaccine. *Curr Opin Investig Drugs* 2005; 6: 155-162.
[77] Ohtaka H, Freire E. Adaptive inhibitors of the HIV-1 protease. *Prog Biophys Mol Biol* 2005; 88: 193-208.
[78] Hartmann H, Vogt MW, Durno AG, et al. Enhanced in vitro inhibition of HIV-1 replication by 3′-fluoro-3′deoxythymidine compard to several other nucleoside analogs. *AIDS Res Hum Retroviruses* 1988; 4: 457-466.
[79] McCormick ML, Denning GM, Reszka KJ, et al. Biological effects of menadione photochemistry: effects of menadione on biological systems may not involve classical oxidant production. *Biochem J.* 2000; 350: 797-804.
[80] Flourie F, Arab K, Gagnieu MC, et al. Redox status in HIV+ patients under HAART. *Ann Biol Clin.* 2004; 62: 713-715.
[81] Repetto M, Reides C, Gomez Carretero ML, et al. Oxidative stress in blood of HIV infected patients. *Clin Chim Acta.* 1996; 255: 107-117.
[82] Jareno EJ, Bosch-Morell F, Fernandez-Delgado R, Donat J, Romero FJ. Serum malondialdehyde in HIV seropositive children. *Free Radic Biol Med.* 1998; 24: 503-506.
[83] LewisW. Mitochondrial dysfunction and nucleoside reverse transcriptase inhibitor therapy: experimental clarifications and persistent clinical questions. *Antiviral Res.* 2003; 58: 189-197.
[84] Cossarizza A, Troiano L, Mussini C. Mitochondria and HIV infection: the first decade. *J Biol Regul Homeost Agents.* 2002; 16: 18-24.
[85] Gil L, Martinez G, Gonzalez I, et al. Contribution to characterization of oxidative stress in HIV/AIDS patients. *Pharmacol Res.* 2003; 47: 217-224.
[86] Schwarz KB. Oxidative stress during viral infection: a review. *Free Radic Biol Med.* 1996; 21: 641-649.
[87] Hulgan T, Morrow J, D'Aquila RT, et al. Oxidant stress is increased during treatment of human immunodeficiency virus infection. *Clin Infect Dis.* 2003; 37: 1711-1717.
[88] Torre D, Pugliese A, Speranza F. Role of nitric oxide in HIV-1 infection: friend or foe? *Lancet Infect Dis.* 2002; 2: 273-280.
[89] Peterhans E. Reactive oxygen species and nitric oxide in viral diseases. *Biol Trace Elem Res.* 1997; 56: 107-116.
[90] Kimura T, Kameoka M, Ikuta K. Amplification of superoxide anion generation in phagocytic cells by HIV-1 infection. *FEBS Lett.* 1993; 326: 232-236.
[91] Elbim C, Prevot MH, Bouscarat F, et al. Impairment of polymorphonuclear neutrophil function in HIV-infected patients. *J Cardiovasc Pharmacol.* 1995; Suppl 2, S66-S70.
[92] Tang AM, Smit E. Oxidative stress in HIV-1-infected injection drug users. *J Acquir Immune Defic Syndr.* 2000; 25 Suppl 1, S12-8.
[93] Jareno EJ, Roma J, Romero B, et al. Serum malondialdehyde correlates with therapeutic efficiency of high activity antiretroviral therapies (HAART) in HIV-1 infected children. *Free Radic Res.* 2002; 36: 341-344.
[94] van Asbeck BS, Georgiou NA, van der Bruggen T, et al. Anti-HIV effect of iron chelators: different mechanisms involved. *J Clin Virol.* 2001; 20: 141-147.

[95] Warso MA, Lands WE. Presence of lipid hydroperoxide in human plasma. *J Clin Invest* 1985; 75: 667-671.

[96] Stief TW. Thrombin generation by hemolysis. *Blood Coagul Fibrinol* 2007; 18: 61-6.

[97] Zhu P, Liu J, Bess J Jr, Chertova E, Lifson JD, Grise H, Ofek GA, Taylor KA, Roux KH. Distribution and three-dimensional structure of AIDS virus envelope spikes. *Nature* 2006; 441: 847-852.

[98] Lenard J, Rabson A, Vanderoef R. Photodynamic inactivation of infectivity of human immunodeficiency virus and other enveloped viruses using hypericin and rose bengal: inhibition of fusion and syncytia formation. *Proc Natl Acad Sci USA* 1993; 90: 58-62.

[99] Prince AM, Pascual D, Meruelo D, Liebes L, Mazur Y, Dubovi E, Mandel M, Lavie G. Strategies for evaluation of enveloped virus inactivation in red cell concentrates using hypericin. *Photochem Photobiol* 2000; 71: 188-95.

[100] Tournaire C, Croux S, Maurette MT, Beck I, Hocquaux M, Braun AM, Oliveros E. Antioxidant activity of flavonoids: efficiency of singlet oxygen (1 delta g) quenching. *J Photochem Photobiol* B 1993; 19: 205-15.

[101] Bensasson RV, Jossang A, Zahir A, Bodo B, Land EJ. Redox regulation of tumor cell toxicity by flavones from Lethedon tannaensis. *Free Radic Biol Med* 1999; 27: 95-9.

[102] Tian B, Sun Z, Xu Z, Hua Y. Chemiluminescence analysis of the prooxidant and antioxidant effects of epigallocatechin-3-gallate. *Asia Pac J Clin Nutr* 2007; 16 Suppl 1: 153-7.

[103] Lee-Hilz YY, Boerboom AM, Westphal AH, Berkel WJ, Aarts JM, Rietjens IM. Pro-oxidant activity of flavonoids induces EpRE-mediated gene expression. *Chem Res Toxicol* 2006; 19: 1499-505.

[104] Fujisawa S, Kadoma Y. Anti- and pro-oxidant effects of oxidized quercetin, curcumin or curcumin-related compounds with thiols or ascorbate as measured by the induction period method. *In Vivo* 2006; 20: 39-44.

[105] Grivennikova VG, Vinogradov AD. Generation of superoxide by the mitochondrial Complex I. *Biochim Biophys Acta* 2006; 1757: 553-61.

[106] Cotelle N, Hapiot P, Pinson J, Rolando C, Vezin H. Polyphenols deriving from chalcones: investigations of redox activities. *J Phys Chem* B 2005; 109: 23720-9.

[107] Sang S, Hou Z, Lambert JD, Yang CS. Redox properties of tea polyphenols and related biological activities. *Antioxid Redox Signal* 2005; 7: 1704-14.

[108] Klöhn PC, Neumann HG. Impairment of respiration and oxidative phosphorylation by redox cyclers 2-nitrosofluorene and menadione. *Chem Biol Interact* 1997; 106: 15-28.

[109] Rahman I, Biswas SK, Kirkham PA. Regulation of inflammation and redox signaling by dietary polyphenols. *Biochem Pharmacol* 2006; 72: 1439-52.

[110] Liu S, Lu H, Zhao Q, He Y, Niu J, Debnath AK, Wu S, Jiang S. Theaflavin derivatives in black tea and catechin derivatives in green tea inhibit HIV-1 entry by targeting gp41. *Biochim Biophys Acta* 2005; 1723: 270-81.

[111] Liu S, Jiang S, Wu Z, Lv L, Zhang J, Zhu Z, Wu S. Identification of inhibitors of the HIV-1 gp41 six-helix bundle formation from extracts of Chinese medicinal herbs Prunella vulgaris and Rhizoma cibotte. *Life Sci* 2002; 71: 1779-91.

[112] Li BQ, Fu T, Dongyan Y, Mikovits JA, Ruscetti FW, Wang JM. Flavonoid baicalin inhibits HIV-1 infection at the level of viral entry. *Biochem Biophys Res Commun* 2000; 276: 534-8.

[113] Reutrakul V, Ningnuek N, Pohmakotr M, Yoosook C, Napaswad C, Kasisit J, Santisuk T, Tuchinda P. Anti HIV-1 Flavonoid Glycosides from Ochna integerrima. *Planta Med* 2007; 73: 683-8.

[114] Song JM, Seong BL. Tea catechins as a potential alternative anti-infectious agent. *Expert Rev Anti Infect Ther* 2007; 5: 497-506.

[115] Veljkovic V, Mouscadet JF, Veljkovic N, Glisic S, Debyser Z. Simple criterion for selection of flavonoid compounds with anti-HIV activity. *Bioorg Med Chem Lett* 2007; 17: 1226-32.

[116] Yu D, Morris-Natschke SL, Lee KH. New developments in natural products-based anti-AIDS research. *Med Res Rev* 2007; 27: 108-32.

[117] Fassina G, Buffa A, Benelli R, Varnier OE, Noonan DM, Albini A. Polyphenolic antioxidant (-)-epigallocatechin-3-gallate from green tea as a candidate anti-HIV agent. *AIDS* 2002; 16: 939-41.

[118] Meragelman KM, McKee TC, Boyd MR. Anti-HIV prenylated flavonoids from Monotes africanus. *J Nat Prod* 2001; 64: 546-8.

[119] Cowan MM. Plant products as antimicrobial agents. *Clin Microbiol Rev* 1999; 12: 564-82.

[120] Mahmood N, Pizza C, Aquino R, De Tommasi N, Piacente S, Colman S, Burke A, Hay AJ. Inhibition of HIV infection by flavanoids. *Antiviral Res* 1993; 22: 189-99.

[121] Váli L, Stefanovits-Bányai E, Szentmihályi K, Fébel H, Sárdi E, Lugasi A, Kocsis I, Blázovics A. Liver-protecting effects of table beet (Beta vulgaris var. rubra) during ischemia-reperfusion. *Nutrition* 2007; 23: 172-8.

[122] Miyoshi T, Matsumoto AH, Shi W. Paradoxical increase in LDL oxidation by endothelial cells from an atherosclerosis-resistant mouse strain. *Atherosclerosis* 2007; 192: 259-65.

[123] Sutherland BA, Rahman RM, Appleton I. Mechanisms of action of green tea catechins, with a focus on ischemia-induced neurodegeneration. *J Nutr Biochem* 2006; 17: 291-306.

[124] Stief TW, Fareed J. The antithrombotic factor singlet oxygen/light ($^1O_2$/hv). *Clin Appl Thromb Hemost* 2000; 6: 22-30.

[125] Kaesemeyer WH, Caldwell RB, Huang J, Caldwell RW. Pravastatin sodium activates endothelial nitric oxide synthase independent of its cholesterol-lowering actions. *J Am Coll Cardiol* 1999; 33: 234-41.

[126] Stief TW. Innovative tests of plasmatic hemostasis. *Laboratory Medicine* 2008; 39: 225-30.

[127] Kalyanaraman B, Feix JB, Sieber F, Thomas JP, Girotti AW. Potodynamic action of merocyanine 540 on artificial and natural cell membranes: involvement of singlet molecular oxygen. *Proc Natl Acad Sci U S A*. 1987; 84: 2999-3003.

[128] Yasui H, Hayashi S, Sakurai H. Possible involvement of singlet oxygen species as multiple oxidants in p450 catalytic reactions. *Drug Metab Pharmacokinet* 2005; 20: 1-13.

[129] Chase MJ, Klebanoff SJ. Viricidal effect of stimulated human mononuclear phagocytes on human immunodeficiency virus type 1. *Proc Natl Acad Sci USA* 1992; 89: 5582-5.

[130] Shuangsuo D, Zhengguo Z, Yunru C, Xin Z, Baofeng W, Lichao Y, Yan'an C. Inhibition of the replication of hepatitis B virus in vitro by emodin. *Med Sci Monit* 2006; 12: BR302-6.

[131] Tanaka N, Okasaka M, Ishimaru Y, Takaishi Y, Sato M, Okamoto M, Oshikawa T, Ahmed SU, Consentino LM, Lee KH. Biyouyanagin A, an anti-HIV agent from hypericum chinense L. var. salicifolium. *Org Lett* 2005; 7: 2997-9.

[132] Miskovsky P. Hypericin--a new antiviral and antitumor photosensitizer: mechanism of action and interaction with biological macromolecules. *Curr Drug Targets* 2002; 3: 55-84.

[133] Lagathu C, Eustace B, Prot M, Frantz D, Gu Y, Bastard JP, Maachi M, Azoulay S, Briggs M, Caron M, Capeau J. Some HIV antiretrovirals increase oxidative stress and alter chemokine, cytokine or adiponectin production in human adipocytes and macrophages. *Antivir Ther* 2007; 12: 489-500.

[134] Ikeda M, Abe K, Yamada M, Dansako H, Naka K, Kato N. Different anti-HCV profiles of statins and their potential for combination therapy with interferon. *Hepatology* 2006; 44: 117-25.

[135] Stief TW, Slenczka W, Renz H, Klenk HD. Singlet oxygen ($^1O_2$) generating chloramines at concentrations that are tolerable for normal hemostasis function inactivate the lipid enveloped vesicular stomatitis virus in human blood. In: *3rd Symposium on the Biology of Endothelial Cells; Pathophysiology of the Endothelium: Vascular and Infectious Diseases*, May 24-26, 2001, Giessen, Germany, Abstr. D10

[136] Stief TW. The physiology and pharmacology of singlet oxygen. *Medical Hypotheses* 2003; 60: 567-72.

[137] De Clercq E. The design of drugs for HIV and HCV. *Nat Rev Drug Discov* 2007; 6: 1001-18.

[138] Pinter A. Roles of HIV-1 Env variable regions in viral neutralization and vaccine development. *Curr HIV Res* 2007; 5: 542-53.

[139] Schiavone M, Quinto I, Scala G. Perspectives for a protective HIV-1 vaccine. *Adv Pharmacol* 2008; 56: 423-52.

[140] Soriano V, Puoti M, Garcia-Gascó P, Rockstroh JK, Benhamou Y, Barreiro P, McGovern B. Antiretroviral drugs and liver injury. *AIDS* 2008; 22: 1-13.

[141] Ahmad N. Molecular mechanisms of HIV-1 vertical transmission and pathogenesis in infants. *Adv Pharmacol* 2008; 56: 453-508.

[142] Hoang V, Withers-Ward E, Camerini D. Nonprimate models of HIV-1 infection and pathogenesis. *Adv Pharmacol* 2008; 56: 399-422.

[143] Semenova EA, Marchand C, Pommier Y. HIV-1 integrase inhibitors: update and perspectives. *Adv Pharmacol* 2008; 56: 199-228.

[144] Mitsuya H, Maeda K, Das D, Ghosh AK. Development of protease inhibitors and the fight with drug-resistant HIV-1 variants. *Adv Pharmacol* 2008; 56: 169-97.

[145] Ilina T, Parniak MA. Inhibitors of HIV-1 reverse transcriptase. *Adv Pharmacol* 2008; 56: 121-67.

[146] Strizki J. Targeting HIV attachment and entry for therapy. *Adv Pharmacol* 2008; 56: 93-120.

[147] Murphy EM, Jimenez HR, Smith SM. Current clinical treatments of AIDS. *Adv Pharmacol* 2008; 56: 27-73.

In: Hemostasis Laboratory Yearbook, Volume 2
Editor: Thomas W. Stief, pp. 39-49
ISBN: 978-1-60741-089-8

DETERMINATION OF ACTIVE ENDOTOXIN IN PLASMA

Thomas W. Stief *

Department of Clinical Chemistry, University Hospital, Giessen & Marburg, Germany

ABSTRACT

There is clinical need for a simple rapid assay that detects active endotoxin (here clinically understood as active lipopolysaccharide (LPS) or active ß-glucan) in blood of patients. Hitherto Limulus-based endotoxin tests cannot be used for plasma testing due to the presence of strong plasmatic serine protease inhibitors of the Limulus clotting system. It was the aim of the present study to destroy these inhibitors without affecting the true content of active endotoxin in plasma.

10 µl citrated or EDTA plasma were oxidized with 10 µl 60 mM chloramine-T® for 10 min (37°C). 10 µl 230 mM methionine without or with 0.63 mg/ml of the LPS inhibitor polymyxin B were added. Then 30 µl Limulus reagent, that contained the factors C,B,G,A and the chromogenic substrate for activated factor A (FAa) Ile-Glu-Gly-Arg-pNA, were added and the increase in absorbance with time was measured.

The normal range is 0.8±0.2 ng/ml LPS reactivity (MV±1SD) and < 0.1 µg/ml ß-glucan reactivity. This method allows to quantify plasmatic LPS reactivities from 0.1 to 1000 ng/ml (about 10-100000 % of normal) and ß-glucan reactivities from 0.1 to 100 µg/ml; e.g. an extreme LPS reactivity of 100 ng/ml means that this plasma behaves in the Limulus assay as if pooled normal plasma with 0.8 ng/ml LPS would have been supplemented with 99.2 ng purified LPS/ml plasma. Only about 1 % of added purified LPS or about 10 % of added purified ß-glucan is free=unbound=active. These new assays will help to diagnose the very early phase of gram-negative or fungal sepsis.

INTRODUCTION

Endotoxin activity circulates in blood of patients with severe sepsis caused by gram-negative germs or by fungi [1]. Free endotoxin, the toxicologically active form of endotoxin, damages the membranes of susceptible human cells. The resulting cell fragments (e.g. phospholipid vesicles or DNA) trigger intrinsic hemostasis, systemic thrombin is generated in excess and disseminated thrombi are formed that can threaten the life of the patient [2,3]. Therefore, severe sepsis has to be diagnosed as early as possible. The biochemical nature of this here clinically defined endotoxin is lipopolysaccharide (LPS) or (1,3)-β-D-glucan, both

---

* Correspondence to: PD Dr. Med. T. Stief, Department of Clinical Chemistry, University Hospital, D-35043 Marburg, Germany; Email: thstief@med.uni-marburg.de; Tel.: +49-6421-58 64471; Fax: +49-6421-58 65594

are derived from the cell walls of gram-negative bacteria or of fungi, respectively. Hitherto endotoxin determinations in plasma are not specific for free = active endotoxin: they determine the total amount of endotoxin, i.e. also endotoxin that is neutralized after binding to endotoxin antibodies, or they are influenced by plasmatic serine protease inhibitors of the Limulus serine proteases [1,4]. The aim of the present work was to develop a new plasma assay that responds only to active endotoxin.

MATERIAL AND METHODS

Limulus Kinetic: Coamatic®-Reagent vs. Pyrochrome®-Reagent

1 ml pooled citrated plasma of patients (0.5 ml 106 mM sodium citrate + 4.5 ml blood, centrifuged at 2800g for 10 min (23°C), containing 1.8 ng/ml LPS reactivity) with normal prothrombin time, APTT, and fibrinogen was supplemented with 0–371 ng/ml LPS (Sigma, Deisenhofen, Germany) and incubated with 1 ml 60 mM chloramine-T® (CT; Sigma) in PBS for 10 min (37°C) in pyrogene-free untreated U-microtiterplates (NUNC, Wiesbaden, Germany). 1 ml 230 mmol/l methionine in H_2O was added (comparable to 3.3 µl plasma + 3.3 µl 60 mM CT + 3.3 µl 230 mM methionine) and after 3 min (room temperature) 10 µl of this mixture were incubated with 10 µl 0 or 5000 U/ml polymyxin B (1 mg=7868 IU; Euro OTC Pharma, Kamen, Germany) in H_2O and 20 µl Pyrochrome®-Reagent (Limulus amoebocyte lyophilizate (LAL) clotting factors/chromogenic substrate (Ile-Glu-Gly-Arg-pNA) colyophilizate; CapeCode, Falmouth, USA) at room temperature (RT; 23°C). The absorption-values were determined after 0 - 44 min (RT) at 405 nm.

10 µl pooled normal citrated plasma, supplemented with 0-100 ng/ml LPS, was incubated with 10 µl 60 mmol/l CT for 10 min at 37°C. 10 µl 200 mmol/l methionine with 2000 U/ml polymyxin B (Sigma) were added and after 3 min RT 30 µl Limulus colyophilizate - reagent Coamatic® (Chromogenix, Mölndal, Sweden) were added and the reaction was incubated at 23°C. Table 1 demonstrates a typical pipetting scheme of the Limulus assay.

Optimization of Chloramine Addition

10 µl sample (pooled normal citrated plasma, pooled plasma plus 3.2 mg/ml K_3 - EDTA, or pooled plasma plus 70 IU/ml heparin (Sarstedt, Nümbrecht, Germany)) supplemented with 0 or 10 ng/ml LPS were incubated with 10 µl 0-133 mmol/l CT in H_2O for 10 min at 37°C. Then 10 µl 200 mmol/l antioxidant (here: sodium ascorbate) and 30 µl Limulus-reagent Coamatic® were added.

10 µl pooled normal citrated plasma, supplemented with 0 or 10 ng/ml LPS or 10 ng/ml LPS + 1 µg/ml zymosan A (Sigma) or 10 µl 7% human albumin (Kabi, Stockholm, Sweden), not supplemented and supplemented with 1 µg/ml zymosan A, were incubated with 10 µl 0-133 mmol/l CT in 100 mmol/l $NaHCO_3$, pH 8.5, for 10 min (37°C). Then 50 µl 200 mmol/l methionine and after 3 min at RT 30 µl Limulus-reagent Coamatic® were added and delta A at 405 nm ($\Delta A_{405\ nm}$) was determined after 93 min at RT.

Comparison of Heat Treatment with Oxidative Treatment in Plasma

a) unsupplemented samples: n=23 unselected EDTA-plasmas of patients were analyzed by means of Coamatic®-Limulus test: they were treated either with heat (10-fold dilution with H_2O, 15 min at 75°C) or with 10 µl 60 mmol/l CT per 10 µl sample (10 min 37°C).

b) supplemented samples: 5 µl 0 or 10 ng/ml LPS in 0.9 % NaCl was freshly prepared and immediately added to EDTA-plasmas of patients, and they were tested in the oxidative assay (n=23) or in the heat treatment version (n=22) with the Coamatic®-reagent.

Comparison of heat treatment with oxidative treatment in purified system

7.5 % human albumin basally containing 0.5 µg/ml zymosan A, supplemented with 0-1000 ng/ml LPS (*E. coli 0111:B4*; purified by gel-filtration; product L 3012-5MG; Sigma) or with + 0-100 µg/ml zymosan A was analyzed as follows:

a. Heat treatment: 20 µl plasma was 10-fold diluted with H_2O and incubated for 15 min at RT or at 75°C (water bath). Then 20 µl heat-treated sample was incubated in duplicate with 20 µl LAL-reagent (Pyrochrome®) at RT and the delta A at 405 nm was determined using a microtiterplate photometer (Milenia-DPC, Los Angeles, USA).
b. Oxidation treatment: 5 µl plasma was incubated in duplicate with 5 µl PBS or 60 mM chloramine-T® in PBS for 10 min at 37°C (water bath). Then 5 µl 230 mM methionine in H_2O was added and after 3 min RT 15 µl LAL-reagent (Pyrochrome®) was added and the delta A at 405 nm (RT) was determined.

RESULTS AND DISCUSSION

Figure 1a demonstrates that usage of 20 µl Limulus-reagent results into a maximal delta A of 470 mA; a delta A of 100 mA (corresponding to about 20 % of the max. delta A) results for 1.7 ng/ml LPS-reactivity in plasma after 37 min RT, for 3.2 ng/ml LPS-reactivity after 32 min RT, for 6.3 ng/ml LPS-reactivity after 26 min RT, for 15.4 ng/ml LPS-reactivity after 24 min RT, for 42.9 ng/ml LPS-reactivity after 23 min RT, for 125 ng/ml LPS-reactivity after 22 min RT, for 371 ng/ml LPS-reactivity after 18 min RT. At a defined reaction time, there is a linear relationship between a pathological standard and dilutions of this standard, if at this time point this patho-standard causes less than 45 % of the maximal obtainable ΔA.

Figure 1b demonstrates that the Coamatic®-reagent has a substantially slower kinetic than the Pyrochrome®-reagent, i.e. Coamatic-reagent might contain less factor C but more chromogenic substrate than Pyrochrome®. Since there is some lot-to-lot variation of the Pyrochrome® reagent that might cause unspecific turbidities, for the below patient studies Coamatic®-reagent was used, because due to a higher concentration of the chromogenic substrate its maximal specific pNA signal is higher than the one measured for Pyrochrome®.

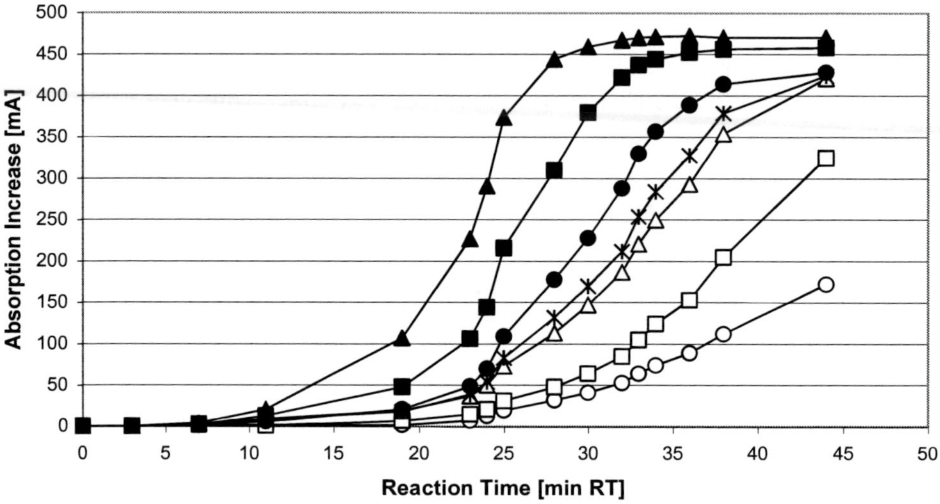

(a)

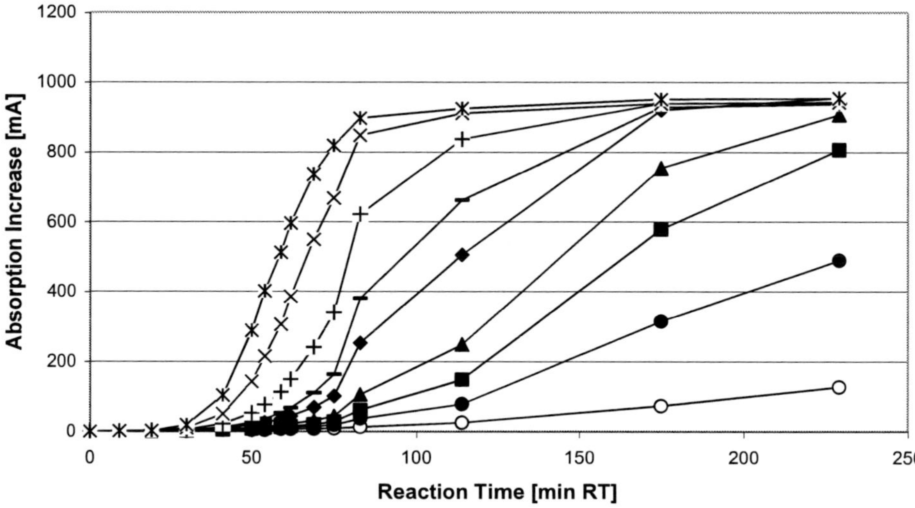

(b)

Figure 1(a). Hyperbolic Limulus kinetic with Pyrochrome®. 1 ml pooled patient plasma (citrated; containing 1.8 ng/ml LPS reactivity) with normal plasmatic coagulation was supplemented with further 0 (O), 1.5 (□), 4.6 (Δ), 13.7 (*), 41.2 (●), 123.5 (■), 371 (▲) ng/ml LPS and was incubated with 1 ml 60 mM chloramine-T® (CT) in PBS for 10 min (37°C). 1 ml 230 mmol/l methionine was added and after 3 min (room temperature; RT) 10 µl of this mixture was incubated with 10 µl H_2O or 5000 U/ml polymyxin B in H_2O and 20 µl Pyrochrome®-Reagent, and the absorption-values were determined after 0-44 min (RT) at 405 nm.

Figure 1(b). Hyperbolic Limulus kinetic with Coamatic®-Reagent. 10 µl pooled normal citrated plasma, supplemented with further 0 (O), 0.8 (●), 1.6 (■), 3.1 (▲), 6.3 (♦), 12.5 (-), 25 (+), 50 (x), 100 (*) ng/ml LPS, was incubated with 10 µl 60 mmol/l CT for 10 min at 37°C. 10 µl 200 mmol/l methionine with 2000 U/ml polymyxin B were added and after 3 min RT 30 µl Limulus-reagent Coamatic® were added and the reaction was incubated at 23°C.

Twenty percent of the max. delta A are about 200 mA; this delta A is reached after 40 min RT for + 100 ng/ml LPS, after 50 min RT for + 50 ng/ml LPS, after 60 min RT for + 25 ng/ml LPS, after 70 min RT for 12.5 ng/ml LPS, after 75 min RT for + 6.3 ng/ml LPS, after 100 min RT for + 3.1 ng/ml LPS, after 120 min RT for + 1.6 ng/ml LPS, after 140 min RT for + 0.8 ng/ml LPS, after about 270 min RT for + 0 ng/ml LPS.

Figure 2a,b for 10 ng/ml LPS supplemented plasmas and for unsupplemented plasmas show that chloramine–concentrations of 40-80 mmol/l are optimal to eliminate plasmatic Limulus inhibitors: without oxidation there is no measurable LPS-reactivity within 50 min RT. 70 IU/ml heparin in the sample *stimulate* the reactivity of 10 ng/ml supplemented LPS in the present oxidative assay about 5-fold, when using an oxidant reagent with ≥ 60 mM CT. Fig. 2a demonstrates that the samples to be analyzed in the present Limulus-assay should contain a similar matrix of calcium complexing compounds.

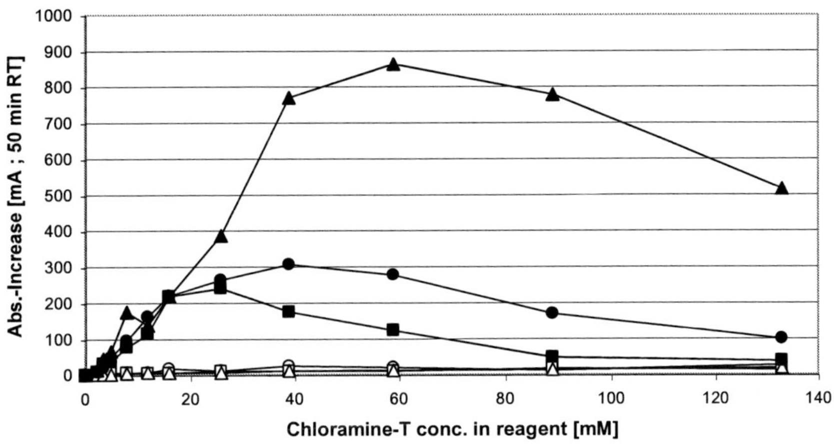

(a)

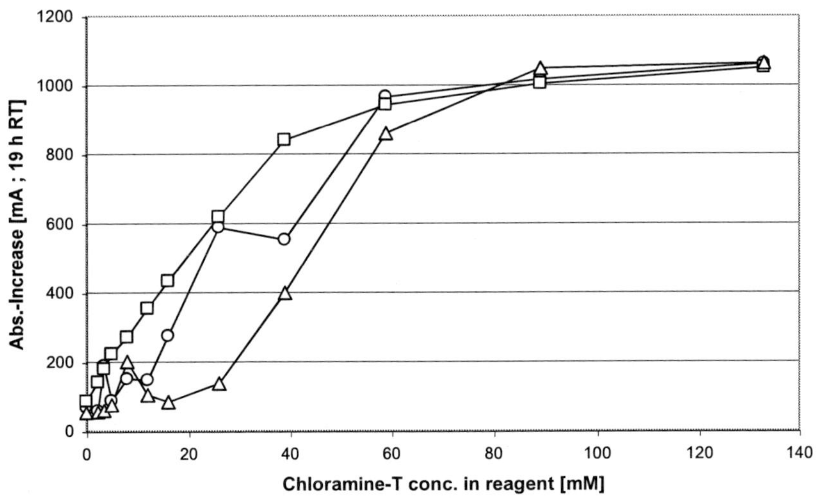

(b)

Figure 2 (a) and (b). Optimization of chloramine addition. 10 µl sample (pooled normal citrated plasma (O,●), pooled plasma plus 3.2 mg/ml EDTA (□,■), or pooled plasma plus 70 IU/ml heparin (Δ,▲)) supplemented with 0 (white symbols) or 10 ng/ml (black symbols) LPS, were incubated with 10 µl 0-133 mmol/l CT in H_2O for 10 min at 37°C. Then 10 µl 200 mmol/l ascorbate and 30 µl Limulus-reagent Coamatic® were added and ΔA after 50 min RT (Fig. 2a) or 19h RT (Fig. 2b) were determined.

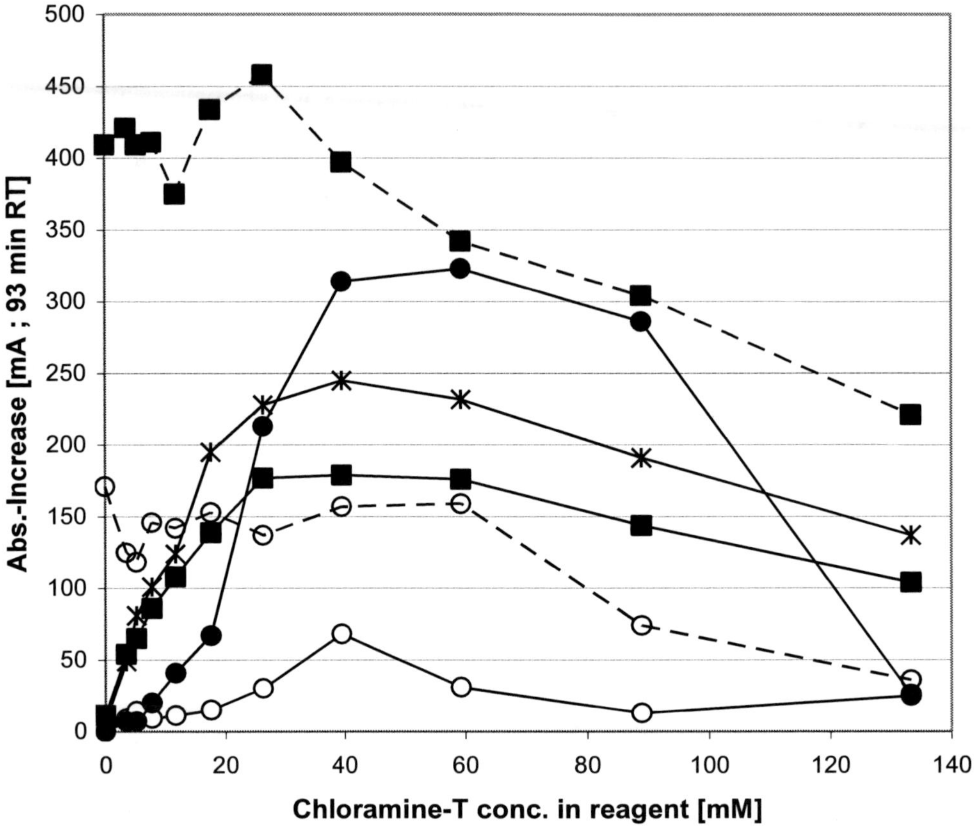

(c)

Figure 2(c). Optimization of chloramine addition. 10 µl pooled normal citrated plasma, supplemented with 0 (O), 10 ng/ml LPS (•), 1 µg/ml zymosan A (■), or 10 ng/ml LPS + 1 µg/ml zymosan A (*), or 10 µl 7% human albumin, not further supplemented (- O -) and further supplemented with 1 µg/ml zymosan A (-■-), were incubated with 10 µl 0-133 mmol/l CT in 100 mmol/l $NaHCO_3$, pH 8.5, for 10 min (37°C). Then 50 µl 200 mmol/l methionine and after 3 min at RT 30 µl Limulus-reagent Coamatic® were added and delta A was determined after 93 min at RT (Fig. 2c).

Without oxidation there is only a Limulus-reactivity of < 100 mA/19 h RT for normal plasma. Addition of 40-80 mM CT increases the reactivity more than 10-fold. At least 60 mM CT in the oxidant reagent are necessary to result into a similar LPS-reactivity in 70 IU/ml heparinized plasma as compared with pooled normal citrated or EDTA plasma.

Figure 2c demonstrates that for pooled normal plasma, unsupplemented and supplemented with LPS or ZyA, there are maximal endotoxin reactivities if the oxidant-reagent contains 40-80 mM CT.

Figure 3 shows that the procedures generate different reactivities (heat treatment: 1.8 ng/ml ± 1.6 ng/ml LPS; CT-treatment: 2.8 ng/ml ± 1.6 ng/ml LPS reactivity; mean value (MV) ± 1 standard deviation (SD); the correlation factor was r= 0.210 (Figure 3a). CT-treatment: from basal 2.8 ± 1.6 ng/ml LPS reactivity in the 10 µl sample after addition of 5 µl 10 ng/ml freshly prepared LPS 6.2 ng/ml ± 3.8 ng/ml LPS reactivity arose, the correlation factor was r = 0.574 (Figure 3b).

Figure 3c shows the results of the heat procedure, in which the addition of 5 µl freshly prepared 10 ng/ml LPS results in 5.8 ± 4.6 ng/ml LPS after prior 1.5 ± 1.1 ng/ml; the correlation factor was only r= 0.024. This correlation factor is substantially smaller than that by oxidation of the samples (r=0.574), i.e. there exists an extreme interindividual deviation in recovery of LPS when testing with the (strongly denaturing) heat treatment in contrast to the oxidation method. 1000 ng/ml LPS after heat treatment acts like 0.1 ng/ml LPS at RT (Figure 4a), i.e. 99.99 % of the active LPS were inactivated by the heat treatment (Figure 4b). Zymosan A is heat resistant. Both the LPS-reactivity (Figure 4c) and the zymosan-reactivity are resistant against oxidation (Figure 4d).

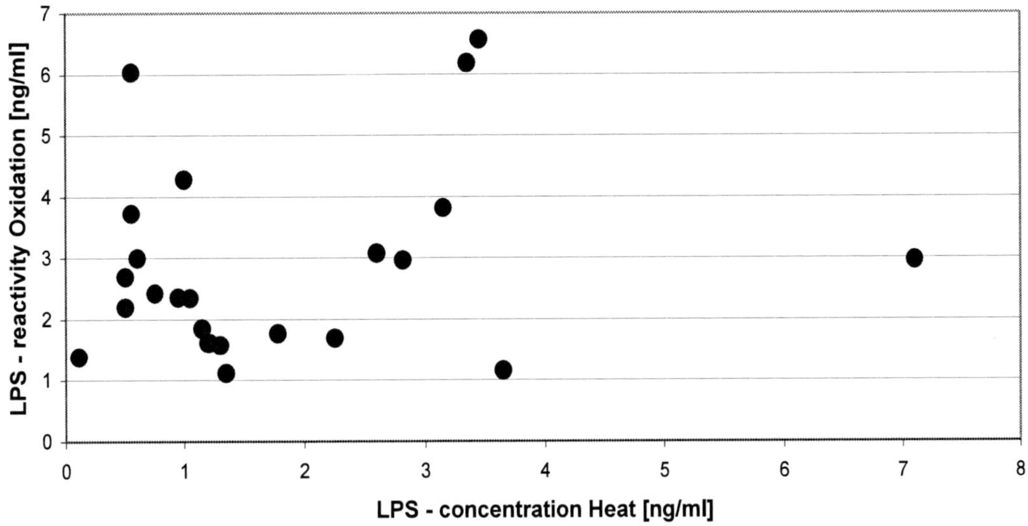

(a)

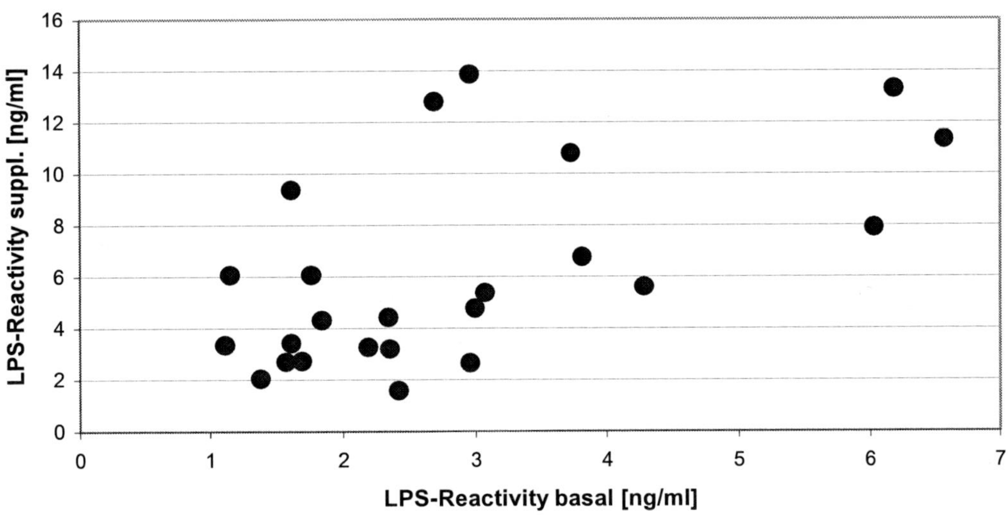

(b)

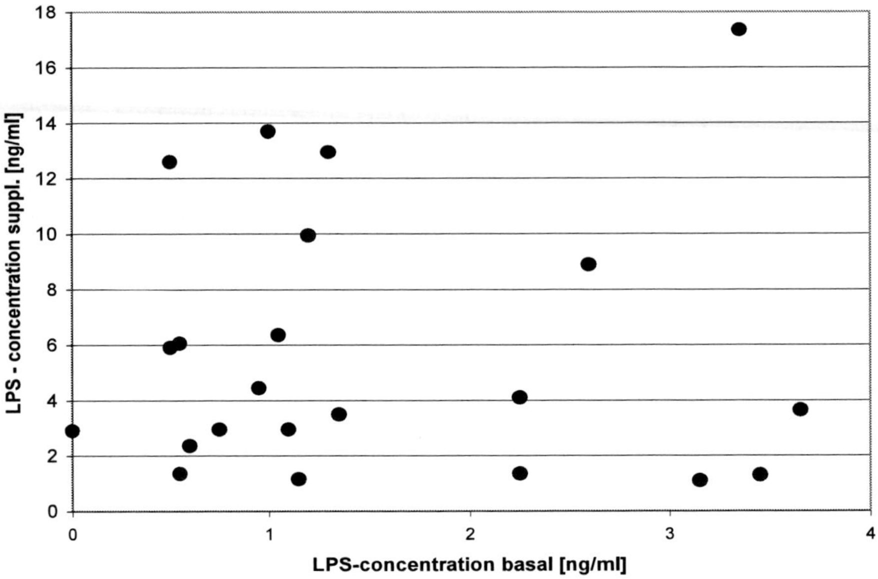

(c)

Figure 3(a). Comparison of heat treatment with oxidative treatment in plasma. Unsupplemented samples. n=23 unselected EDTA-plasmas of patients were analyzed by means of Coamatic®-Limulus test: they were treated either with heat (10-fold dilution with H_2O, 15 min at 75°C) or with 10 µl 60 mmol/l chloramine-T® per 10 µl sample.

Figure 3 (b) and (c) Supplemented samples. 5 µl 0 or 10 ng/ml LPS were added to EDTA-samples of patients and they were tested in the oxidative assay (Fig. 3b; n=24) or in the heat treatment version (Fig. 3c; n=22) with the Coamatic®-reagent.

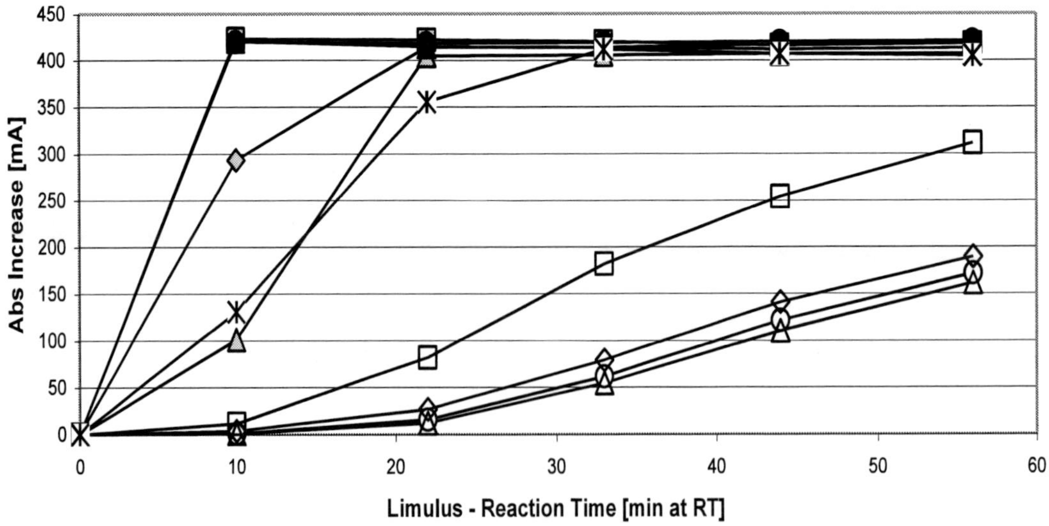

(a)

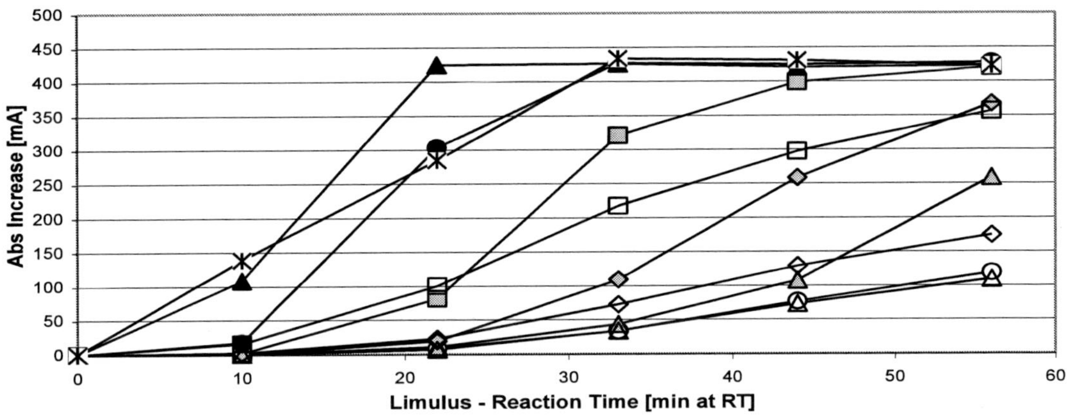

(b)

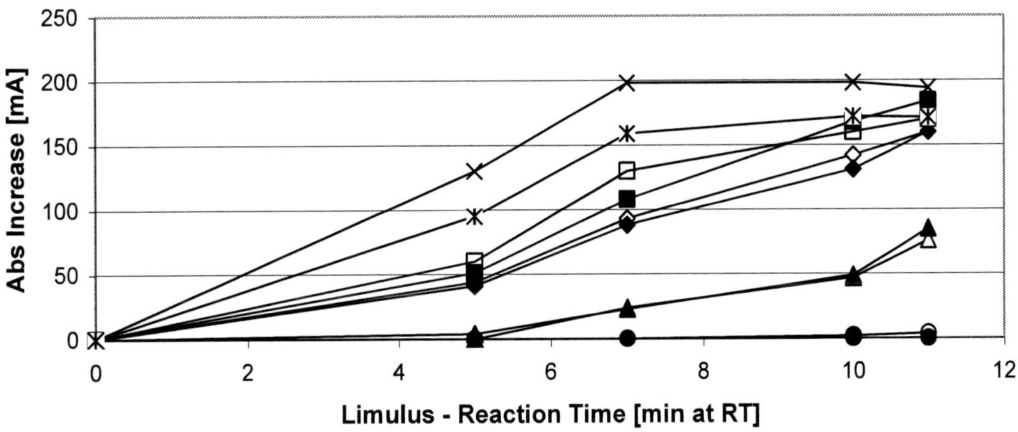

(c)

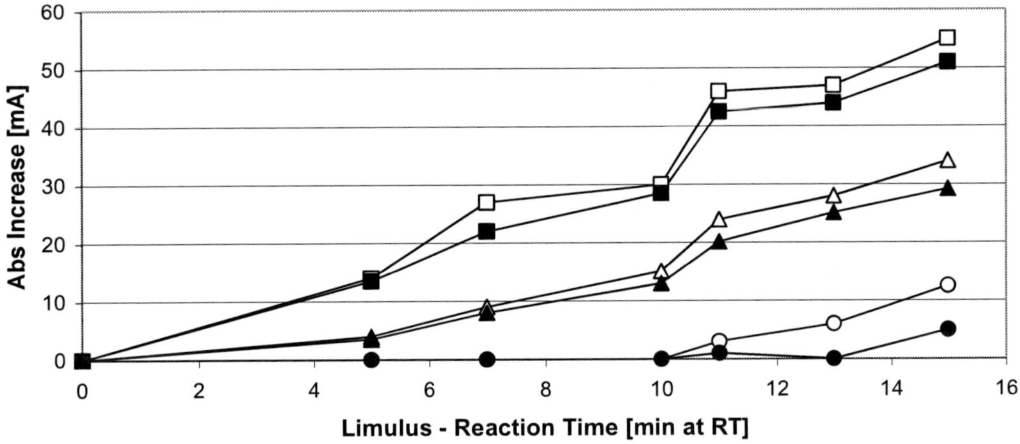

(d)

Figure 4(a). Comparison of heat treatment with oxidative treatment in purified system.
Figure 4(a) and (b): 23°C vs. 75°C. 7.5 % human albumin containing 0.5 μg/ml zymosan A, supplemented with 0-1000 ng/ml LPS or with 0-100 μg/ml zymosan A was analyzed without further treatment (Fig. 4a) or with heat treatment of endotoxins (Fig. 4b). 20 μl sample was 10-fold diluted

with H_2O and incubated for 15 min at 23°C or at 75°C (water bath). Then 20 µl heat-treated sample was incubated with 20 µl Limulus-reagent (Pyrochrome®) at RT and ΔA at 405 nm was determined; samples supplemented by: + 0 ng/ml LPS (O), + 0.1 ng/ml LPS (grey Δ), + 1 ng/ml LPS (grey ◊), +10 ng/ml LPS (grey □), +100 ng/ml (•), +1000 ng/ml LPS (▲), +0.1 µg/ml ZyA (Δ), +1 µg/ml ZyA (◊), +10 µg/ml ZyA (□), +100 µg/ml ZyA (*).
Figure 4 (c). 0 vs. 60 mM CT for LPS. 5 µl 7.5 % human albumin containing 0.5 µg/ml zymosan A, supplemented with 0 (O,•), 0.1 (Δ,▲), 1 (◊,♦), 10 (□,■), 100 ng/ml (x,*) LPS was incubated with 5 µl PBS (white symbols) or 60 mM chloramine-T® in PBS (black symbols) for 10 min at 37°C. Then 5 µl 230 mM methionine in H_2O was added and after 3 min RT 15 µl Limulus-reagent (Pyrochrome®) was added and ΔA at 405 nm (RT) was determined.
Figure 4 (d). 0 vs. 60 mM CT for ß-glucan. 5 µl 7.5 % human albumin containing 0.5 µg/ml zymosan A, supplemented with further 0.1 (O,•), 1 (Δ,▲), 10 (□,■) µg/ml ß-glucan, was incubated with 5 µl PBS (white symbols) or 60 mM chloramine-T® in PBS (black symbols) for 10 min at 37°C. Then 5 µl 230 mM methionine in H_2O was added and after 3 min RT 15 µl Limulus-reagent (Pyrochrome®) was added and ΔA at 405 nm (RT) was determined.

LPS reactivity increases up to the range of 100fold in patients with severe sepsis, e.g. by *Neisseria meningitidis* [6]. LPS reactivities of 2-3 ng/ml or ß-glucan reactivities of about 0.5 µg/ml might be considered as threshold concentrations to cause phospholipase A2 activation and cell fragmentation, leading to pathologic disseminated intravascular coagulation (PDIC) with elevated plasmatic thrombin activities [2,5,7].

The present technique allows the quantification of active endotoxin in plasma within about 30 min (37°C). Of special interest for each individual patient would be the early diagnosis of sepsis, i.e. the very early phase of sepsis with LPS reacitivities in the range of 2-3 ng/ml or ß-glucan reactivities in the range of 0.2-0.5 µg/ml. With a very early diagnosis the adequate treatment can start in time.

Table 1a. Test for plasmatic active endotoxin (here: LPS+ß-glucan).

10 µl plasma (EDTA or citrate) or standards (1, 10, 100, 1000 ng/ml LPS reactivity) 10 µl 60 mM chloramine-T® in 50 mM sodium citrate, pH 7.8
10 min (37°C)
10 µl 230 mM methionine
2 min (37°C)
30 µl Limulus-reagent (Limulus factors + chromogenic substrate)
0, 10, 30 min (37°C)
Absorbance at 405 nm

Table 1b. Test for plasmatic active ß-glucan.

10 µl plasma (EDTA or citrate) or standards (0, 1, 10, 100 µg/ml ß-glucan reactivity) 10 µl 60 mM chloramine-T® in in 50 mM sodium citrate, pH 7.8
10 min (37°C)
10 µl 230 mM methionine, 0.63 mg/ml (4957 IU/ml) polymyxin B
2 min (37°C)
30 µl Limulus-reagent (Limulus factors + chromogenic substrate)
0, 10, 30 min (37°C)
Absorbance at 405 nm

LPS reactivity [mA/t] = endotoxin reactivity [mA/t] minus β-glucan reactivity [mA/t]

Reactivity examples:

- 10 ng/ml LPS reactivity corresponds to the LPS reactivity of normal plasma containing 1 ng/ml LPS that had been supplemented with additional 9 ng/ml purified LPS.
- 10 µg/ml ß-glucan reactivity corresponds to the ß-glucan reactivity of normal plasma containing < 0.1 µg/ml ß-glucan that had been supplemented with 10 µg/ml purified ß-glucan.

REFERENCES

[1] Hurley JC. Endotoxemia: methods of detection and clinical correlates. *Clin Microbiol Rev* 1995; 8: 268-92.

[2] Stief TW. Coagulation activation by lipopolysaccharides. *Clin Appl Thrombosis/ Hemostasis* Dec 26, 2007 doi: 10.1177/1076029607309256

[3] Stief TW. Thrombin generation by exposure of blood to endotoxin: a simple model to study disseminated intravascular coagulation. *Clin Appl Thromb Hemost* 2006; 12: 137-61.

[4] Roth RI, Levin FC, Levin J. Optimization of detection of bacterial endotoxin in plasma with the Limulus test. *J Lab Clin Med* 1990; 116: 153-61.

[5] Stief TW, Ijagha O, Weiste B, Herzum I, Renz H, Max M. Analysis of hemostasis alterations in sepsis. *Blood Coagul Fibrinolysis.* 2007; 18: 179-86.

[6] Brandtzaeg P, Bjerre A, Øvstebø R, Brusletto B, Joø GB, Kierulf P. Neisseria meningitidis lipopolysaccharides in human pathology. *J Endotoxin Res* 2001; 7: 401-20.

[7] Zayat M, Lichtenberger LM, Dial EJ. Pathophysiology of LPS-induced gastrointestinal injury in the rat: role of secretory phospholipase A2. *Shock.* 2007 Dec 20 [Epub ahead of print]

In: Hemostasis Laboratory Yearbook, Volume 2
Editor: Thomas W. Stief, pp. 51-58

ISBN: 978-1-60741-089-8

ACTIVE ENDOTOXIN IN SEPSIS

Thomas W. Stief [1,*] ***and Martin Max*** [2]

[1]Department of Clinical Chemistry, University Hospital, Giessen & Marburg, Germany
[2]Department of Intensive Care Medicine, Centre Hospitalier de Luxembourg, Luxembourg

ABSTRACT

Background

Early diagnosis and rapid treatment are important for survival in patients with severe sepsis. However, conventional microbiological techniques are time consuming. Therefore, new plasma methods have been developed to accelerate diagnosis and to permit rapid evaluation of the antibiotic treatment. Active endotoxin (here clinically understood as free lipopolysaccharide (LPS) or free ß-glucan) is proposed to indicate the diagnosis and severity of sepsis syndrome and the patient´s risk to develop infection-associated severe complications such as pathologic disseminated intravascular coagulation (PDIC).

Material and Methods

Active plasmatic endotoxin is measured via a modified *Limulus* test: 10 µl EDTA-plasma of 63 patients with severe sepsis at their first day in intensive care unit and of 48 healthy donors and plasmatic reactivity standards supplemented with 0-1000 ng/ml purified LPS or with 0-100 µg/ml purified Zymosan A (a ß-glucan) were incubated with 5 µl 106 mM sodium citrate, pH 7.4, and with 10 µl 60 mM chloramine-T® for 10 min (37°C). 10 µl 230 mM methionine without (testing for active LPS + active ß-glucan) or with 0.63 mg/ml polymyxin B (testing only for active ß-glucan) were added. Then 30 µl *Limulus* factors / Ile-Glu-Gly-Arg-pNA reagent were added and the increase in absorbance with time was measured. An exemplary LPS reactivity of 20.8 ng/ml means that this plasma is as active as pooled normal plasma (with 0.8 ng/ml LPS reactivity) that had been supplemented with additional 20 ng/ml purified LPS.

* Correspondence to: Priv.-Doz. Dr. Med. T. Stief, Department of Clinical Chemistry, University Hospital, D-35043 Marburg, Germany; Email: thstief@med.uni-marburg.de; Tel. : +49-6421-58 64471; FAX: +49-6421-58 65594

Results

The patients with severe sepsis had ≥ 3 ng/ml LPS reactivity or ≥ 0.5 µg/ml ß-glucan reactivity, or both. 81 % of the patients had a LPS reactivity ≥ 3 ng/ml: these had 25.3±19.1 ng/ml, range 3.9-98 ng/ml (normal range: 0.8±0.2 ng/ml). Thus, LPS reactivity increases up to about 100fold in patients with severe sepsis. 75 % of the patients had a ß-glucan reactivity ≥ 0.5 µg/ml: these had 6.3±7.5 µg/ml, range 0.5-36.2 µg/ml (normal range: < 0.1 µg/ml). Dividing the ß-glucan reactivity [ng/ml] by 300 and adding the LPS reactivity [ng/ml] gives the total endotoxin reactivity of plasma [ng/ml]. The sepsis-associated organ failure assessment (SOFA) score displayed significantly positive correlations with active LPS ($p = 0.03$), active ß-glucan ($p = 0.035$), and active total endotoxin ($p = 0.0004$).

Discussion

Plasmatic LPS reactivities of about 2-3 ng/ml or plasmatic ß-glucan reactivities of about 0.5 µg/ml are considered as threshold concentrations to cause severe hemostasis complications such as PDIC. These new plasma assays for active LPS or active ß-glucan could help to diagnose the very early phase of gram-negative or fungal sepsis.

Key words: Endotoxin, lipopolysaccharide, ß-glucan, sepsis, DIC

INTRODUCTION

Gram-negative bacteria have cell walls of lipopolysaccharide (LPS), fungi have cell walls of ß-glucan. LPS and ß-glucan can both clinically act as endotoxin that causes severe sepsis: endotoxin activates certain membrane proteins of suspectible cells of the blood stream, e.g. membraneous phospholipase A_2 of monocytes [1-3]. Normally, about 99 % of LPS or about 90 % of ß-glucan, that enters the circulating blood, is neutralized by plasma proteins, e.g. by immunoglobulins. Unbound (= free = active) endotoxin is of great pathological importance: it destroys susceptible cells, and the resulting cell fragments trigger a pathologic disseminated intravascular coagulation (PDIC) [4]. The aim of the present work was to investigate the feasibility to measure active endotoxin in plasma of septic patients by new tests that respond only to active LPS or to active ß-glucan. Thereby these tests could offer new possibilities regarding the diagnosis of the severity of sepsis and the risk to develop complications such as PDIC.

PATIENTS, MATERIAL AND METHODS

Plasma samples from intensive care patients

After approvement by the ethical committee, 2.6 ml venous blood anticoagulated by tri-potassium salt of ethylene diamine tetra acetic acid (1.6 mg K_3-EDTA/ ml blood) was taken from 63 septic patients upon admission to the intensive care unit. The blood was transported immediately into the central laboratory, where it was centrifuged at 2800g for 10 min (23°C), and 100 µl aliquots of EDTA-plasma were frozen at -80°C [5].

All patients were admitted to our Intensive Care Unit for the treatment of newly developed severe sepsis. Patient characteristics are displayed in table 1.

Table 1a. Patient characteristics.

	n (%)
Male Gender	41 (65.1)
Septic focus	
Pneumonia	30 (47.6)
Peritonitis	19 (30.2)
Other	14 (22.2)
Intensive care unit (ICU) mortality	23 (36.5)
Hospital mortality	28 (44.4)
Renal replacement therapy	33 (52.4)

Table 1b. Patient characteristics.

	Mean ± 1 SD
Age [years]	62.9 ± 12.8
Length of stay in ICU [days]	17.2 ± 11.5
Length of stay in hospital [days]	33.5 ± 26.4
Duration of mechanical ventilation [days]	13.3 ± 11.9
SAPS II	45.1 ± 16.6
SOFA score at day 1	9.7 ± 4.3
Number of organ failures at day 1	1.8 ± 1.2

Limulus assay

Active LPS and active (1,3)-beta-D-glucan (here clinically understood as plasmatic reactivity of endotoxin) were functionally determined by singlet oxygen – mediated destruction of plasmatic inhibitors of the *Limulus polyphemus* clotting factors cascade and performance of the chromogenic *Limulus* assay [3]. The standards were pooled normal citrated plasma supplemented with 0–1000 ng/ml LPS (*Escherichia coli* 055:B5, purified by gel filtration, protein content < 1 %; Sigma, Deisenhofen, Germany; article nr. L 2637-5MG) or supplemented with 0–100 µg/ml Zymosan A (*Saccharomyces cerevisiae*; Sigma; article nr. Z 4250). 15 min (23°C) after endotoxin supplementation, 3.2 mg/ml K_3-EDTA were added. Normal plasma inhibits about 99 % of added LPS and about 90 % of added ß-glucan. 10 µl standard or EDTA-plasma of patients were incubated in duplicate in untreated polystyrol flat bottom wells (F-wells; Polysorp®, NUNC, Wiesbaden, Germany; article nr. 446140) with 5 µl 106 mM sodium citrate, pH 7.4, and 10 µl 60 mM chloramine-T® (Sigma) in 0.9 % NaCl for 10 min (37°C). 10 µl 230 mM methionine in H_2O without (= reactivity assay of LPS+ß-glucan) or with (= reactivity assay of ß-glucan) 0.63 mg/ml polymyxin B (PMB; Sigma-Fluka) were added. This PMB concentration inhibits a plasmatic LPS reactivity up to 1000 ng/ml. After 3 min at 23°C, 30 μl *Limulus* amebocyte lysate reagent in 0.2 M Tris, pH 8, containing the *Limulus* factors C, B, G, A and the chromogenic substrate for activated factor A Ile-Glu-Gly-Arg-pNA (*Limulus* factors/ chromogenic substrate co-lyophilizate) (Coamatic®Chromo-LAL; Chromogenix, Mölndal, Sweden) were added. The hyperbolic rate assay was followed at 405 nm for 0-120 min (23°C), using a microtiterplate reader with a 1 mA resolution (Milenia; DPC, Los Angeles, USA). The normal range of endotoxin reactivity as determined by analysis of plasma samples of 48 healthy donors is 100 ± 25 % of normal (mean value (MV) ± 1 standard deviation (SD); 100 % = 0.8 ng/ml) LPS reactivity and < 0.1 μg/ml ß-glucan reactivity in EDTA plasma. A LPS reactivity of e.g. 10 ng/ml means, that this plasma is as active as pooled normal plasma that has been supplemented with additional 9.2 ng/ml purified LPS; a ß-glucan reactivity of e.g. 3 μg/ml means, that this plasma is as active as pooled normal plasma that has been supplemented with 3 μg/ml purified Zymosan A (ß-glucan).

Statistical analyses of interactions between patients characteristics and active endotoxin in plasma were performed using t-test when two groups were compared and ANOVA when multiple groups were compared. Correlations were tested using Pearson´s coefficient.

RESULTS AND DISCUSSION

Figure 1 demonstrates that 81 % of the patients (51/63) had a pathologic LPS reactivity with 25.3 ± 19.1 (range 3.9-98) ng/ml, which is 3163 ± 2388 % of normal, i.e. the LPS reactivity can increase up to about 100fold in patients with severe sepsis. This is in agreement with the in the range of 100fold increase of LPS in patients with *Neisseria meningitidis* sepsis [6], 75 % of the patients (47/63) had a pathologic ß-glucan reactivity with 6.3 ± 7.5 (range 0.5-36.2) μg/ml ß-glucan reactivity. 54 % of the patients (34/63) had a combined gram-negative/fungal septicemia with 25.7 ± 19.2 (range 3.9-98) ng/ml LPS reactivity and 4.6 ± 4.6 (range 0.5-21.1) μg/ml ß-glucan reactivity. LPS is about 300fold more potent than ß-glucan, as derived from the pathophysiological concentrations of active endotoxin. However, the ß-glucan pathology should not be underestimated, since fungi might grow rapidly. In figure 2 the total plasma load of active endotoxin has been calculated by division of the ß-glucan reactivities [ng/ml] by 300.

LPS reactivities of about 2-3 ng/ml or ß-glucan reactivities of about 0.5 μg/ml might be considered as threshold concentrations to cause membraneous phospholipase A_2 (PLA_2) activation and cell fragmentation, which leads to pathologic disseminated intravascular coagulation (PDIC) with elevated plasmatic thrombin activities [5]. Of pathophysiologic importance is the binding of free endotoxin to membrane enzymes, particularly to cellular phospholipases (especially PLA_2 and PLC) or to membraneous phospholipids. Susceptible cells (e.g. the monocytes) are activated or fragmented, depending on the amount of free endotoxin that interacts with the cell membrane; cell activation means PLA_2 and PLC activation, arachidonic acid is released by PLA_2 and intra-cellular messengers are released by PLC; cyclooxygenases and lipoxygenases transform arachidonic acid to eicosanoids (e.g. prostaglandins/thromboxanes or leukotrienes), that mediate inflammation [7-33]. The oxidative burst (generation of ·OH or $^1O_2$) of phagocytes is activated that might be offensive (radicalic, procoagulant) in the case of monocytes but defensive (nonradicalic, profibrinolytic) in the case of granulocytes [34].

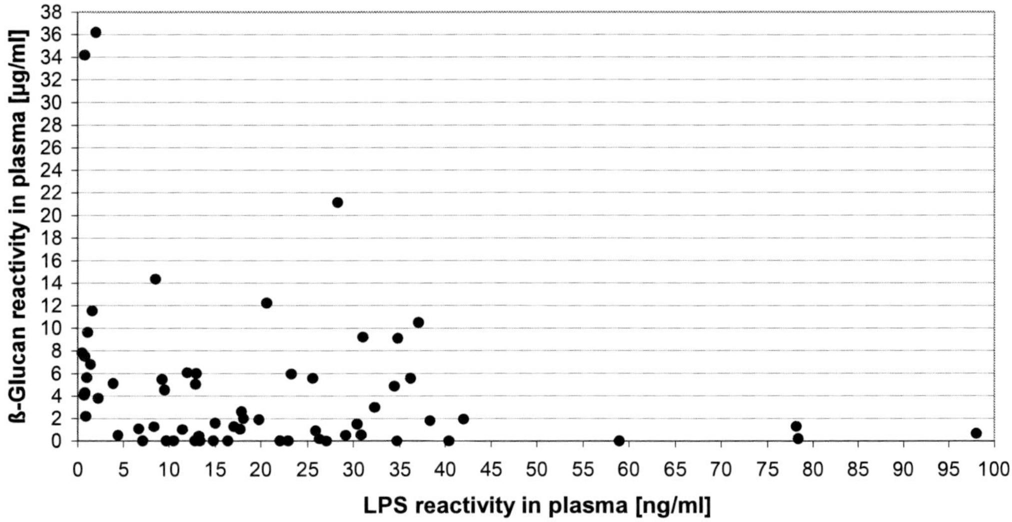

Figure 1. Active LPS and active ß-glucan in plasma. 63 patients with severe sepsis at the time point of admission to the intensive care unit were tested for LPS reactivity and ß-glucan reactivity. The patients had 20.7 ± 19.6 ng/ml LPS reactivity and 4.6 ± 7.0 µg/ml ß-glucan reactivity (MV ± 1 SD; r= - 0.255); e.g. 20.8 ng/ml LPS reactivity means that this plasma is as active as pooled normal EDTA-plasma, that had been supplemented with 20 ng/ml purified LPS, or e.g. 4 µg/ml ß-glucan reactivity means that this plasma is as active as pooled normal EDTA-plasma, that had been supplemented with 4 µg/ml purified ß-glucan.

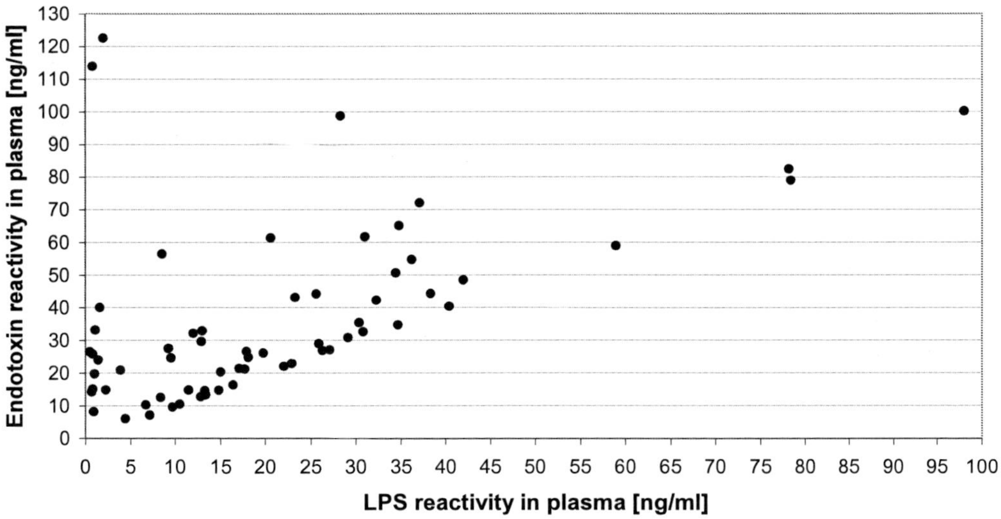

Figure 2. Active endotoxin in plasma. The ß-glucan reactivities (4.6 ± 7.0 µg/ml) of Fig. 1 were divided by 300 and added to the respective LPS-reactivities (20.7 ± 19.6 ng/ml) to obtain total endotoxin reactivities (36.1 ± 26.3 ng/ml) (r=0.521).

There were no differences in LPS-, ß-glucan- or total endotoxin reactivity depending on ICU or hospital survival, gender, the use of renal replacement therapy or localisation of the septic focus. In contrast, SAPS (simplified acute physiology score) II showed a correlation with active ß-glucan ($p = 0.006$) as well as total active endotoxin ($p = 0.004$), but not with active LPS, while SOFA (sepsis-associated organ failure assessment) score at day 1 of ICU displayed positive correlations with all three parameters (active ß-glucan: $p = 0.035$, active LPS: $p = 0.03$, active total endotoxin: $p = 0.0004$). Thus, the SOFA score indicates that it is of pathophysiologic importance to calculate the total blood load of active endotoxin of the patient as:

- *Endotoxin reactivity [ng/ml] = LPS reactivity [ng/ml] + ß-glucan reactivity [ng/ml]/300*

Instead of calculating the ß-glucan reactivity in ng/ml divided by 300 the ß-glucan reactivity in µg/ml can also be multiplied by 3.33.

The new *Limulus* technique allows the quantification of active endotoxin in plasma within about 20-30 min (37°C). Of special interest for each individual patient would be the very early diagnosis of sepsis, i.e. the very earliest phase of sepsis with LPS reacitivities in the range of 2 ng/ml or ß-glucan reactivities in the range of 0.2 µg/ml. With a diagnosis as early as possible the adequate treatment can start in time.

REFERENCES

[1] Hurley JC. Endotoxemia: methods of detection and clinical correlates. *Clin Microbiol Rev* 1995; 8: 268-92.

[2] Stief TW. Thrombin generation by exposure of blood to endotoxin: a simple model to study disseminated intravascular coagulation. *Clin Appl Thromb Hemost* 2006; 12: 137-61.

[3] Stief TW. Coagulation activation by lipopolysaccharides. *Clin Appl Thrombosis/ Hemostasis* Dec 26, 2007 doi: 10.1177/1076029607309256

[4] Bick RL. Disseminated intravascular coagulation: a review of etiology, pathophysiology, diagnosis, and management: guidelines for care. *Clin Appl Thromb Hemost* 2002; 8: 1-31.

[5] Stief TW, Ijagha O, Weiste B, Herzum I, Renz H, Max M. Analysis of hemostasis alterations in sepsis. *Blood Coagul Fibrinolysis.* 2007; 18: 179-86.

[6] Brandtzaeg P, Bjerre A, Øvstebø R, Brusletto B, Joø GB, Kierulf P. Neisseria meningitidis lipopolysaccharides in human pathology. *J Endotoxin Res* 2001; 7: 401-20.

[7] Zayat M, Lichtenberger LM, Dial EJ. Pathophysiology of LPS-induced gastrointestinal injury in the rat: role of secretory phospholipase A2. *Shock* 2007; Dec 20 [Epub ahead of print]

[8] Ruipérez V, Casas J, Balboa MA, Balsinde J. Group V phospholipase A2-derived lysophosphatidylcholine mediates cyclooxygenase-2 induction in lipopolysaccharide-stimulated macrophages. *J Immunol* 2007; 179: 631-8.

[9] Kikuchi M, Endo S, Inada K, Inoue Y, Wakabayashi G, Ishikura H, Tanaka T. Assessment of inflammatory mediators in patients with generalized peritonitis. *J Med* 1999; 30: 245-58.

[10] Cuschieri J, Billgren J, Maier RV. Phosphatidylcholine-specific phospholipase C (PC-PLC) is required for LPS-mediated macrophage activation through CD14. *J Leukoc Biol* 2006; 80: 407-14.

[11] Slomiany BL, Slomiany A. Cytosolic phospholipase A2 activation in Helicobacter pylori lipopolysaccharide-induced interference with gastric mucin synthesis. *IUBMB Life* 2006; 58: 217-23.

[12] Kim YS, Kim GY, Kim JH, You HJ, Park YM, Lee HK, Yu HC, Chung SM, Jin ZW, Ko HM, Cho BH. Glutamine inhibits lipopolysaccharide-induced cytoplasmic phospholipase A2 activation and protects against endotoxin shock in mouse. *Shock* 2006; 25: 290-4.

[13] Balzary RW, Cocks TM. Lipopolysaccharide induces epithelium- and prostaglandin E(2)-dependent relaxation of mouse isolated trachea through activation of cyclooxygenase (COX)-1 and COX-2. *J Pharmacol Exp Ther* 2006; 317: 806-12.

[14] Luo Induction of cytosolic phospholipase A2 by lipopolysaccharide in canine tracheal smooth muscle cells: involvement of MAPKs and NF-kappaB pathways. *Cell Signal* 2006; 18: 1201-11.

[15] Touqui L, Paya M, Thouron F, Guiyoule A, Zarantonelli ML, Leduc D, Wu Y, Taha MK, Alonso JM. Neisseria meningitidis pili induce type-IIA phospholipase A2 expression in alveolar macrophages. *FEBS Lett* 2005; 579: 4923-7.

[16] Akundi RS, Candelario-Jalil E, Hess S, Hüll M, Lieb K, Gebicke-Haerter PJ, Fiebich BL. Signal transduction pathways regulating cyclooxygenase-2 in lipopolysaccharide-activated primary rat microglia. *Glia* 2005; 51: 199-208.

[17] Santamaría C, Larios S, Quirós S, Pizarro-Cerda J, Gorvel JP, Lomonte B, Moreno E. Bactericidal and antiendotoxic properties of short cationic peptides derived from a snake venom Lys49 phospholipase A2. *Antimicrob Agents Chemother* 2005; 49: 1340-5.

[18] Won JS, Im YB, Khan M, Singh AK, Singh I. Involvement of phospholipase A2 and lipoxygenase in lipopolysaccharide-induced inducible nitric oxide synthase expression in glial cells. *Glia* 2005; 51: 13-21.

[19] Woodruff TM, Arumugam TV, Shiels IA, Newman ML, Ross PA, Reid RC, Fairlie DP, Taylor SM. A potent and selective inhibitor of group IIa secretory phospholipase A2 protects rats from TNBS-induced colitis. *Int Immunopharmacol* 2005; 5: 883-92.

[20] Sapirstein A, Saito H, Texel SJ, Samad TA, O'Leary E, Bonventre JV. Cytosolic phospholipase A2alpha regulates induction of brain cyclooxygenase-2 in a mouse model of inflammation. *Am J Physiol Regul Integr Comp Physiol* 2005; 288: R1774-82.

[21] Schaloske RH, Provins JW, Kessen UA, Dennis EA. Molecular characterization of the lipopolysaccharide/platelet activating factor- and zymosan-induced pathways leading to prostaglandin production in P388D1 macrophages. *Biochim Biophys Acta* 2005; 1687: 64-75.

[22] Jackson SK, Parton J. Lysophospholipid acyltransferases in monocyte inflammatory responses and sepsis. *Immunobiology* 2004; 209: 31-8.

[23] Andrei C, Margiocco P, Poggi A, Lotti LV, Torrisi MR, Rubartelli A. Phospholipases C and A2 control lysosome-mediated IL-1 beta secretion: Implications for inflammatory processes. *Proc Natl Acad Sci U S A* 2004; 101: 9745-50.

[24] Constantin D, Cordenier A, Robinson K, Ala'Aldeen DA, Murphy S. Neisseria meningitidis-induced death of cerebrovascular endothelium: mechanisms triggering transcriptional activation of inducible nitric oxide synthase. *J Neurochem* 2004; 89: 1166-74.

[25] Hong J, Bose M, Ju J, Ryu JH, Chen X, Sang S, Lee MJ, Yang CS. Modulation of arachidonic acid metabolism by curcumin and related beta-diketone derivatives: effects on cytosolic phospholipase A(2), cyclooxygenases and 5-lipoxygenase. *Carcinogenesis* 2004; 25: 1671-9.

[26] Rosenberger TA, Villacreses NE, Hovda JT, Bosetti F, Weerasinghe G, Wine RN, Harry GJ, Rapoport SI. Rat brain arachidonic acid metabolism is increased by a 6-day intracerebral ventricular infusion of bacterial lipopolysaccharide. *J Neurochem* 2004; 88: 1168-78.

[27] Ivanov AI, Romanovsky AA. Prostaglandin E2 as a mediator of fever: synthesis and catabolism. *Front Biosci* 2004; 9: 1977-93.

[28] Balboa MA, Shirai Y, Gaietta G, Ellisman MH, Balsinde J, Dennis EA. Localization of group V phospholipase A2 in caveolin-enriched granules in activated P388D1 macrophage-like cells. *J Biol Chem* 2003; 278: 48059-65.

[29] Lee SC, Han JS, Seo JK, Cha YN. Modulation of cyclooxygenase-2 expression by phosphatidylcholine specific phospholipase C and D in macrophages stimulated with lipopolysaccharide. *Mol Cells* 2003; 15: 320-6.

[30] Beck GCh, Hermes WC, Yard BA, Kaszkin M, von Zabern D, Schulte J, Haak M, Prem K, Krimsky W, van Ackern K, van der Woude FJ, Yedgar S. Amelioration of endotoxin-induced sepsis in rats by membrane anchored lipid conjugates. *Crit Care Med* 2003; 31: 2015-21.

[31] Jiang YJ, Lu B, Choy PC, Hatch GM. Regulation of cytosolic phospholipase A2, cyclooxygenase-1 and -2 expression by PMA, TNFalpha, LPS and M-CSF in human monocytes and macrophages. *Mol Cell Biochem* 2003; 246: 31-8.

[32] Dieter P, Scheibe R, Kamionka S, Kolada A. LPS-induced synthesis and release of PGE2 in liver macrophages: regulation by CPLA2, COX-1, COX-2, and PGE2 synthase. *Adv Exp Med Biol* 2002; 507: 457-62.

[33] Touqui L, Alaoui-El-Azher M. Mammalian secreted phospholipases A2 and their pathophysiological significance in inflammatory diseases. *Curr Mol Med* 2001; 1: 739-54.

[34] Martins PS, Brunialti MK, Martos LS, Machado FR, Assuncao MS, Blecher S, Salomao R. Expression of cell surface receptors and oxidative metabolism modulation in the clinical continuum of sepsis. *Crit Care* 2008; 12: R25 [Epub ahead of print]

In: Hemostasis Laboratory Yearbook, Volume 2 ISBN: 978-1-60741-089-8
Editor: Thomas W. Stief, pp. 59-73

PLASMATIC FIBRINOLYSIS IN SEPSIS

Thomas W. Stief [1,*]***, Korinna Ulbricht*** [1]***, Harald Renz*** [1]
and Martin Max [2]

[1]Department of Clinical Chemistry, University Hospital Giessen & Marburg, Germany
[2]Department of Anesthesia and Intensive Care Medicine, University Hospital Giessen & Marburg, Germany

ABSTRACT

The aim of this laboratory study was to test new assays that focus on fibrinolysis alterations in septic patients, aberrance of the results from normal values, and correlation to coagulation markers.

For the present work, samples of potassium-ethylene-diamine-tetraacetic acid (K_3-EDTA)-plasma and citrated plasma were collected from n=48 intensive care patients with a clinical diagnosis of sepsis. Additionally, a subset of K_3-EDTA-plasma was stabilized 1+1 with 2.5 M arginine, pH 8.6, to conserve the real state of fibrinolysis activation in unstable plasma samples as e.g. from critically ill patients.

At admission to the intensive care unit the patients had 127±118% (mean value ± 1 standard deviation) (normal range (N)=100±20%) amidolytic plasmatic plasmin activity, 43±18% (N=100±20%) plasminogen function, 130±53% (N=100±20%) antiplasmin activity, 12.5±7.9 (N=1.1±0.7) anti-urokinase units/ml PAI-1, 3.05±2.52 (N=0.049±0.025) µg/ml D-dimer, 371±142% (N=100±30%) plasmin-antiplasmin complex, 20±14% (N=100±15%) fibrinolysis parameters assay (FIPA) activity, 1.06±0.28 (N=1.0±0.1) fibrinogen function/fibrinogen antigen ratio, and 0.58±0.59 (N=0.44±0.14) nmol/l prothrombin fragment F1+2. The intra-assay coefficients of variation of all functional or antigenic tests were < 5% or < 10%, respectively. Most patients showed a significantly decreased plasmatic fibrinolytic state, when compared with healthy individuals; amidolytic plasmin activity in EDTA-1.25 M arginine-stabilized plasma presented large aberrations in some septic patients. The FIPA mean values approximately doubled within about 1 week in the intensive care unit. The results will be the basis of further clinical studies.

Key words: Sepsis, plasmin, fibrinolysis, arginine

---

[*] Send correspondence to: Priv.-Doz. Dr. Med. T. Stief, Department of Clinical Chemistry, University Hospital, D-35033 Marburg, Germany; Email: thstief@med.uni-marburg.de; Tel. : +49-6421-58 64471; FAX: +49-6421-58 65594; present address of Prof. Max: Department of Intensive Care Medicine; Centre Hospitalaire de Luxembourg

1. Introduction

Sepsis results in serious alterations of hemostasis: coagulation might be pathologically activated and fibrinolysis pathologically inhibited; consequently, multiple disseminated micro-thrombi may occur in all organs. The rapid diagnosis of pathologic disseminated intravascular coagulation (PDIC) is therefore a major challenge of each hemostasis laboratory. PDIC diagnosis is difficult, e.g. primary hyperfibrinolysis must be differentiated from PDIC [1-3]. Recently we demonstrated that pathologic thrombin activities in septic patients can reliably be measured [4]. Plasma of septic patients is rather unstable, especially freezing/thawing procedures alters the plasma level of important hemostatic markers artefactually. Therefore, we stabilized plasma 1+1 with 2.5 M arginine, pH 8.6. The aim of the present work was to test new chromogenic assays to analyze alterations of fibrinolysis in septic patients and correlations to other hemostasis parameters.

2. Patients, Material and Methods

The local ethic committee approved this study (54/04). After informed consent, 1.6 mg/ml K_3-EDTA blood (Sarstedt monovettes, Nümbrecht, Germany) and citrated blood (0.5 ml 106 mM sodium citrate + 4.5 ml venous blood) of 48 septic patients (additional to them in [4]) was transported immediately after blood drawing (always at 8 a.m.) from the intensive care unit to the central laboratory of our university hospital. Sepsis syndrome was diagnosed when systemic signs of inflammation (e.g. tachycardia, hypotension) due to a known or suspected infection (e.g. perforation of viscus, radiographic and clinical evidence of pneumonia). Plasma was obtained by blood centrifugation at 2800 g for 10 min at 23°C.

To stabilize EDTA-plasma of the critical ill patients (0-10 days stay in intensive care unit), one part EDTA–plasma was immediately mixed with one part of 2.5 M arginine, pH 8.6. Aliquots of 200 µl of EDTA-1.25 M arginine-plasma, 100 µl EDTA-plasma, or 500 µl of citrated plasma were frozen at -80°C until performance of the respective test. Within a total storage time of less than 30 min (23°C) the plasma samples were frozen. Active plasminogen activators circulate in blood at plasma concentrations inferior to 10 ng/ml. The mean concentration of active PAI-1 is about 10fold higher in septic patients, i.e. artificial fibrinolysis changes by preanalytic complexation of urokinase (u-PA) or t-PA with PAI-1 are minimal.

To avoid in vitro changes of the sample during the first incubation in the respective enzyme immuno assays (EIAs) the reaction between the antigen in EDTA-arginine-plasma and capture antibody was performed in presence of 500-625 mM arginine, pH 8.7, because arginine at this concentration completely inhibits hemostasis activation [5,6]. Upon dilution of 2.5 M arginine, pH 8.6, its pH value increases slightly.

The amidolytic activities of plasmatic plasmin (Pli) or plasmatic thrombin (IIa) were determined, incubating 50 µl EDTA-1.25 M arginine patient plasma, 100 % of normal pooled EDTA-arginine plasma, or 1.6 mg/ml EDTA, 1.25 M arginine, pH 8.7, with 50 µl 0 or 0.77 mM chromogenic plasmin substrate HD-alanyl-cyclohexyltyrosyl-lysyl-paranitro-anilide·2AcOH (Ala-HHT-Lys-pNA; MW=626.8; Km= about 0.127 mM (at pH 7.4)) or chromogenic thrombin substrate HD-cyclohexylglycyl-alanyl-arginyl-paranitroanilide

·2AcOH (CHG-Ala-Arg-pNA;MW=624.7; Km= about 0.016 mM (at pH 7.4)) (both substrates from Pentapharm, Basel, Switzerland) in 1.25 M arginine, pH 8.7, in untreated U-well polystyrol microtiter plates (NUNC, Wiesbaden, Germany; article nr. 268152) at 37°C [6]. 10 μmoles lyophilized chromogenic substrate were dissolved in 650 μl H_2O and then diluted with 650 μl 2.5 M arginine, pH 8.6, and 11.7 ml 1.25 M arginine, pH 8.7. ΔA at 405 nm /h was determined for IIa activity (100 % of normal = about 50 specific mA/h = 5.5 mIU/ml thrombin) and ΔA/d (100 % of normal = about 17 specific mA/d = 0.05 mU/ml = 0.2 mIU/ml plasmin) was determined for Pli activity. The photometer used was a microtiter plate photometer with a 1 mA resolution (Milenia; Diagnostics Products Corporation, Los Angeles, USA). The specific ΔA values had been corrected by the spontaneous decay of both chromogenic substrates in 1.25 M arginine, pH 8.7, which was 0.5 mA/h (37°C). Ultra-sensitive photometers might detect pathological plasmatic plasmin activities within one hour. The normal range is 100 ± 20 % (mean value (MV) ± 1 standard deviation (SD)).

In the global fibrinolysis test **FIPA** (=fibrinolysis parameters assay) 40 μl patient plasma or pooled normal citrated plasma (100 % of normal FIPA) were incubated with 4 μl 100 IU/ml urokinase (medac, Hamburg, Germany), 6 mM tranexamic acid (Bayer, Leverkusen, Germany), 6 % human albumin, PBS (urokinsae-reagent) in U-wells for 10 min (FIPA-10 = main value) or for 30 min (FIPA-30) fibrinolysis reaction time (FRT) at 37°C. 100 μl 2.5 M arginine, pH 8.6, 0.144 % Triton X 100® and 25 μl 1.5 mM Val-Leu-Lys-pNA (Chromogenix, Mölndal, Sweden) in 1.5 M arginine, pH 8.7, 1.5 M KCl (plasmin substrate reagent) were added, the plate was intensely shaked, and the increase in absorbance with time (ΔA/t) was measured. 100 % of normal FIPA-10 results into a ΔA/t value of about 100 mA/h RT, FIPA-30 ΔA/t values are about twice that of FIPA-10; the maximal ΔA is about 1400 mA, the ΔA range is nearly linear within 0 - 40 % of the maximal ΔA. The present FIPA-10 version in nearly undiluted plasma correlates with r=0.908 with the FIPA version in 1+1 diluted plasma and 20 min FRT [7]. The principle of the FIPA is urokinase-mediated activation of plasmatic plasminogen to plasmin in presence of tranexamic acid at 0.55 mM, which is a sufficiently low concentration that only partially inhibits the action of plasmatic α_2-antiplasmin. The normal range of FIPA-10 is 100±15 % (MV±1SD) that of FIPA-30 is 100±20 % (MV±1SD).

Plasminogen was functionally determined (Berichrom Plasminogen, DadeBehring, Marburg, Germany) according to the manufacturer's instructions, however with 1.5 M arginine, pH 8.7 in the chromogenic plasmin detection phase. The normal range is 100±20 % (MV±1SD).

α_2-Antiplasmin (AP = plasmin-inhibitor (PI)) was functionally determined (Berichrom α_2-Antiplasmin, DadeBehring) according to the manufacturer's instructions, however with 1.5 M arginine, pH 8.7 in the chromogenic plasmin detection phase. The normal range is 100±20 % (MV±1SD).

Plasminogen Activator Inhibitor – 1 (PAI-1) was functionally determined via oxidative inactivation of plasmin-inhibitor (Berichrom PAI, DadeBehring): 4 μl citrated plasma or PAI-1 standards containing about 0, 5.2, or 14 U/ml PAI-1 were incubated in the PAI-1/u-PA reaction phase with 8 μl 10 IU/ml urokinase (2 ml - urokinase reagent of the commercial kit additionly supplemented with 20 μl 500 IU/ml (10 IU) urokinase; medac, Hamburg, Germany), 100 mM Tris, 0.1 % Triton X 100®, 1 % polygeline, pH 8.4 for 5 min (37°C) in polystyrol U-wells. Then 16 μl 15 CTA-U (0.375 mg)/ml Glu-plasminogen in 100 mM Tris, pH 8.4, and 16 µl 6.4 mM chloramine-T®, 3 mM tranexamic acid were added. After 5 min (37°C) 100 µl 2.5 M arginine, pH 8.6, 0.1 % Triton X 100® and 10 µl 3 mM HD-NVA-CHA-Lys-pNA were added, the plate was intensely shaked, and the linear ΔA/t at 405 nm was determined. PAI-1 activities up to 14 U/ml resulted into a linear decrease of u-PA activity. Plasmas with PAI-1 activities > 14 U/ml were diluted with PAI depleted plasma (the 0 calibrator) and assayed again. The normal range is 1.1±0.7 U (urokinase inhibiting units)/ml (MV±1SD).

Plasmin-Antiplasmin-complex (PAP) was determined by EIA (IMUCLONE® PAP; american diagnostica). 50 µl sample buffer and 50 µl EDTA-1.25 M arginine, pH 8.7–stabilized patient plasma or EDTA-arginine-stabilized pooled normal plasma were assayed according to the manufacturer´s instructions. The normal range is 100±30 % (MV±1 SD).

D-Dimer (DD) testing was performed by EIA (IMUCLONE® D-Dimer; american diagnostica, Stamford, USA) according to the manufacturer´s instructions, however with the antigen/antibody reaction in presence of 500 mM arginine. The normal range is 0.049±0.025 µg/ml (MV±1 SD).

Fibrinogen function (FIFTA) [8] or fibrinogen antigen (FIATA) [9] were tested by new microtiter plate assays in polystyrol microtiter plates with flat bottom (F-wells; NUNC, Wiesbaden, Germany, article Nr. 446140). In the FIFTA 40 µl citrated plasma is incubated with 80 µl 300 mIU/ml thrombin, 400 µg/ml polybrene®, 6 % albumin and the fibrin-related turbidity increase at 405 nm is measured after 5 min (23°C) or 2 min (37°C). In the FIATA 20 µl citrated plasma is incubated with 40 µl phosphate buffered saline (PBS) and 40 µl 4.4 mM vancomycin in PBS. The turbidity increase / 2 min RT is measured. Vancomycin precipitates fibrinogen like molecules. The FIFTA/FIATA ratio (FI ratio) was calculated (normal range=1.0±0.1, MV±SD); a FI ratio > 1.1 indicates the presence of over-reactive fibrinogen (e.g. soluble fibrin might be a "crystallization point" for nascending fibrin), and a FI ratio < 0.9 indicates the presence of under-reactive fibrinogen (e.g. dysfibrinogens or fibrinogen degradation products). The normal range is for both new fibrinogen tests 100±20% (MV±1 SD).

Protein C (PC) function was determined via Protac® activation (Berichrom Protein C; DadeBehring). The normal range is 100±15% (MV±1 SD).

Antithrombin III (AT3) function was determined in citrated plasma that was only diluted by 20 % (20 µl plasma + 4 µl thrombin reagent) in the thrombin/AT3 reaction. The thrombin reagent is prepared by dissolving 130 IU lyophilized bovine thrombin (DadeBehring, Marburg, Germany, article nr. B4233-25) in 0.25 ml 6 % human albumin, PBS; after 3 min (23°C) 0.5 ml 20 % human albumin (BAXTER, Unterschleißheim, Germany) and 1.5 ml 2.4 M arginine, pH 7.4, (Sigma, Deisenhofen, Germany) were added; the dissolved thrombin was then given into a heparin-monovette (Sarstedt) containing 4.9*25 =122.5 IU heparin. In the thrombin/AT3 reaction phase 20 µl citrated plasma or standards (100 % of the norm pooled plasma and this plasma diluted with 0.9 % NaCl) were incubated with 4 µl thrombin reagent = 58 IU/ml (final 9.7 IU/ml) thrombin, 6 % human albumin, 54.4 IU/ml (9.1 IU/ml final) unfractionated heparin, 1600 mM (267 mM final) arginine, pH 7.4) in F-wells. Sample or standard dilutions with AT deficient plasma (american diagnostica) resulted in identical results as dilutions with 0.9 % NaCl; the thrombin/AT3 reaction phase was 45 s (at 23°C which is equivalent to about 15-20 s at 37°C, a short incubation time is important to detect possible heparin-binding site deficiencies; manual pipetting of one 96 well microtiter plate takes about 45 seconds). Then, 100 µl 2.5 M arginine, pH 8.6, 0.124 % Triton X 100® (Sigma) were added to stop the thrombin/AT3 reaction. After 3 min (23°C) the thrombin detection phase started with addition of 25 µl 1 mM (0.17 mM final) chromogenic thrombin substrate HD-CHG-Ala-Arg-pNA (Pentapharm, Basel, Switzerland) in 1.25 M (1.93 final) arginine, pH 8.7. ΔA/t at 405 nm was determined. The normal MV±1 SD of functional AT3 is 100±15 %. In n=83 samples of unselected patients this method in nearly undiluted plasma was compared with a commercial method employing 61fold diluted plasma (Berichrom AntithrombinIII; DadeBehring BCT®): 1 µl citrated plasma was incubated with 60 µl thrombin reagent (bovine thrombin, heparin, aprotinin, 100 mM Tris, 0.87 % NaCl, pH 8.2) for 3 min at 37°C. 10 µl substrate reagent (4 mM tosylglycyl-L-prolyl-L-arginyl-5-amino-2-nitrobenzoic acid-isopropylamide) were added and $\Delta A_{405\ nm}$/min was measured. Both methods correlated with r=0.823.

Thrombin-Antithrombin-complex (TAT) was determined by EIA (Enzygnost® TAT micro; DadeBehring) in presence of 625 mM arginine, pH 8.7. The normal range is 1.3±0.4 ng/ml (MV±1 SD). **Prothrombin fragment F1+2 (F1+2)** was also determined by an EIA (Enzygnost® F1+2 micro; DadeBehring) that was similar to the TAT-assay: 50 µl sample buffer (100 mM Tris, 1 % Tween 20®, 37 g/l EDTA) and 50 µl EDTA-1.25 M arginine, pH 8.7 – stabilized plasma reacted with the immobilized capture antibody (rabbit antibodies against human F1.2) for 2 h (RT) and were determined according to the manufacturer's instructions, using peroxidase conjugated detection antibody. The normal range for F1.2 is 0.44±0.14 nmol/l (MV±1 SD).

Tissue factor (TF) was determined by EIA (IMUBIND® Tissue Factor; american diagnostica). 50 µl sample buffer containing 2 % human albumin and 50 µl EDTA-1.25 M arginine plasma or 100 % of normal standards (containing 140 pg/ml TF) supplemented with additional 0-1000 pg/ml TF were incubated with the immobilized murine monoclonal anti-human TF antibody for 3 h (RT) and were assayed according to the manufacturer's instructions. Normal range =140±42 pg/ml (MV±1SD).

Soluble intercellular adhesion molecule – 1 (sICAM-1) was measured by EIA (R&D, Wiesbaden, Germany) according to the manufacturer's instructions, however with the antigen/antibody reaction in presence of 500 mM arginine. Normal range = 0.19±0.04 µg/ml (MV±1SD).

Statistics

The precision of all tests was determined by 10fold determination of pooled normal plasma (100 % of norm standard), and of standards of about 200 % and about 50 % of norm. The intra-assay coefficients of variation (CV) were calculated: CV = SD/MV * 100 %. The tests were performed in duplicate. The photometric enzyme assays had intra- and inter- assay CV values < 5 %, the CV values of the immunologic tests were < 10 %.

The reference ranges are given as ±1SD of the mean value because subtle pathologic changes of critical hemostasis parameters are better identified at a normal range that is MV±1SD than at one MV±2SD. The healthy donors were n=48 medical students. They generated Gaussian distributions. The measured values of the patients were compared with the normal mean values and tested for significance ($p < 0.05$) by two-fold Yates-corrected chi-square comparison against the control-mean ($X^2\bar{x}$ Test) [9].

3. Results

Table 1 demonstrates parameters of fibrinolysis activation and of basal fibrinolysis in patients at admission to the intensive care unit. The patients had a significantly decreased plasminogen function and a significantly increased PAI-1 activity. The global fibrinolysis assay (FIPA) - activity is significantly decreased. The antiplasmin activity was elevated. Some patients had increased others had normal or decreased plasmatic plasmin activity. The concentrations of PAP and of DD were significantly increased, the FIFTA/FIATA ratio is pathologically elevated. Table 2 shows the results of several other coagulation parameters.

Table 1. Fibrinolysis parameters in 48 patients with clinical diagnosis of sepsis upon admission to ICU.

Parameter	**Normal range** MV±1SD [% of normal]	**Patients with clinical diagnosis of sepsis** Median [% of normal]	**Patients with clinical diagnosis of sepsis** MV±1SD [% of normal]
Plasmin activity	100 ± 20	98	127 ± 118
Plgen activity	100 ± 20	40	43 ± 18
AP activity	100 ± 20	114	130 ± 53
PAI-1 activity	100 ± 64	945	1136 ± 718
DD conc.	100 ± 40	5245	6224 ± 5143
PAP conc.	100 ± 30	340	371 ± 142
FIPA-10	100 ± 15	18	20 ± 14
FIPA-30	100 ± 20	14	18 ± 20
Fbgen-function	100 ± 20	176	178 ± 51
Fbgen-antigen	100 ± 20	176	173 ± 46
Fbgen-ratio	100 ± 10	100	106 ± 28

Table 2. Coagulation parameters in 48 patients with clinical diagnosis of sepsis upon admission to ICU.

Parameter	**Normal range** MV±1SD [% of normal]	**Patients with clinical diagnosis of sepsis** Median [% of normal]	**Patients with clinical diagnosis of sepsis** MV±1SD[% of normal]
Thrombin activity	100 ± 20	148	147 ± 37
AT3 activity	100 ± 15	48	47 ± 27
TF concentration	100 ± 30	203	239 ± 123
TAT concentration	100 ± 30	508	815 ± 738
F_{1+2} concentration	100 ± 32	77	132 ± 134
Protein C function	100 ± 15	65	70 ± 29
sICAM-1 conc.	100 ± 21	700	863 ± 653

Plasmatic plasmin activity correlated slightly with the DD concentration (Figure 1a). There was nearly no correlation between DD and PAP (Figure 1b). Plasminogen function is decreased and α2-antiplasmin activity is increased (Figure 2a). The PAI-1 activity correlated inversely with the FIPA-10 activity (Figure 2b). The two assay versions of FIPA with 10 min and 30 min fibrinolysis reaction time correlated strongly (r=0.858) (Figure 2c).

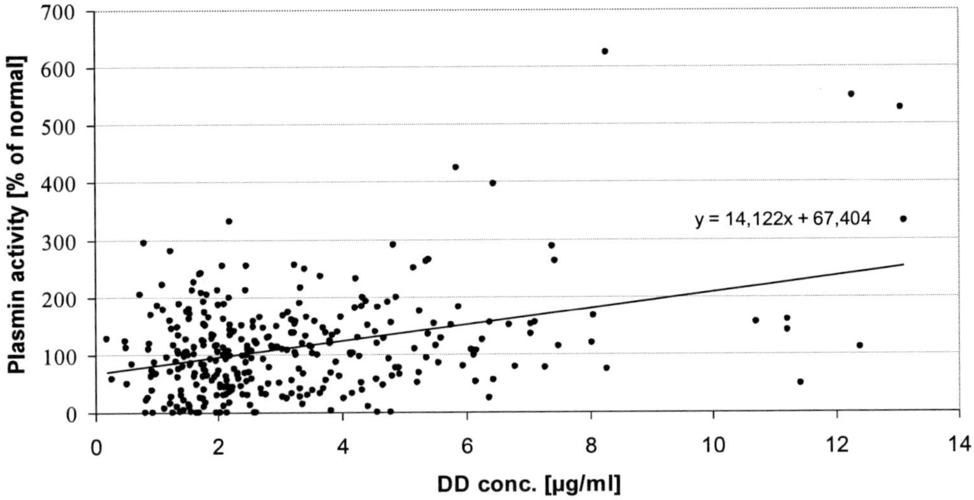

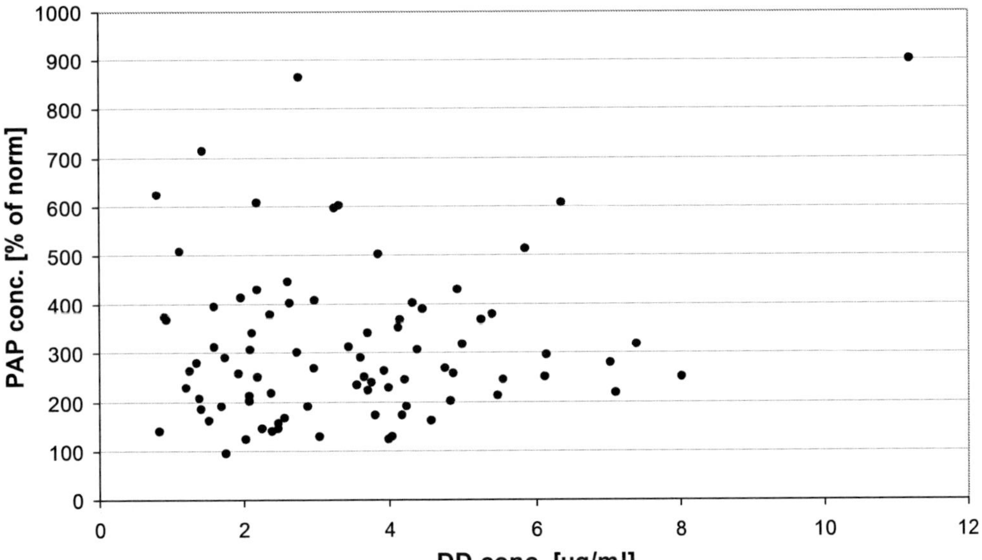

Figure 1. Fibrinolysis activation markers in sepsis. Figure 1a: Comparison of plasmatic plasmin activity (112±85 %) with DD concentration (3.16±2.18 µg/ml) (r=0.365) in 319 samples of patients with a stay in the intensive care unit of up to 10 days. Figure 1b: Comparison of DD concentration (3.44±1.88 µg/ml) with PAP concentration (312±160 %) (r=0.171) in 84 intensive care patient samples.

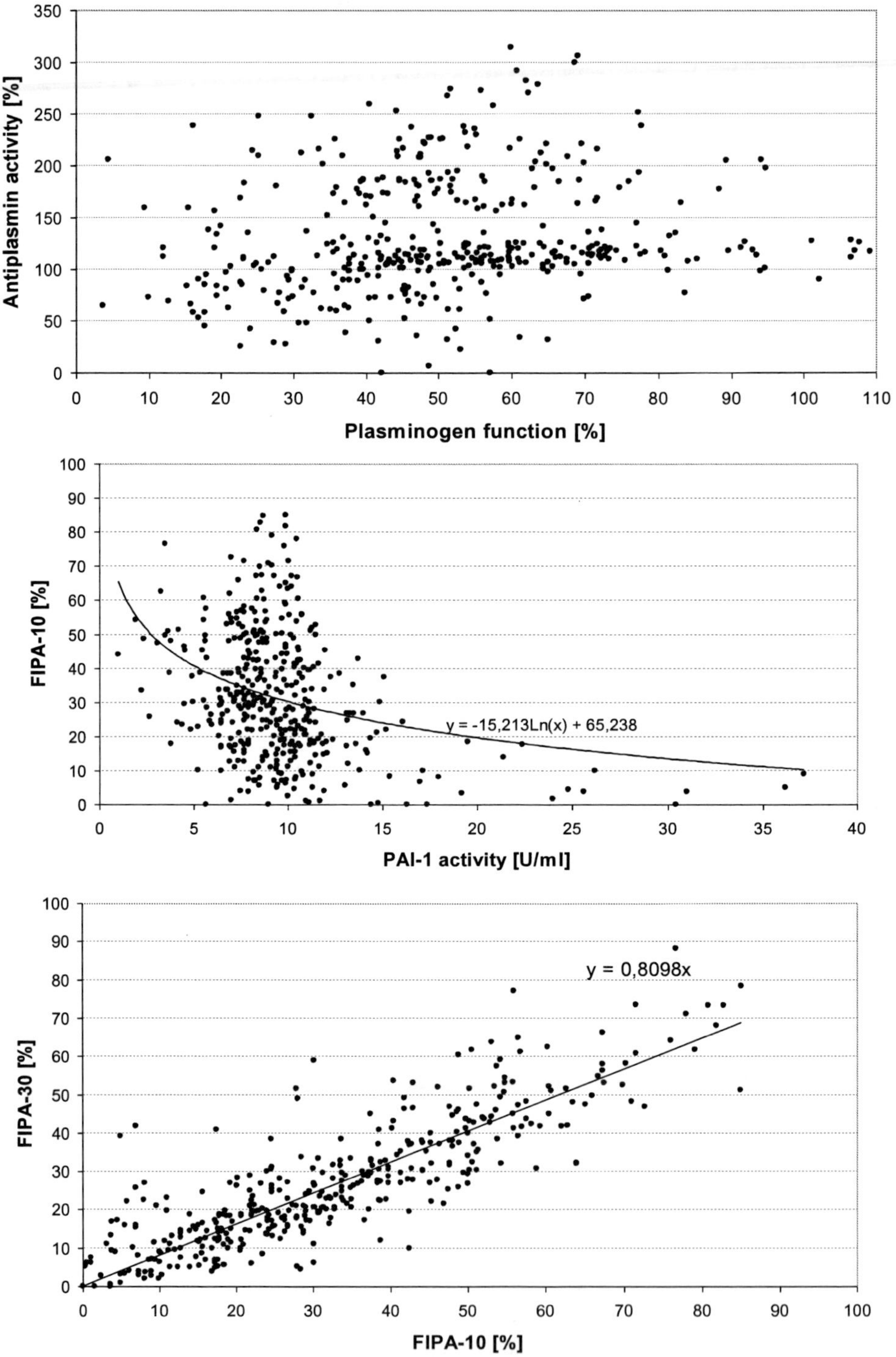

Figure 2. Basal fibrinolysis parameters in sepsis. Figure 2a: Comparison of plasminogen function (50.8±19.2 %) with antiplasmin activity (131.4±56.4 %) (r=0.161) in 404 samples of patients within the first 10 days of stay in the intensive care unit. Figure 2b: Comparison of PAI-1 activity (9.6±4.0 U/ml) with FIPA-10 activity (32.0±18.6 %) (r= - 0.335). Figure 2c: Comparison of FIPA-10 with FIPA-30 (26.3±16.7 %) (r=0.858).

In figure 3a the fibrinogen function is compared with the fibrinogen antigen, the r-value is about 0.7. The here tested samples of 48 patients during the first 10 days in the intensive care unit had a FI ratio of 1.10±0.21. The fibrinogen antigen tends to correlate inversely with the FI ratio (Figure 3b).

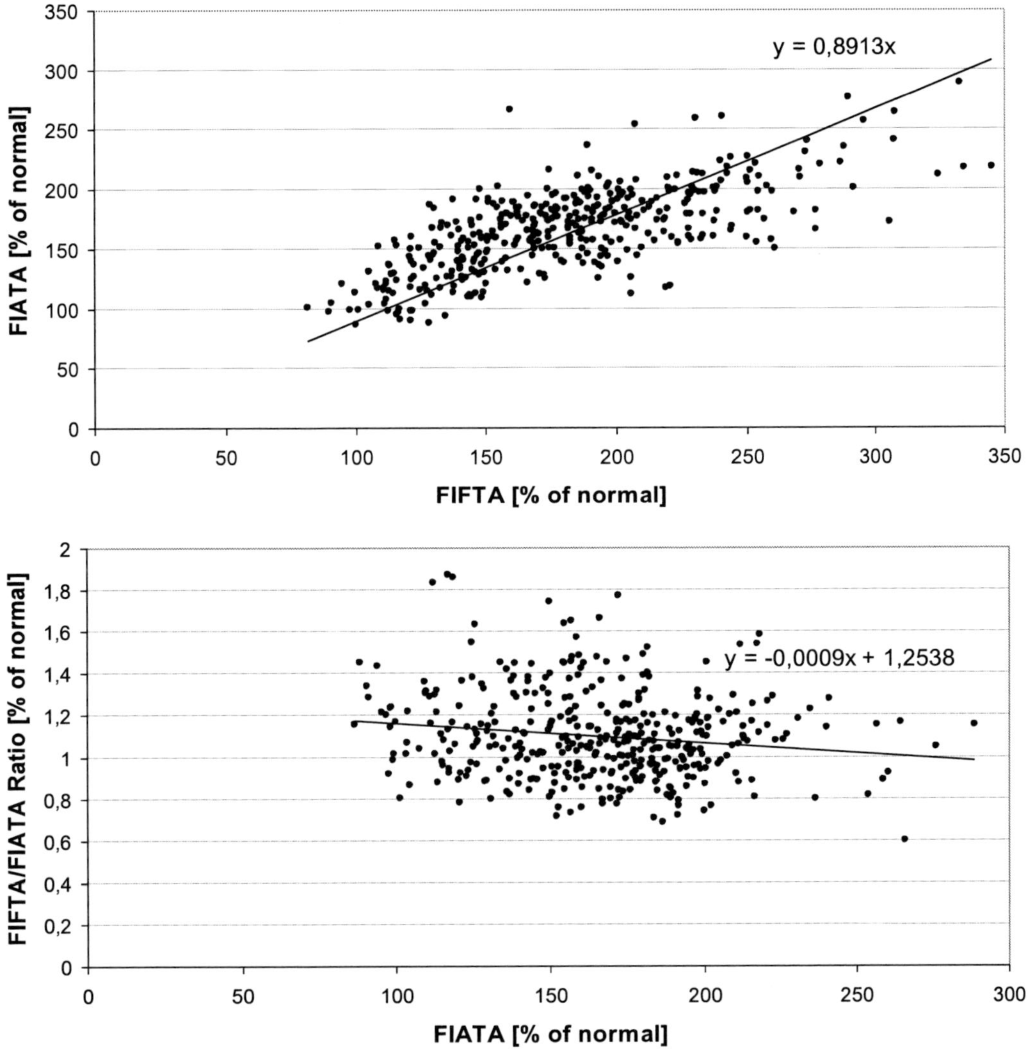

Figure 3. Fibrinogen in sepsis. Figure 3a: Comparison of fibrinogen function (FIFTA) (181±47 % of normal) with fibrinogen antigen (FIATA) (166±35 % of normal) (r=0.698) in 400 samples of patients within the first 10 days of stay in the intensive care unit. Figure 3b: Comparison of fibrinogen antigen to the FIFTA/FIATA ratio (1.10±0.21) (r= - 0.157).

Figure 4a demonstrates the distribution of the basal coagulation parameters antithrombin and protein C. The coagulation activation markers TAT and F1+2 are compared in figure 4b and TF and F1+2 in figure 4c. No correlation appeared between plasmatic thrombin and TAT or F1+2.

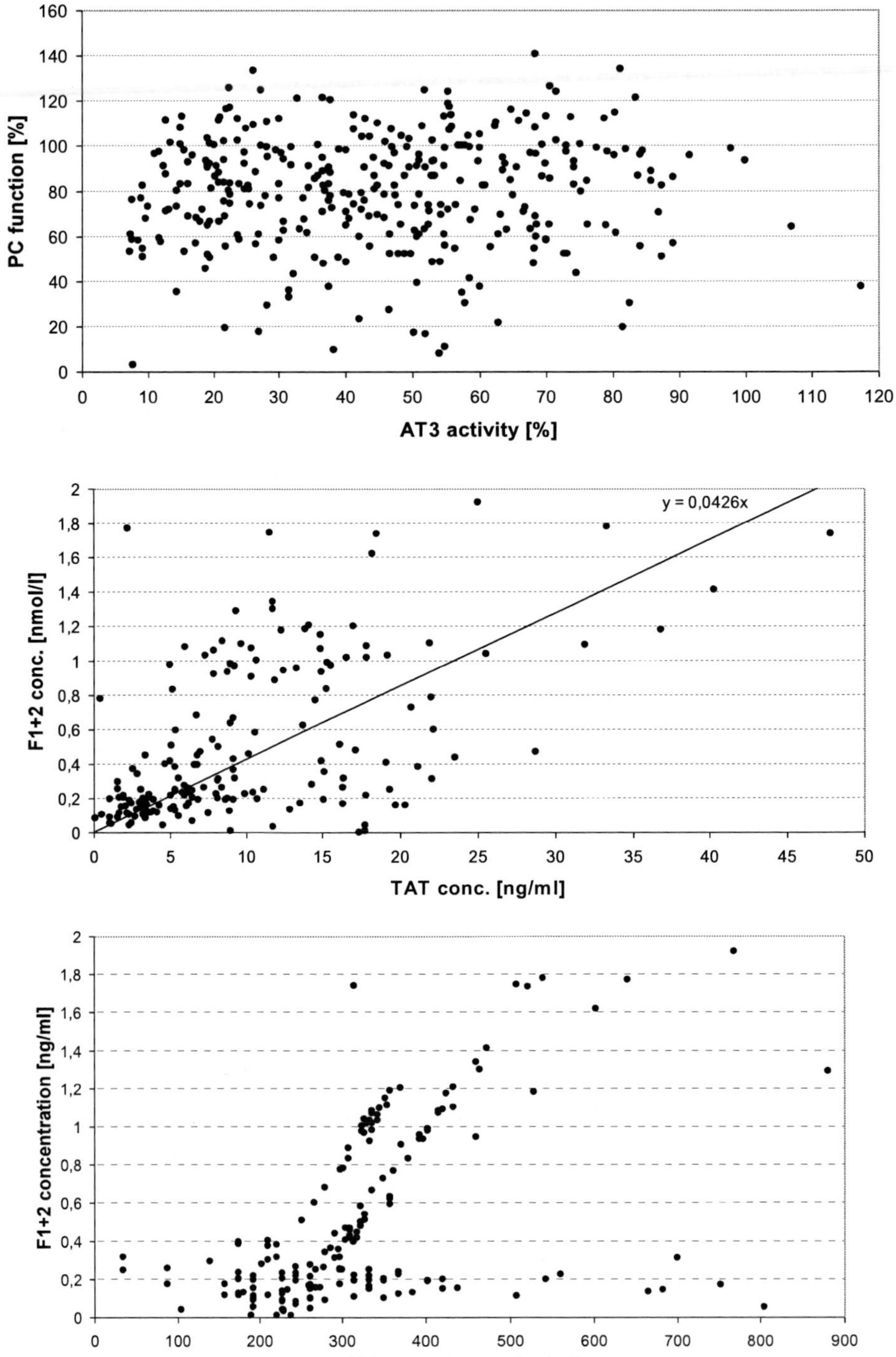

Figure 4. Coagulation parameters in sepsis. Figure 4a: Comparison of antithrombin activity (44.8±22.1 % of normal) with protein C function (80.1±24.8 % of normal) (r=0.047) in 340 samples of patients within the first 10 days of stay in the intensive care unit. Figure 4b: Comparison of TAT concentration (10.0±7.9 ng/ml) with F1+2 concentration (0.50±0.45 nmol/l) (r= 0.538) in 176 samples of intensive care patients. Figure 4c: Comparison of TF concentration (323±132 pg/ml) with F1+2 concentration (r=0.484), n=176.

Soluble ICAM-1 correlated slightly with the DD concentration (Figure 5a). There appeared a slightly inverse correlation between soluble ICAM-1 and the FIFTA/FIATA ratio (Figure 5b).

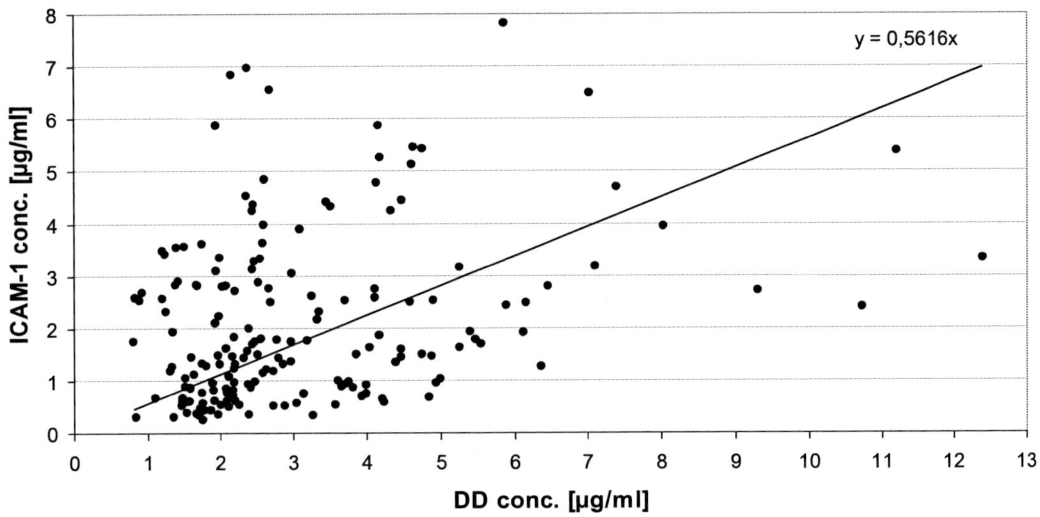

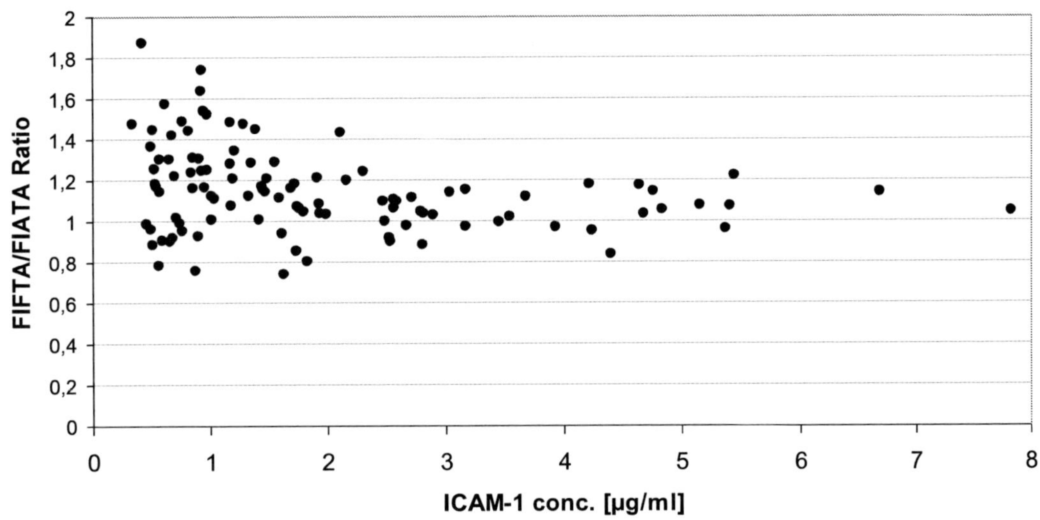

Figure 5. Endothelial damage and plasmatic hemostasis in sepsis. Figure 5a: Comparison of DD concentration (3.09±1.87 µg/ml) with soluble ICAM-1 concentration (2.09±1.50 µg/ml) (r=0.302) in 176 samples of patients within the first 10 days of stay in intensive care unit. Figure 5b: Comparison of soluble ICAM-1 concentration (1.96±1.52 µg/ml) with FIFTA/FIATA ratio (1.15±0.20) (r= - 0.282) in 106 samples of intensive care patients.

Figure 6 demonstrates the mean values of the measured parameters during the first 8 days of stay in intensive care unit (ICU). Of particular interest is the approximately two-fold increase in global plasmatic fibrinolysis activity, measured by the FIPA-10.

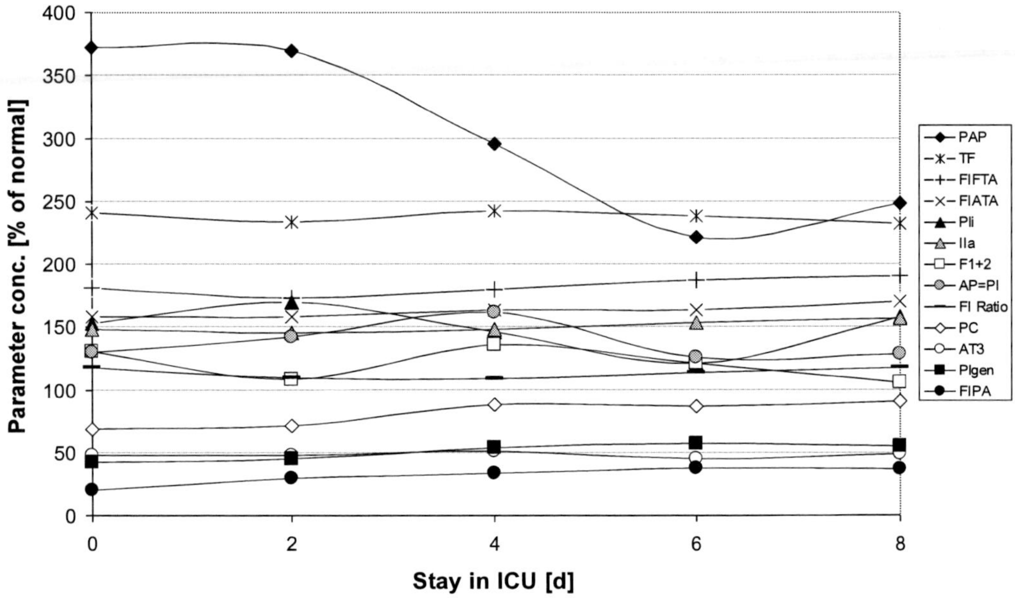

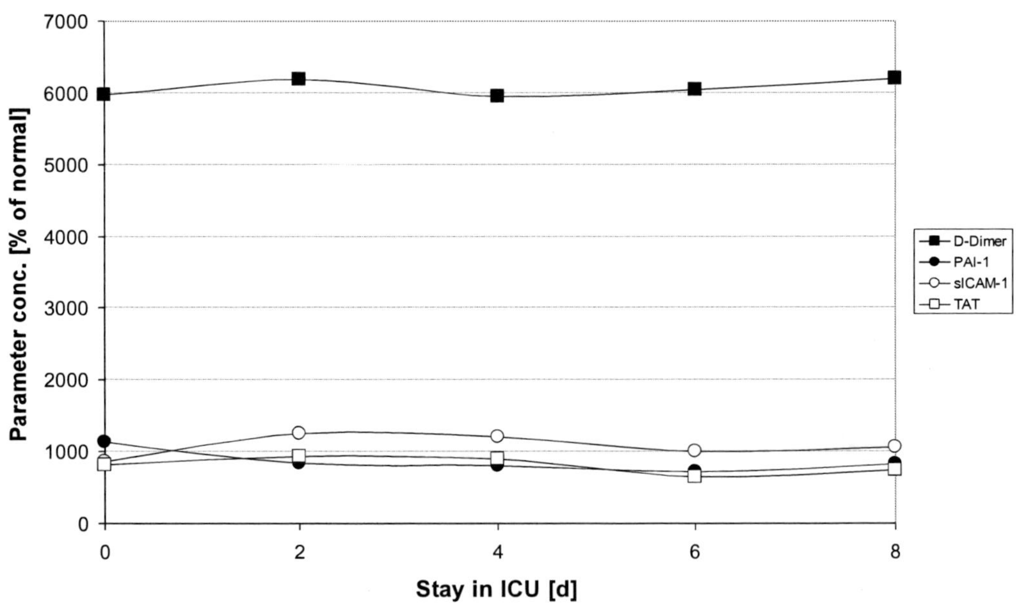

Figure 6. Mean concentrations of hemostasis parameters in intensive care patients.
Plasma samples of 48 intensive care patients were analyzed for: FIFTA = fibrinogen function, FIATA = fibrinogen antigen, FIFTA/FIATA ratio = FI ratio, AP = α2-antiplasmin = plasmin inhibitor (PI), Plgen = plasminogen function, FIPA = global fibrinolysis parameters assay with 10 min reaction time (•), AT3 = antithrombin III = antithrombin activity, PC = protein C function, TF = tissue factor antigen, PAP = plasmin antiplasmin complex, F1+2 = prothrombin fragment F 1+2, Pli = plasmin activity, and IIa = thrombin activity (Figure 6a); PAI-1 = plasminogen activator inhibitor–1 activity, sICAM-1 = soluble intercellular adhesion molecule - 1, TAT = thrombin antithrombin complex (Figure 6b). The mean values of the results were calculated and expressed in % of normal.

4. Discussion

The present data further underline that hemostasis activation in sepsis tends more to be an activation of coagulation than one of fibrinolysis. The global fibrinolysis assay FIPA reflects well the fibrinolysis depression of septic patients. FIPA-10 is the main assay version of FIPA, 10 min reaction time is preferable because within 10 min reaction time (37°C) the PAI-1 reactivity is complete and there appears no plasminogen exhaustion. A prolongation of the reaction time to 30 min might favour the reactivity of PAI-2 if present, so FIPA-30 might be of special interest in gynaecology: the more the FIPA results decreases from FIPA-10 to FIPA-30 the greater the PAI-2 activity. Coagulation markers in septic patients could be found at similar concentrations as previously reported [4]. The elevated FIFTA/FIATA ratio indicates presence of over-reactive fibrinogen, e.g. by soluble fibrin, a low ratio indicates presence of under-reactive fibrinogen, e.g. by fibrinogen degradation products or dysfunctional fibrinogen. The more fibrinogen antigen is present in plasma the more likely it seems that the antigen is dysfunctional fibrinogen than over-reactive fibrinogen (Figure 3b). Especially low endothelial damage (soluble ICAM-1 moderately elevated) tends to result in over-reactive fibrinogen (Figure 5b).

In PDIC susceptible cells (such as the monocytes) fragment into triggers of intrinsic or extrinsic hemostasis activation [2,10,11]. Microvascular thrombosis becomes generalized, and extensive tissue ischaemia may cause organ failure. The microvascular thrombi occur e.g. in the kidneys, liver, lung, gut, adrenals, and brain; the degree of organ insufficiency is related to the quantity of thrombi. PDIC therapies should inhibit coagulation or promote fibrinolysis to reduce organ failure [12,13]. Inhibition of thrombin action decreases the blood levels of F1+2, TAT, DD, and PAI-1 [14-17]. The thrombin + factor XIIIa + plasmin product DD is an unspecific marker of hemostasis activation of whatever nature: DD does not discriminate between coagulation activation and fibrinolysis activation. Therapeutic inhibition of fibrinolysis seems to be of limited benefit for PDIC patients [18].

There is a need for pathobiochemical plasma markers that are available in clinical practice who can help to differentiate primary hyperfibrinolysis from PDIC [19-23], e.g. in liver disease less hemostasis factors such as α2-antiplasmin (plasmin-inhibitor) are synthesized and less activated factors such as plasminogen activators or plasmin are cleared from the blood stream. The present laboratory study demonstrates that analysis of arginine-stabilized EDTA plasma and of citrated plasma results in highly reproducible fibrinolysis results in septic patients: known fibrinolysis activation parameters are PAP or DD [3,24]. Unfortunately, DD is rather unspecific and PAP (like TAT) sometimes does not correlate with the degree of hemostasis activation, e.g. the blood concentrations of the serine protease/serine protease inhibitor complexes PAP and TAT depend also on the liver function of the patient. PAI-1 function is an interesting marker for endothelial dysfunction [25] and sICAM-1 [26,27] one for endothelial destruction. Interestingly, the decrease of antithrombin function (median value = 48 %) is significantly more pronounced in septic patients than that of protein C (median value = 65 %) (Figure 4a). The present study demonstrates that the determination of plasmatic plasmin activity, the fibrinogen function/antigen ratio, and FIPA-10 might add pathophysiological information. In conclusion, the present study investigates the use of a wide range of mainly fibrinolysis related biochemical markers in septic patients. The results will be the basis of further clinical studies.

Plasminogen (Plgen), α2-antiplasmin (AP; plasmin-inhibitor), plasminogen activator inhibitor (PAI)- 1, D-dimer (DD), plasmin/antiplasmin complex (PAP), fibrinolysis parameters assay with 10 min and 30 min reaction time (FIPA-10 and FIPA-30), fibrinogen (Fbgen); *median = [value at n/2 + value at n/2 + 1] / 2* with n values in increasing order.

Antithrombin III (AT3), tissue factor (TF), thrombin/antithrombin complex (TAT), prothrombin fragment F1+2 (F1+2), soluble intercellular adhesion molecule (sICAM) - 1.

ACKNOWLEDGMENT

This work is part of the academic thesis (MD) of Korinna Ulbricht.

REFERENCES

[1] Francis CW, Marder VJ. Physiologic regulation and pathologic disorders of fibrinolysis. *Hum Pathol* 1987; 18: 263-74.

[2] Levi M. Disseminated intravascular coagulation: what´s new ? *Crit Care Clin* 2005; 21: 449-467.

[3] Takahashi H, Hanano M, Takizawa S, Tatewaki W, Shibata A. Plasmin - alpha 2-plasmin inhibitor complex in plasma of patients with disseminated intravascular coagulation. *Am J Hematol* 1988; 28: 162-6.

[4] Stief TW, Ijagha O, Weiste B, Herzum I, Renz H, Max M. Analysis of hemostasis alterations in sepsis. *Blood Coagul Fibrinolysis* 2007; 18: 179-86.

[5] Stief TW, Weippert M, Kretschmer V, Renz H. Arginine inhibits hemostasis activation. *Thromb Res* 2001; 104: 265-274.

[6] Stief TW. Specific determination of plasmatic plasmin activity. *Blood Coagul Fibrinolysis* 2007; 18: 213.

[7] Stief TW, Hinz F, Kurz J, Doss MO, Kretschmer V. A simple screening assay for certain fibrinolysis parameters (FIPA). *Thromb Res* 2000; 97: 231-7.

[8] Stief TW. The fibrinogen functional turbidimetric assay (FIFTA). *Clin Appl Thromb Hemost* 2008; 14: 84-96.

[9] Stief TW. The fibrinogen antigenic turbidimetric assay (FIATA). The $X^2\bar{x}$ Test: the corrected chi-square comparison against the control mean. *Clin Appl Thromb Hemost* 2007; 13: 73-100.

[10] Niewland R, Berckmans RJ, Reni C. et al. Cell-derived microparticles generated in patients during cardiopulmonary bypass are highly procoagulant. *Circulation* 1997; 96: 3534-3541.

[11] Evans TJ. The role of macrophages in septic shock. Immunobiology 1996; 195: 655-9.

[12] Vallet B. Microthrombosis in sepsis. *Minerva Anestesiol* 2001; 67: 298-301.

[13] Dixon B. The role of microvascular thrombosis in sepsis. *Anaesth Intensive Care* 2004; 32: 619-29.

[14] Leitner JM, Firbas C, Mayr FB, Reiter RA, Steinlechner B, Jilma B. Recombinant human antithrombin inhibits thrombin formation and interleukin 6 release in human endotoxemia. *Clin Pharmacol Ther* 2006; 79: 23-34.

[15] Iba T, Kidokoro A. High-dose antithrombin therapy for sepsis: mechanisms of action. *Shock* 2002; 5: 389-394.

[16] Fouassier M, Moreau D, Thiolliere F, Frere C, Marques-Verdier A, Souweine B. Evolution of thrombin formation and fibrinolysis markers, including thrombin-activatable fibrinolysis inhibitor, during severe meningococcemia. *Pathophysiol Haemost Thromb* 2005; 34: 284-7.

[17] Wiedermann CJ, Kaneider NC. A systematic review of antithrombin concentrate use in patients with disseminated intravascular coagulation of severe sepsis. *Blood Coagulation & Fibrinolysis* 2006; 17: 521-526.

[18] Renckens R, Weijer S, de Vos AF, Pater JM, Meijers JC, Hack CE, Levi M, van der Poll T. Inhibition of plasmin activity by tranexamic acid does not influence inflammatory pathways during human endotoxemia. *Arterioscler Thromb Vasc Biol* 2004; 24: 483-8.

[19] Amitrano L, Guardascione MA, Brancaccio V, Balzano A. Coagulation disorders in liver disease. *Semin Liver Dis* 2002; 22: 83-96.

[20] Oudijk EJ, Nieuwenhuis HK, Bos R, Fijnheer R. Elastase mediated fibrinolysis in acute promyelocytic leukemia. *Thromb Haemost* 2000; 83: 906-8.

[21] Basili S, Ferro D, Violi F. Endotoxaemia, hyperfibrinolysis, and bleeding in cirrhosis. *Lancet* 1999; 353: 1102.

[22] Duran I, Tannock IF. Disseminated intravascular coagulation as the presenting sign of metastatic prostate cancer. *J Gen Intern Med* 2006; 21: C6-8.

[23] Matsumoto T, Wada H, Nobori T, Nakatani K, Onishi K, Nishikawa M, Shiku H, Kazahaya Y, Sawai T, Koike K, Matsuda M. Elevated plasma levels of fibrin degradation products by granulocyte-derived elastase in patients with disseminated intravascular coagulation. *Clin Appl Thromb Hemost* 2005; 11: 391-400.

[24] Iba T, Kidokoro A, Fukunaga M, Sugiyama K, Sawada T, Kato H. Association between the severity of sepsis and the changes in hemostatic molecular markers and vascular endothelial damage markers. *Shock* 2005; 23: 25-9.

[25] Madoiwa S, Nunomiya S, Ono T, Shintani Y, Ohmori T, Mimuro J, Sakata Y. Related plasminogen activator inhibitor 1 promotes a poor prognosis in sepsis-induced disseminated intravascular coagulation. *Int J Hematol* 2006; 84: 398-405.

[26] Weigand MA, Schmidt H, Pourmahmoud M, Zhao O, Martin E, Bardenheuer HJ. Circulating intercellular adhesion molecule – 1 as an early predictor of hepatic failure in patients with septic shock. *Crit Care Med* 1999; 27: 2656-2661.

[27] Horstmann LL, Jy W, Jimenez JJ, Ahn YS. Endothelial microparticles as markers of endothelial dysfunction. *Front Biosci* 2004; 9: 1118-1135.

In: Hemostasis Laboratory Yearbook, Volume 2
Editor: Thomas W. Stief, pp. 75-100
ISBN: 978-1-60741-089-8

MODULATION OF GRANULOCYTE-MEDIATED THROMBOLYSIS

Thomas W. Stief*
[1]Department of Clinical Chemistry, University Hospital Giessen & Marburg, Germany

ABSTRACT

Polymorphonuclear granulocytes (PMN = neutrophils) lyse thrombi. To study this important cellular part of fibrinolysis, 50 µl plasma-clots (without and with 0.5 µmoles chloramine) were incubated with the possible PMN modulator and with 50 µl PMN-rich citrated plasma. The turbidity decrease was measured at 405 nm and the approximate effective doses were determined (microtiter plate clot lysis assay with PMN-rich plasma = PMN-CLA).

G-CSF had an approximate 50% stimulatory concentration (SC50) of 1.5 µg/ml, 50 % thrombolysis occured within 1d. The prooxidative SC50 of G-CSF was 0.5 µg/ml. Singlet oxygen ($^1\Delta O_2$) generator chloramine stimulated thrombolysis of unoxidized or oxidized clots (SC50 = 5 mM or 2 mM). 1.4 mM vancomycin was the SC50 against oxidized clots. The approximate inhibitory concentrations 50% (IC50) for unoxidized clots were: 12 mM glucose, 51 µg/ml vitamin K_1 (phytomenadione=2-methyl-3-phytyl-1,4-naphtoquinone), 2 µg/ml doxycyclin, 3.4 mg/ml hydrocortisone, 0.06 mg/ml dexamethasone, > 20 IU/ml heparin, 25 IU/ml dalteparin, 4 IU/ml certoparin, 56 µg/ml pentosanpolysulphate, 0.26 mM tranexamic acid, 1.2 mM epsilon-amino-caproid-acid, 9.3 KIU/ml aprotinin, 52 mM arginine. Vitamin K_1 and dexamethasone also stimulated thrombolysis at 10-20fold higher concentrations. Plasmin in unoxidized clot supernatants increased from 2 mU/ml to 10 mU/ml within 4.5d. Plasmin in oxidized clot supernatants increased 5-10fold. After 18 h (37°C) maximally about 0.16 mM chloramine was generated by 245 PMN/µl that were stimulated by 3 µg/ml G-CSF. This means that about 10000 activated PMN/µl could generate 5-10 mM chloramine. PMN enhance fibrinolysis by activation of their $^1\Delta O_2$ generating respiratory burst.

It is suggested to diagnose the cellular fibrinolysis by means of the present PMN-CLA in each individual patient, and to treat a patient with with hypo- or hyper-reactive PMN with an adequate PMN modulator.

* Send correspondance to: Priv.-Doz. Dr. Med. T. Stief, Department of Clinical Chemistry, University Hospital, D-35043 Marburg, Germany, FAX: +49-6421-5865594, Email: thstief@med.uni-marburg.de

Abbreviations

A, absorbance; AMCHA, aminomethylcyclohexanoic acid (tranexamic acid); AP, α2-antiplasmin=plasmin-inhibitor; CT, chloramine-T®; CV, coefficient of variation; ΔA, increase in absorbance; Δt, time interval; EACA, epsilon-amino-caproic acid; ED50, effective dose 50 % (can be IC50 or SC50); ET50, effective time point 50 % ; g, centrifugal force; G-CSF, granulocyte-colony stimulating factor; IC50, inhibitory concentration 50 %; IU, international units; KIU, kallikrein inhibiting units; LDH, lactate dehydrogenase; mA, milliabsorbance units; MW, molecular weight; NADPH, nicotine amide adenine dinucleotide phosphate reduced; PBS, phosphate buffered saline; physiol. NaCl; 0.9 % NaCl; Pli, plasmin; PMN, polymorphonuclear neutrophils; r, correlation factor; rr, rotating radius in cm; rpm, rotations per minute; RT, room temperature; SC50, stimulatory concentration 50 %; Stop-CS-reagent, 1.6 M arginine, pH 8.7, 1.2 M KCl, 0.75 mM Val-Leu-Lys-pNA; Val-Leu-Lys-pNA, valine-leucine-lysine-paranitroanilide; TF, tissue factor; t-PA, tissue type plasminogen activator; u-PA, urokinase; WBC, white blood cells; CLA, microwell clot lysis assay.

1. Introduction

Thrombi are destroyed by the fibrinolytic system, which is also called tertiary hemostasis (primary hemostasis = platelets, secondary hemostasis = plasmatic coagulation). Fibrinolysis is of plasmatic [1] and of cellular nature [2-11]. The neutrophil granulocytes (PMN) are the main cells of cellular fibrinolysis. Whereas the determination of plasmatic fibrinolysis is rather easy, the measurement of cellular fibrinolysis is complicated [12,13]. Recently, we described a new test for cellular fibrinolysis: the microtiter plate clot lysis assay with polymorphonuclear granulocytes (CLA-PMN). Here the masses of plasmatic clots are determined via their turbidity [14]. PMN produce urokinase (u-PA), elastase, and chloramines that generate nonradical excited singlet oxygen ($^1\Delta O_2$). PMN bind to fibrin, get activated, and release reactive oxygen species [15-20]. An activated phagocyte, especially an activated PMN, has a peri-cellular thrombolysis zone, whose diameter is severalfold that of the activated cell (e.g. in right upper corner of figure 4B of [7] or in figure 3B of [8]).

The cellular part of fibrinolysis seems to be more important than the plasmatic one, e.g. total plasminogen deficiency might not result into thrombosis [9], whereas neutropenia is prothrombotic [20]. The rationale of the present work is to find out the stimulatory and inhibitory concentrations 50 % of different modulators of PMN in an assay system that imitates physiological cellular fibrinolysis. Of clinical interest is the enhancement of cellular fibrinolysis in blood (against e.g. atherothrombosis [21,22]) or its inhibition (against diseases caused by hyperactivated phagocytes [23], e.g. re-bleeding after subarachnoidal hemorrhage [40]).

2. Material and Methods

2.1. Cellular fibrinolysis enhancement by G-CSF

10 ml pooled unfrozen (≤ 6 h RT old) normal plasma were recalcified by 100 μl 1563 mM $CaCl_2$ and immediately given in 50 μl portions to a flat bottom-microtiter plate (NUNC PolySorp, Wiesbaden, Germany) using a multipette. After 60 min (37°C) the 50 μl clots were incubated in duplicate with 20 μl 25 mM chloramine-T® (CT; Sigma, Deisenhofen, Germany) in physiol. NaCl for 30 min (37°C); unoxidized control clots were incubated without CT. 50 μl diluted buffy coat were added. The diluted buffy coat was prepared by pooling the after routine analysis remaining buffy coats of n=28 normal citrated 4.5 ml blood samples (1 part 106 mM sodium citrate + 9 parts of venous blood; centrifugation at 2500g for 5 min and cautious transferring of the white cells into pooled fresh normal plasma). The so obtained diluted buffy coat had 2360 white blood cells (WBC)/μl, 1490 PMN/μl, 700 lymphocytes/μl, 110 monocytes/μl, 50 eosinophils/μl, 10 basophils/μl, 10000 erythrocytes/μl, and 90000 platelets/μl (automatically counted by MAXM analyzer, Beckman-Coulter, Krefeld, Germany).

10 μl 0 - 300 μg/ml G-CSF (Neupogen®, Amgen, Munich, Germany) in 0.9 % NaCl were added and the absorbance of the clots were determined at 405 nm after 0 – 3.5 d (37°C), using a microtiter plate photometer with a 1 mA resolution (Milenia; DPC, Los Angeles, USA). The main clot turbidity was considered that after 2.5 d, 100 % clot turbidity of unoxidized clots was that after 1 d, 100 % clot turbidity of oxidized clots was that after 0 h; 0 % clot was that after 8 d (37°C) in unoxidized clots and corresponded to the turbidity of nonrecalcified plasma + PBS + PMN modulator + diluted buffy coat; in lysed oxidized clots the 0 % clot turbidity was about 10 % higher than in lysed unoxidized clots. (0 % unoxidized clot = 413 mA, 0 % oxidized clot = 454 mA; 100 % unoxidized clot = 902 mA; 100 % oxidized clot = 919 mA; the coefficients of variation of 100 % clot were < 5 %)

Calculation of clot mass and clot lysis

Clot mass and clot lysis were calculated using the following formulas:

- Clot mass = (main turbidity – 0 % clot turbidity)/(100 % clot turbidity – 0 % clot turbidity) x 100 %
- Clot lysis = 100 % minus clot mass

2.1.1. Plasmin activity in dependence of G-CSF amount

50 μl supernatant of unoxidized clots and of oxidized clots after 3.5 d (37°C) of above were incubated with 50 μl 1.5 M arginine, pH 8.7 and 50 μl Stop-CS-reagent (1.6 M arginine (Sigma), 1.2 M KCl, 0.75 mM Val-Leu-Lys-pNA (Chromogenix, Mölndal, Sweden), pH 8.7). The standard was 100 μl 0.5 U/ml plasmin in 50 % plasma, 750 mM arginine, pH 8.7 [24] (resulting in 12.5 mA/min RT; maximal ΔA=1000 mA, valid linear ΔA range= 0-400 mA; 1 U/ml plasmin = maximally inducible plasmin activity in pooled normal plasma).

2.1.2. Generation of chloramine-like oxidants by activated PMN

20 μl of pooled PMN-rich plasma (normal citrated blood (n=12), 6 h room temperature (RT) old, centrifuged at 1500 rpm for 2 min) were incubated in duplicate with 5 μl 0-120

μg/ml G-CSF in 6.7 % human albumin for 0 h (zero control) or 18 h (37°C). 200 μl 4 M KI in PBS (Sigma) were added and the absorbance at 405 nm was determined [25]. The standard was 20 μl 1.18 mM chloramine-T® in H_2O (ΔA=566 ± 16 mA). For matrix control, 20 μl pooled PMN-rich plasma + 5 μl 6.7 % human albumin were added to 200 μl 4 M KI in PBS that had been reacted with 2 μl 1 mM or 10 mM chloramine-T®. The generated absorbance (23°C) decreased by 0 % or about 1 % of the initial value, without presence of plasma or with presence of plasma, respectively.

2.1.3. Clinical-chemical parameters during PMN activation

PMN-rich plasma was centrifuged at 2860g (4000 rpm) for 3 min, the obtained PMN-deprived plasma was incubated for 0 or 18 h (37°C). 1000 μl PMN-rich plasma were supplemented with 20 μl 0 or 120 μg/ml G-CSF in 6.7 % human albumin (final conc.: 0 or 2.4 μg/ml G-CSF) and were incubated for 18 h (37°C). WBC and platelets were determined automatically before and after 18 h (37°C) incubation. The respective plasma samples were analyzed for functional fibrinogen (modified Clauss-Method; Behring Coagulation Timer, DadeBehring, Marburg, Germany), K^+, glucose, lactate, and lactate dehydrogenase (Hitachi 917, Roche, Basel, Switzerland). For control, destroyed PMN were analyzed in the Hitachi 917: PMN-rich plasma was centrifuged at 2500g for 3 min, the plasma was separated from the cells, H_2O was added that replaced the plasma, the cells were dissolved again, frozen at -32°C and thawed at 23°C.

2.2. Cellular Clot Lysis modulation

10 ml pooled normal plasma (-80°C frozen/thawed under shaking for 3 min at 37°C) were recalcified with 100 μl 1563 mM $CaCl_2$. 50 μl portions were immediately pipetted into microtiter plates with flat bottom. After 45 min (37°C) 20 μl 0 or 25 mM CT in PBS were added and incubated for 45 min (37°C). 10 μl PMN modulator in 6 % human albumin-PBS were added:

- Vancomycin: 0-50 mM (final conc.: 0-6.25 mM); Lilly, Giessen, Germany.
- Glucose: 0-1000 mM (final conc.: 0-125 mM); Merck, Darmstadt, Germany
- Vitamin K_1 (Phytomenadione=2-methyl-3-phytyl-1,4-naphtoquinone): 0-10 mg/ml (final conc.: 0-1250 μg/ml); Roche, Basel, Switerland
- Doxycyclin: 0-20 mg/ml (final conc.: 0-2500 μg/ml); ratiopharm, Ulm, Germany
- Hydrocortisone: 0-80 mg/ml (final conc.: 0-10 mg/ml); Pfizer, Karlsruhe, Germany
- Dexamethasone: 0-10 mg/ml (final conc.: 0-1.25 mg/ml); Merck, Darmstadt, Germany
- Heparin : 0-5000 IU/ml (final conc.: 0-625 IU/ml); Roche, Basel, Switzerland
- Dalteparin (Fragmin P®): 0-12500 IU/ml (final conc.: 0-1563 IU/ml), Pharmacia and Upjohn, Erlangen, Germany
- Certoparin (Monoembolex®): 0-3000 IU/ml (final conc.: 0-375 IU/ml), Sandoz, Nürnberg, Germany
- Pentosanpolysulfate (Fibrezym®): 0-100 mg/ml (final conc.: 0-12.5 mg/ml), bene Arzneimittel GmbH, Germany

- Tranexamic acid (AMCHA, Ugurol®): 0-637 mM (final conc.: 0-80 mM), Bayer, Leverkusen, Germany
- ϵ-amino-caproic acid (EACA): 0-637 mM (final conc.: 0-80 mM), Sigma, Deisenhofen, Germany
- Aprotinin: 0-10000 KIU/ml (final conc.: 0-1250 KIU/ml), Bayer, Leverkusen, Germany
- Arginine: 0-1000 mM (final conc.: 0-125 mM), Braun, Melsungen, Germany.

50 µl diluted buffy coat in pooled fresh normal plasma were added. The diluted buffy coat contained 240 PMN/µl (390 WBC/µl, 110 lymphocytes/µl, 30 monocytes/µl, 10 eosinophils/µl, no erythrocytes, 98000 platelets/µl). The clot turbidity was determined after 0-5.5 d (37°C). The main clot turbidity was considered that after 2.5 d, 100 % clot turbidity was that after 0 h, 0 % clot in unoxidized clots corresponded to that of nonrecalcified plasma + PBS + PMN modulator + diluted buffy coat, in lysed oxidized clots the 0 % clot turbidity was about 10 % higher than in lysed unoxidized clots.

When using the $^1\Delta O_2$ - generator chloramine 10 µl 0 – 150 mM (0-18.8 mM final) chloramine-T® (CT) in 0.9 % NaCl were added after addition of diluted buffy coat.

2.2.1. Plasmin, α2-antiplasmin, and urokinase in clot supernatants

Arginine-stabilization of clot supernatants

10 µl clot supernatant of unoxidized and 0.5 µmoles CT-oxidized clots without addition of a PMN modulator (control: 10 µl 6 % human albumin in PBS (Kabi, Stockholm, Sweden)) were withdrawn in duplicate from the clots after 0 – 4.5 d (37°C; incubator). 10 µl 1.5 M arginine, pH 8.7, were added and the so stabilized clot supernatant was frozen at -20°C in a U-well microtiter plate. The arginine-stabilized clot supernatants were thawn, 5 µl of them were withdrawn and analyzed for α2-antiplasmin (AP; plasmin-inhibitor) activity; the remaining 15 µl were analyzed for plasmin (Pli) activity.

Determination of plasmin (Pli) activity in clot supernatants

15 µl 0.75 M arginine-stabilized clot supernatant were incubated with 10 µl 75 mM chloramine-T® in PBS for 60 min (RT). 50 µl 1.6 M arginine, pH 8.7, 1.2 M KCl, 0.75 mM Val-Leu-Lys-pNA (Stop-CS-reagent) and 125 µl 5 % human albumin-PBS were added and ΔA at 405 nm (RT=23°C; Δt=18h) was measured by a microtiter plate reader (Milenia, DPC, Los Angeles, USA). The Pli standard was 0.5 U/ml plasmin in pooled normal plasma (plasma that had reacted for 30 min with 1000 IU/ml urokinase (medac, Hamburg, Germany); 1+1 diluted with 1.5 M arginine, pH 8.7), that resulted into a linear ΔA of 302 mA/h (RT).

Determination of α2-antiplasmin (AP) activity in clot supernatants

5 µl 0.75 M arginine-stabilized clot supernatant were incubated in duplicate with 20 µl 10 µg/ml plasmin in 7 % human albumin-PBS, freshly prepared from an aliquoted stock solution of 125 µg/ml active plasmin (Chromogenix, Mölndal, Sweden; MW=85000) in 20 % glycerol-PBS for 8 min (RT). 50 µl Stop-CS-reagent and 50 µl 5 % human albumin-PBS were added ΔA at 405 nm (RT; Δt=2h) was measured by the Milenia-microtiter plate reader. The AP standards were: pooled normal plasma, undiluted (100 % AP standard) and diluted 1+1, 1+2, 1+3, 1+4, 1+5, 1+6, 1+7, 1+8, 1+9, and 1+14 with 6 % human albumin-PBS, or

albumin-PBS instead of plasma (0 % AP standard), all stabilized 1+1 with 1.5 M arginine, pH 8.7; the 100 % AP (= plasmin-inhibitor) standard resulting into a ΔA of 21 mA/2h (RT), the 0 % AP standard resulting into a ΔA of 112 mA/2h (RT).

Determination of u-PA antigen in clot supernatant

Total urokinase antigen was determined by a commercial test kit (Technoclone®, Vienna, Austria), the final incubation time was prolonged 3fold (60 min RT) resulting in a calibration curve that was linear up a specific absorbance increase of 848 mA at 450 nm after addition of H_2SO_4 or 156 mA at 405 nm before addition of H_2SO_4), the 100 % of norm value (pooled normal citrated plasma) was 6 ng/ml u-PA.

3. Pre-analytic Generation of PMN-Rich Plasma

Pooled citrated blood (n=24 individual 4 ml samples) (1 part 106 mM citrate + 9 parts venous blood; after 12 h at 4°C) was aliquoted into 4 ml aliquots that were centrifuged for 2-15 min at 700-2500 rpm (Megafuge 1.0R, Heraeus, Hanau, Germany); $G = 0.00001118 \cdot$ rotating radius (rr) $\cdot$ rotations per minute $(\text{rpm})^2$. The obtained plasma was analyzed by a MAXM hematology analyzer (Beckman Coulter, Krefeld, Germany) and controlled microscopically after hematoxylin-eosin-staining.

4. Cellular Lysis of Tissue Factor - or Contact-Phase Generated Micro-Clots

50 µl pooled normal plasma (4 h RT old) were incubated with 5 µl 10 % Thromborel-S ® (10 % = 16 ng/ml human placental tissue factor (TF) without polybrene®; DadeBehring), 250 mM $CaCl_2$ or 5 µl Pathromtin-SL® (DadeBehring), 250 mM $CaCl_2$ for 40 min (37°C). 20 µl pooled PMN-rich plasma from n=9 citrated normal blood samples centrifuged at 1500 rpm for 2 min were added to the generated micro-clots. 5 µl 0-30 µg/ml G-CSF in 6 % human albumin were added and the turbidity of the wells was determined at 405 nm.

5. Statistics

The intra-assay coefficients of variation (CV), as defined as standard deviation divided by mean value ($MV=\bar{x}$) and multiplied by 100 %, of the CLA values (at least duplicate determinations) were < 10 %. Critical 14fold results were compared with respective 14fold controls and tested for significance ($p< 0.05$), using the non-categorical values to categorical values transformed two-fold Yates-corrected chi-square comparison against the control-mean ($X^2\bar{x}$ Test) [26].

6. RESULTS

G-CSF

G-CSF enhances clot lysis. Figs. 1a,c show that an unoxidized plasma-clot is lysed to 50 % after 2.5 d (37°C), if clot lysis is stimulated by about 1.5 μg/ml = approx. ED50= approx. SC50. Oxidized clots do not respond as well to PMN stimulation by G-CSF, the respective ED50 increases more than 10fold when compared to unoxidized clots (Fig. 1b). The unoxidized clot without G-CSF addition lyses only by about 30 % after 2.5 d and lyses by about 50 % after 3d. The oxidized clot without G-CSF lyses by about 40 % after 2.5 d and lyses by about 60 % after 3d. The plasmin activity observed after 4.5 d increases proportional to the added G-CSF amount. 0 μg G-CSF added results in about 10 mU/ml plasmin, 1.5 μg G-CSF added (about 19 μg/ml G-CSF in the clot supernatant) in about 18 mU/ml plasmin in unoxidized and oxidized clots (Fig. 1d).

Fig. 1e demonstrates the generation of chloramine-like oxidants by PMN: after 18 h (37°C) maximally about 0.16 mM active chloramine is generated, when the cells are stimulated by 3 μg/ml G-CSF. 50 % of this chloramine maximum is reached at 0.5 μg/ml G-CSF.

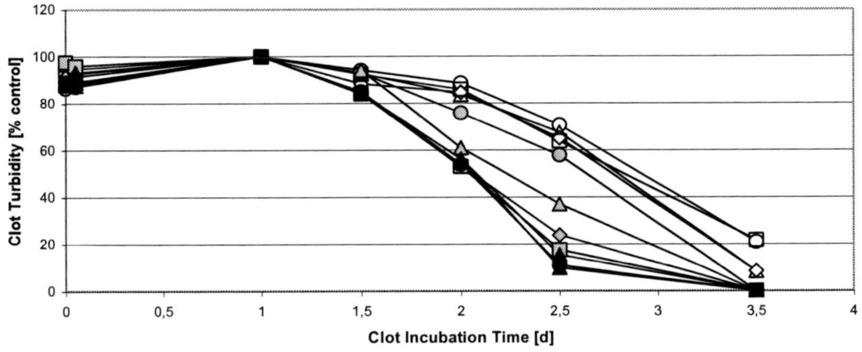

Figure 1a.

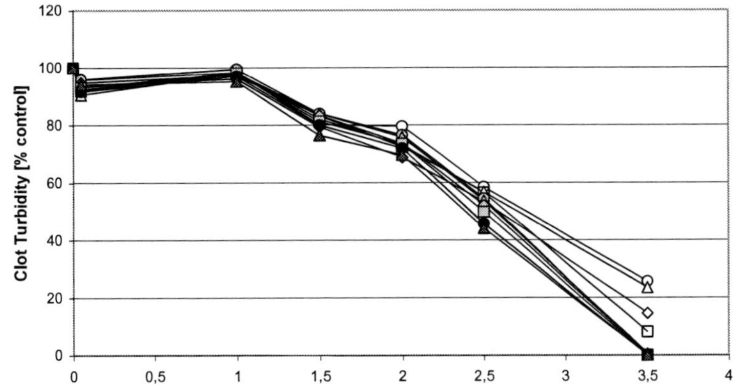

Figure 1b.

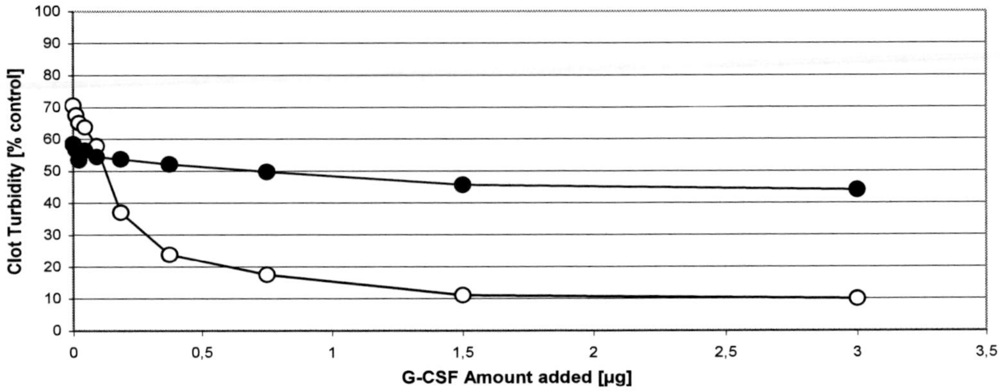

Figure 1c.

Figure 1a-c. Cellular fibrinolysis enhancement by G-CSF. 50 µl clots of pooled unfrozen (≤ 6 h RT old) normal plasma were incubated with 20 µl physiol. NaCl (Fig. 1a) or 25 mM chloramine-T® in 0.9 % NaCl (Fig. 1b) for 30 min (37°C). 50 µl diluted buffy coat containing 1490 PMN/µl and 10 µl G-CSF in 0.9 % NaCl were added and the absorbance of the clots were determined at 405 nm after 0–3.5 d (37°C). The added G-CSF amounts were 0 µg (O), 0.01 µg (Δ),0.03 µg (◊), 0.05 µg (□), 0.1 µg (grey O), 0.19 µg (grey Δ), 0.38 µg (grey ◊), 0.75 µg (grey □), 1.5 µg (●), and 3 µg (▲)
The ED50 of G-CSF on fibrinolysis was determined after 2.5 d (37°C) (Fig. 1c).

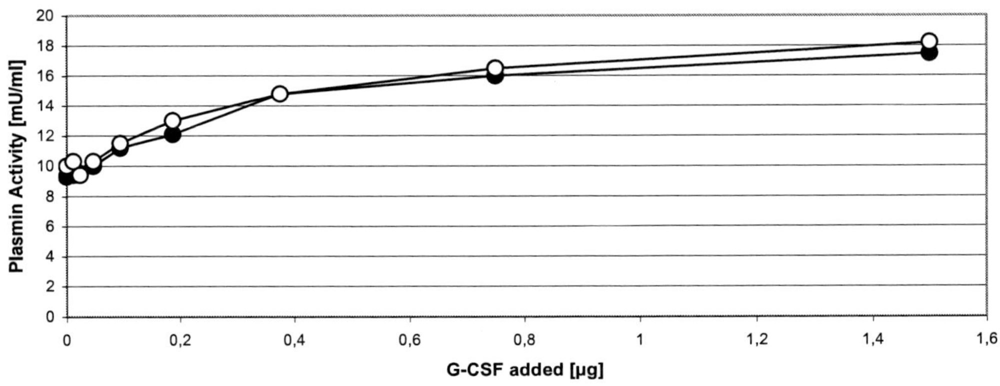

Figure 1d. Plasmin-activity increase in dependence of G-CSF amount. 50 µl supernatant of unoxidized clot (O) and of oxidized clot (●) after 3.5 d (37°C) of Fig. 1a,b were incubated with 50 µl 1.5 M arginine, pH 8.7 and 50 µl Stop-CS-reagent. The standard was 100 µl 0.5 U/ml plasmin in 50 % plasma, 750 mM arginine, pH 8.7 (resulting in 12.5 mA/min RT; max. delta A=1000 mA).

The concentration of active fibrinogen was 4.1 g/l in PMN-rich plasma incubated for 18 h (37°C) without addition of G-CSF and 4.3 g/l in presence of 2.4 µg/ml G-CSF. Pooled plasma incubated for 0 or 18 h (37°C) had 4.3 g/l or 3.9 g/l active fibrinogen, respectively. These differences in fibrinogen function were not statistically significant. Originally the PMN-rich plasma had 245 PMN/µl and 466000 platelets/µl. After 18 h (37°C) the PMN-rich plasma without G-CSF had 200 PMN/µl and 288000 platelets/µl; the PMN-rich plasma with 2.4 µg/ml G-CSF had 190 PMN/µl and 290000 platelets/µl, i.e. there appears only a 18 % or 22 % loss in PMN during 18 h (37°C), respectively.

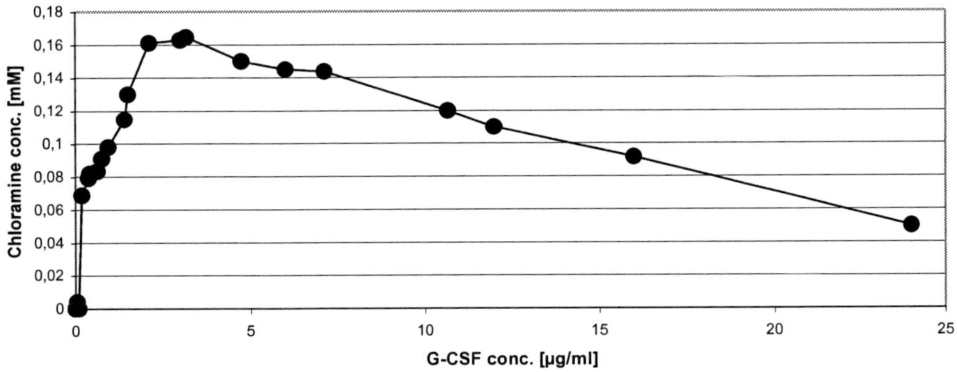

Figure 1e. Chloramine-generation in dependence of G-CSF concentration. 20 µl of pooled normal PMN-rich citrated plasma were incubated with 5 µl 0-120 µg/ml G-CSF in 6.7 % human albumin for 18 h (37°C). 200 µl 4 M KI or H_2O (blank control) were added and the absorbance at 405 nm was determined.

Initially, the pooled plasma had 3.4 mM K^+, 79 mg/dl glucose, 5.6 mM lactate, and 238 U/l LDH. After 18 h (37°C) pooled plasma had 3.4 mM K^+, 70 mg/dl glucose, 5.0 mM lactate, and 196 U/l LDH. PMN-rich plasma without G-CSF had 3.4 mM K^+, 53 mg/dl glucose, 6.4 mM lactate, and 213 U/l LDH; PMN-rich plasma with 2.4 µg/ml G-CSF had 3.4 mM K^+, 54 mg/dl glucose, 6.4 mM lactate, and 211 U/l LDH, i.e. the 245 PMN/µl consumed 16.5 mg/dl (0.92 mM) glucose, resulting into an increase of 1.4 mM lactate during 18 h (37°C), the LDH increase was < 10 %. There was no change in K^+. Destroyed PMN had 750 U/l LDH.

$^1\Delta O_2$ generator chloramine

Fig. 2 demonstrates that the singlet oxygen-generator chloramine stimulates cellular clot lysis (approx. SC50=5 mM for unoxidized clots or 2 mM for oxidized clots). The approximate 50% effective time point (ET50) for 4.7 mM chloramines is 2.4 d for unoxidized clots and 1d for oxidized clots.

The plasmin activity in the clot supernatants at begin of incubation is about 2 mU/ml; it increases about 5fold within 4.5 d (37°C) in unoxidized and in oxidized clots (Fig. 2d,e). The α2-antiplasmin activity decreases from an initial value of about 60 - 70 % (of norm, when compared to pooled normal plasma) to about 20 - 30 % after 1.5 d (37°C), i.e. about 30-40 % of initial AP is still present after 1.5 d (Fig. 2f,g). At this time point (1.5 d) about 30 % of the unoxidized or oxidized clots and are lysed (Fig. 2a,b). The plasmin activity in $^1\Delta O_2$ treated clot supernatant after 1.5 d (37°C) increases 5-10fold in dependence of chloramine-concentration: 0 mM chloramine → 3 mU/ml plasmin, 30 mM chloramine → 18 mU/ml plasmin. The respective AP activity after 1.5 d decreases from about 40 % of norm (0 mM CT) to about 25 % of norm (8 mM CT). 9.4 mM CT in the supernatant of clots primarily not oxidized by 0.5 µmoles of CT results into about 20 % clot lysis after 1.5 d, the respective plasmin and plasmin-inhibitor values are 7 mU/ml and 23 % of norm. There appears no change in urokinase antigen in the clot supernatants.

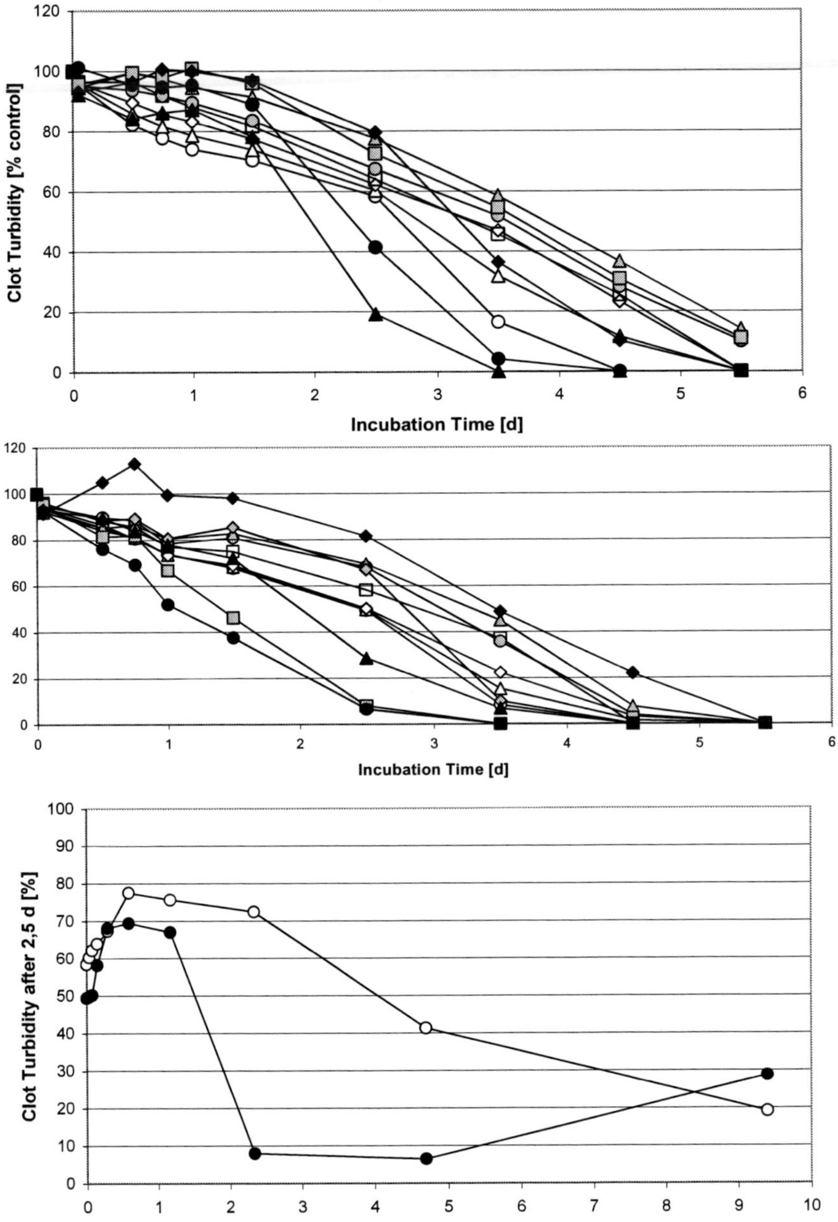

Figure. 2. Cellular Clot Lysis stimulation by chloramine. 50 µl clots of frozen/thawed pooled normal plasma were incubated with 20 µl 0 or 25 mM chloramine-T® (CT) in PBS for 45 min (37°C). 10 µl PMN modulator in 6 % human albumin-PBS and 50 µl diluted buffy coat containing 240 PMN/µl in pooled unfrozen normal plasma were added. The clot turbidity was determined after 0-4.5 d (37°C) (100% clot = 700 mA, 0% clot = 282 mA). Fig. 2a Unoxidized clots, Fig. 2b Oxidized clots, Fig. 2c ED50 determination of chloramines after 2.5 d (37°C). The final CT concentrations were: 0 mM (O), 0.04 mM (Δ), 0.08 mM (◊), 0.15 mM (□), 0.3 mM (grey O), 0.6 mM (grey Δ), 1.2 mM (grey ◊), 2.4 mM (grey □), 4.7 mM (●), 9.4 mM (▲), and 18.8 mM (♦). Fig. 2c is the ED50 determination for unoxidized (O) and oxidized clots (●). The aprox. ED50 was 5 mM (O) or 2 mM (●). The approx. ET50 at 4.7 mM CT was 2.4 d for unoxidized and 1 d for oxidized clots.

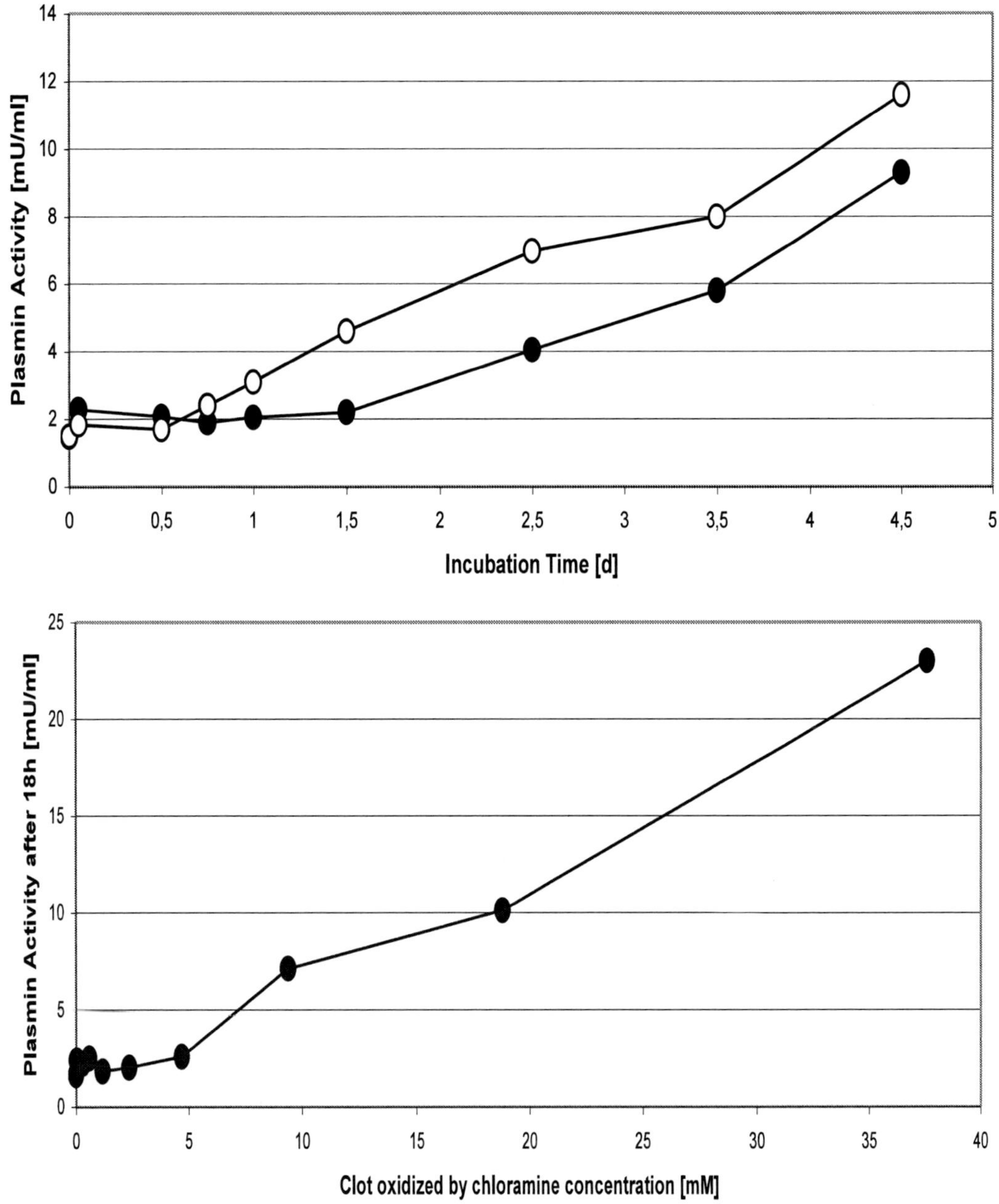

Figure 2d,e. Plasmin - activity in clot supernatants. 15 µl arginine-stabilized clot supernatant of Fig. 2a,b with PBS-control as PMN modulator were incubated with 10 µl 75 mM chloramine-T® in PBS for 60 min (RT). 50 µl 1.6 M arginine, pH 8.7, 1.2 M KCl, 0.75 mM Val-Leu-Lys-pNA (Stop-CS-reagent) and 125 µl 5 % human albumin-PBS were added and ΔA at 405 nm (RT; Δt=18h) was measured (Fig. 2d). Analysis of the clot supernatants of Fig. 2a after 18 h (37°C) (Fig. 2e).

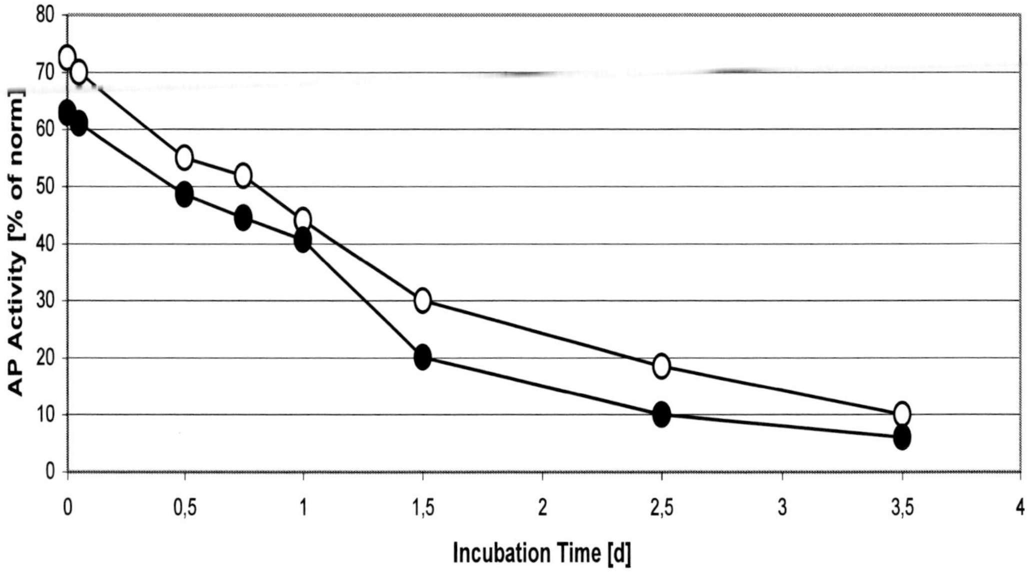

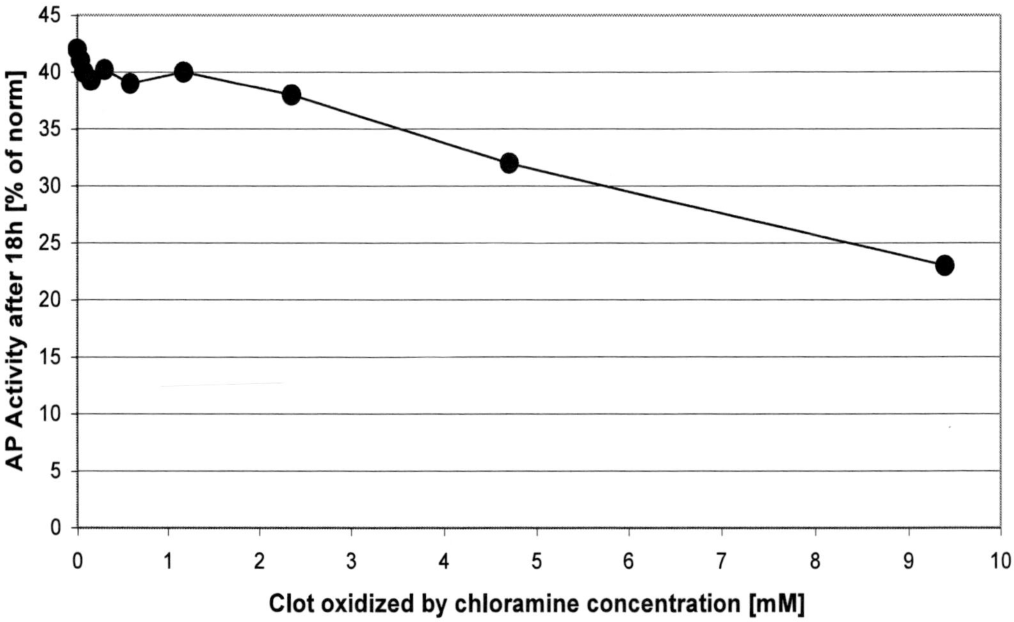

Figure 2 f,g. α2-Antiplasmin - activity in clot supernatants. 5 µl arginine-stabilized clot supernatant of Fig. 2a,b with PBS-control as PMN modulator were incubated with 20 µl 10 µg/ml plasmin in 7 % human albumin-PBS. 50 µl Stop-CS-reagent and 50 µl 5 % human albumin-PBS were added ΔA at 405 nm (RT; Δt=2h) was measured (Fig. 2f). Analysis of the clot supernatants of Fig. 2a after 18 h (37°C) (Fig. 2g).

Other PMN-modulators

Table 1 shows a comparison of ED50 data of the PMN-modulators tested. Vancomycin stimulates lysis of oxidized micro-clots with an SC50 of 1.4 mM (Fig. 3)

Table 1. Approximate ED50 values of different PMN-modulators on cellular fibrinolysis.

	IC50 unox. clot	IC50 ox. clot	SC50 unox. clot	SC50 ox. clot
G-CSF			1.5 μg/ml	40 μg/ml
Chloramine			5 mM	2 mM
Vancomycin	3 mM			1.4 mM
Glucose	12 mM	1.4 mM		
Vitamin K	51 μg/ml	62 μg/ml	550 μg/ml	500 μg/ml
Doxycyclin	2 μg/ml	2 μg/ml		
Hydrocortisone	3.4 mg/ml	0.25 mg/ml		
Dexamethasone	0.06 mg/ml	0.06 mg/ml	1.1 mg/ml	1 mg/ml
Heparin	> 20 IU/ml	0.64 IU/ml		
Dalteparin	25 IU/ml	130 IU/ml		
Certoparin	4 IU/ml	64 IU/ml		
Pentosanpolysulfate	56 μg/ml	937 μg/ml		
Tranexamic acid	0.26 mM	0.26 mM		
εAminocaproic acid	1.2 mM	1.2 mM		
Aprotinin	9.3 KIU/ml	4.6 KIU/ml		
Arginine	52 mM	3 mM		

50 % effective dose (ED50), 50 % inhibitory concentration (IC50), 50 % stimulatory concentration (SC50), unoxidized (unox.) clot = 0 μmol chloramine added to 50 μl clots, oxidized (ox.) clot = 0.5 μmoles chloramine added to 50 μl clots.

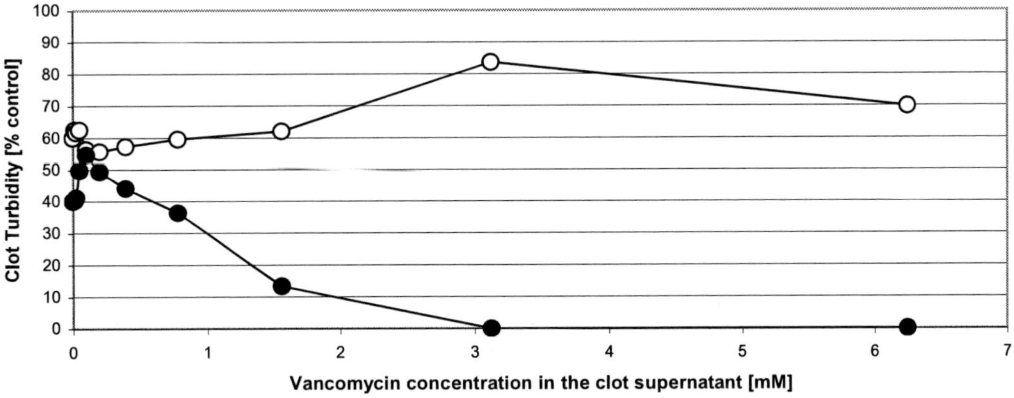

Figure 3. PMN-stimulator = Vancomycin. The cellular clot lysis assay was performed in presence of 0-6.3 mM (final concentration) vancomycin. There appeared a 50 % stimulatory concentration of 1.4 mM for oxidized clots (•); lysis of unoxidized clots (O) was not stimulated by vancomycin.

Additional **glucose** inhibits clot lysis by PMN: the IC50 is 12 mM for unoxidized clots and 1.4 mM for oxidized ones (Fig. 4).

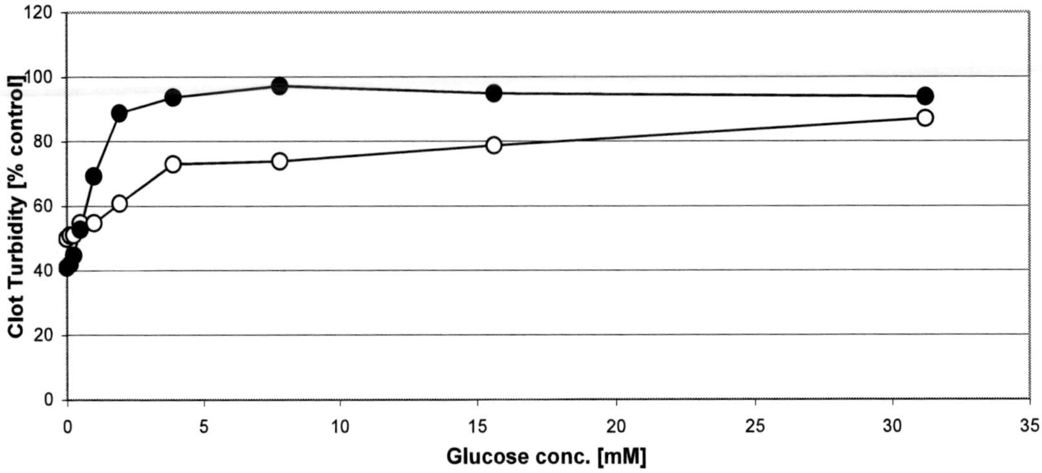

Figure 4. PMN-modulator = Glucose. The cellular clot lysis assay was performed in presence of 0-31 mM (final conc.) glucose. The approx. IC50 was 12 mM for unoxidized clots (O) or 1.4 mM (●) for oxidized clots.

Vitamin K first inhibits cellular clot lysis (IC50=51 or 62 µg/ml), increasing concentrations stimulate cellular clot lysis (SC50= about 0.5 mg/ml) (Fig. 5).

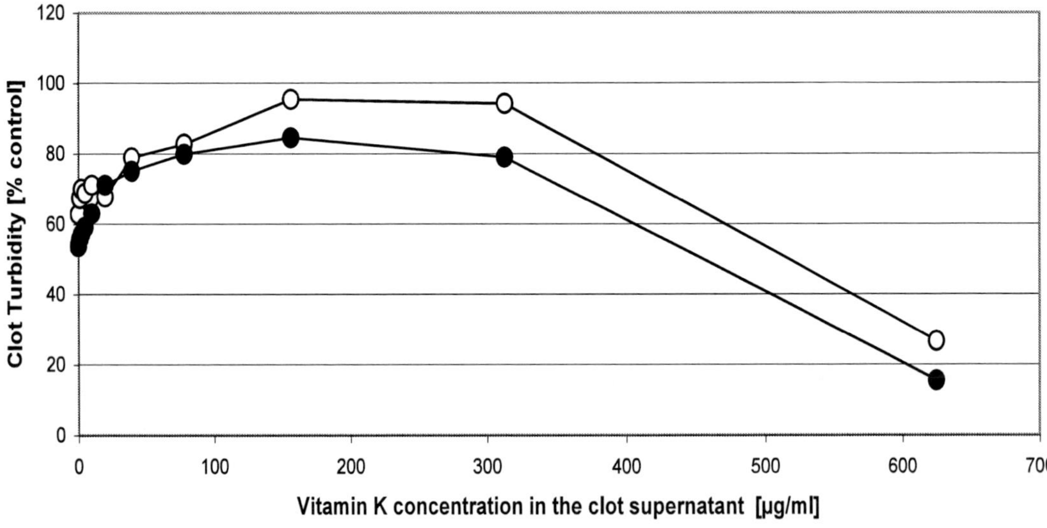

Figure 5. PMN-modulator = vitamin K (phylloquinone). The cellular clot lysis assay was performed in presence of 0-625 µg/ml (final concentration) vitamin K. The approx. IC50 is 51 µg/ml for unoxidized clots (O) or 62 µg/ml (●) for oxidized clots; there appeared also an approx. 50 % stimulatory concentration of 550 µg/ml for unoxidized and 500 µg/ml for oxidized clots.

Doxycyclin inhibits cellular clot lysis (approx. IC50=2 µg/ml) (Fig. 6).

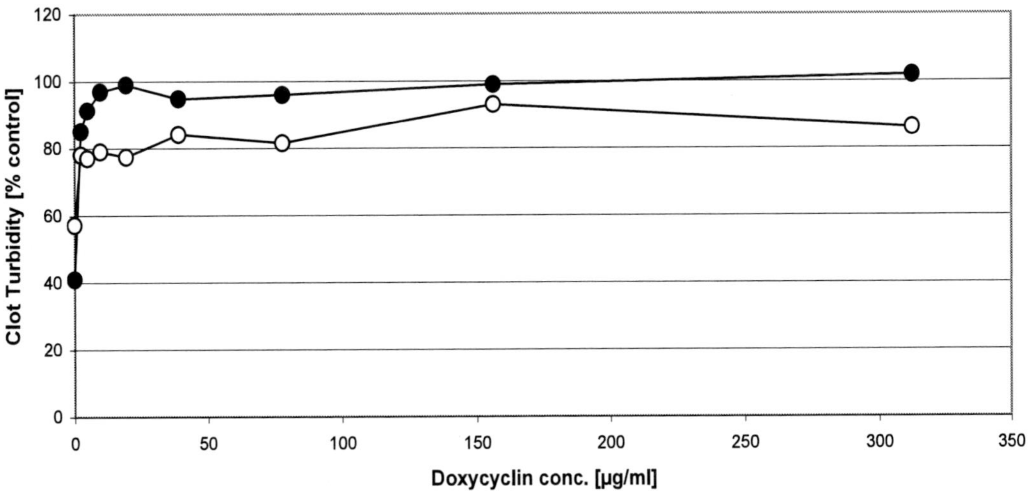

Figure 6. PMN-modulator = doxycyclin. The cellular clot lysis assay was performed in presence of 0-313 µg/ml (final conc.) doxycyclin. The approx. IC50 was 2 µg/ml both for unoxidized clots (O) or for oxidized clots (•).

Glucocorticoids inhibit cellular clot lysis: **hydrocortisone** has an IC50 of 3.4 mg/ml or 0.25 mg/ml, the IC50 values of **dexamethasone** are 0.06 mg/ml for both types of clots. However, dexamethasone at higher concentrations stimulates cellular clot lysis: SC50= about 1 mg/ml (Fig. 7).

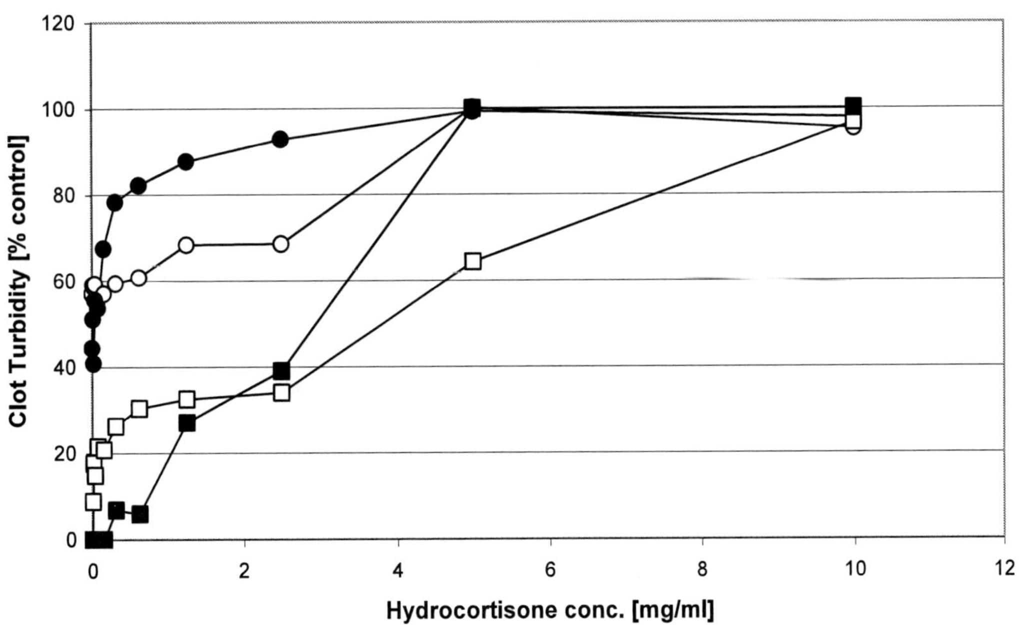

Figure 7. (Continues on next page).

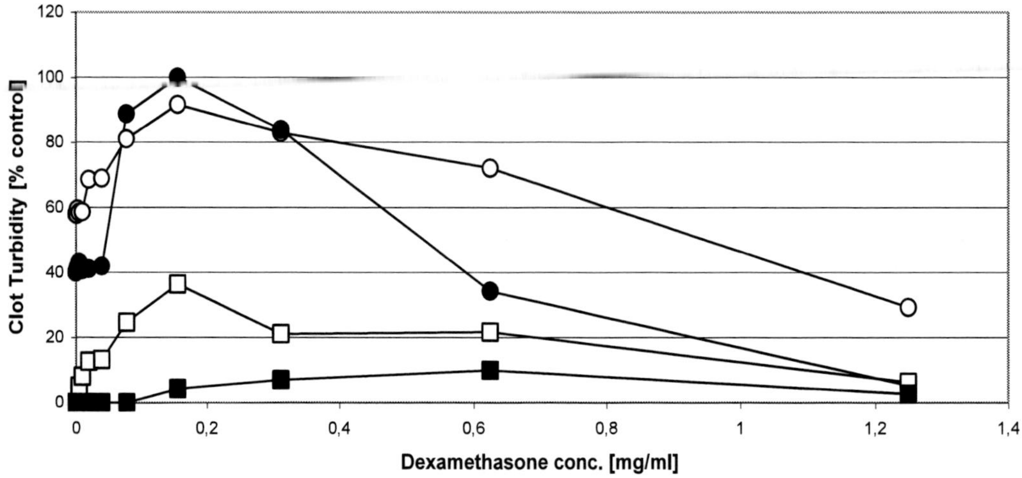

Figure 7. PMN-modulator = glucocorticoids. The cellular clot lysis assay was performed in presence of 0-10 mg/ml (final conc.) hydrocortisone. The approx. IC50 was 3.4 mg/ml for unoxidized clots (O) or 0.25 mg/ml (●) for oxidized clots (Fig. 7a). 5.5 d (37°C) instead of 2.5 d (37°C): unoxidized clots (□), oxidized clots (■). The cellular clot lysis assay was also performed in presence of 0-1.25 mg/ml (final conc.) dexamethasone. The approx. IC50 was 0.06 mg/ml for both types of clots; there appeared also an approx. ED50 of 1.1 mg/ml for unoxidized clots and 1 mg/ml for oxidized clots (Fig. 7b). 5.5 d (37°C) instead of 2.5 d (37°C): unoxidized clots (□), oxidized clots (■).

Sulfated glycosaminoglycans inhibit cellular clot lysis: the IC50 of **heparin** is > 20 IU/ml for unoxidized clots or 0.64 IU/ml for oxidized clots, the two low molecular weight heparins **dalteparin** and **certoparin** IC50s of 25 IU/ml and 130 IU/ml vs. 4 IU/ml and 64 IU/ml. **Pentosanpolysulfate** had approx. IC50s of 56 μg/ml and 937 μg/ml (Fig. 8).

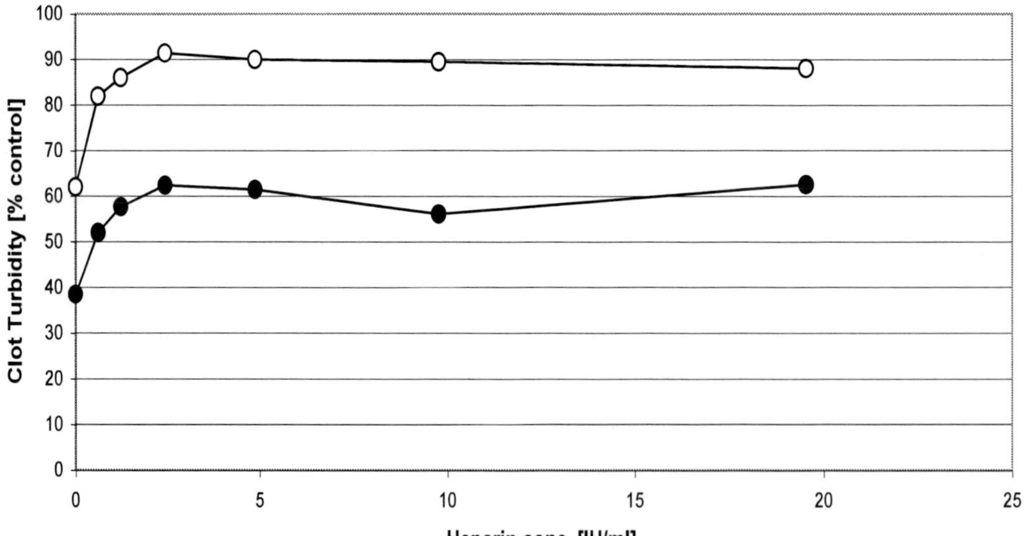

Figure 8. (Continues on next page).

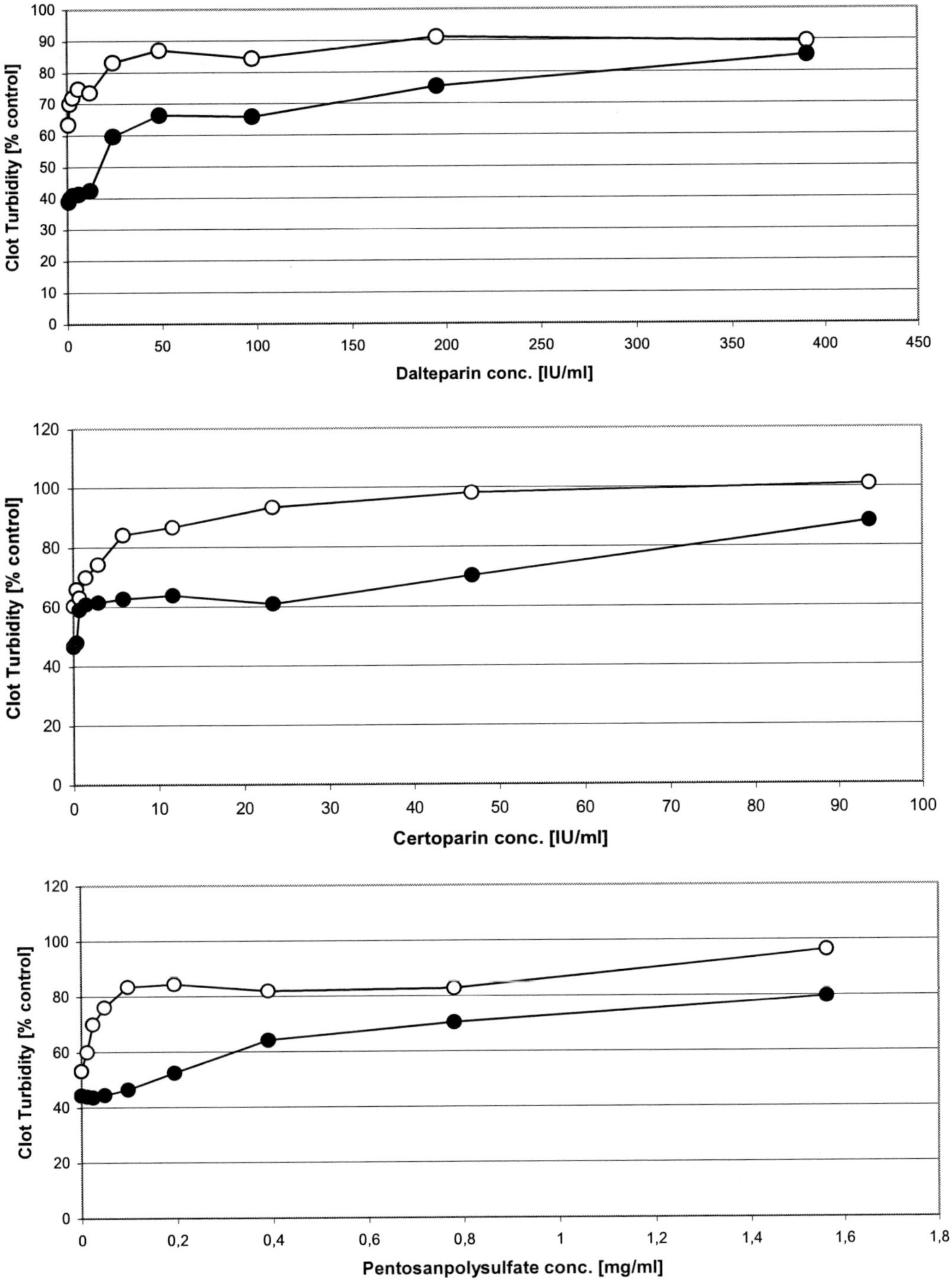

Figure 8. PMN-modulator = glycosaminoglycans. The cellular clot lysis assay was performed in presence of 0-20 IU/ml (final conc.) heparin. The approx. IC50 is > 20 IU/ml for unoxidized clot (O) and 0.64 IU/ml for oxdized clots (•) (Fig. 8a). 0-391 IU/ml dalteparin gave an approx. IC50 of 25 or 130 IU/ml (Fig. 8b). 0-94 IU/ml certoparin gave an approx. IC50 of 4 or 64 IU/ml (24 or 384 µg/ml) (Fig. 8c). 0-1.56 mg/ml pentosanpolysulfate gave an approx. IC50 of 56 or 937 µg/ml (Fig. 8d).

The **antifibrinolytics** tested inhibit cellular clot lysis: approx. IC50 of **AMCHA** = 0.26 mM for both types of clots, approx. IC50 of **EACA** = 1.2 mM for both types of clots, and approx. IC50 of **aprotinin** = 9.3 or 4.6 KIU/ml for unoxidized or oxidized clots, respectively (Fig. 9).

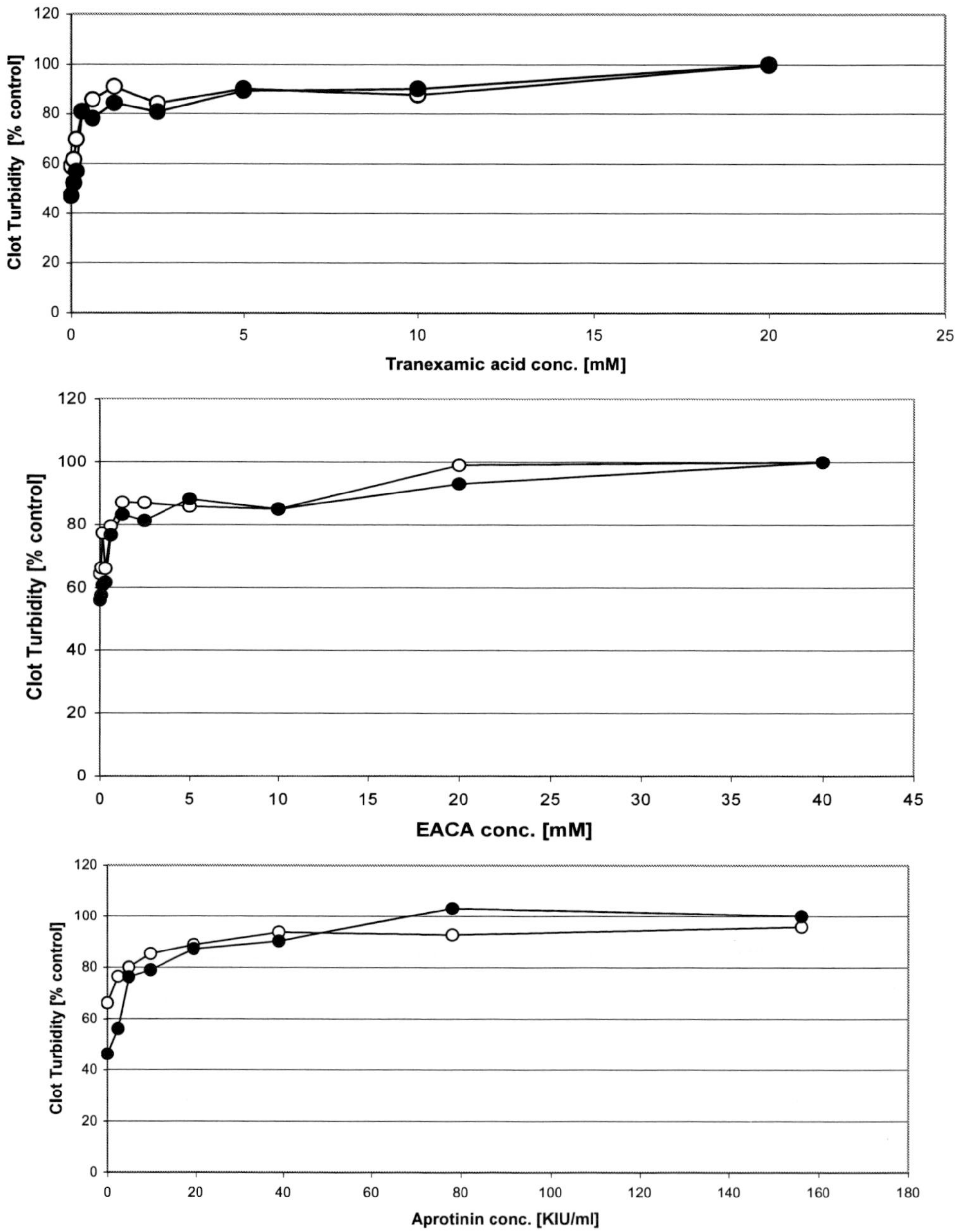

Figure 9. PMN-modulator = antifibrinolytics. The cellular clot lysis assay was performed in presence of 0-20 mM tranexamic acid (AMCHA). The approx. IC50 is 0.26 mM for both types of clots (Fig. 9a). 0-40 mM epsilon-aminocaproic acid (EACA) gave an approx. IC50 of 1.2 mM for both types of clots (Fig. 9b). 0-156 KIU/ml aprotinin gave an approx. IC50 of 9.3 or 4.6 KIU/ml for unoxidized or oxidized clots, respectively (Fig. 9c).

Arginine inhibits cellular clot lysis with IC50 of 52 and 3 mM for unoxidized or oxidized clots, respectively (Fig. 10). Final arginine concentrations > 20 mM seem to partially dissolve an oxidized clot.

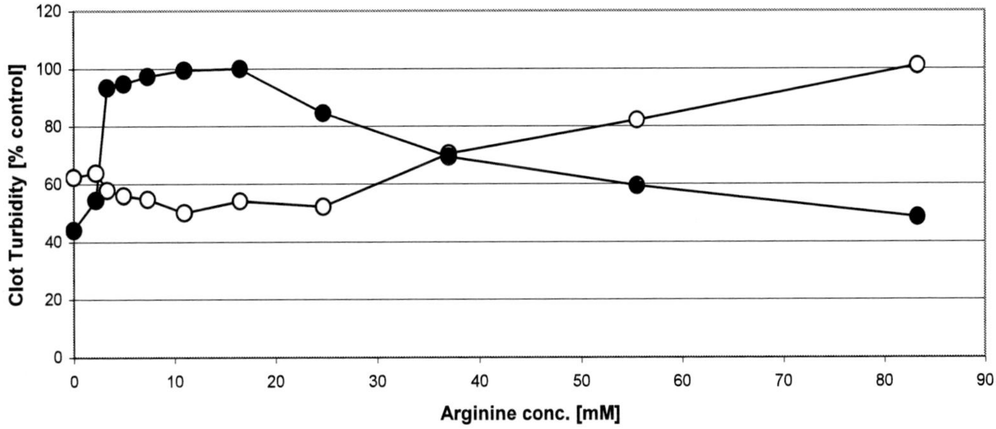

Figure 10. PMN-modulator = arginine. The cellular clot lysis assay was performed in presence of 0-83 mM arginine. The approx. IC50 was 52 mM or 3 mM for unoxidized or oxidized clots, respectively.

A possible centrifugation procedure to obtain PMN-rich plasma is 1500 rpm (about 400g) for 2-3 min (Fig. 11a). This results in about 300 PMN/µl plasma of pooled citrated blood. Also centrifugation at 700 rpm for 9 min (88g) results in 300-400 PMN/µl (Fig. 11b). Microscopic control of the cells found by the automatic analyzer in plasma showed that > 95 % of WBC were PMN, many PMN were automatically counted as lymphocytes.

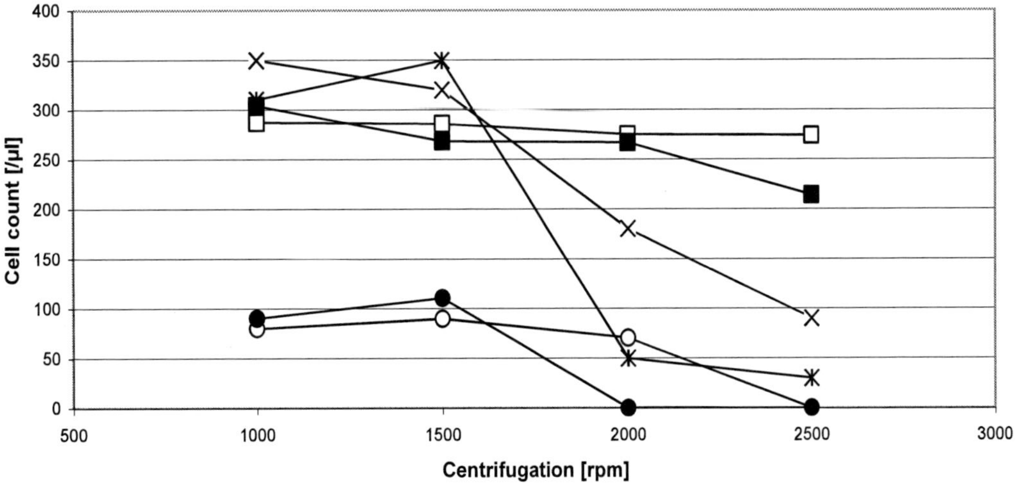

Figure 11. (Continues on next page)

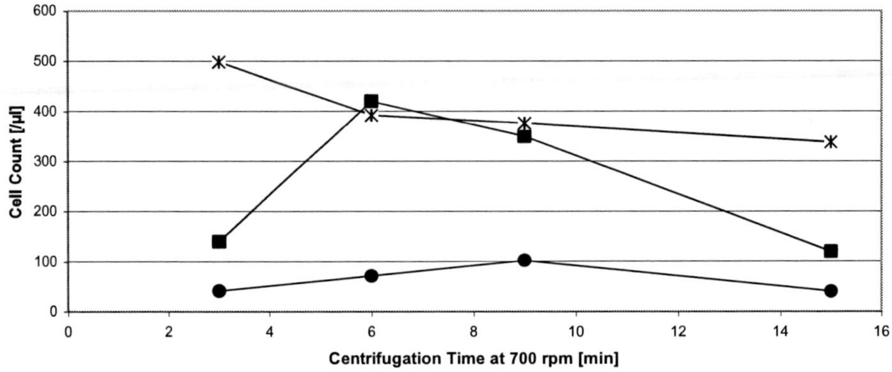

Figure 11. Generation of PMN-rich plasma by blood centrifugation. Pooled citrated blood of n=24 patients was aliquoted into 4 ml aliquots that were centrifuged for 2 or 3 min at 700-2500 rpm. The obtained plasma was analyzed by an automatic hematology analyzer. Leukocytes (WBC; squares), neutrophils (PMN; circles), platelets (crosses); open symbols: 2 min centrifugation time, filled symbols: 3 min centrifugation time (Fig. 11a). The blood aliquots were also centrifuged for 2-15 min at 700 rpm (Fig. 11b). The optimal centrifugation modus for this purpose is 2 min at about 1500 rpm = about 400g. By microscopic analysis, the WBC were to > 95 % PMN.

Fig. 12 shows the lysis of micro-clots of fresh pooled normal plasma by TF-triggered or contact phase-triggered clotting. TF-triggered clotting occurs within 5 min (37°C). Lysis enhancement is optimal by addition of about 0.04 µg G-CSF (about 1.6 µg/ml final conc.). Higher amounts of G-CSF result into a decrease of clot lysis.

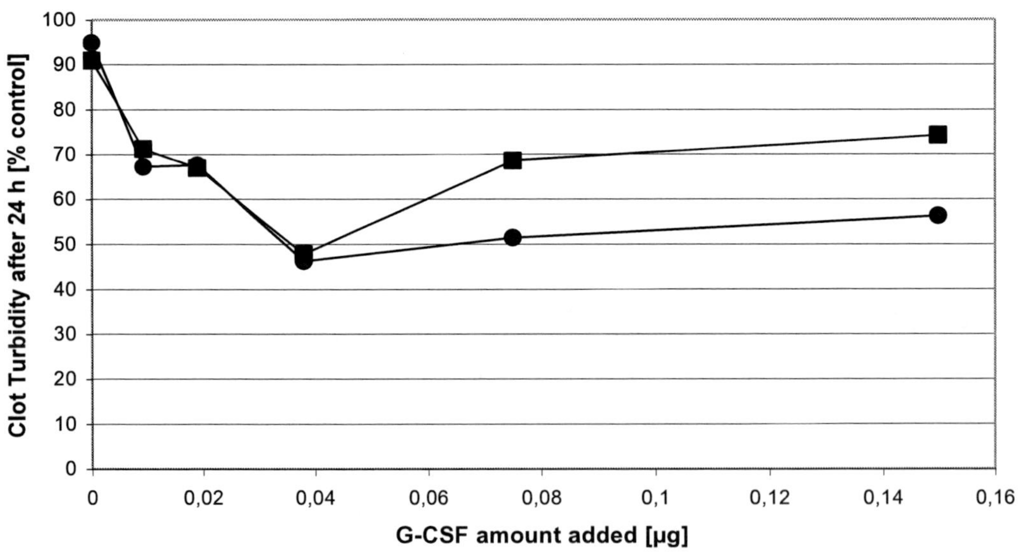

Figure 12. Enhancement of cellular lysis of TF- or contact-phase generated clots by G-CSF. 50 µl pooled normal plasma (4 h RT old) were incubated with 5 µl 10 % Thromborel-S ®, 250 mM $CaCl_2$ (●) or 5 µl Pathromtin-SL®, 250 mM $CaCl_2$ (■) for 40 min (37°C). 20 µl pooled PMN suspension (from n=9 citrated blood samples centrifuged at 1500 rpm for 2 min) were added to the generated micro-clots. 5 µl 0-30 µg/ml G-CSF in 6 % human albumin were added and the turbidity of the wells was determined at 405 nm.

7. Discussion

The present study shows the adaptation of a new assay technique to study plasmatic clot lysis for investigations of cellular clot lysis. PMN are the most important cells in cellular clot lysis. An assay condition that is as similar as possible to the in vivo milieu in blood is the most physiological approach to study PMN-mediated clot lysis. Here micro-clots of plasma were subjected to cellular fibrinolysis. These 50 µl micro-clots were either unoxidized or oxidized by 0.5 µmoles of chloramine. 0.5 µmoles of chloramines / 50 µl means a final chloramine concentration in the range of about 10 mM, which is a chloramine- concentration that can be reached in the microambience of activated PMN [43]. Therefore, the experiment imitates the attack of PMN against unoxidized thrombi, which is of major importance, and it imitates the attack of PMN against already inflamed fibrin rich tissue.

PMN purifications (e.g. by gradient centrifugation) often result into an unphysiologic PMN milieu. Here the buffy coats of citrated blood samples were pooled, centrifuged again, and the pooled buffy coats (without major contamination by erythrocytes) transferred into pooled unfrozen normal citrated plasma, obtaining a diluted buffy coat with about 200-1000 PMN/µl. An easier possibility to obtain PMN-rich plasma might be to centrifuge citrated blood at 400-520g (1500-1700 rpm) for 2 min (23°C). Buffy coat contains PMN, thrombocytes, and other leukocytes; when microscopically checked, PMN-rich plasma, obtained by centrifugation at about 500g, only contains PMN and thrombocytes. Since diluted buffy coat and PMN-rich plasma behaves similarly with respect to lysis of micro-clots, it might be assumed that lymphocytes do not significantly influence cellular fibrinolysis. Slightly activated thrombocytes in citrated plasma might activate PMN, and consequently would act pro-inflammatory and pro-fibrinolytic [41].

There is a plasmatic part and a cellular part of fibrinolysis: more than 50 % of the thrombolytic power of PMN-rich plasma is due to cellular fibrinolysis, less than 50 % is due to plasmatic fibrinolysis [14].

An excellent PMN activator is G-CSF [27]. The approximate ED50 of G-CSF to stimulate PMN mediated clot lysis is 1.5 µg/ml, at about 0.5 µg/ml G-CSF the PMN generate halfmaximal amount of singlet oxygen; these concentrations are 10-100fold the normal plasma concentration, they correspond to the approximate concentration in severe bacterial infections [28]. In the TF-assay version, which is the assay form without interference of artefactual changes of the contact phase of coagulation, about 1.6 µg G-CSF/ml results into the best enhancement of clot lysis. Higher amounts might inhibit respiratory burst or lysis to some extent, similarly as elevated concentrations of glucose: the cells could be over-stimulated, resulting in partial cell auto-destruction. It might be concluded that about 1-5 mg G-CSF given i.v. to a patient of 75 kg could dramatically improve his cellular fibrinolytic capacity.

Cellular fibrinolysis is of selective nature: clot lysis is achieved without total consumption of α2-antiplasmin (plasmin-inhibitor). The PMN generate plasmin that is bound to membrane receptors and protected against α2-antiplasmin and lyses peri-cellular fibrin. PMN are specifically activated by fibrin and do not degrade normal circulating fibrinogen. Thus, the serious bleeding complications of therapeutic plasmatic thrombolysis might not occur, if the PMN are selectively activated without loss of α2-antiplasmin activity. 245 stimulated PMN/µl generate maximally 0.16 mM active chloramines, without change in oxidation-sensible fibrinogen molecules [29]. Only about 5 % of chloramine can be found active in plasma after 3h (37°C) because about 95 % react with methionines and cysteines of plasmatic proteins [30]. The total generation of chloramines by PMN seems to be about 4-20 mM in the cellular microenvironment, which corresponds well to the IC50 values of 2-12 mM methionine measured after 2.5-3.5 d (37°C) in clot lysis assay with PMN rich plasma (PMN-CLA) [14].

245 activated PMN/µl = 4900 activated PMN in 20 µl generated 0.16 mM = 3200 pmoles chloramines = 0.65 pmoles chloramine / single cell, which means that an activated PMN can generate chloramine-concentrations of about 10-20 mM in his cell surrounding, that might be severalfold the PMN diameter. 10000 activated PMN/µl might generate 5-10 mM chloramine.

The different fibrinolytic activities of the PMN seem to be caused primarily by different activation of the oxidative respiratory burst of the cells and not by increased synthesis of u-PA, which is the main plasminogen activator in normal blood and the main plasminogen activator of PMN. The PMN lyse thrombi by synergistic action of singlet oxygen ($^1O_2$) and u-PA. The $^1O_2$ generator chloramine behaves as a PMN-activator.

The IC50 of plasminogen activator inhibitor – 2 (PAI-2; macrophage type PAI) is about 1-2 u-PA inhibiting units (U) / ml [14]. The normal u-PA activity of plasma, after full activation of pro-urokinase, is about 0.6 IU/ml [34]. An u-PA activity of about 1 IU/ml is 50 % inhibited by about 1 U/ml PAI-2, i.e. in the above described experiments of PMN-mediated thrombolysis about 1 IU/ml u-PA is acting. After maximal clot oxidation by about 10-20 mM chloramine, about 1 IU/ml u-PA lyses a micro-clot by about 10 % within about 6h (37°C) [13], i.e. 1 IU/ml u-PA together with maximal amounts of $^1O_2$ can lyse a plasmatic micro-clot by 50 % within 1-2d (37°C).

Many of the substances tested here inhibit cellular clot lysis: of clinical relevance seems to be the inhibition of cellular clot lysis by glucocorticoids [31,32]: hydrocortisone with an IC50 of 3.4 mg/ml is an about 100fold weaker inhibitor of cellular clot lysis than dexamethasone with an IC50 of 0.06 mg/ml, which would be within the normal therapeutic range of dexamethasone; however dexamethasone with its organically bound F-atom stimulates cellular clot lysis at mg/ml concentrations. A similar biphasic effect could be observed for vitamin K, a physiologic quinone, i.e. a potential redoxcycler and thus generator of singlet oxygen [21], the usual therapeutic plasma concentrations are only in the range of about 1 µg/ml. Doxycyclin (usual therapeutic plasma concentrations in the range of about 10 µg/ml), another potential redox cycler, did not substantially improve cellular clot lysis at the concentrations tested. However, these in vitro data on fibrinolysis stimulation might not reflect the in vivo situation, since the liver is a very important cytochrome P450 rich organ, that might metabolize a pro-redox cycler into the real redox-cycler.

The fibrinolysis enhancement by vancomycin might be explained by a vancomycin mediated change in fibrin(ogen) folding that particularly in the case of oxidized fibrin(ogen) activates PMN e.g. by binding to membraneous CD11b/18.

About 5-10 KIU/ml was the measured IC50 of aprotinin, the therapeutic plasma concentrations are in the range of 30-300 KIU/ml [33]. This IC50 is about 5-10fold lower than the approximate IC50 of aprotinin against plasmatic clot lysis by about 350 IU/ml urokinase [45]. Therapeutically, urokinase is given at plasma activities of up to about 35 IU/ml (350 ng/ml) [34], the plasmatic plasmin activities in therapeutic thrombolysis are about 0.1-0.2 U/ml [35].

The omega-amino-carboic acids AMCHA and EACA inhibit cellular clot lysis with IC50s of 0.26 and 1.2 mM, respectively. The usual therapeutic plasma concentration of AMCHA is about 1 mM. Thus, these antifibrinolytics tested might be of clinical interest for patients with hyperactivated phagocytes, e.g. in re-bleeding after subarachnoidal bleeding (i.e. too early lysis of a physiologic micro-thrombus [40]) or multiple sclerosis.

Elevated glucose concentrations inhibit cellular clot lysis: one of the most important PMN enzymes in singlet oxygen biogenesis is the NADPH-oxidase, an enzyme that uses as cofactor NADPH, and phosphorylated glucose is an important donor of hydrogen-atoms. But NADPH might also directly neutralize singlet oxygen. The observed inhibition of cellular clot lysis by glucose might contribute to atherothrombotic complications in diabetes mellitus or to disseminated clotting in sepsis [36]. The normal blood glucose concentration is about 5 mM. Increasing this concentration to about 15 mM during a short time might be of interest to inhibit hyper-activated phagocytes.

All the sulphated glycosaminogylcans tested acted as inhibitors of granulocyte-mediated fibrinolysis [37]. The heparins had IC50s against unoxidized clots that were >10fold above the usual therapeutic concentrations. It seems that the pro-fibrinolytic action of heparins is more due to easier lysis of a clot that has been generated by less thrombin than normal [14,38,39] than due a direct stimulatory action on PMN.

The present date give evidence that PMN infiltration into fibrin [42,43] is a physiologic response to -and not the cause of- pathologic fibrin deposits on endothelium. Unfortunately, coagulation activation is sometimes so dramatically increased that the PMN action against pathologic fibrin results insufficient (frustrane fibrinolysis). The present investigation suggests that it is possible to test individual clot lysis and to modulate cellular fibrinolysis [44,45] to treat diseases caused by hypo- or hyper-activated PMN. Cellular clot lysis might also be enhanced by a physiological PMN activator such as G-CSF to treat thrombosis or atherothrombosis.

References

[1] Collen D, Lijnen HR. The fibrinolytic system in man. *Crit Rev Oncol Hematol.* 1986; 4: 249-301.

[2] Kwaan HC, Astrup T. Demonstration of cellular fibrinolytic activity by the histochemical fibrin slide technique. *Lab Invest.* 1967; 17: 140-5.

[3] Langleben D, Moroz LA. Interspecies variation in the cellular phase of blood fibrinolytic activity. *Proc Soc Exp Biol Med.* 1991; 196: 270-2.

[4] Gonzalez-Gronow M, Stack S, Pizzo SV. Plasmin binding to the plasminogen receptor enhances catalytic efficiency and activates the receptor for subsequent ligand binding. *Arch Biochem Biophys.* 1991; 286: 625-8.

[5] Plow EF, Felez J, Miles LA. Cellular regulation of fibrinolysis. *Thromb Haemost.* 1991; 66: 32-6.

[6] Humphries JE, Vasudevan J, Gonias SL. Fibrinogenolytic and fibrinolytic activity of cell-associated plasmin. *Arterioscler Thro*mb. 1993; 13: 48-55.

[7] Merhi Y, King M, Guidoin R. Acute thrombogenicity of intact and injured natural blood conduits versus synthetic conduits: neutrophil, platelet, and fibrin(ogen) adsorption under various shear-rate conditions. *J Biomed Mater Res* 1997; 34: 477-85.

[8] Stief TW, Fareed J. The antithrombotic factor singlet oxygen/light ($^1O_2$/hv). *Clin Appl Thromb Hemost.* 2000; 6: 22-30.

[9] Dempfle CE, Pfitzner SA, Schott D, Niessen KH, Heene DL. Fibrinogen heterogeneity in homozygous plasminogen deficiency type I: further evidence that plasmin is not involved in formation of LMW- and LMW'-fibrinogen. *Thromb Haemost.* 1997; 77: 879-83.

[10] Stief TW. In vitro - simulation of therapeutic thrombolysis by microtiter plate clot-lysis-assay. *Clin Appl Thromb Hemost* 2006; 12: 21-32.

[11] Hoffman M, Monroe DM. Coagulation 2006: a modern view of hemostasis. *Hematol Oncol Clin North Am* 2007; 21: 1-11.

[12] Gallimore MJ, Harris SL, Tappenden KA, Winter M, Jones DW. Urokinase induced fibrinolysis in thromboelastography: a model for studying fibrinolysis and coagulation in whole blood. *J Thromb Haemost* 2005; 3: 2506-13.

[13] Stief TW. Singlet oxygen potentiates thrombolysis. *Clin Appl Thromb Hemost* 2007; 13: 259-78.

[14] Stief TW, Fröhlich S, Renz H. Determination of the global fibrinolytic state. *Blood Coagul Fibrinolysis* 2007; 18: 479-87.

[15] Loike JD, Sodeik B, Cao L, Leucona S, Weitz JI, Detmers PA, Wright SD, Silverstein SC. CD11c/CD18 on neutrophils recognizes a domain at the N terminus of the A alpha chain of fibrinogen. *Proc Natl Acad Sci USA* 1991; 88: 1044-8.

[16] Ryan TJ, Lai L, Malik AB. Plasmin generation induces neutrophil aggregation: dependence on the catalytic and lysine binding sites. *J Cell Physiol* 1992; 151: 255-61.

[17] Cao D, Mizukami IF, Garni-Wagner BA, Kindzelskii AL, Todd RF 3rd, Boxer LA, Petty HR. Human urokinase-type plasminogen activator primes neutrophils for superoxide anion release. Possible roles of complement receptor type 3 and calcium. *J Immunol* 1995; 154: 1817-29.

[18] Gross TJ, Leavell KJ, Peterson MW. CD11b/CD18 mediates the neutrophil chemotactic activity of fibrin degradation product D domain. *Thromb Haemost* 1997; 77: 894-900.

[19] Moir E, Booth NA, Bennett B, Robbie LA. Polymorphonuclear leucocytes mediate endogenous thrombus lysis via a u-PA-dependent mechanism. *Br J Haematol* 2001; 113: 72-80.

[20] Varma MR, Varga AJ, Knipp BS, Sukheepod P, Upchurch GR, Kunkel SL, Wakefield TW, Henke PK. Neutropenia impairs venous thrombosis resolution in the rat. *J Vasc Surg* 2003; 8:1090-8.

[21] Stief TW. Regulation of Hemostasis by Singlet-Oxygen ($^1\Delta O_2$*). *Curr Vasc Pharmacol* 2004; 2: 357-62.

[22] Stief T. G-CSF enhances cellular fibrinolysis. *Clin Appl Thromb Hemost* 2006; 12: 122.

[23] Stief TW, Schorlemmer HU, Beck-Speier I, Doss MO. PAI-2 inhibits the chemiluminescence of phagocytes and suppresses autoimmunity. *Fibrinolysis & Proteolysis* 1999; 13: 245-51.

[24] Stief TW, Richter A, Bünder R, Maisch B, Renz H. Functional determination of plasmin in arginine-stabilized plasma. *Clin Appl Thromb Hemost* 2005; 11: 303-9.

[25] Witko V, Nguyen AT, Descamps-Latscha B. Microtiter plate assay for phagocyte-derived taurine-chloramines. *J Clin Lab Anal*. 1992; 6: 47-53.

[26] Stief TW. The fibrinogen antigenic turbidimetric assay (FIATA). The $X^2\bar{x}$ test: the corrected chi-square comparison against the control-mean. *Clin Appl Thromb/Hemost* 2007; 13: 73-100.

[27] Kitagawa S, Yuo A, Souza LM, Saito M, Miura Y, Takaku F (1987). Recombinant human granulocyte colony-stimulating factor enhances superoxide release in human granulocytes stimulated by the chemotactic peptide. *Biochem Biophys Res Commun*; 144: 1143-6.

[28] Kawakami M, Tsutsumi H, Kumakawa T, Abe H, Hirai M, Kurosawa S, Mori M, Fukushima M (1990). Levels of serum granulocyte colony – stimulating factor in patients with infections. *Blood*; 76: 1962-4.

[29] Stief TW, Kurz J, Doss MO, Fareed J. Singlet oxygen ($^1O_2$) inactivates fibrinogen, factor V, factor VIII, factor X, and platelet aggregation of human blood. *Thromb Res* 2000; 97: 473-80.

[30] Stief TW. Singlet oxygen inactivates plasmatic protein C. (this issue)

[31] Coleman PL, Barouski PA, Gelehrter TD. The dexamethasone-induced inhibitor of fibrinolytic activity in hepatoma cells. A cellular product which specifically inhibits plasminogen activation. *J Biol Chem*. 1982; 257: 4260-4.

[32] Langleben D, Moroz LA, Schlesinger RD. Cellular-phase fibrinolysis and coronary reperfusion during acute myocardial infarction: a study in patients receiving intravenous streptokinase-methylprednisolone therapy. *Thromb Res*. 1990; 59: 247-58.

[33] Donahue MA, Price PM. Aprotinin: antifibrinolytic and anti-inflammatory mechanisms of action in cardiac surgery with cardiopulmonary bypass. *Dynamics*. 2002; 13:16-23.

[34] Stief TW, Stief MH, Ehrenthal W, Darius H, Martin E. Nonradical oxidants of the phagocyte type induce the activation of plasmatic single chain- urokinase. *Thromb Res* 1991; 64: 597-610.

[35] Stief TW, Richter A, Maisch B, Renz H. Monitoring of Functional Plasminogen in Blood of Patients Receiving Fibrinolytics. *Clin Appl Thromb Hemost* 2007 Dec 26; [Epub ahead of print]

[36] Das, U. N. Current advances in sepsis and septic shock with particular emphasis on the role of insulin. *Med Sci Monit* 9[8], RA181-RA192. 2003.

[37] Dawes J. Interactions of heparins in the vascular environment. *Haemostasis*. 1993;23 Suppl 1:212-9.

[38] Fareed J, Jeske W, Hoppensteadt D, Clarizio R, Walenga JM. Low-molecular-weight heparins: pharmacologic profile and product differentiation. *Am J Cardiol* 1998; 10; 82: 3L-10L.

[39] Wolberg AS. Thrombin generation and fibrin clot structure. *Blood Rev* 2007; 21: 131-42.

[40] Toyoda O, Nakajima H, Nukui H. Changes in coagulation and fibrinolysis and effects of ticlopidine and cisternal drainage in the acute phase following aneurysm rupture. *Neurol Med Chir* (Tokyo) 1990; 30: 670-5.

[41] Kulkarni S, Woollard KJ, Thomas S, Oxley D, Jackson SP. Conversion of platelets from a proaggregatory to a proinflammatory adhesive phenotype: role of PAF in spatially regulating neutrophil adhesion and spreading. *Blood* 2007; 110: 1879-86.

[42] Brown KA, Brain SD, Pearson JD, Edgeworth JD, Lewis SM, Treacher DF. Neutrophils in development of multiple organ failure in sepsis. *Lancet* 2006; 368: 157-69.

[43] Langer F, Spath B, Haubold K, Holstein K, Marx G, Wierecky J, Brümmendorf TH, Dierlamm J, Bokemeyer C, Eifrig B. Tissue factor procoagulant activity of plasma microparticles in patients with cancer-associated disseminated intravascular coagulation. *Ann Hematol* 2008; 87: 451-7.

[44] Weiss SJ. Tissue destruction by neutrophils. *N Engl J Med* 1989; 320: 365-76.

[45] Stief TW. In vitro simulation of thrombolysis inhibition. *Clin Appl Thromb/Hemost* 2008; 14: 234-40.

In: Hemostasis Laboratory Yearbook, Volume 2
Editor: Thomas W. Stief, pp. 101-106

ISBN: 978-1-60741-089-8

ENTRAPMENT OF PLASMA COMPONENTS IN A CLOT

Thomas W. Stief *

[1]Department of Clinical Chemistry, University Hospital Giessen & Marburg, Germany

ABSTRACT

Knowledge of the composition and protein release pattern of human thrombi is of importance to understand hemostasis. 9 ml pooled normal human citrated plasma were recalcified. The generated clots (about 2x10cm) were incubated in duplicate with 41 ml 0.9% NaCl or H_2O. After 0-4d (37°C) the clot supernatants and the unclotted plasma were analyzed for routine clinical-chemical analytes. Plasmin was determined by incubation of 50 µl sample with 100 µl 1.5 M arginine, pH 8.7, and 150 µl 0.93 mM HD-Val-Leu-Lys-pNA, 938 mM KCl. About 50-60 % of all plasma components are initially entrapped in a plasma clot with a large surface. After 1-6 h still about 30-40 % of plasmatic proteins or cholesterol, triglycerides are entrapped in the clot. After 24 h the entrapment is only about 20 %. Active plasmin in the supernatants was < 1 mIU/ml at 0-24h, plasmin activity in the supernatants after 4d was about 5 mIU/ml. The here demonstrated plasma entrapment in a clot within the first 3h (37°C) after clot generation facilitates the study of lysis of blood thrombi, e.g. by replacing radioactive markers by gamma-glutamyl transferase (GGT) or pseudocholine esterase.

Key words: thrombus, fibrin, plasma, coagulation, fibrinolysis, clinical biochemistry

INTRODUCTION

The exact composition of a human thrombus is of interest. The basic matrix of a plasmatic thrombus consists of fibrin, that is generated by thrombin-mediated cleavage of fibrinogen [1]. In contrast to the water-soluble fibrinogen, fibrin precipitates in an aqueous milieu. The aim of the present study was to find out to which degree the plasma components are entrapped in a clot and if they are released to the supernatant in a function of time.

---

* Send correspondance to: T. W. Stief, M.D., Priv.-Doz., Department of Clinical Chemistry, Philipps-University Hospital, D-35043 Marburg, Germany; Tel. +49-6421-5864471; Fax: +49-6421-5865594; Email: thstief@med.uni-marburg.de.

MATERIAL AND METHODS

Normal human plasma clots were prepared, adding in 4fold 90 µl 1563 mM $CaCl_2$ (140.7 µmol Ca^{++}, 281.3 µmol Cl^-) to 9 ml of pooled normal human citrated (1 part 106 mM sodium citrate + 9 parts venous blood, centrifuged for 10 min at 2800g (23°C)) plasma. The final Ca^{++} concentration was about 16 mM. 50 ml H_2O-rinsed polypropylene tubes with the clotting plasma were nearly horizontally positioned (the liquid not reaching the top of the tubes). After 20 min at 37°C the generated snail-like clots (about 2 x 10 cm) were separated carefully from the wall of the 50 ml tubes, using new pipette tips. Expelling of fluid was kept to an absolute minimum. Then, 41 ml of either 155.2 mM (0.9 %) NaCl or H_2O were added in duplicate. The experiment was performed with 0.9 % NaCl or with H_2O as clot supernatant because NaCl is the more physiological ion matrix, but H_2O is more suitable for analysis of certain analytes, e.g. Na^+ or Cl^- ions. At 0 h (within 5 min room temperature), 1 h, 3 h, 6 h, 24 h, and 4 d (37°C) the approximate weights of the clots were determined after careful decanting the supernatant into other H_2O-rinsed 50 ml tubes without expelling clot-water. Then, the supernatants were added again and 1 ml aliquots of the supernatants were withdrawn. These supernatants, the unclotted plasma pool, mouse serum (BALB/c mice; Harlan Winkelmann, Borchen, Germany), and 37°C storage controls consisting of 9 ml + 41 ml 0.9 % NaCl or H_2O stored for 0-4 d were analyzed for Na^+, K^+, Ca^{++}, Mg^{++}, PO_4^{3-}, Cl^-, alcaline phosphatase (AP), gamma-glutamyl transferase (GGT), lactate dehydrogenase (LDH), creatine kinase (CK), pancreas amylase, pseudo-cholinesterase (PCHE), glucose, creatinine, urea, uric acid, cholesterol, triglycerides, albumin, immunoglobulin G (IgG), and total protein in a Hitachi 917 automatic clinical chemistry analyzer (Roche, Basel, Switzerland). Considering a mean haematocrit of 44, the analyte concentrations in pooled citrated plasma (1 volume citrate + 9 volumes blood) have to be multiplied by 1.2 to obtain real in vivo plasma concentrations. The total amounts of each substance in the supernatants were calculated (correcting for the analyte amounts in the previously drawn 1 ml aliquots), expressed in µmol, µg, or mg and compared with that of the 9 ml aliquots of the plasma pool that had been converted into clots. The intention of the present study was to use the same (9+41 ml) approach for the analysis of the plasma parameters.

Creatine kinase and alkaline phosphatase is only stable up to 4d (37°C), glucose is only stable for 1d (37°C). Mouse serum concentrations for albumin and IgG are not valid, because the used monoclonal antibody is of murine origin.

Plasmin was determined by incubation of 50 µl sample with 100 µl 1.5 M arginine, pH 8.7, and 150 µl 0.93 mM HD-Val-Leu-Lys-pNA (Chromogenix, Mölndal, Sweden), 938 mM KCl, at 37°C. The resulting linear absorbance increase/time ($\Delta A/t$) was determined by a microtiter plate reader with a 1 mA resolution (Milenia; DPC, Los Angeles, USA). The standards were 5 µl freshly prepared 1 µg/ml plasmin (Haemochrom, Essen, Germany) in 6 % bovine serum albumin, 25 % glycerol and 5 µl 0.5 U/ml plasmatic plasmin in 0.75 M arginine, pH 8.7, incubated with 100 µl 1.5 M arginine, pH 8.7, 45 µl 0.9 % NaCl and 150 µl chromogenic plasmin substrate; 45 mg/l plasmin = 0.53 µmol/l = 1 U/ml = 4 IU/ml [2].

In a control experiment with high molecular weight plasma proteins 4 x 1 ml aliquots of plasma-pool in 5 ml polystyrol tubes were clotted by addition of 4 x 10 µl 1563 mM $CaCl_2$ and incubation for 20 min (37°C). After clotting, the thrombi were separated from the walls of the vertically positioned tubes (Ø=1 cm). The supernatants were separated from the clots, the weight of the clots was determined, and the supernatants were analyzed for the above analytes and for the high molecular weight proteins α2-macroglobulin, IgM, and ferritin. Patient pool and supernatants were also subjected to agarose gel-electrophoresis (Sebia, Fulda, Germany).

RESULTS AND DISCUSSION

Table 1 demonstrates the concentrations of the analytes in the plasma-pool and in mouse serum and the calculated amounts of each analyte in the plasma clot. Interestingly, there appeared no GGT activity in mouse samples.

Table 1. Clinical chemistry of citrated plasma-pool and mouse-serum.

Analyte	Citr.Plasma-Pool Concentration	Mouse-Serum Concentration	Citr.Plasma-Pool Amount in 9 ml Unclotted Plasma
Na^+	162 mM	149 mM	1458 μmol
K^+	3.3 mM	4.4 mM	29.7 μmol
Ca^{++}	1.8 mM	2.2 mM	16,2 +141 μmol
Mg^{++}	0.7 mM	1.0 mM	6.3 μmol
PO_4^{3-}	0.9 mM	2.0 mM	8,1 μmol
Cl^-	85 mM	110 mM	765 + 281 μmol
Glucose	90 mg/dl	118 mg/dl	8100 μg
Urea	31 mg/dl	64 mg/dl	2790 μg
Uric Acid	3.6 mg/dl	2.4 mg/dl	324 μg
Creatinine	0.88 mg/dl	0.16 mg/dl	79.2 μg
Cholesterol	161 mg/dl	96 mg/dl	14490 μg
Triglycerides	102 mg/dl	138 mg/dl	9180 μg
AP	67 U/l	196 U/l	603 mU
GGT	11 U/l	< 1 U/l	99 mU
LDH	161 U/l	368 U/l	1449 mU
CK	33 U/l	56 U/l	297 mU
Pancreas-Amylase	41 U/l	2620 U/l	369 mU
PCHE	4344 U/l	4616 U/l	39096 mU
Albumin	29 g/l	-	261 mg
IgG	8.2 g/l	-	73.8 mg
Protein	58 g/l	27 g/l	522 mg

Table 2a shows the amounts of the analytes in the NaCl-supernatants of the clots in a function of incubation time at 37°C. Table 2b demonstrates the amounts of the analytes in the H_2O-supernatants of the clots in a function of incubation time at 37°C. Especially the data about Na^+ and Cl^- can be better interpreted with H_2O supernatant. From the data (Table 2a, 2b: 0 h values) it can be concluded that about 50-60 % of all plasma components – even low molecular substances - are initially entrapped in a plasma clot with a large surface, a small volume/surface ratio, and a large surface/liquid contact area (the respective analyte amounts in the supernatants are about 40-50%). After 1-6 h (37°C) still about 30-40 % of plasmatic proteins or hydrophobic agents as cholesterol or triglycerides are entrapped in the clot (the respective analyte amounts in the supernatant are about 60-70 %). After 24 h (37°C) the entrapment decreases to about 20% (analyte amounts in the supernatant ≥ 80 %). Active plasmin conc. in the supernatants or in pooled normal plasma was < 10 ng/ml (< 1 mIU/ml) at 0-24h (37°C). Active plasmin conc. in the supernatants at day 4 was 52 ± 7 ng/ml (about 5 mIU/ml). The concentrations of all low-molecular (<5000 Dalton) analytes (except cholesterol with 92%) in the non-entrapped water (=undiluted supernatants) are ≥ 95% of the analyte concentrations of the unclotted plasma-pool, i.e. the plasmatic matrix of the clot is nearly identical to plasma or serum. The total protein concentration of the supernatant was 89 % of that of the plasma-pool, due to the fibrinogen of plasma that has been converted to fibrin in the clot, and due to some proteins such as α2-macroglobulin, LDH, CK, transferrin, IgG, IgA, or IgM, whose concentration in the supernatant is 90-92 % of the concentration in the plasma-pool. The electrophoresis pattern of the supernatant is identical to that of pooled plasma, except the ß-peak of plasmatic fibrinogen that is absent in the supernatant.

Table 2a. Analyte amounts in % of the total amounts in the supernatants of plasma clots with 0.9 % NaCl supernatant after Δt.

Analyte	0 h	1 h	3 h	6 h	24 h	4 d
Na^+	-	-	-	-	-	-
K^+	60	87	87	88	89	91
Ca^{++}	43	68	71	76	79	80
PO_4^{3-}	56	56	57	57	94	100
Cl^-	-	-	-	-	-	-
Glucose	51	79	80	81	86	-
Urea	65	80	92	93	94	94
Uric Acid	42	63	65	76	78	81
Creatinine	52	67	72	83	85	87
Cholesterol	41	55	60	63	79	90
Triglycerides	49	60	61	62	83	96
AP	45	65	71	72	85	86
GGT	44	61	69	75	85	90
LDH	44	57	60	66	82	86
CK	45	59	60	71	86	90
Pancr-Amyl.	37	60	64	78	80	91
PCHE	45	63	67	72	86	87
Albumin	36	65	65	66	81	83
IgG	49	65	71	72	87	89
Protein	43	59	66	67	74	83
Clot weight	4.88 g	4.32 g	4.08 g	4.04 g	3.84 g	3.43 g

Table 2b. Analyte amounts in % of the total amounts in the supernatants of plasma clots with H_2O supernatant after Δt.

Analyte	0 h	1 h	3 h	6 h	24 h	4 d
Na^+	54	84	87	90	92	93
K^+	43	74	75	76	78	81
Ca^{++}	39	67	65	73	79	82
PO_4^{3-}	56	56	56	66	94	100
Cl^-	67	77	79	82	95	100
Glucose	45	81	81	86	87	-
Urea	62	80	90	91	92	93
Uric Acid	41	68	65	77	80	81
Creatinine	44	73	77	73	74	85
Cholesterol	45	59	64	69	80	83
Triglycerides	45	61	62	67	84	92
AP	43	62	68	75	82	85
GGT	45	65	70	74	88	89
LDH	47	61	67	73	81	88
CK	45	59	60	72	88	89
Pancr-Amyl.	49	63	64	80	89	91
PCHE	46	68	69	77	80	95
Albumin	50	64	64	79	83	86
IgG	47	69	69	74	87	90
Protein	43	63	65	74	82	91
Clot weight	4.69 g	4.49 g	4.28 g	4.48 g	3.89 g	3.36 g

The plasma entrapment demonstrated here in a clot during the first 3h after generation of the clot might be important to study thrombolysis in vitro or in vivo, replacing harmful radioactive markers in animal studies [3,4] by high concentrations of e.g. triglycerides or enzymes such as GGT or PCHE, and measuring the release of them within 6h out of a thrombus. Although cholesterol is well entrapped in the hydrophobic plasma clot, it might not be an ideal marker candidate, since it inhibits singlet oxygen [5], one of the main triggers of granulocyte - mediated fibrinolysis [6,7].

REFERENCES

[1] Weisel JW. Structure of fibrin: impact on clot stability. *J Thromb Haemost* 2007; 5 Suppl 1: 116-24.

[2] Stief TW, Bünder R, Richter A, Maisch B, Renz H, Fareed J. In vitro simulation of therapeutic plasmatic fibrinolysis. *Clin Appl Thrombosis/Hemostasis* 2003; 9: 211-220.

[3] Stief TW, Fareed J. The antithrombotic factor singlet oxygen/light ($^1O_2/h\nu$). *Clin Appl Thrombosis/Hemostasis* 2000; 6: 22-30.

[4] Lijnen HR, Collen D. Fibrinolytic agents: mechanisms of activity and pharmacology. *Thromb Haemost* 1995; 74: 387-90.

[5] Foote CS, Clennan EL. Properties and reactions of singlet oxygen. In: Foote CS, Valentine JS, Greenberg A, Liebman JF, eds. *Active oxygen in chemistry*. London: Blackie Academic and Professional, 1995: 105-41.

[6] Stief TW, Fröhlich S, Renz H. Determination of the global fibrinolytic state. *Blood Coagul Fibrinolysis* 2007; 18: 479-87.

[7] Weiss SJ. Tissue destruction by neutrophils. *N Engl J Med*; 1989: 320, 365-76.

In: Hemostasis Laboratory Yearbook, Volume 2
Editor: Thomas W. Stief, pp. 107-116
ISBN: 978-1-60741-089-8

POLYCATIONS NEUTRALIZE PLASMATIC PAI-1

Thomas W. Stief *

Department of Clinical Chemistry,
University Hospital, Giessen & Marburg, Germany

ABSTRACT

Activated phagocytes are important cells in hemostasis and inflammation. Essential phagocyte mediators are urokinase (u-PA), singlet oxygen ($^1\Delta O_2$), and cationic proteins/polypeptides (polycations). The aim of the present work was to study the interaction of u-PA, $^1O_2$, and polycations with plasmatic fibrinolysis.

0-60 µg poly-L-lysine (PLL; MW=60 kDa) were incubated with 0.5 IU u-PA in 100 µl 100 mM Tris, 25 mM sodium citrate, 63 mM NaCl, 1 % polygelin, 0.1 % Triton X 100®, pH 7.7 (assay buffer) for 0-3 h (37°C). Then 25 µl plasminogen activator inhibitor (PAI)–1 depleted citrated plasma and pooled plasma with 5.7 U (u-PA inhibiting units)/ml PAI–1 or with 5.7 U/ml PAI-2 were added. After 10 min (37°C) the remaining u-PA activity was determined by addition of plasminogen, $^1\Delta O_2$ generating chloramine, and chromogenic plasmin substrate.

The activity of 0.5 IU u-PA preincubated for 3h (37°C) with 25 µg PLL in 100 µl assay buffer was about 40 % higher than that of untreated u-PA. Plasmatic PAI-1 lost function when it was incubated with u-PA/PLL: the approximate 50 % inhibitory concentration (IC50) was 0.2-0.3 mg/ml for PLL of 60 kDa and 3h (37°C) u-PA/PLL preincubation. Polycations neutralize the function of PAI-1 and enhance that of PAI-2 in plasma.

Activated phagocytes release large amounts of polycations (cationic proteins or defensins). Therefore, the interactions between polycations and u-PA and that between polycations and PAI modulate inflammation, enhancing (→PAI-1) or inhibiting (→PAI-2) plasmin generation in the microenvironment of activated phagocytes.

Keywords: Phagocytes, cationic proteins, urokinase, singlet oxygen, PAI-1, plasma, fibrinolysis, inflammation

* Department of Clinical Chemistry, University Hospital, D-35043 Marburg, Germany; Tel. +49-6421-58 64471; Fax + 49-6421-58 65594; Email: thstief@med.uni-marburg.de.

ABBREVIATIONS

PMN, polymorphonuclear neutrophils = granulocytes; MØ, macrophages; PAI, plasminogen activator inhibitor; $^1O_2$, singlet oxygen; PLL, poly-L-lysine; PDL, poly-D-lysine; u-PA, urinary plasminogen activator (u-PA=urokinase); tranexamic acid, trans-4-aminomethyl-cyclohexanecarboxylic acid; Tris, tris-hydroxymethyl-aminomethane; Triton X 100®, t-octylphenoxy-polyethoxyethanol; IU, international units; pNA, para-nitroanilide; ΔA/t, increase in absorbance with time; chloramine T®, N-chloro-p-toluenesulfonamide sodium salt; PF4, platelet factor 4; MW, molecular weight; kDa kilo Dalton, NADPH, reduced nicotineamide-adenine-dinucleotide-phosphate.

INTRODUCTION

Activated phagocytes (granulocytes=polymorphonuclear neutrophils (PMN) or macrophages (MØ)) are important inflammatory cells. The granules of phagocytes contain:

1. myeloperoxidase
2. proteases (e.g. urokinase, elastase, collagenase)
3. cationic proteins/polypeptides
4. lactoferrin
5. membrane proteins (e.g. NADPH-oxidase parts [1] or CD11b/18)

The substances of 1.2.3. might be components of the same granule [2-5]. Phagocytes generate large amounts of cationic proteins/polypeptides, e.g. the macrophage/neutrophil/ eosinophil cationic proteins [6] or the defensins [7-14]. Upon phagocyte activation, many granules are transported to the cell membrane, and their content is released to the surrounding or to the membrane of the cell. NADPH-oxidase and myeloperoxidase generate together reactive oxygen species: first, H_2O_2 is generated that is the origin for

a. radicalic oxidants of the type of hydroxyl-radical (·OH)
b. nonradicalic oxidants of the type of singlet oxygen ($^1\Delta O_2$);

in physiologic (=adequate=defensive) inflammation, $^1\Delta O_2$ might be the predominant oxidant, in pathologic (=excessive=offensive) inflammation, it might be ·OH. H_2O_2 can also be generated by redox-cycling, i.e. reversible repetitive reduction-oxidation-reduction cycles of quinone like molecules [15,16]. The interaction of $^1\Delta O_2$, proteases, and polycations is therefore of eminent physiological importance in inflammation [17]. $^1\Delta O_2$ generating PMN are also the main effectors of cellular fibrinolysis [16]. The aim of the present study was therefore to imitate the interaction of $^1\Delta O_2$, urokinase, and polycations in plasma.

Material and Methods

Human two chain urokinase (u-PA; 80 % high molecular weight form), polygelin, and Berichrom® PAI were from Behringwerke, Marburg, Germany. Poly-L-lysine (MW = 60 kDa or 239 kDa), Poly-D-lysine (190 kDa), Tris (tris(hydroxymethyl) aminomethane), Triton X 100® (t-octylphenoxypolyethoxyethanol), chloramine T® (N-chloro-p-toluene-sulfonamide sodium salt), tranexamic acid (trans-4-(aminomethyl)-cyclohexanecarboxylic acid), polybrene® (hexadimethrine bromide), methionine, and arginine were purchased from Sigma, Deisenhofen, Germany. Plasminogen activator inhibitor (PAI)-2 (unglycosylated) was from Calbiochem-Behring, Frankfurt, Germany. HD-Nva-CHA-Lys-pNA was from Pentapharm, Basel, Switzerland, Glu-plasminogen from Chromogenix, Mölndal, Sweden. PF4 was from Stago, Asnieres, France, protamine from Roche, Basel, Switzerland.

Neutralization of Plasmatic PAI-1 by Poly-L-lysine (PLL)

0.5 IU u-PA were incubated with 0 , 12.5, or 25 µg of PLL (60 kDa) in 100 µl 100 mM Tris, 25 mM sodium citrate, 63 mM NaCl, 1 % polygelin, 0.1 % Triton X 100®, pH 7.7 (assay buffer) for 0–3 h at 37 °C. 25 µl of PAI depleted plasma or of 5.7 units/ml PAI-1 plasma were added, incubated for 10 min (37 °C), and the remaining PAI-1 activity was determined by addition of plasminogen/chloramine/chromogenic plasmin substrate (Berichrom PAI®): 100 µl of 2.78 µM (0.256 g/l) Glu-plasminogen and 100 µl of 8 mmol/l chloramine T®, 3 mM tranexamic acid were added; after 5 min (37 °C), 500 µl 0.6 mM chromogenic plasmin substrate HD-Nva-CHA-Lys-pNA, 480 mM KCl was added and $\Delta A/t$ was measured, using an Eppendorf photometer.

Interaction between Plasmatic PAI-1 or PAI-2 and Urokinase/PLL

0.5 IU urokinase (u-PA) were incubated in duplicate with 0-60 µg poly-L-lysine (PLL) (MW= 60 kDa) in 100 µl assay buffer for 3 h at 37°C. The basal turbidity at 405 nm was measured. Then 25 µl of human plasmas containing 5.7 (u-PA inhibiting) units/ml PAI-1 or 5.7 (u-PA inhibiting) units/ml PAI-2 were added. After an incubation of 10 min at 37°C, the remaining PAI-activity was determined, using the amplifying plasminogen/chloramine/ chromogenic plasmin substrate system.

PLL and Equimolar Concentrations of U-PA / PAI-1

5.7 IU/ml u-PA were preincubated for 3 h (37°C) with 0-0.5 mg/ml PLL (60 kDa) in assay buffer. 50 µl thereof were incubated in duplicate with 50 µl PAI deficient plasma or pooled plasma with 5.7 U/ml PAI-1. After 10 min (37°C) the remaining u-PA activity was determined, using 200 µl plasminogen reagent, 200 µl chloramine-T®, tranexamic acid reagent, and 500 µl chromogenic substrate reagent with 0.6 M KCl.

Various Polycations

25 µg of a) purified human PF4, b) protamine, c) PLL (60 kDa), d) PLL (239 kDa), e) PDL (190 kDa) in assay buffer, f) polybrene®, or g) assay buffer (control) were incubated with 0.5 IU u-PA in 100 µl assay buffer for 3 h (37°C). 25 µl of 0 or 14.4 U/ml PAI-1 plasma were added and incubated for 10 min (37°C). The remaining u-PA activity was determined via addition of plasminogen/chloramine/chromogenic substrate.

Results

Cationic polypeptides/proteins interact with u-PA and neutralize plasmatic PAI-1. After incubating 0.5 IU u-PA with 25 µg PLL for 3 h (37°C), the plasmatic PAI-1 activity decreased to about 40 % of the initial value. Lower concentrations of PLL or decreased incubation times resulted in diminished anti-PAI-1 activity (Fig. 1). PLL concentrations > 0.6 mg/ml resulted in an increase of basal turbidity, i.e. PLL precipitated susceptible plasma proteins. Therefore, the experiments on u-PA/polycations were performed at final polycation concentrations ≤ 0.6 mg/ml. The activity of 0.5 IU u-PA preincubated for 3h (37°C) with 25 µg PLL in 100 µl assay buffer was about 40 % higher than that of untreated u-PA.

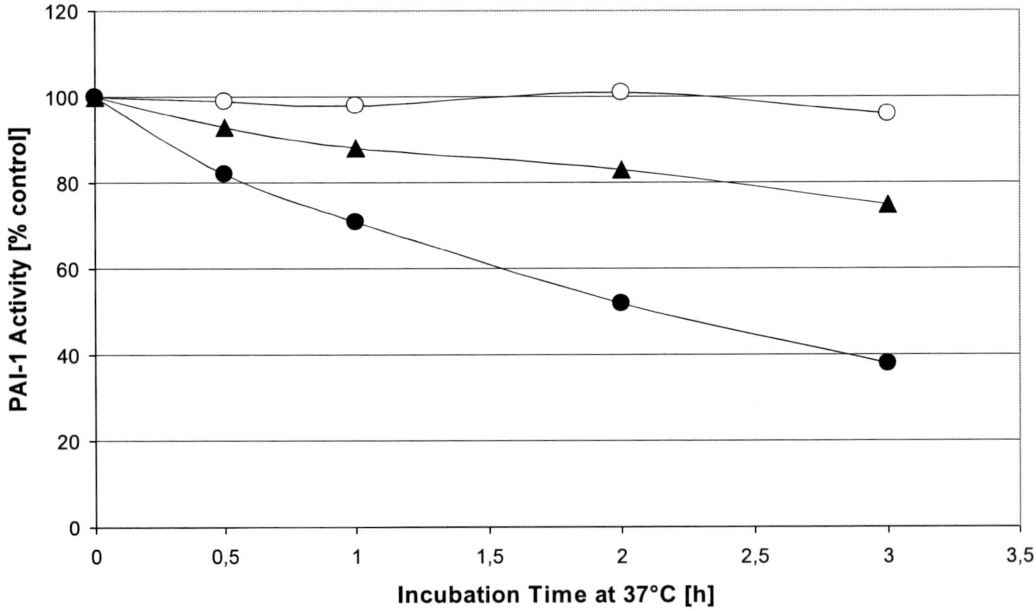

Figure 1. Neutralization of plasmatic PAI-1 by poly-L-lysine (PLL). 0.5 IU u-PA were incubated with 0 µg (O), 12.5 µg (▲), or 25 µg (•) of PLL (60 000 Da) in 100 µl assay buffer for 0–3 h at 37 °C. 25 µl of PAI deficient plasma or of 5.7 units/ml PAI-1 plasma were added, incubated for 10 min (37 °C), and the remaining PAI-1 activity was determined by addition of plasminogen/chloramine/chromogenic plasmin substrate.

Figure 2 demonstrates that the approximate 50 % inhibitory concentration (IC50) of PLL (60 kDa; 3h 37°C preincubated with 5.7 IU/ml u-PA; equimolar concentrations of u-PA and

PAI-1) on plasmatic PAI-1 is 0.3 mg/ml, if relatively smaller amounts of plasma are used, the IC50 is about 0.2 mg/ml (Fig. 3). PAI-2 is not inhibited by polycations, the in this work used low molecular weight PAI-2 is slightly stimulated by polycations (Fig. 3).

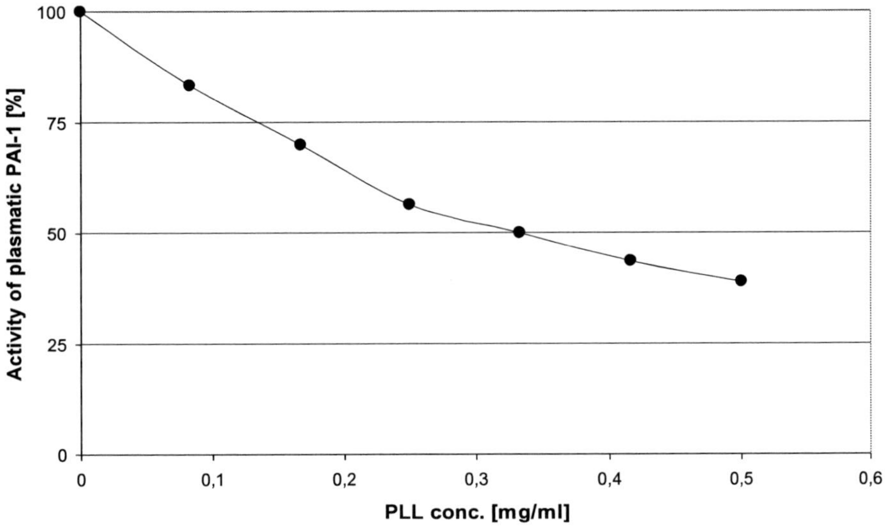

Figure 2. Poly-L-lysine (PLL) and equimolar concentrations of u-PA / PAI-1. 5.7 IU/ml u-PA were preincubated for 3 h (37°C) with 0-0.5 mg/ml PLL (60 kDa) in assay buffer. 50 µl thereof were incubated in duplicate with 50 µl PAI deficient plasma or pooled plasma with 5.7 U/ml PAI-1. After 10 min (37°C) the remaining u-PA activity was determined.

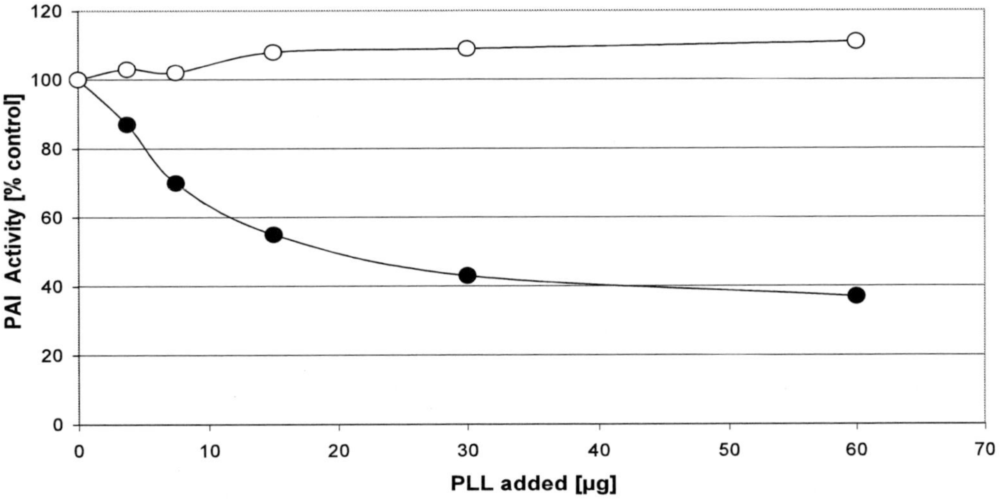

Figure 3. Interaction between plasmatic PAI-1 or PAI-2 and u-PA/PLL. 0.5 IU u-PA were incubated with increaing amounts of poly-L-lysine (PLL; 60 kDa) in 100 µl assay buffer for 3 h (37 °C). 25 µl of plasmas with 5.7 units/ml PAI-1 (•) or with 5.7 units/ml PAI-2 (O) were added. After an incubation period of 10 min (37°C) the remaining PAI activity was determined (100 % control: PAI activity without addition of PLL).

Polylysines of the L or the D configuration of about 200 kDa are more effective than PLL of lower MW: 0.2 mg/ml (final conc.) of PLL (239 kDa) or PDL (190 kDa) decreased the plasmatic PAI-1 activity by about 70 %; PF4, protamine, polybrene®, or PLL (60 kDa) decreased the plasmatic PAI-1 activity by about 60 %.

Discussion

The main control enzymes of fibrinolysis are u-PA and t-PA, that are regulated by PAI [18,54]. Phagocytes are the cells of cellular fibrinolysis. Activated phagocytes release u-PA, oxidants, and cationic proteins/polypeptides that in concert destroy pathogenic material in the surrounding of the activated phagocyte [16,19-25]. The present work demonstrates that polycations neutralize the action of plasmatic PAI-1 via:

A) Modulation of plasmatic PAI-1 stabilizers
B) Interaction with u-PA

While reaction A) is of immediate nature, reaction B) proceeds within hours of incubation at 37°C. Polycations can enhance the activity of plasminogen activators [26,27], the u-PA/polycation interaction might change the folding of the u-PA molecule.

Human PAI-1 binds to stabilizing plasma proteins [28]. The major PAI-1 stabilizer is vitronectin (S-protein of complement) [29]. Vitronectin has a positively charged heparin binding site, that binds the terminal components of the complement pathway [30,31]. Polycationic proteins antagonize this C5b-9/vitronectin interaction and enable the membrane attack complex to act unopposed.

With u-PA and polycations being present in the same granule, the polycations might attach to u-PA molecules, that so become resistant against plasmatic PAI-1. The u-PA/polycations interaction might involve negatively charged structures of the u-PA molecule, e.g. the P3′-P4′ (Glu-Glu) region of the plasmin cleavage site that might be important in u-PA/PAI-1 interaction.

Polycations discriminate between PAI-1 and PAI-2 in plasma. Polycations shift the global plasmatic PAI activity in favour of PAI-2. Polycations stimulate PAI-2 [32]. Normally, functional PAI tests measure only PAI-1 or PAI-1 + PAI-2 [33-36]. Basing on the present data, a rapid functional assay for plasmatic PAI-2 might be developed that imitates the physiologic peri-phagocytic microambiance of inflammation, containing oxidants, proteases, and cationic proteins. These agents interact with each other and enhance the inflammatory response [16,25,31,37-39]. PAI-1 is the endothelial fibrinolysis inhibitor, PAI-2 is of macrophage (and placental) origin, that controls inflammation [40]. In normal pregnancy, PAI-2 increases to > 20 U/ml. A placenta insufficiency results in pathologically decreased blood concentrations of PAI-2 [41]. Since PAI-1, in contrast to PAI-2, is susceptible to inactivation by singlet oxygen [42-44] and polycations, plasmatic PAI-2 might be measured directly, if PAI-1 is inactivated by singlet oxygen and/or polycations.

The assay system used in the present study imitates the oxidative phagocyte attack towards inflamed (=activated) tissue: polycations might selectively neutralize plasmatic PAI-1 and not plasmatic PAI-2. Physiological polycations (e.g. platelet factor 4, phagocyte cationic proteins or defensins) could be of physiological importance in the microenvironment of aggregating platelets or of activated phagocytes. Although the plasma concentration of polycations is low (e.g. PF4 conc. = about 10 ng/ml), in defined micro-areas of inflammation the polycation concentration can increase drastically (e.g. PF4 conc. = about 25 μg/ml [45]). Even polycation concentrations in the range of 10 mg/ml in the micro-ambience of an activated phagocyte might be possible. By generation of oxidants, polycations, and u-PA the activated phagocytes might peri-cellularly destroy pathogens, e.g. bacteria, fungi, or fibrin [17,46].

Macrophages are important defence cells. After destruction of the endothelial barrier, macrophage-derived tissue factor might generate a physiological micro-thrombus that prevents bleeding complications. This micro-clot is digested by the fibrinolytic system, when the damaged endothelium and tissue have been repaired: the macrophages might then switch from pro-thrombinic to pro-plasminic. Especially the latter ones might call for fibrinolysis amplification by activation of PMN [47]. If fibrinolysis starts too early, the patient might suffer from re-bleeding, e.g. into the brain [48]. PMN are far less thrombin generators and far better plasmin / $^{1}\Delta O_2$ generators than MØ that express tissue factor and PAI-2 [49-56].

REFERENCES

[1] Babior BM. NADPH oxidase. *Curr Opin Immunol* 2004; 16: 42-7.

[2] Borregard N. Development of neutrophil granule diversity. *Annals of the New York Academy of Sciences* 1997; 832: 62-68.

[3] Faurschou M, Kamp S, Cowland JB, Udby L, Johnsen AH, Calafat J, Winther H, Borregaard N. Prodefensins are matrix proteins of specific granules in human neutrophils. *J Leukoc Biol* 2005; 78: 785-93.

[4] Moraes TJ, Zurawska JH, Downey GP. Neutrophil granule contents in the pathogenesis of lung injury. *Curr Opin Hematol* 2006; 13: 21-7.

[5] Selsted ME, Ouellette AJ. Defensins in granules of phagocytic and non-phagocytic cells. *Trends Cell Biol* 1995; 5: 114-9.

[6] Sawyer JG, Martin NL, Hancock RE. Interaction of macrophage cationic proteins with the outer membrane of Pseudomonas aeruginosa. *Infect Immun* 1988; 56: 693-8.

[7] Kulinsky VI. Biochemical aspects of inflammation. *Biochemistry* 2007; 72: 595-607.

[8] de Leeuw E, Lu W. Human defensins: turning defense into offense? *Infect Disord Drug Targets* 2007; 7: 67-70.

[9] Pazgier M, Hoover DM, Yang D, Lu W, Lubkowski J. Human beta-defensins. *Cell Mol Life Sci* 2006; 63: 1294-313.

[10] Chen H, Xu Z, Peng L, Fang X, Yin X, Xu N, Cen P. Recent advances in the research and development of human defensins. *Peptides* 2006; 27: 931-40.

[11] Schneider JJ, Unholzer A, Schaller M, Schäfer-Korting M, Korting HC. Human defensins. *J Mol Med* 2005; 83: 587-95.

[12] Duits LA, Ravensbergen B, Rademaker M, Hiemstra PS, Nibbering PH. Expression of beta-defensin 1 and 2 mRNA by human monocytes, macrophages and dendritic cells. *Immunology* 2002; 106: 517-25.

[13] Ryan LK, Rhodes J, Bhat M, Diamond G. Expression of beta-defensin genes in bovine alveolar macrophages. *Infect Immun* 1998; 66: 878-81.
[14] Hiemstra PS, van Furth R. Antimicrobial mechanisms: antimicrobial polypeptides of mononuclear phagocytes. *Immunol Ser* 1994; 60: 197-202.
[15] Afanas'ev IB, Korkina LG, Suslova TB, Soodaeva SK. Are quinones producers or scavengers of superoxide ion in cells? *Arch Biochem Biophys* 1990; 281: 245-50.
[16] Stief TW, Fareed J. The antithrombotic factor singlet oxygen/light ($^1O_2$/hv). *Clin Appl Thromb Hemost* 2000; 6: 22-30.
[17] Henson PM, Johnston RB. Tissue injury in inflammation: oxidants, proteinases, and cationic proteins. *J Clin Invest* 1987; 79: 669-74.
[18] Collen D, Lijnen HR. The fibrinolytic system in man. *Crit Rev Oncol Hematol* 1986; 4: 249-301.
[19] Granelli-Piperano A, Vassalli JD, Reich E. Secretion of plasminogen activator by human polymorphonuclear leukocytes. Modulation by glucocorticoids and other effectors. *J Exp Med* 1977; 146: 1693-1706.
[20] Desrochers PE, Mookhtiar K, Van Wart HE Proteolytic inactivation of alpha 1-proteinase inhibitor and alpha 1-antichymotrypsin by oxidatively activated human neutrophil metalloproteinases. *J Biol Chem* 1992; 267: 5005-12.
[21] Reddy VY, Pizzo SV, Weiss SJ. Functional inactivation and structural disruption of human alpha 2-macroglobulin by neutrophils and eosinophils. *J Biol Chem* 1989; 264: 13801-9.
[22] Weiss SJ, Peppin G, Ortiz X, Ragsdale C, Test ST. Oxidative autoactivation of latent collagenase by human neutrophils. *Science* 1985; 227: 747-9.
[23] Weiss SJ, Curnutte JT, Regiani S. Neutrophil-mediated solubilization of the subendothelial matrix: oxidative and nonoxidative mechanisms of proteolysis used by normal and chronic granulomatous disease phagocytes. *J Immunol* 1986; 136: 636-41.
[24] Weiss SJ, Regiani S. Neutrophils degrade subendothelial matrices in the presence of alpha-1-proteinase inhibitor. Cooperative use of lysosomal proteinases and oxygen metabolites. *J Clin Invest* 1984; 73: 1297-303.
[25] Weiss SJ. Tissue destruction by neutrophils. N Engl J Med 1989; 320: 365-76.
[26] Allen RA. An enhancing effect of poly-lysine on the activation of plasminogen. *Thromb Haemostas* 1982; 47: 41-5.
[27] Dahl R, Venge P. Enhancement of urokinase-induced plasminogen activation by the cationic protein of human eosinophil granulocytes. *Thromb Res* 1979; 14: 599-608.
[28] Chmielewska J, Carlsson T, Urden G, Wiman B. On the relationship between different molecular forms of the fast inhibitor of tissue plasminogen activator. *Fibrinolysis* 1987; 1: 67-73.
[29] Declerck PJ, de Mol M, Alessi MC et al. Purification and characterization of a plasminogen activator inhibitor 1 binding protein from human plasma. Identification as multimeric form of S protein (vitronectin). *J Biol Chem* 1988; 263: 15454-15461.
[30] Jenne D, Stanley KK. Molecular cloning of S-protein, a link between complement, coagulation and cell-substrate adhesion. *EMBO J* 1985; 4: 3153-3157.
[31] Baker PJ, Lint TF, Mc Leod BC, Behrends CL, Gewurz H. Studies on the inhibition of C56-induced lysis (reactive lysis) VI. Modulation of C56- induced lysis by polyanions and polycations. *J Immunol* 1975; 114: 554-558.

[32] Leung KC, Byatt JA, Stephens RW. Poly-D-Lysine dependent inactivation of tissue plasminogen activator by a class PAI-2 inhibitor (minactivin). *Thromb Res* 1987; 46: 767-777.

[33] Chmielewska J, Ranby M, Wiman B. Evidence for a rapid inhibitor to tissue plasminogen activator in plasma. *Thromb Res* 1983;31:427-36.

[34] Nilsson IM, Felding P, Lecander I, Lenner C, Astedt B. Different types of plasminogen activator inhibitors in plasma and platelets in pregnant women. *Br J Haematol* 1986; 62: 215-220.

[35] Kruithof EKO, Tran-Thang C, Gudinchet A, Hauert J, Nicoloso G, Genton C, Welti H, Bachmann F. Fibrinolysis in pregnancy: a study of plasminogen activator inhibitors. *Blood* 1987; 49: 460-466.

[36] Stief TW, Lenz P, Becker U, Heimburger N. Determination of plasminogen activator inhibitor (PAI) capacity of human plasma in presence of oxidants. *Thromb Res* 1988; 50: 559-73.

[37] Rosen H, Klebanoff SJ. Formation of singlet oxygen by the myeloperoxidase-mediated antimicrobial system. *J Biol Chem* 1977;252:4803-10.

[38] Hampton MB, Kettle AJ, Winterbourn CC. Inside the neutrophil phagosome: oxidants, myeloperoxidase, and bacterial killing. *Blood* 1998; 92: 3007-17.

[39] Vogt W. Complement activation by myeloperoxidase products released from stimulated human polymorphonuclear leukocytes. *Immunobiol* 1996; 195: 334-6.

[40] Kinnby B, Matson L, Astedt B. Aggravation of gingival inflammatory symptoms during pregnancy associated with the concentration of plasminogen activator inhibitor type 2 (PAI-2) in gingival fluid. *J Periodontal Res* 1996;31: 271-7.

[41] Kruithof EKO, Tran-Thang C, Gudinchet A, Hauert J, Nicoloso G, Genton C, Welti H, Bachmann F. Fibrinolysis in pregnancy: a study of plasminogen activator inhibitors. *Blood* 1987; 69: 460-6.

[42] Lawrence DA, Loskutoff DJ. Inactivation of plasminogen actvator inhibitor by oxidants. *Biochemistry* 1986; 25: 6351-5.

[43] Stief TW, Martin E, Caso F, Rodriguez JM. Oxidation susceptibility of plasminogen activator inhibitors of human plasma. *Thromb Res* 1990; 60: 177-80.

[44] Baker MS, Green SP, Goss N, Katrantzis M, Doe WF. Plasminogen activator inhibitor 2 (PAI-2) is not inactivated by exposure to oxidants which can be released from activated neutrophils. *Biochem Biophys Res Commun* 1990;166: 993-1000.

[45] Maione TE, Gray GS, Petro J, Hunt AJ, Donner AL, Bauer SI, Carson HF, Sharpe RJ. Inhibition of angiogenesis by recombinant human platelet factor-4 and related peptides. *Science* 1990; 247: 77-79.

[46] Kulkarni S, Woollard KJ, Thomas S, Oxley D, Jackson SP. Conversion of platelets from a proaggregatory to a proinflammatory adhesive phenotype: role of PAF in spatially regulating neutrophil adhesion and spreading. *Blood* 2007; 110: 1879-86.

[47] Daniels RH, Finnen MJ, Hill ME, Lackie JM. Recombinant human monocyte IL-8 primes NADPH-oxidase and phospholipase A_2 activation in human neutrophils. *Immunology* 1992; **75:** 157–163.

[48] Hoff JT, Xi G. Brain edema from intracerebral hemorrhage. *Acta Neurochir Suppl.* 2003; 86: 11-5.

[49] Østerud B. Tissue factor in neutrophils: no. *J Thromb Haemost* 2004; 2: 218-20.

[50] Nathan CF. Secretory products of macrophages. *J Clin Invest* 1987; 79: 319-26.

[51] Test ST, Weiss SJ. Assay of the extracellular hydrogen peroxide pool generated by phagocytes. *Methods Enzymol* 1986; 132: 401-6.

[52] Weiss SJ, Lampert MB, Test ST. Long-lived oxidants generated by human neutrophils: characterization and bioactivity. *Science* 1983; 222: 625-8.

[53] Paul R, Winkler F, Bayerlein I, Popp B, Pfister HW, Koedel U. Urokinase-type plasminogen activator receptor regulates leukocyte recruitment during experimental pneumococcal meningitis. *J Infect Dis* 2005; 191: 776-82.

[54] Stief TW. Singlet oxygen enhances intrinsic thrombolysis: the intrinsic oxidative clot lysis assay (INOXCLA). *Clin Appl Thromb Hemost* 2007; 13: 369-83.

[55] Wygrecka M, Markart P, Ruppert C, Petri K, Preissner KT, Seeger W, Guenther A. Cellular origin of pro-coagulant and (anti)-fibrinolytic factors in bleomycin-injured lungs. *Eur Respir J* 2007; 29: 1105-14.

[56] Nicholl SM, Roztocil E, Davies MG. Plasminogen activator system and vascular disease. *Curr Vasc Pharmacol* 2006; 4: 101-16.

In: Hemostasis Laboratory Yearbook, Volume 2
Editor: Thomas W. Stief, pp. 117-122
ISBN: 978-1-60741-089-8

TISSUE FACTOR IS RESISTANT TO SINGLET OXYGEN

Thomas W. Stief*

Department of Clinical Chemistry, University Hospital, Giessen & Marburg, Germany

ABSTRACT

Tissue factor (TF) triggers extrinsic hemostasis. Monocytes/macrophages (MØ) contain high amounts of pre-TF or TF. Upon MØ activation these cells generate large concentrations of singlet oxygen ($^1\Delta O_2$). The question arises, if TF is resistant against this important oxidant.

150 µl 2.3 ng/ml placental TF in 6 % human albumin, PBS was incubated at 37°C at final chloramineT®-concentrations of 0-20 mM for 10 min. Then 150 µl 258 mM methionine were added. After 15 min (23°C) 30 µl 2.75 M $CaCl_2$ were added. 5 µl of this oxidized 1 ng/ml TF, 239 mM Ca^{++} were incubated with 50 µl unfrozen pooled normal citrated plasma and the extrinsic coagulation activity assay (EXCA) was performed. For control 1, plasmatic fibrinogen was oxidized similarly and the fibrinogen function turbidimetric assay (FIFTA) was performed. For control 2, the FIFTA-reagent (0.3 IU/ml thrombin in 6 % human albumin, PBS) was oxidized similarly and the FIFTA was performed with pooled normal citrated plasma.

1-2 mM chloramine enhance the TF activity by about 40 %. The approximate 50 % inhibitory concentration (IC50) of chloramine-T® against TF is 17 mM, which is comparable to that of thrombin that is resistant to oxidation (IC50=16 mM). Plasmatic fibrinogen is sensible to singlet oxygen: the approximate IC50 of its generator chloramine is 2 mM.

The TF-resistance against $^1\Delta O_2$ might be of importance in inflammatory areas, where MØ might generate both, TF and $^1\Delta O_2$. TF causes coagulation and $^1\Delta O_2$ prevents the generation of fibrin that would limitate the inflammatory focus.

INTRODUCTION

Tissue factor (TF) triggers extrinsic coagulation [1]. Monocytes are the main cells of the blood stream that contain pre-TF or TF, some TF seems to be also in the platelets [2-7]. Monocytes/macrophages (MØ) are important inflammatory cells. Wheras MØ upon activation express high TF amounts [8-10], neutrophil granulocytes do not generate TF [11,12]. Since MØ express membrane bound TF and generate reactive oxygen species, the question arises, if TF is resistant to singlet oxygen ($^1O_2$). The aim of the present study was to

* Send correspondance to: Department of Clinical Chemistry, University Hospital, D-35043 Marburg, Germany; Tel. +49-6421-58 64471; Fax + 49-6421-58 65594; Email: thstief@med.uni-marburg.de

compare the 50 % inhibitory concentrations (IC50) of chloramine (which is an important in vivo generator of $^1O_2$) against TF with that of fibrinogen and thrombin, known $^1O_2$ sensible and resistant hemostasis factors, respectively.

Material and Methods

Tissue Factor and Singlet Oxygen

150 µl 2.3 ng/ml tissue factor (TF; placental Thromborel S®, Behringwerke, Marburg, Germany; one with 10 ml reconstituted vial contains 160 ng/ml TF, as assayed by the TF enzyme immuno assay from American Diagnostica, Greenwich, USA) in 6 % human albumin (Kabi, Stockholm, Sweden) with phosphate buffered saline (PBS) was incubated at 37°C with 15 µl 0-220 mM chloramine-T® (Sigma, Deisenhofen, Germany) in 0.9 % NaCl, obtaining final chloramine-concentrations of 0-20 mM, in U-well microtiter plates (Greiner, Frickenhausen, Germany; article nr. 650161, lot nr. 05281161). After 10 min, 150 µl 258 mM methionine (Sigma) were added. After 15 min (23°C), 30 µl 2.75 M $CaCl_2$ were added. 5 µl portions of this oxidized 1 ng/ml TF, 239 mM Ca^{++} were withdrawn and pipetted into U-wells, using 0.9 % NaCl-rinsed new tips of an Eppendorf-multipette®. 50 µl unfrozen pooled normal plasma were added in duplicate and the extrinsic coagulation activity assay (EXCA) was performed [13,25]: after 1 min (37°C) coagulation reaction time (CRT), 50 µl 2.5 M arginine, pH 8.6, 0.16 % Triton X 100® were added. After 3 min (23°C), 25 µl 1 mM HD-CHG-Ala-Arg-pNA in 1.25 M arginine, pH 8.7, were added and $\Delta A_{405\ nm}/t$ (23°C) was determined by a microtiter plate photometer with a 1 mA resolution (Milenia, DPC, Los Angeles, USA). The standard was 1 IU/ml bovine thrombin (DadeBehring) in 6.7 % human albumin.

For $^1O_2$ – sensible-hemostasis-factor-control plasmatic fibrinogen was chosen: 50 µl pooled normal plasma were oxidized with 5 µl 0-220 mM chloramine-T® in 0.9 % NaCl for 10 min (37°C). 50 µl 258 mM methionine were added. After 15 min (23°C), 50 µl 0.3 IU/ml thrombin in 6 % human albumin, PBS were added in duplicate, and ΔA/t (13 min 23°C) was measured (modified fibrinogen function turbidimetric assay (FIFTA) [14].

For $^1O_2$ – resistant-hemostasis-factor-control thrombin was chosen: 100 µl FIFTA-reagent with 0.3 IU/ml thrombin in 6 % human albumin, PBS were oxidized with 10 µl 0-220 mM chloramine-T® for 10 min (37°C). 100 µl 258 mM methionine were added. After 15 min (23°C), 50 µl pooled normal plasma were added in duplicate, and ΔA/t (13 min 23°C) was determined.

EXCA-trigger and Singlet Oxygen

5 µl EXCA-trigger (1 ng/ml TF in 6 % human albumin, PBS, 250 mM $CaCl_2$) were incubated in triplicate with 5 µl 0-20 mM chloramine-T®, 0.9 % NaCl in U-well microtiter plates for 10 min (37°C). 5 µl 230 mM methionine were added. After 15 min (23°C), 50 µl unfrozen pooled normal citrated plasma or citrated plasma of two healthy donors were added and the EXCA was performed.

RESULTS AND DISCUSSION

Figure 1 demonstrates that final chloramine concentrations of 1-2 mM enhance the TF activity by about 40 %. The approximate IC50 of chloramine-T® against TF is 17 mM. This corresponds well to the approximate IC50 of chloramine against thrombin, which is 16 mM (Fig. 1). There is some 20 % increase in thrombin activity by about 4 mM chloramine. Fibrinogen behaves as sensible to singlet oxygen: its approximate IC50 is 2 mM chloramine (Fig. 1).

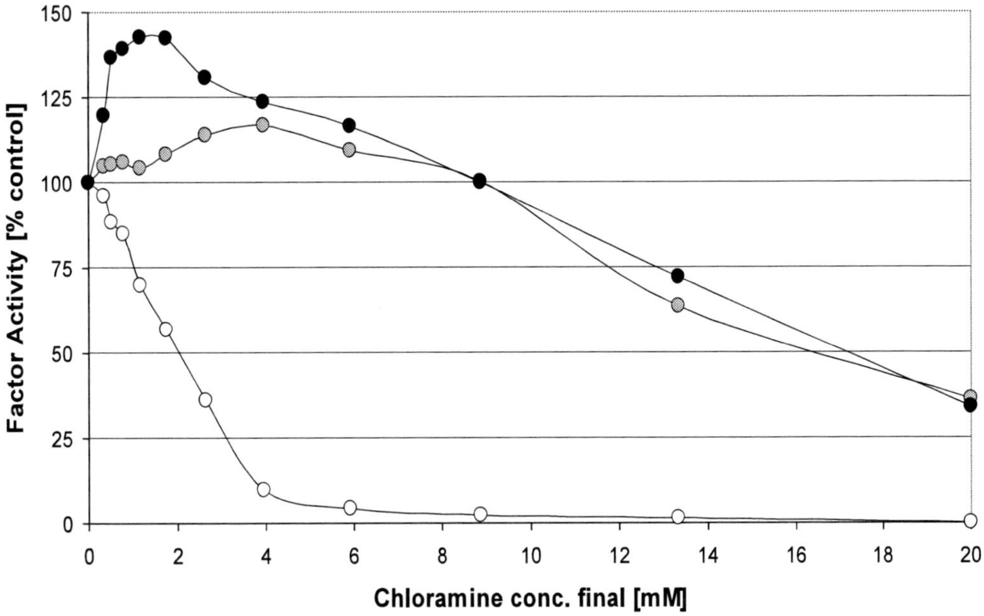

Figure 1. Tissue factor (TF) and singlet oxygen ($^1O_2$). 150 µl 2.3 ng/ml TF in 6 % human albumin, PBS was incubated at 37°C at final chloramine-T® concentrations of 0-20 mM. After 10 min, 150 µl 258 mM methionine were added. After 15 min (23°C), 30 µl 2.75 M $CaCl_2$ were added. With 5 µl of this oxidized 1 ng/ml TF, 239 mM Ca^{++} (●) and 50 µl pooled normal plasma the extrinsic coagulation activity assay (EXCA) was performed; 100 % control = thrombin generation of 0.5 IU/ml. For control 1, plasmatic fibrinogen (O) in 50 µl samples of pooled normal plasma was similarly oxidized and a modified fibrinogen function turbidimetric assay (FIFTA) was performed with 50 µl FIFTA-reagent; 100 % = 93 mA. For control 2, thrombin (greyO) in the 100 µl FIFTA reagent was similarly oxidized and a modified FIFTA was performed with 50 µl pooled normal plasma; 100 % = 185 mA.

If TF is not oxidized in a physiologic matrix but 1+1 diluted in presence of 125 mM final concentration Ca^{++}, the approximate 50 % inhibitory amount of chloramine decreases about 3fold (Fig. 2).

Singlet oxygen modulates hemostasis: its action is anti-thrombotic and pro-fibrinolytic [15-17]. Some hemostasis factors are especially sensible to singlet oxygen: thrombocytes, fibrinogen, factors V, VIII, X, and plasmin-inhibitor have IC50 values of about 1-2 mM chloramine. Other hemostasis factors are resistant to oxidation, eg. factors II, VII, IX [18].

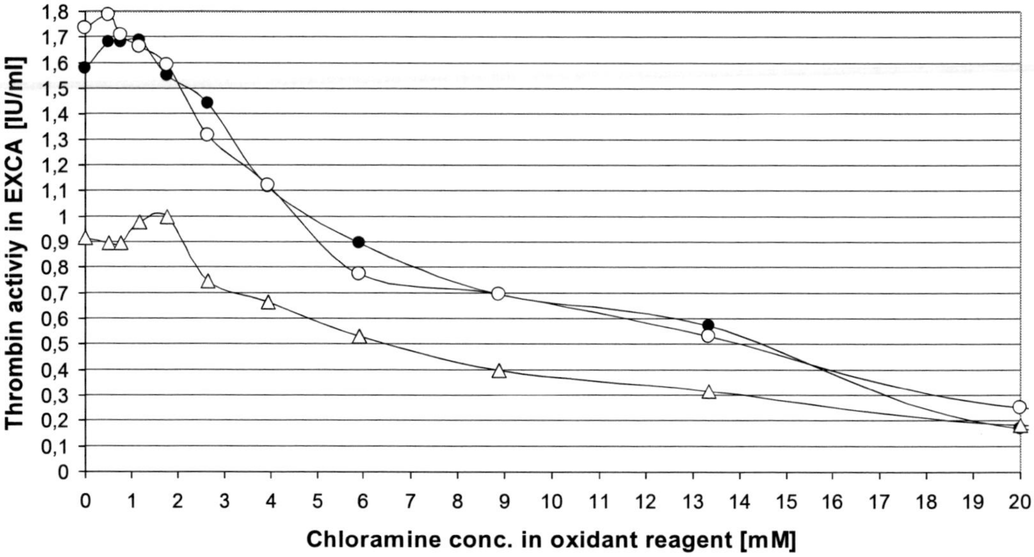

Figure 2. EXCA-trigger and $^1O_2$. 5 µl EXCA-trigger (1 ng/ml TF in 6 % human albumin, PBS, 250 mM $CaCl_2$) were incubated with 5 µl 0-20 mM chloramine-T®, 0.9 % NaCl in U-well microtiter plates for 10 min (37°C). 5 µl 230 mM methionine were added. After 5 min (23°C), 50 µl pooled normal plasma (●) or plasma of two healthy donors (O,Δ) were added. The EXCA was performed: after 1 min (37°C), 50 µl 2.5 M arginine, pH 8.6, 0.16 % Triton X 100® were added. After 3 min (23°C), 25 µl 1 mM HD-CHG-Ala-Arg-pNA in 1.25 M arginine, pH 8.7, were added and $\Delta A_{405\ nm}/t$ (23°C) was determined.

The present work demonstrates that also TF is $^1O_2$ resistant. Low $^1O_2$ concentrations even stimulate the TF activity by about 40 %. Oxidative activation of TF has already been described [19-21], singlet oxygen might oxidize critical methionine or cysteine residues of the protein [22]. With TF being $^1O_2$ resistant and fibrinogen being $^1O_2$ sensible, thrombin generated in the micro-ambience of activated MØ does not act as a clotting enzyme. Instead, thrombin might be modulated in a pro-fibrinolytic [23] or in a pro-inflammatory sense [24]. Ultra-specific, ultra-sensitive thrombin generation assays help to diagnose the true hemostasis state of the individual patient [25].

References

[1] Houston DS. Tissue factor - a therapeutic target for thrombotic disorders. *Expert Opin Ther Targets* 2002; 6: 159-74.

[2] Nojima J, Masuda Y, Iwatani Y, Suehisa E, Futsukaichi Y, Kuratsune H, Watanabe Y, Takano T, Hidaka Y, Kanakura Y. Tissue factor expression on monocytes induced by anti-phospholipid antibodies as a strong risk factor for thromboembolic complications in SLE patients. *Biochem Biophys Res Commun* 2008; 365: 195-200.

[3] Panasiuk A, Zak J, Panasiuk B, Prokopowicz D. Increase in expression of monocytic tissue factor (CD142) with monocytes and blood platelet activation in liver cirrhosis. *Blood Coagul Fibrinolysis* 2007; 18: 739-44.

[4] Sovershaev MA, Egorina EM, Gruber FX, Olsen JO, Osterud B. High tissue factor-expressing human monocytes carry low surface CD36: application to intersubject variability. *J Thromb Haemost* 2007; 5: 2453-60.

[5] Sakamoto T, Ishibashi T, Maruyama Y. Role of Ca^{2+} influx in tissue factor expression in monocyte adhesion to endothelial cells. *J Atheroscler Thromb* 2007; 14: 109-15.

[6] Recalde H, Miranda GR. A method of analyzing procoagulant activity in monocytes at single cell level. *Haematologica* 2003; 88: 44-53.

[7] Siddiqui FA, Desai H, Amirkhosravi A, Amaya M, Francis JL. The presence and release of tissue factor from human platelets. *Platelets* 2002; 13: 247-53.

[8] Geisbert TW, Young HA, Jahrling PB, Davis KJ, Kagan E, Hensley LE. Mechanisms underlying coagulation abnormalities in ebola hemorrhagic fever: overexpression of tissue factor in primate monocytes/macrophages is a key event. *J Infect Dis* 2003; 188: 1618-29.

[9] Bouwman JJ, Visseren FL, Bosch MC, Bouter KP, Diepersloot RJ. Procoagulant and inflammatory response of virus-infected monocytes. *Eur J Clin Invest* 2002; 32: 759-66.

[10] Meisel SR, Xu XP, Edgington TS, Dimayuga P, Kaul S, Lee S, Fishbein MC, Cercek B, Shah PK. Differentiation of adherent human monocytes into macrophages markedly enhances tissue factor protein expression and procoagulant activity. *Atherosclerosis* 2002; 161: 35-43.

[11] Østerud B, Rao LVM, Olsen JO. Induction of tissue factor expression in whole blood: lack of evidence for the presence of tissue factor expression in granulocytes. *Thromb Haemostas* 2000; 83: 861-7.

[12] Østerud B. Tissue factor in neutrophils: no. *J Thromb Haemost* 2004; 2: 218-20.

[13] Stief TW. The efficiency of anti-activated factor X and anti-activated factor II anticoagulants. *Blood Coagul Fibrinolysis* 2007; 18: 265-9.

[14] Stief TW. The fibrinogen functional turbidimetric assay. *Clin Appl Thromb Hemost.* 2008; 14: 84-96.

[15] Stief TW, Fareed J. The antithrombotic factor singlet oxygen/light ($^1O_2$/hv). *Clin Appl Thromb Hemost* 2000; 6: 22-30.

[16] Stief TW. The blood fibrinolysis/deep-sea analogy: a hypothesis on the cell signals singlet oxygen/photons as natural antithrombotics. *Thromb Res* 2000; 99: 1-20.

[17] Stief TW. Regulation of hemostasis by singlet-oxygen ($^1\Delta O_2$*). *Curr Vasc Pharmacol* 2004; 2: 357-62.

[18] Stief TW, Kurz J, Doss M, Fareed J. Singlet oxygen inactivates fibrinogen, factor V, factor VIII, factor X, and platelet aggregation of human blood. *Thromb Res* 2000; 97: 473-80.

[19] Reinhardt C, von Brühl ML, Manukyan D, Grahl L, Lorenz M, Altmann B, Dlugai S, Hess S, Konrad I, Orschiedt L, Mackman N, Ruddock L, Massberg S, Engelmann B. Protein disulfide isomerase acts as an injury response signal that enhances fibrin generation via tissue factor activation. *J Clin Invest* 2008 Feb 14; [Epub ahead of print]

[20] Versteeg HH, Ruf W. Tissue factor coagulant function is enhanced by protein-disulfide isomerase independent of oxidoreductase activity. *J Biol Chem* 2007; 282: 25416-24.

[21] Chen VM, Ahamed J, Versteeg HH, Berndt MC, Ruf W, Hogg PJ. Evidence for activation of tissue factor by an allosteric disulfide bond. *Biochemistry* 2006; 45: 12020-8.

[22] Shechter Y, Burstein Y, Patchornik A. Selective oxidation of methionine residues in proteins. *Biochemistry* 1975; 14: 4497-503.

[23] Stief TW, Kretschmer V, Kosche B, Doss MO, Renz H. Thrombin converts singlet oxygen ($^1O_2$) - oxidized fibrinogen into a soluble t-PA cofactor. *Ann Hematol* 2001; 80: 189-94.

[24] Bokarewa MI, Morrissey JH, Tarkowski A. Tissue factor as a proinflammatory agent. *Arthritis Res* 2002; 4: 190-5.

[25] Stief TW. Innovative tests of plasmatic hemostasis. *Laboratory Medicine* 2008; 39: 225-30.

In: Hemostasis Laboratory Yearbook, Volume 2
Editor: Thomas W. Stief, pp. 123-131
ISBN: 978-1-60741-089-8

SINGLET OXYGEN INACTIVATES PLASMATIC PROTEIN C

Thomas W. Stief*
Department of Clinical Chemistry; University Hospital Giessen & Marburg, Germany

ABSTRACT

Activated granulocytes respond to foci of inflammation or of fibrin with the generation of millimolar concentrations of chloramines that are generators of nonradical singlet oxygen ($^1\Delta O_2$). Protein C and antithrombin are the main down-regulators of plasmatic thrombin activity. Here the interaction between chloramines and these important coagulation regulators was investigated.

Pooled normal human citrated plasma (pH 7.4) was oxidized with the nonradicalic oxidant chloramine-T® for 20 min at 37°C. Then the activities of protein C and antithrombin were chromogenically tested. For control, also plasmin inhibitor was functionally determined and the global plasmatic fibrinolysis parameters assay (FIPA) was performed. Oxidative inactivation of protein C at pH 7.4 by 1.5 mM chloramine-T® is quenched by 21 mM of the $^1\Delta O_2$ - inhibitor methionine and is not affected by 21 mM or 75 mM of the hydroxyl radical (·OH)- inhibitor mannitol. Chloramine-consumption in plasma was tested by supplementation of citrated plasma with chloramine-T®. Remaining chloramine was photometrically determined at 405 nm after addition of 200 µl 4 M KI in phosphate buffered saline (PBS) to 20 µl oxidized plasma.

The approximate inhibitory concentrations 50% (IC50) of chloramine-T® against protein C, antithrombin, or plasmin-inhibitor were 2 mM, 3 mM, or 1.5 mM, respectively; 1.5 mM chloramine enhanced FIPA by 50 %. Chloramines might inactivate $^1\Delta O_2$-susceptible hemostasis factors via oxidation of critical methionines or cysteines. About 1 mM chloramine had a plasma half life of less than 1 minute. $^1\Delta O_2$ generators down-regulate the inhibition of coagulation and of fibrinolysis and possibly facilitate inflammation.

Key words: Singlet oxygen, chloramines, protein c, hemostasis

* Send correspondence to: PD Dr. med. T. Stief, Department of Clinical Chemistry, University Hospital, D-35043 Marburg, Germany; Email: thstief@med.uni-marburg.de; Tel. +49-6421-5864471; FAX: +49-6421-5865594

INTRODUCTION

Activated polymorphonuclear neutrophils (PMN) are important cells of inflammation. Activated PMN can generate high concentrations (1-10 mM) of nonradical oxidants of the chloramine-type, that are generators of singlet molecular oxygen ($^1O_2$) [1-3]. Since PMN - oxidants can alter hemostasis (coagulation + fibrinolysis) [4-9], here the modulatory action of $^1O_2$ on protein C and antithrombin, important down-regulators of hemostasis, was investigated.

MATERIAL AND METHODS

Plasma Oxidation

1 ml unfrozen pooled normal citrated plasma or 6 % phosphate buffered human albumin (HA; Kabi, Stockholm, Sweden) was incubated for 20 min (37°C) with 100 µl 0-114 mM N-chloro-p-toluenesulfonamide (chloramine-T® trihydrate sodium salt; CT; MW=282; Sigma, Deisenhofen, Germany) in 0.9 % NaCl, resulting in final concentrations (conc.) of 0-10.4 mM CT.

Oxidative Inactivation of Plasmatic Protein C

2 µl pre-oxidized plasma or albumin were incubated in duplicate with 20 µl Protac® (extract of the venom of Agkistrodon contortix) in 25 mM HEPES, pH 8.25, 2.5 g/l polyethylene glycol, 30 mM (5 g/l) CsCl (Berichrom Protein C; DadeBehring, Marburg, Germany; Cs^+ ions are chaotropic: they inhibit unspecific protein-protein interactions) for 5 min (37°C) in polystyrol microtiter plates with round bottomed wells (U-wells; Nunc, Wiesbaden, Germany). 10 µl 2.5 M (final 676 mM) arginine, pH 8.6 (Sigma) and 5 µl 2.4 mM (final 0.65 mM) chromogenic substrate for activated protein C pyro-Glu-Pro-Arg-methoxynitroanilide were added and the linear ΔA/t (23°C) was measured with a microtiter plate photometer with a 1 mA resolution (Milenia; DPC, Los Angeles, USA).

Oxidative Inactivation of Plasmatic Antithrombin

The antithrombin activity was determined in duplicate as follows: the thrombin reagent was prepared by dissolving 130 IU lyophilized bovine thrombin (DadeBehring, Marburg, Germany, article nr. B4233-25) in 0.25 ml 6 % human albumin; after 3 min (23°C) 0.5 ml 20 % human albumin (BAXTER, Vienna, Austria) and 1.5 ml 2.4 M arginine, pH 7.4, (Sigma) were added; the dissolved thrombin was then given into a heparin-monovette (Sarstedt, Nümbrecht, Germany) containing 4.9*25 =122.5 IU heparin. In the AT3/thrombin reaction phase 20 µl pre-oxidized plasma or albumin, and standards (100 % of the norm pooled plasma and this plasma diluted with 0.9 % NaCl) were incubated with 4 µl thrombin reagent = 58 IU/ml (final 9.6 IU/ml) thrombin, 6 % human albumin, 54.4 IU/ml (9.1 IU/ml final) unfractionated heparin, 1600 mM (267 mM final) arginine, pH 7.4 for 30s (23°C) in microtiter plates with flat bottom (F-wells). 100 µl 2.5 M arginine, pH 8.6, 0.124 % Triton X 100® (Sigma) were added. After 3 min (23°C) the thrombin detection phase started with addition of 25 µl 1 mM (0.17 mM final) chromogenic thrombin substrate HD-CHG-Ala-Arg-pNA (Pentapharm, Basel, Switzerland) in 1.25 M (1.89 M final) arginine, pH 8.7. ΔA/t at 405 nm was determined. The normal range (MV±1SD) of functional AT3 is 100±15 %. Thrombin activity added to oxidized human albumin did not change significantly.

Oxidative Inactivation of Plasmatic Plasmin Inhibitor (PI)

2 µl pre-oxidized plasma or albumin and 0.9 % NaCl were incubated in duplicate in the PI/plasmin reaction phase with 50 µl 0.1 CTA-U (about 2.5 µg)/ml plasmin, 25 % glycerol, 0.9 g/l NaCl, 100 mM KH_2PO_4, pH 7.5 for 1 min (37°C) in U-wells. In the plasmin-detection phase 100 µl 2.5 M (1.54 M final) arginine, pH 8.6, 0.152 % Triton X 100® and 10 µl 3 mM (0.19 mM final) HD-NVA-CHA-Lys-pNA in H_2O were added, the plate was intensely shaked, and the linear ΔA/t at 405 nm was measured. The normal range is 100±20 % (MV±1SD). The activity of plasmin when added to oxidized 6% human albumin did not change significantly.

Oxidative Activation of Plasmatic Fibrinolysis

The global fibrinolysis test FIPA (=fibrinolysis parameters assay [10,11]) was performed in duplicate with 40 µl pre-oxidized samples that were incubated with 4 µl 100 IU/ml urokinase (medac, Hamburg, Germany), 6 mM tranexamic acid (Bayer, Leverkusen, Germany), 6 % human albumin (urokinsae-reagent) in U-wells for 10 min (FIPA-10) or for 30 min (FIPA-30) fibrinolysis reaction time (FRT) at 37°C. 100 µl 2.5 M arginine, pH 8.6, 0.144 % Triton X 100® and 25 µl 1.5 mM (0.22 mM final) Val-Leu-Lys-pNA (Chromogenix, Mölndal, Sweden) in 1.5 M (1.49 M final) arginine, pH 8.7, 1.5 M KCl (plasmin substrate - reagent) were added, the plate was intensely shaked, and the increase in absorbance with time (ΔA/t) was measured. 100 % of normal FIPA-10 results into a ΔA/t value of about 100 mA/h RT, FIPA-30 ΔA/t values are about twice that of FIPA-10; the maximal ΔA is about 1400 mA, the ΔA range is nearly linear within 0 - 40 % of the maximal ΔA.

Chloramine Inhibition by Methionine

To show that physiologic concentrations of chloramines under physiologic conditions in plasma (pH about 7.4) act as generators of nonradicalic $^1O_2$ and not of oxygen radicals, pooled normal citrated plasma supplemented with 21 mM methionine (a quencher of $^1O_2$; Sigma), with 21 mM or 75 mM mannitol (a quencher of hydroxyl radicals; Sigma), with 21 mM alanine (control: an amino acid without oxidizable sulphur; Sigma), or unsupplemented was oxidized at 0 or 1.5 mM chloramine-T® (20 min 37°C). Then the protein C function was determined 24fold.

Consumption of Chloramines in Plasma

900 µl pooled unfrozen normal citrated plasma were supplemented with 100 µl 0-200 mM chloramine-T® (CT) in 0.9 % NaCl. After 0.5–72 h (37°C) 20 µl plasma samples or chloramine standards (0-5 mM CT in 0.9 % NaCl) were incubated in duplicate in flat bottom wells (F-wells; Nunc) with 200 µl 4 M KI in PBS and the ΔA at 405 nm was determined by a microtiterplate photometer. To measure consumption of chloramines (R-N-Cl) within the first 30 min reaction time, 20 µl samples of citrated plasma were incubated in duplicate with 2 µl 10 mM CT or 100 mM CT in 0.9 % NaCl for 1-32 min (37°C or 23°C). Then 200 µl 4 M KI in PBS were added and ΔA_{405nm} was immediately determined. For matrix control, 20 µl pooled plasma were added to 200 µl 4 M KI in PBS that had been reacted with 2 µl 10 mM CT and A_{405nm} was immediately determined. The present KI-assay for R-N-Cl has been derived from the test of taurine-chloramine that has been previously described [12]. In the present R-N-Cl test there appears a strictly linear ΔA response to the chloramine concentration in the standards, 1 mM chloramine resulting in a ΔA_{405nm} of about 500 mA. The abbreviation R-N-Cl stands for R-NH-Cl or R=N-Cl.

Statistics

The intra- and inter- assay coefficients of variation (CV) were calculated: CV = SD/MV * 100 %. The chromogenic assays had CV values < 5 %. The obtained values of oxidized plasma samples were compared with the control values of normal plasma supplemented with 0.9 % NaCl instead of chloramine in 0.9 % NaCl. All tests were performed in duplicate, the critical values in the $^1O_2$ quenching experiment were tested for significance ($p < 0.05$) by two-fold Yates-corrected chi-square comparison of the 24fold measured assay results against the control-mean ($X^2\bar{x}$ test): the chi-squared mean value test transforms non-categorical results that are quantitative into categorical results that are qualitative (to be or not to be above $\bar{x}$), and compares them by the X^2 test after 2fold Yates-correction of the 4fields-table (adding or subtracting 2*0.5 = 1 to the numbers of the 4fields-table towards insignificance), the $p < 0.05$ limit at $X^2 = 3.841$, the $p < 0.01$ limit at $X^2 = 6.635$ [13].

Results and Discussion

Activated protein C (PCa) inactivates factor Va and VIIIa, the most important accelerators of blood coagulation. Protein C in human plasma is inactivated by chloramines that act via singlet oxygen. The inhibitory concentration 50 % (IC50) is about 2 mM (Fig. 1).

Another important down-regulator of thrombin generation is antithrombin: the IC50 of chloramines against antithrombin is about 3 mM (Fig. 1). The serine protease inactivator (serpin) antithrombin forms 1:1 complexes with thrombin, the central enzyme in coagulation.

The central enzyme in fibrinolysis is plasmin that is inactivated by the serpin plasmin inhibitor, which is also a protein that is susceptible to chloramine: the IC50 is about 1.5 mM (Fig. 1). At this plasma concentration plasmatic fibrinolysis in FIPA is enhanced by about 50 %; 4 mM chloramine accelerate plasmatic fibrinolysis in FIPA about 3 fold (Fig. 2).

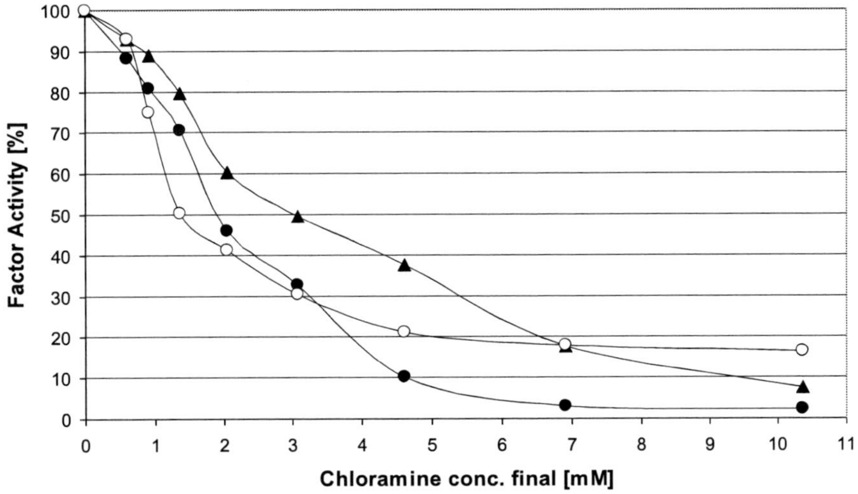

Figure 1. Oxidative inactivation of plasmatic protein C. 1 ml pooled normal citrated plasma was incubated for 20 min (37°C) with 100 µl 0-172 mM chloramine-T® in 0.9% NaCl. Then the activity of protein C (●), antithrombin (▲), and plasmin-inhibitor (O) was determined.

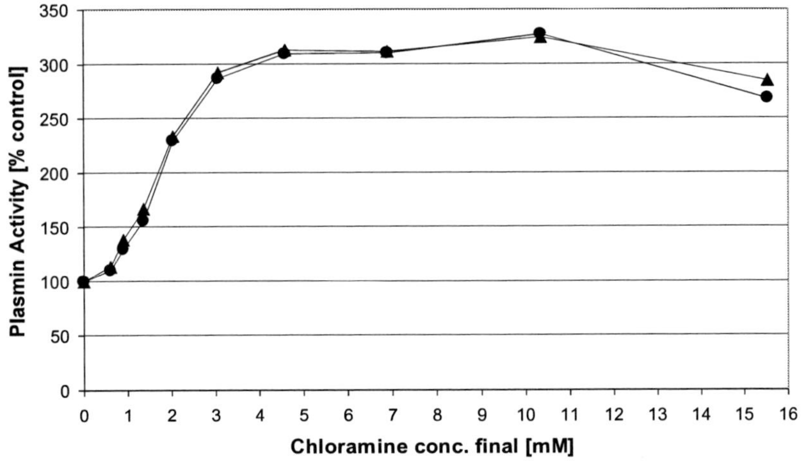

Figure 2. Oxidative activation of plasmatic fibrinolysis. 1 ml pooled normal citrated plasma was incubated for 20 min (37°C) with 100 µl 0-172 mM chloramine-T® in physiol. NaCl. Then the FIPA-10 (●) or the FIPA-30 (▲) activity (global plasmatic fibrinolysis parameters assay with 10 or 30 min reaction time) was determined by urokinase activation of plasma and subsequent plasmin detection by 0.22 mM (final) chromogenic substrate for plasmin in presence of 1.49 M (final) arginine.

21 mM methionine, a quencher of singlet oxygen, completely neutralizes the inactivation of protein C by 1.5 mM chloramine in human plasma, 21 mM alanine (amino acid control), 21 mM or 75 mM mannitol, a quencher of hydroxyl radicals, does not inhibit the action of

chloramine (Table 1). Thus, at physiologic conditions chloramines act as singlet oxygen generators and not as generators of oxygen radicals. Chloramines might attack critical methionines or cysteines susceptible proteins like protein C [14,17].

Table 1. Quenching of chloramine by methionine.

Protein C-Activity [%] after addition of	0.9 % NaCl	21 mM Alanine	21 mM Mannitol	75 mM Mannitol	21 mM Methionine
0 mM Chloramine	100±6.8	103.5±5.8	117.6±10.2	110±5.2	96.3±5.6
1.5 mM Chloramine	80.3±2.8	78.7±7.5	81.6±7.2	67.1±8.1	107.1±9.6

mean values ± 1 standard deviation of 24 fold determinations.

The Yates-corrected X^2 values for unoxidized vs. oxidized plasma are 11.111 ($p < 0.01$) for supplementation with a) 0.9 % NaCl, b) alanine, or c) mannitol. There are no significant differences between the results on unoxidized vs. oxidized plasma that contains methionine.

Figure 3 demonstrates that the half life of chloramines in human plasma is extremely short. After an oxidation time of 30 min (37°C) up to about 2 mM supplemented chloramine were nearly completely consumed, about 10 % CT remains after addition of 4.5 mM CT, about 20 % CT remained after addition of 9 mM CT, and about 25 % CT remained after addition of 18 mM CT (Fig. 3a). After an oxidation time of 3 h (37°C) only about 5 % of added CT remained (Fig. 3a). After an oxidation time of 22 h (37°C) less than 0.4 % of added CT remained: 18 mM CT became 0.07 mM and 9 mM CT became 0.01 mM. After 72 h (37°C) 0.02 mM (0.1 %) chloramine remained from initially 18 mM. Within 1 min reaction time (37°C) about 40 % of 9.1 mM CT added is consumed in human plasma (Fig. 3b).

Especially a chloramine-concentration of about 1 mM is of special interest as potential new therapy against lipid-enveloped viruses. Of initial 0.91 mM CT 60-70 % are consumed when plasma is incubated at 37°C and about 50 % is consumed when incubated at 23°C within 1 min. For 70 % chloramine consumption about 7 min at 23°C are necessary. Ninety percent chloramine consumption is achieved by 8 min (37°C) or 32 min (23°C).

Decreased PCa results in increased thrombin activity in blood. However, in an oxidative ambience thrombin cannot act as the normal fibrinogen→fibrin clotting enzyme, because chloramine-oxidized fibrinogen cannot polymerize (IC50=2 mM [15,16]): Thrombin - instead of generating a fibrin clot- produces soluble oxidized fibrin monomer, a strong stimulator of tissue - plasminogen activator [22]. In peri-cellular areas, the clotting cascade might still generate factor Xa or thrombin [18], but the fibrinogen→fibrin polymerization is abolished by singlet oxygen. Consequently, singlet oxygen might antagonize a restriction of the inflammatory response [12,19,20]. The content of oxidized fibrinogen molecules and that of clotting proteases in inflammatory fluid might be of pathophysiological interest [20-23]. Whereas singlet oxygen at plasmatic concentrations of about 5-10 mM might strongly favour inflammation, singlet oxygen at plasmatic concentrations of about 0.5-1 mM might be beneficial against thrombotic diseases or against lipid-enveloped viruses.

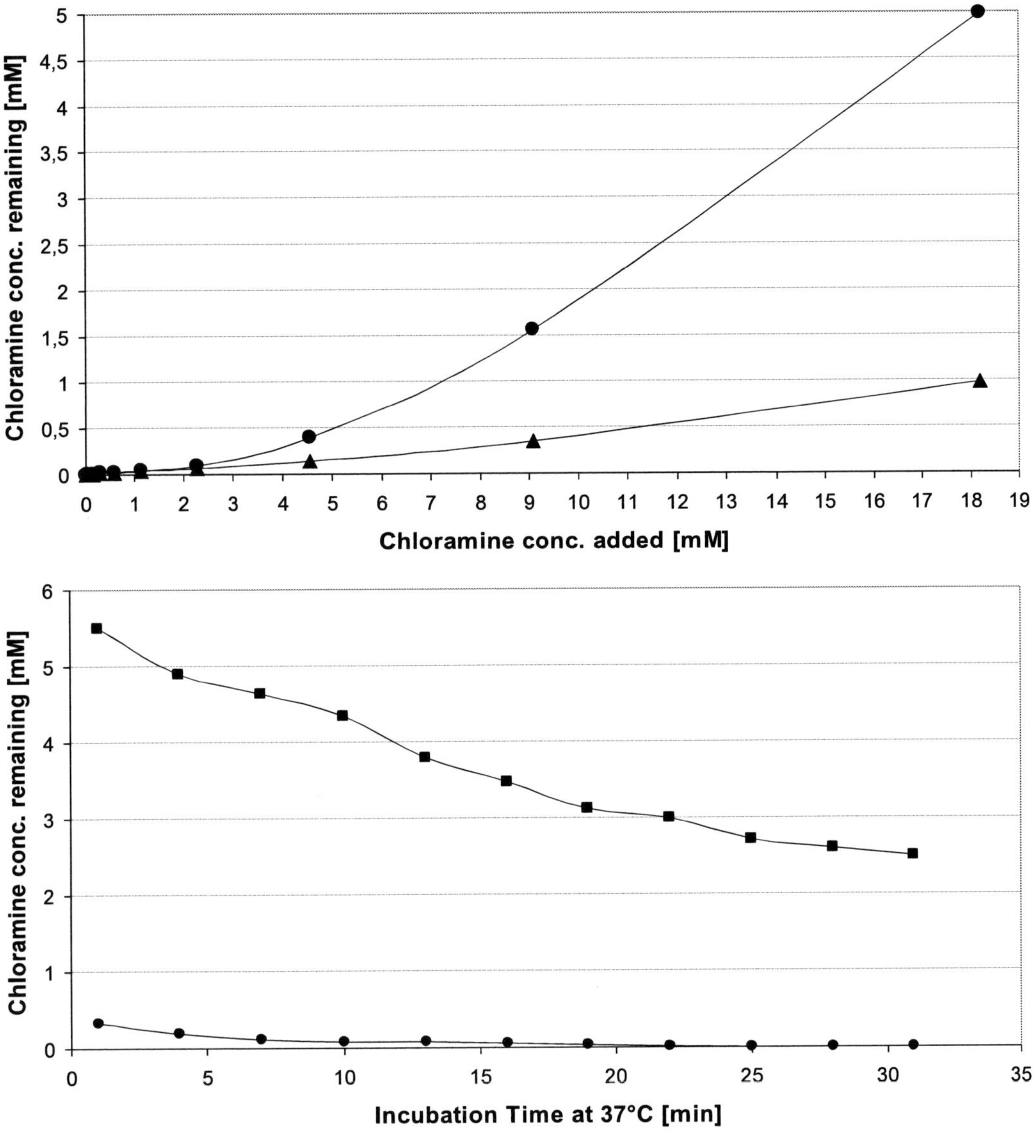

Figure 3. Consumption of chloramines (R-N-Cl) in plasma. Pooled unfrozen normal citrated plasma was supplemented with chloramine-T® (CT). After increasing oxidation times at 37°C, 20 µl plasma samples or 1 mM chloramine standard were incubated with 200 µl 4 M KI in PBS and the ΔA at 405 nm was determined. Fig. 3a: R-N-Cl consumption after 30 min (●) or after 3 h (▲). Fig. 3b: R-N-Cl consumption in dependence of short incubation times (37°C);plasma supplementation with 0.91 mM CT (●),9.1 mM CT (■).

REFERENCES

[1] Rosen H, Klebanoff SJ. Formation of singlet oxygen by the myeloperoxidase-mediated antimicrobial system. *J Biol Chem* 1977; 252: 4803-10.

[2] Weiss SJ. Tissue destruction by neutrophils. *N Engl J Med* 1989; 320: 365-76.

[3] Stief TW. Regulation of hemostasis by singlet-oxygen ($^1\Delta O_2$*). *Curr Vasc Pharmacol* 2004; 2: 357-62.

[4] Deng X, Luyendyk JP, Zou W, Lu J, Malle E, Ganey PE, Roth RA. Neutrophil interaction with the hemostatic system contributes to liver injury in rats cotreated with lipopolysaccharide and ranitidine. *J Pharmacol Exp Ther* 2007; 322: 852-61.

[5] Zarbock A, Polanowska-Grabowska RK, Ley K. Platelet-neutrophil-interactions: linking hemostasis and inflammation. *Blood Rev* 2007; 21: 99-111.

[6] Gerasimov IG, Ignatov DY. Blood coagulation initiates respiratory burst in neutrophils. *Bull Exp Biol Med* 2005; 140: 77-9.

[7] Eilertsen KE, Osterud B. The role of blood cells and their microparticles in blood coagulation. *Biochem Soc Trans* 2005; 33: 418-22.

[8] Guo RF, Ward PA. Role of C5a in inflammatory responses. *Annu Rev Immunol* 2005; 23: 821-52.

[9] Vogt W, Hesse D. Oxidants generated by the myeloperoxidase-halide system activate the fifth component of human complement, C5. *Immunobiology* 1994; 192: 1-9.

[10] Stief TW, Hinz F, Kurz J, Doss MO, Kretschmer V. A simple screening assay for certain fibrinolysis parameters (FIPA). *Thromb Res* 2000; 97: 231-7.

[11] Stief TW, Fröhlich S, Renz H. Determination of the global fibrinolytic state. *Blood Coagul Fibrinolysis* 2007; 18: 479-87.

[12] Witko V, Nguyen AT, Descamps-Latscha B. Microtiter plate assay for phagocyte-derived taurine-chloramines. *J Clin Lab Anal* 1992; 6: 47-53.

[13] Stief TW. The fibrinogen antigenic turbidimetric assay (FIATA). The $X^2_{\bar{x}}$ test: the corrected chi-square comparison against the control-mean. *Clin Appl Thromb Hemost* 2007; 13: 73-100.

[14] Shechter Y, Burstein Y, Patchornik A. Selective oxidation of methionine residues in proteins. *Biochemistry* 1975; 14: 4497-503.

[15] Inada Y, Hessel B, Blomback B. Photooxidation of fibrinogen in the presence of methylene blue and its effect on polymerization. *Biochim Biophys Acta* 1978; 532: 161-70.

[16] Stief TW, Kurz J, Doss MO, Fareed J. Singlet oxygen inactivates fibrinogen, factor V, factor VIII, factor X, and platelet aggregation of human blood. *Thromb Res* 2000; 97: 473-80.

[17] Heeb MJ, Bischoff R, Courtney M, Griffin JH. Inhibition of activated protein C by recombinant alpha 1-antitrypsin variants with substitution of arginine or leucine for methionine358. *J Biol Chem* 1990; 265: 2365-9.

[18] Bhattacharjee G, Ahamed J, Pawlinski R, Liu C, Mackman N, Ruf W, Edgington TS. Factor Xa Binding to Annexin 2 Mediates Signal Transduction via Protease-Activated Receptor 1. *Circ Res* 2008 Jan 3; [Epub ahead of print]

[19] Lawrence DA, Loskutoff DJ. Inactivation of plasminogen activator inhibitor by oxidants. *Biochemistry* 1986; 25: 6351-5.

[20] Henschen AH. Human fibrinogen--structural variants and functional sites. *Thromb Haemost* 1993; 70: 42-7.

[21] Manadan AM, Block JA. Rheumatoid Arthritis: Beyond Tumor Necrosis Factor-alpha Antagonists, B Cell Depletion, and T Cell Blockade. *Am J Ther* 2008; 15: 53-8.

[22] Stief TW, Kretschmer V, Kosche B, Doss MO, Renz H. Thrombin converts singlet oxygen ($^1O_2$)-oxidized fibrinogen into a soluble t-PA cofactor. A new method for preparing a stimulator for functional t-PA assays. *Ann Hematol* 2001; 80: 189-94.

[23] Stief TW, Fareed J. The antithrombotic factor singlet oxygen/light ($^1O_2$/hv). *Clin Appl Thromb Hemost* 2000; 6: 22-30.

In: Hemostasis Laboratory Yearbook, Volume 2
Editor: Thomas W. Stief, pp. 133-139
ISBN: 978-1-60741-089-8

LOSS OF ANTICOAGULANT ACTION BY ULTRA-LOW-DOSE HEPARIN

Thomas W. Stief**, Salem Ajib and Harald Renz
Institute of Clinical Chemistry, University Hospital, Giessen & Marburg, Germany

ABSTRACT

The aim of the present study was to compare ultra low doses of heparin and of the low molecular weight heparin enoxaparin, when the anticoagulants were added to plasma directly out of the original siliconized glass vial to obtain the final plasma concentration without further plasma dilution steps. This imitates the continuous administration of these heparins. The recalcified coagulation activity assay (RECA) was performed with n=10 citrated plasmas of healthy donors and with n=32 citrated plasmas of patients without hemostasis alterations, 50 µl plasma being supplemented with 2 µl 0, 2.6, 26, or 260 mIU/ml heparin or enoxaparin, generating final concentrations of 0, 0.1, 1, or 10 mIU/ml. Venous blood had been collected in polypropylene tubes, recalcified thrombin generation with 40 min (37°C) coagulation reaction time was performed in polystyrol microwells with flat bottom.

0.1 mIU/ml enoxaparin decreased the thrombin generation by about 30-60 %, when compared with unsupplemented plasma; the thrombin generation in plasma with 0.1 mIU/ml heparin was nearly identical or even about 20 % higher than that in unsupplemented plasma. The data demonstrate that ultra low concentrations of heparin, as e.g. occurring in the end of heparin infusions, might be dangerous especially for some susceptible patients. It is suggested to replace heparin by enoxaparin or to "bridge" the end of a heparin infusion with administration of enoxaparin, and to monitor the correct dosage of enoxaparin in each individual patient by means of a specific thrombin generation assay.

INTRODUCTION

Glycosaminoglycans are the main physiologic anticoagulants [1-12]. Heparin and low molecular weight heparins, such as enoxaparin, are the most common used anticoagulants for patients within hospitals. Unfortunately, some patients are especially susceptible to unfractionated heparin, they might develop a paradoxical hemostasis activation. Heparins can be given in bolus or continuously per infusion or subcutaneous injection. Bolus

* Send correspondence to: T. W. Stief, MD, Priv.-Doz.; Department of Clinical Chemistry, University Hospital of Giessen & Marburg, D-35043 Marburg, Germany; FAX: +49-6421-586 5594; Email: thstief@med. uni-marburg.de.

administration is imitated in [13], where heparin has been added in very high concentrations (> 10 IU/ml) to plasma directly out of the original drug vial. Heparin or enoxaparin, when added in very high plasmatic concentrations and subsequently diluted, acts about 3fold stronger (as derived from respective 50 % inhibitory concentrations [13]), when compared with direct low supplementation of the drug into plasma, as e.g. shown in the present study. The aim of the present study was to compare ultra low doses of heparin and enoxaparin, when the anticoagulants were added to plasma directly out of the original vial to obtain the final plasma concentration without further plasma dilution steps, which imitates the continuous infusion or the subcutaneous administration of these anticoagulants.

Material and Methods

After informed consent, samples of citrated blood (0.5 ml 106 mM sodium citrate + 4.5 ml venous blood in polypropylene monovettes, Sarstedt, Nümbrecht, Germany) of n=10 normal donors were taken, within 2 h (23°C) centrifuged at 2800g for 10 min (23°C). Additionly, n=32 plasmas of patients not on hemostasis therapy with normal prothrombin time (international normalized ratio (INR) 0.9-1.1; Thromborel S®, DadeBehring, Marburg, Germany), normal activated partial thromboplastin time (APTT < 36s; Pathromtin SL®, DadeBehring), normal fibrinogen (2.1-3.5g/l; modified Clauss method, DadeBehring; all routine assays performed on a Behring Coagulation Timer®) were analyzed in the present study, when they were about 5 h old (stored at 23°C), i.e. at the time point when the routine citrated samples are usually thrown away.

In the recalcified coagulation activity assay (RECA) 50 µl samples were pipetted in duplicate by means of a Multipette® (Eppendorf AG, Hamburg, Germany) with 0.9 % NaCl-rinsed and completely emptied new polypropylene tips into polystyrol microtiterplates with flat bottom (F-wells, NUNC, Wiesbaden, Germany, article nr. 446140). 2 µl 0-260 mIU/ml unfractionated heparin (ratiopharm, Ulm, Germany) in 0.9 % NaCl or 2 µl 0-260 mIU/ml low molecular weight heparin enoxaparin (Aventis, Frankfurt, Germany) in 0.9 % NaCl (both heparins in siliconized glass bottles, DadeBehring, Marburg, Germany, article nr. OVKE49) were added to generate final anticoagulant concentrations of 0, 0.1, 1, and 10 mIU/ml, starting with the lowest concentration. The plates were intensely shaken for 10s. After 10 min (23°C) 5 µl 250 mM $CaCl_2$ (RECA-trigger) were added. After intense shaking for 10s, the plates were brought into a 37°C digitally controlled water-bath. After 40 min (main value) or 45 min (control value) at 37°C, 100 µl 2.5 M arginine, pH 8.6, 0.16 % Triton X 100® were added. After 3 min 25 µl 1 mM chromogenic thrombin substrate CHG-Ala-Arg-pNA (Pentapharm, Basel, Switzerland) in 1.25 M arginine, pH 8.7, were added, and the linear increase of absorbance with time at 23°C (ΔA/t) was measured (linear range: up to 40 % of maximal ΔA (900 mA)). The results were standardized against 1 IU/ml bovine thrombin (DadeBehring) in 6.7 % human albumin (Kabi, Stockholm, Sweden), that replaced the plasma sample, and resulted in about 16 mA/min (23°C). The basal thrombin activity in citrated plasma prior to any CRT was also determined, this about 10 mIU/ml basal thrombin activity was substracted from all IIa values measured in RECA. The plasmas were analyzed in the RECA with a coagulation reaction time (CRT) of 40 min (37°C) (= RECA-40). 40 min reaction time was chosen for these lots of polypropylene blood sampling tubes and of microwells [untreated U-well polystyrol plates (e.g. Brand, Wertheim, Germany, article nr.

701300) might be less anticoagulant], because at 40 min CRT the thrombin generation was still ascending, i.e. the ratio between (thrombin activity at 40 min CRT) and (thrombin activity at 45 min CRT) in unsupplemented plasmas was less than 1.

STATISTICS

The intra- and inter-assay coefficients of variation (CV) (=standard deviation divided by mean value and multiplied by 100 %) of the thrombin generation values in the RECA were < 10 %. The data points were compared with the respective controls and tested for significance ($p < 0.05$), using the two-fold Yates-corrected chi-square comparison against the control-mean ($X^2\bar{x}$ Test) [14].

RESULTS AND DISCUSSION

Figure 1 demonstrates that heparin or enoxaparin at final plasma concentrations > 1 mIU/ml result into > 50 % decrease of thrombin generation in RECA. The decrease of thrombin generation at 10 mIU/ml anticoagulant is more pronounced for heparin than for enoxaparin, i.e. at this concentration heparin is a stronger anticoagulant than enoxaparin. In contrast, 0.1 mIU/ml heparin does not decrease thrombin generation in RECA, instead it even increases it by about 20 %, whereas 0.1 mIU/ml enoxaparin significantly decreases thrombin generation in RECA by about 30 %.

Figure 2 shows a similar action of these heparins in normal plasma of patients not on anticoagulation: 0.1 mIU/ml heparin decreases thrombin generation by only about 10 %, whereas 0.1 mIU/ml enoxaparin decreases it by about 55 %. At 10 mIU/ml anticoagulant heparin is at least as efficient as enoxaparin. The slight differences between Fig. 1c and 2c might be due to

1. different storage time of healthy donor samples and patient samples, which might result in different generation of procoagulant microparticles [15],
2. different lots of polypropylene blood tubes with polypropylene tops, that might contain different amounts of pro-or anti-heparinic plastic material [16],
3. different lots of polystyrol microtiter plates, which might also contain different amounts of pro- or anti-heparinic plastic material, especially if the plates are gamma-irradiated [17].

Heparin is a 10,000 to 20,000 Dalton sized polynegative molecule that not only activates antithrombin III (AT3) but also pre-kallikrein; kallikrein initiates the intrinsic phase of hemostasis: thrombin is formed, that activates FV and FVIII, the two main accelerators of hemostasis. Small heparin derivatives of about 6000 Dalton, such as the low molecular weight heparin enoxaparin, still activate AT3 but they do not seem to significantly trigger intrinsic hemostasis [18]. Therefore, heparin looses function at 23°C (temperatures lower than 37°C favour contact activation) and therefore, heparin looses function in ultra low concentrations, where the ability of contact activation might be superior to the ability of AT3 activation. Thus, especially in the end of a therapy with unfractionated heparin one should be aware of this possible complication in susceptible patients. Enoxaparin does not show this phenomenon, wherefore enoxaparin might be the clinically preferred drug to avoid these complications of heparin. It is suggested to monitor the correct dosage of enoxaparin for each individual patient [19,20] by means of ultra-specific thrombin generation assays.

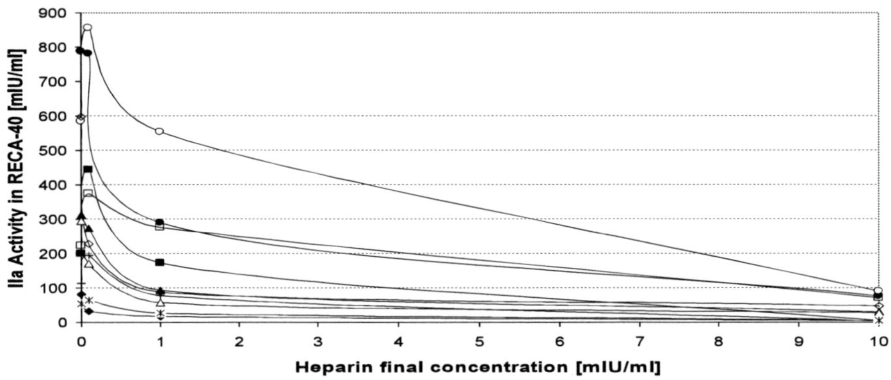

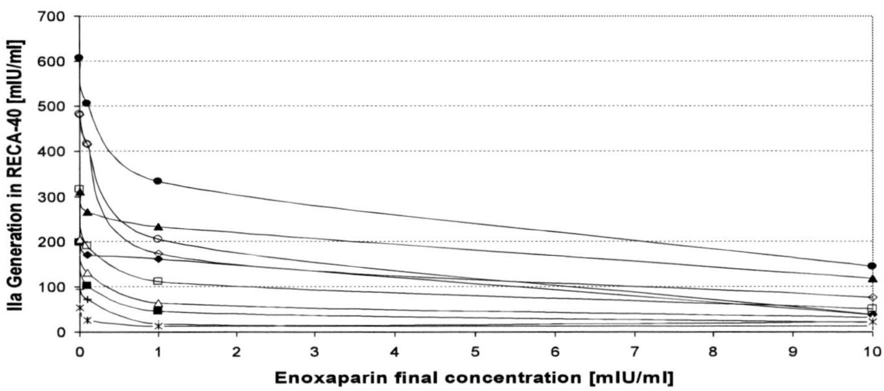

Figure 1 (Continues).

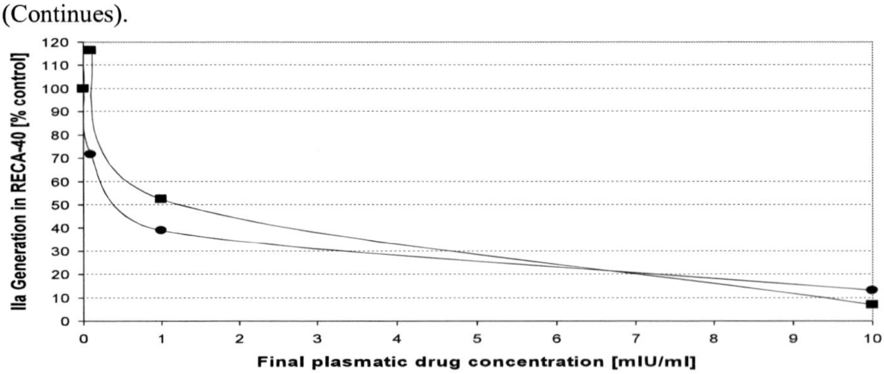

Figure 1. RECA inhibition by heparins. 50 µl citrated plasma of n=10 healthy donors (each donor has an individual symbol) in flat bottomed polystyrol microwells were supplemented with 0-10 mIU/ml heparin (Fig. 1a) or 0-10 mIU/ml enoxaparin (Fig. 1b). 5 µl 250 mM $CaCl_2$ were added. After 40 min at 37°C 100 µl 2.5 M arginine, pH 8.6, 0.16 % Triton X 100® and 25 µl 1 mM CHG-Ala-Arg-pNA in 1.25 M arginine, pH 8.7, were added, and ΔA/t was measured. Fig. 1c shows the mean values for heparin (■; 100 % control (no heparin) = 325 ± 250 mIU/ml thrombin (IIa)) and enoxaparin (●; 100 % control (no enoxaparin) = 295 ± 180 mIU/ml thrombin).

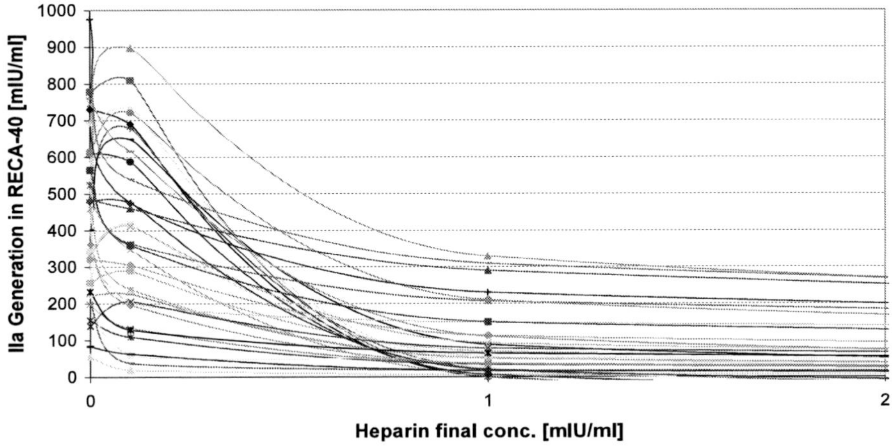

Figure 2 (Continues).

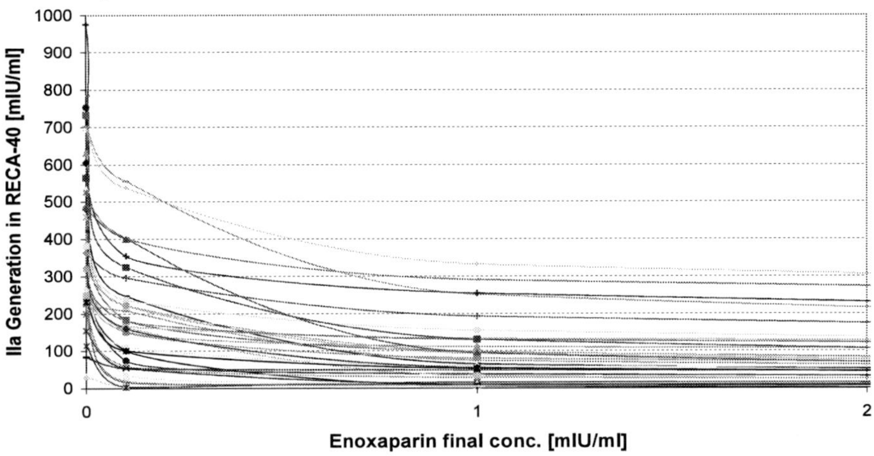

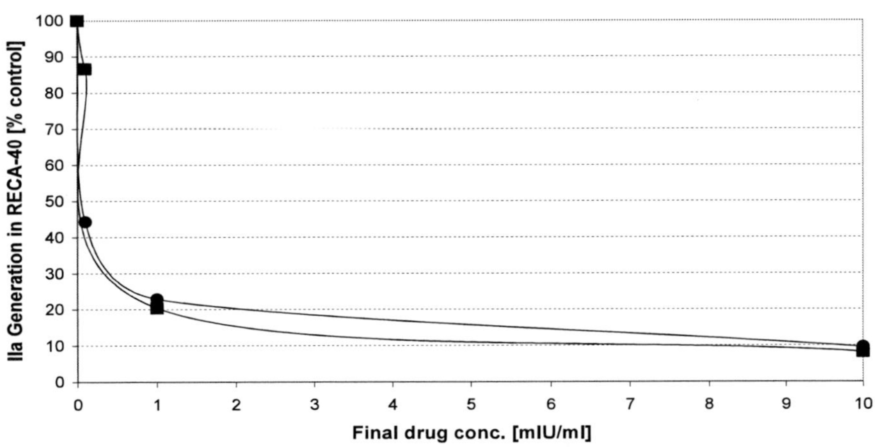

Figure 2. RECA inhibition by heparins. 50 µl citrated plasma of n=32 patients with normal PT, APTT, and fibrinogen and without hemostatic therapy (each patient has an individual symbol) in flat bottomed polystyrol microwells were supplemented with heparin (Fig. 2a) or enoxaparin (Fig. 2b). 5 µl 250 mM $CaCl_2$ were added. After 40 min at 37°C 100 µl 2.5 M arginine, pH 8.6, 0.16 % Triton X 100® and 25 µl 1 mM CHG-Ala-Arg-pNA in 1.25 M arginine, pH 8.7, were added, and ΔA/t was measured. Fig. 2c shows the mean values for heparin (■; 100 % control (no heparin) = 449 ± 239 mIU/ml thrombin) and enoxaparin (●; 100 % control (no enoxaparin) = 413 ± 227 mIU/ml thrombin (IIa).

ACKNOWLEDGMENT

This work is part of the academic thesis (MD) of Salem Ajib.

REFERENCES

[1] Mukherjee D, Eagle KA. The use of antithrombotics for acute coronary syndromes in the emergency department: considerations and impact. *Prog Cardiovasc Dis* 2007 ; 50: 167-80.

[2] Shorr AF. The pharmacoeconomics of deep vein thrombosis treatment. *Am J Med* 2007; 120 (Suppl 2): S35-41.

[3] Malowany JI, Knoppert DC, Chan AK, Pepelassis D, Lee DS. Enoxaparin use in the neonatal intensive care unit: experience over 8 years. *Pharmacotherapy* 2007; 27: 1263-71.

[4] Schmidt-Lucke C, Schultheiss HP. Enoxaparin injection for the treatment of high-risk patients with non-ST elevation acute coronary syndrome. *Vasc Health Risk Manag* 2007; 3: 221-8.

[5] Lee S, Gibson CM. Enoxaparin in acute coronary syndromes. *Expert Rev Cardiovasc Ther* 2007; 5: 387-99.

[6] Tribout B, Colin-Mercier F. New versus established drugs in venous thromboprophylaxis: efficacy and safety considerations related to timing of administration. *Am J Cardiovasc Drugs* 2007; 7: 1-15.

[7] Spinler SA, Wittkowsky AK, Nutescu EA, Smythe MA. Anticoagulation monitoring part 2: Unfractionated heparin and low-molecular-weight heparin. *Ann Pharmacother* 2005; 39: 1275-85.

[8] Kane-Gill SL, Feng Y, Bobek MB, Bies RR, Pruchnicki MC, Dasta JF. Administration of enoxaparin by continuous infusion in a naturalistic setting: analysis of renal function and safety. *J Clin Pharm Ther* 2005; 30: 207-13.

[9] Siddiqui MA, Wagstaff AJ. Enoxaparin: a review of its use as thromboprophylaxis in acutely ill, nonsurgical patients. *Drugs* 2005; 65: 1025-36.

[10] Sandercock P, Counsell C, Stobbs SL. Low-molecular-weight heparins or heparinoids versus standard unfractionated heparin for acute ischaemic stroke. *Cochrane Database Syst Rev* 2005; (2):CD000119.

[11] Fareed J, Leong WL, Hoppensteadt DA, Jeske WP, Walenga J, Wahi R, Bick RL. Generic low-molecular-weight heparins: some practical considerations. *Semin Thromb Hemost* 2004; 30: 703-13.

[12] Iqbal O, Aziz S, Hoppensteadt DA, Ahmad S, Walenga JM, Bakhos M, Fareed J. Emerging anticoagulant and thrombolytic drugs. *Expert Opin Emerg Drugs* 2001; 6: 111-35.

[13] Stief TW. Inhibition of thrombin generation in recalcified plasma. *Blood Coagul Fibrinolysis* 2007; 18: 751-60.

[14] Stief TW. The fibrinogen antigenic turbidimetric assay (FIATA). The $X^2\bar{x}$ test: the corrected chi-square comparison against the control-mean. *Clin Appl Thromb/Hemost* 2007; 13: 73-100.

[15] Sinauridze EI, Kireev DA, Popenko NY, Pichugin AV, Panteleev MA, Krymskaya OV, Ataullakhanov FI. Platelet microparticle membranes have 50- to 100-fold higher specific procoagulant activity than activated platelets. *Thromb Haemost* 2007; 97: 425-34.

[16] Stief TW. Influence of the surface on thrombin generation. *Int J Lab Hemat* (in press)

[17] Stief TW. Inhibition of intrinsic thrombin generation. *Drug Targets Insights* 2006; 2: 6-11.

[18] Stief TW. The anticoagulant capacity of plasmatic unfractionated heparin decreases at 23°C. *Blood Coagul Fibrinolysis* 2007; 18: 209-12.

[19] Fareed J, Walenga JM, Lassen M, Borris L, Hoppensteadt D, Murphy R, Ahsan A, Weber S, Jorgensen LN, Hauch O, et al. Pharmacologic profile of a low molecular weight heparin (enoxaparin): experimental and clinical validation of the prophylactic antithrombotic effects. *Acta Chir Scand Suppl* 1990; 556: 75-90.

[20] Dawes J. Comparison of the pharmacokinetics of enoxaparin (Clexane) and unfractionated heparin. *Acta Chir Scand Suppl* 1990; 556: 68-74.

In: Hemostasis Laboratory Yearbook, Volume 2
Editor: Thomas W. Stief, pp. 141-155

ISBN: 978-1-60741-089-8

The Sensibility of Individual Plasma to Heparins

Thomas W. Stief*, Salem Ajib and Harald Renz
Department of Clinical Chemistry, University Hospital, Giessen & Marburg, Germany

Abstract

Background

The activity of low-molecular-weight-heparin (LMWH) or unfractionated heparin towards individual plasmatic thrombin (IIa) generation is clinically important. Here the individual anticoagulant efficiency of heparins was determined, imitating their continuous administration.

Methods

To 50 µl citrated plasma of 51 healthy donors or of 213 patients (without anticoagulation therapy; with normal PT and APTT) in polystyrol microwells 2 µl of the anticoagulants in 0.9 % NaCl were added directly out of a siliconized glass vial, resulting in final plasma concentrations of 0-1 IU/ml of the heparins without further plasma dilutions. After 10 min (23°C) the extrinsic coagulation activity assay (EXCA) was performed. Pooled unfrozen normal plasma supplemented with these heparins was simultaneously analyzed for APTT and EXCA.

Results and Discussion

The approximate 50 % inhibitory concentration (IC50) of heparin in EXCA is 0.08 IU/ml, the approximate IC50 of enoxaparin is 0.14 IU/ml. 0.1 IU/ml heparin or enoxaparin in individual normal plasmas results in a thrombin generation of 43±16 % or 57±12 % of normal, respectively (MV±1SD) of the unsupplemented plasma control; 0.2 IU/ml enoxaparin results in a thrombin generation of 42±11 % of normal. Normal thrombin generation at 0.1 IU/ml heparin correlates only slightly to normal thrombin generation at 0.1 IU/ml enoxaparin (r= 0.334). 0.01 IU/ml heparin or enoxaparin reduce normal thrombin generation by about 10 % or 20 %, respectively. At 1 IU/ml enoxaparin

* Send correspondence to: T. W. Stief, MD, Priv.-Doz. Department of Clinical Chemistry, University Hospital of Giessen & Marburg, D-35043 Marburg, Germany; FAX: +49-6421-586 5594; Email: thstief@med.uni-marburg.de

there is still approximately 13 % of normal thrombin generation, whereas at 1 IU/ml heparin there is nearly no thrombin generation. Thus, heparin at concentrations in the range of 0.01 IU/ml might be too weak, at concentrations in the range of 1 IU/ml heparin might be too strong. About 5-10 % of samples are partially resistant to heparin or enoxaparin: a thrombin generation > MV+1SD of normal indicates plasmatic resistance against heparin or LMWH; a thrombin generation < MV–1SD of normal indicates plasmatic hyper-responsiveness to heparin or LMWH. The APTT in pooled normal plasma is 1.5fold or 2fold prolonged by 0.11 IU/ml of 0.15 IU/ml heparin, respectively, which corresponds to about 40 % or 20 % of normal thrombin generation in EXCA; the plasmatic LMWH concentration that is prophylactic (about 40 % of normal EXCA) or therapeutic (about 10-20 % of normal EXCA) is about 0.3 IU/ml enoxaparin or about 0.6–1 IU/ml enoxaparin, respectively. The LMWH dosage of each patient should be adjusted with an ultra-specific thrombin generation assay.

INTRODUCTION

Low molecular weight heparins (LMWH) and unfractionated heparin are usual clinical anticoagulants [1-6]. The anticoagulant efficiency of unfractionated heparin can be measured by the activated partial thromboplastin time (APTT); however, the APTT is too blunted to monitor the anticoagulant efficiency of LMWH [7]. Recently, we presented new chromogenic thrombin generation assays for the extrinsic or intrinsic coagulation activity (EXCA or INCA) [8,9]. Heparins might be about 3fold more efficient when given as a bolus than when infused continuously, as derived from the respective 50 % inhibitory concentrations (IC50) [10]. The aim of the present study was to measure the individual anticoagulant efficiency of heparin and of the LMWH enoxaparin, imitating continuous infusion / subcutaneous administration of these heparins.

MATERIAL AND METHODS

APTT and EXCA in Pooled Normal Plasma

500 µl samples of unfrozen pooled normal plasma were supplemented with 20 µl 0-26 IU/ml unfractionated heparin (ratiopharm, Ulm, Germany) in 0.9 % NaCl or with 20 µl 0-26 IU/ml of the low-molecular-weight-heparin (LMWH) enoxaparin (Aventis, Frankfurt, Germany) in 0.9 % NaCl. After 90 min at 23°C the samples were assayed for activated partial thromboplastin time (APTT; Pathromtin SL®, Behring Coagulation Timer (BCT), DadeBehring, Marburg, Germany); the control value was that of 0 IU/ml final drug concentration in plasma.

Exactly at the same time point, these samples were also analyzed in the extrinsic coagulation activity assay (EXCA): 50 µl plasma in polystyrol U-wells (Greiner, Frickenhausen, Germany; article nr. 650161, lot nr. 05281161) were activated after 90 min pre-incubation at 23°C with 5 µl EXCA-trigger, that was added by means of a Multipette® with NaCl-rinsed polypropylene-tips. The EXCA-triggers were 1 ml aliquots of once frozen/thawed 1 ng/ml tissue factor without polybrene® (Thromborel S®, Behringwerke, Marburg, Germany), 250 mM $CaCl_2$, 5 % human albumin (Kabi, Stockholm, Sweden) in siliconized 15 ml glass vials (DadeBehring, Marburg, Germany, article nr. OVKE49). After intense shaking for 5s, the plates were brought into a 37°C digitally controlled water-bath. After 1 min or 2 min at 37°C, the plates were taken out of the water-bath and 100 µl 2.5 M arginine, pH 8.6, 0.16 % Triton X 100® were added. The coagulation reaction time (CRT) of 1 min (37°C) is the main value = EXCA-1, the CRT of 2 min is the control value = EXCA-2 (the EXCA-1/EXCA-2 ratio was always < 1, i.e. thrombin generation at 1 min CRT was always in the increasing part of the thrombin generation curve). After 3 min at 23°C, 25 µl 1 mM chromogenic thrombin substrate CHG-Ala-Arg-pNA (Pentapharm, Basel, Switzerland) in 1.25 M arginine, pH 8.7, were added, and the linear increase of absorbance with time at 23°C (ΔA/t) was measured (linear range: up to 40 % of maximal ΔA, which is about 1050 mA, by a microtiter plate photometer with a 1 mA resolution (Milenia; DPC, Los Angeles, USA). The results were standardized with 1 IU/ml bovine thrombin (DadeBehring) in 6.7 % human albumin that replaced the plasma sample, and resulted in about 16 mA/min (23°C). The basal thrombin activity [11] in citrated plasma prior to any CRT was also determined by first addition of the arginine reagent and then addition of the tissue factor reagent. This basal thrombin activity was substracted from all thrombin values measured in EXCA, transforming the thrombin activity values into thrombin generation values. The basal thrombin activity in citrated patient plasmas was 8.0±2.4 mIU/ml (100±30%). Basal IIa in citrated plasmas of healthy donors was 7.3±2.0 mIU/ml (100±27%). Since the basal IIa activity in pooled normal EDTA-plasma is 5.5 mIU/ml [11], hemostasis in the citrated samples was only minimally pre-activated.

EXCA in Normal Plasma and Patient Plasma

Samples of citrated plasma (0.5 ml 106 mM sodium citrate + 4.5 ml venous blood in polypropylene monovettes (Sarstedt, Nümbrecht, Germany), centrifuged at 2800g for 10 min (23°C=RT)) of n=51 healthy donors taken after informed consent (2h RT old, after routine analysis) and of n=213 patients without hemostasis therapy with normal prothrombin time (PT; international normalized ratio (INR) = 0.85-1.2; Thromborel S®, DadeBehring) and normal APTT (≤ 36s) (5h RT old, remaining samples after routine analysis, at the time point of throwing away the routine samples) were analyzed in duplicate in the extrinsic coagulation activity assay (EXCA): 50 µl samples were pipetted with a Multipette® (Eppendorf AG, Hamburg, Germany) with 0.9 % NaCl-rinsed and completely emptied new polypropylene tips into polystyrol microwells with round bottom (U-wells; Greiner) 2 µl 0-26 IU/ml unfractionated heparin in 0.9 % NaCl or 2 µl 0-26 IU/ml enoxaparin in 0.9 % NaCl (both heparins in siliconized 15 ml glass vials) were added to generate final anticoagulant concentrations of 0, 0.01, 0.1, 0.2, 0.5, and 1 IU/ml, starting with the lowest concentration. The plates were intensely shaken for 5s. After 10 min (23°C) the EXCA was performed as described above.

Comparison of Routine Parameters with EXCA

The EXCA 1 values were compared with the routinely measured values for INR (Thromborel S®), APTT (Pathromtin SL®; Behring Coagulation Timer (BCT); DadeBehring), fibrinogen (modified Clauss-Method; BCT; DadeBehring), thrombocytes count (SysmexXE2100, Hamburg, Germany), and C reactive protein (CRP; Beckman, Krefeld, Germany). Samples with CRP values < 5 mg/l were pooled, the pool was analyzed with an ultrasensitive assay for CRP, resulting in 2 mg/l CRP. All CRP results < 5 mg/l were attributed to 2 mg/l.

STATISTICS

The intra-assay coefficients of variation (CV) (=standard deviation divided by mean value and multiplied by 100 %) of the thrombin generation values in the EXCA were < 5 %. Results were tested for significance ($X^2 > 3.841 = p < 0.05$ or $X^2 > 6.635 = p < 0.01$), using the non-categorical → categorical transformation of the 2fold Yates-corrected chi-square test [12].

RESULTS

Figure 1a demonstrates the known blunted nature of the APTT against low molecular weight heparin: 0.5 IU/ml enoxaparin are necessary to increase the APTT of pooled normal plasma from 29s to about 40s; the same APTT increase results by only 0.1 IU/ml unfractionated heparin. The 1.5fold, 2fold, or 3fold prolongation of the 100 % value (29s) is caused by about 0.11 IU/ml, 0.15 IU/ml, or 0.25 IU/ml heparin, respectively. 0.11 IU/ml, 0.15 IU/ml, or 0.25 IU/ml heparin correspond to about 40 %, 20 %, or 10 % of normal thrombin generation in the EXCA, respectively, in pooled normal plasma that was assayed simultaneously to the APTT (Fig. 1b). This prophylactic (about 40 % of normal EXCA) or therapeutic (about 10-20 % of normal EXCA) heparinization occurs at about 0.3 IU/ml or about 0.6 - 1 IU/ml enoxaparin (Fig. 1b).

In 51 normal donors the mean approximate 50 % inhibitory concentration (IC50) of heparin is 0.08 IU/ml, the mean IC50 of enoxaparin is 0.14 IU/ml (Fig. 2a). 0.01 IU/ml enoxaparin reduces normal thrombin generation by about 17 % whereas 0.01 IU/ml heparin reduces normal thrombin generation only by about 9 %. At 1 IU/ml enoxaparin there is still about 13 % of normal thrombin generation, whereas with 1 IU/ml heparin the normal thrombin generation is nearly completely inhibited. 0.1 IU/ml heparin in individual normal plasmas results in a thrombin generation of 43±16 % of the respective unsupplemented plasma control, i.e. a thrombin generation > 59 % of normal indicates plasmatic resistance against 0.1 IU/ml heparin, a thrombin generation < 27 % of normal indicates plasmatic hyper-responsiveness to 0.1 IU/ml heparin (Fig. 2b). There is nearly no correlation (r=0.227) between normal IIa generation [mIU/ml] at 0 IU/ml heparin and IIa generation [% of normal] at 0.1 IU/ml heparin.

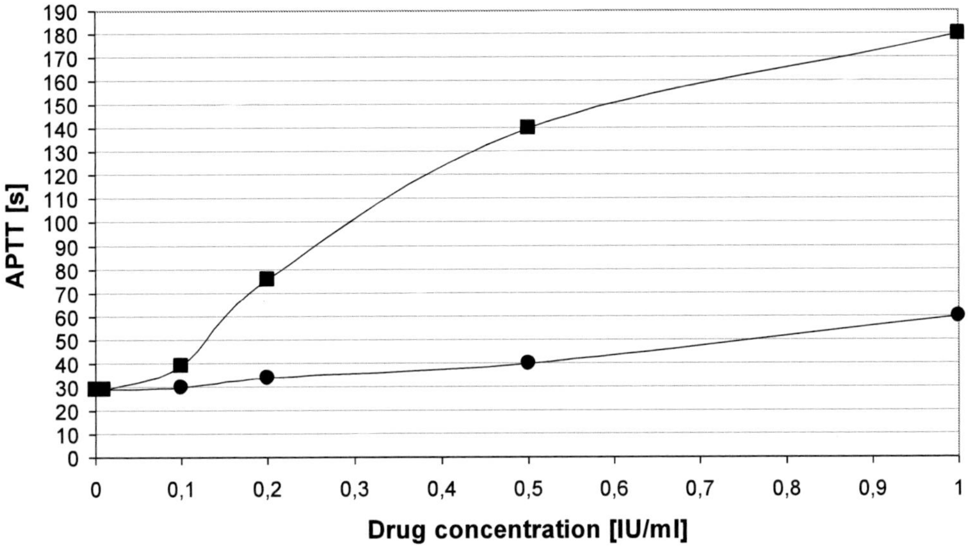

Figure 1. APTT in pooled normal plasma. Unfrozen pooled normal plasma was supplemented with heparin (■) or with the low-molecular-weight-heparin (LMWH) enoxaparin (●). After 90 min at 23°C the samples were assayed for APTT (Pathromtin SL®, BCT); control (0 IU/ml drug) = 29s. 1.5fold the control value = 43s is reached at 0.11 IU/ml heparin, 2fold the control value = 58s is reached at 0.15 IU/ml heparin.

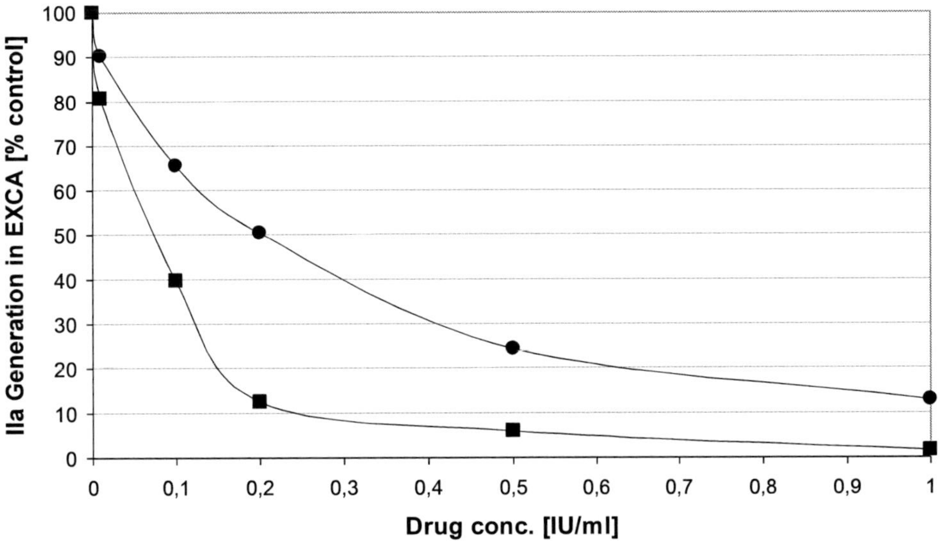

Figure 1b. EXCA in pooled normal citrated plasma. The extrinsic coagulation activity assay (EXCA) was performed as described in Methods with the same samples of Fig. 1a (heparin(■), enoxaparin (●)) simultaneously to the APTT determination after exactly the same preincubation time of 90 min (23°C); 100 % EXCA = generation of 462±23 mIU/ml (mean value ± 1 standard deviation) thrombin (IIa) within 1 min (37°C) in unsupplemented control; 1.5 fold prolongation of the normal APTT corresponds to about 40 % EXCA, 2fold prolongation of the normal APTT corresponds to about 20 % EXCA.

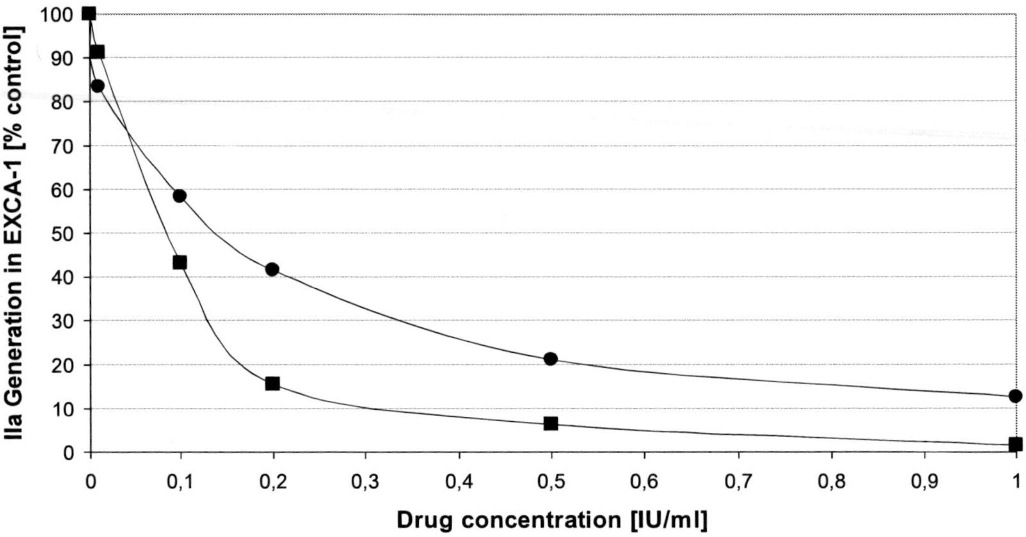

Figure 2a. EXCA inhibition by heparins in normal plasmas. Citrated plasma samples of n=51 normal donors were supplemented with heparin (■) or with enoxaparin (●). The EXCA was performed (main value = 1 min incubation at 37°C = EXCA-1). Shown are the mean values [% of unsupplemented control]. The approximate 50 % inhibitory concentrations (IC50) were 0.08 IU/ml heparin and 0.14 IU/ml enoxaparin.

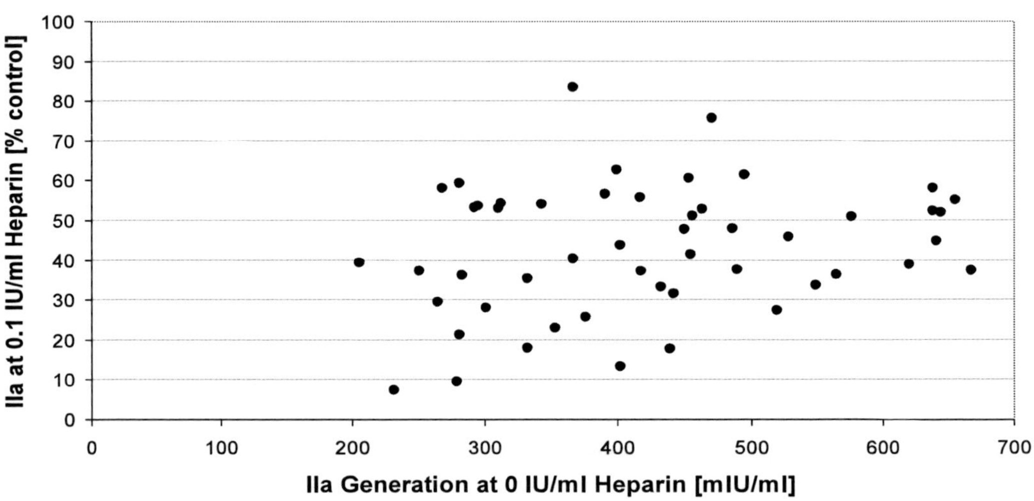

Figure 2b. IIa generation in normal plasmas with 0 IU/ml or with 0.1 IU/ml heparin. Thrombin (IIa) generation in EXCA [% unsupplemented control] was measured in n=51 normal plasmas that had been supplemented with 0 IU/ml (423±127 mIU/ml = 100 % IIa generation) or with 0.1 IU/ml heparin, r= 0.227.

0.1 IU/ml enoxaparin in individual normal plasmas results in a thrombin generation of 57±12 % of the respective unsupplemented plasma control, i.e. a thrombin generation > 69 % of normal indicates plasmatic resistance against 0.1 IU/ml enoxaparin, a thrombin generation < 45 % of normal indicates plasmatic hyper-responsiveness against 0.1 IU/ml enoxaparin (Fig. 2c). There is no correlation between normal IIa generation [mIU/ml] at 0 IU/ml enoxaparinn and IIa generation [% of normal] at 0.1 IU/ml enoxaparin.

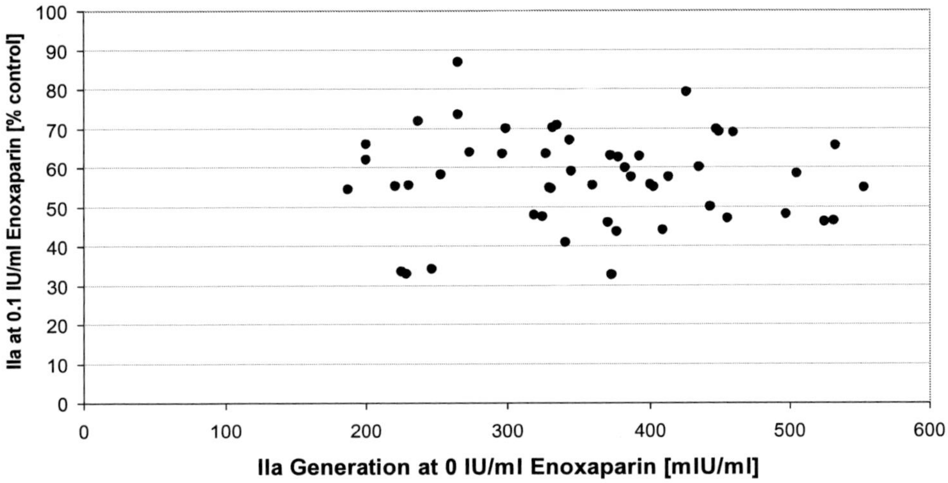

Figure 2c. IIa generation in normal plasmas with 0 IU/ml or with 0.1 IU/ml LMWH. IIa generation in EXCA [% unsupplemented control] was measured in n=51 normal plasmas that had been supplemented with 0 IU/ml (358±96 mIU/ml = 100 % IIa generation) or with 0.1 IU/ml enoxaparin, r= - 0.026.

There is only a slight correlation (r=0.334) between normal thrombin generation at 0.1 IU/ml heparin and normal thrombin generation at 0.1 IU/ml enoxaparin (Fig. 2d), i.e. an individual patient might respond completely different to heparin or to enoxaparin.

0.2 IU/ml enoxaparin results in 42±11 %, 0.5 IU/ml enoxaparin in 21±10 %, and 1 IU/ml in 13±7 % of normal IIa generation. The respective values for heparin are 16±10 %, 6±4 %, and 2±3 %.

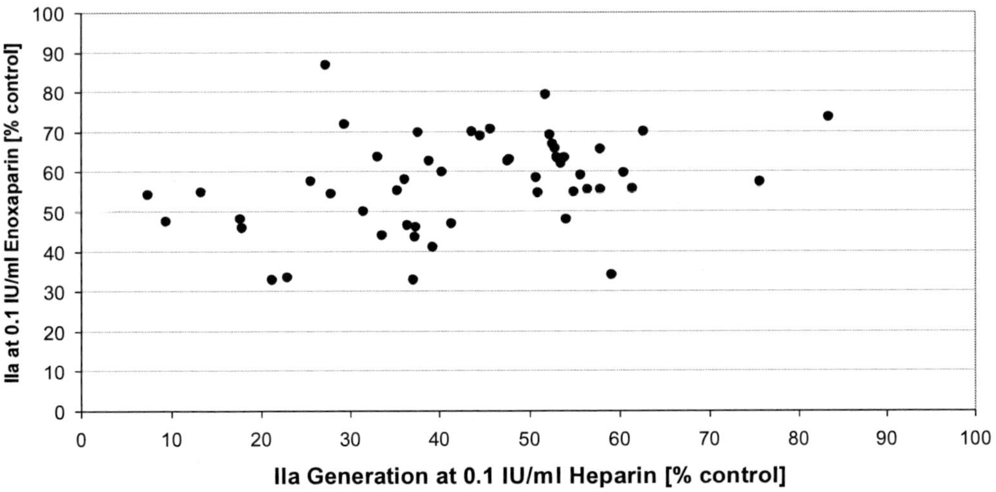

Figure 2d. IIa generation in normal plasmas with 0.1 IU/ml heparin or with 0.1 IU/ml LMWH. IIa generation in EXCA [% unsupplemented control] was measured in n=51 normal plasmas that had been supplemented with 0.1 IU/ml heparin or with 0.1 IU/ml enoxaparin, r= 0.334.

In the n=213 plasma samples of patients here tested the mean IC50 of heparin is 0.09 IU/ml, the mean IC50 of enoxaparin is 0.16 IU/ml (Fig. 3a). The superior anticoagulant efficiency of 0.01 IU/ml enoxaparin (MV=84 %) when compared with 0.01 IU/ml heparin (MV=93 %) is statistically significant (X^2corr = 8.58, p< 0.01).

There appears nearly no correlation between IIa generation [mIU/ml] at 0 IU/ml heparin and IIa generation [% of control] at 0.1 IU/ml heparin (Fig. 3b). The higher IIa generation [mIU/ml] in plasma samples of patients when compared to that of healthy donors might be attributed to a) pre-analytic differences (longer pre-analytic time interval of till analysis), and b) some procoagulant tendencies in blood of patients when compared with healthy donors.

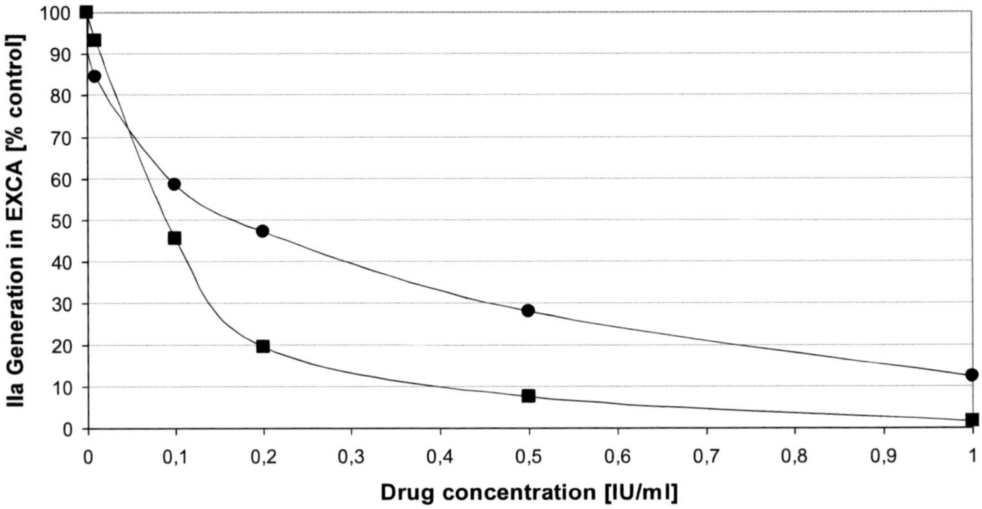

Figure 3a. EXCA inhibition by heparins in patient plasmas. Citrated plasma samples of n=213 patients without hemostasis therapy and with normal prothrombin time and APTT were supplemented with heparin (■) or with enoxaparin (●). The EXCA was performed (main value = 1 min incubation at 37°C = EXCA-1). Shown are the mean values [% of unsupplemented control]. The approximate 50 % inhibitory concentrations (IC50) were 0.09 IU/ml heparin and 0.16 IU/ml enoxaparin.

0.1 IU/ml heparin in individual patient plasmas results in a thrombin generation of 46±14% of the respective unsupplemented plasma control, i.e. a thrombin generation > 60 % of control indicates plasmatic resistance against 0.1 IU/ml heparin; a thrombin generation < 32 % of control indicates hyper-responsiveness against 0.1 IU/ml plasmatic heparin (Fig. 3b). 0.2 IU/ml enoxaparin in individual patient plasmas results in a thrombin generation of 47±13% of the respective unsupplemented plasma control, i.e. a thrombin generation > 60 % of control indicates plasmatic resistance against 0.2 IU/ml enoxaparin, a thrombin generation < 34 % of control indicates plasmatic hyper-responsiveness against 0.2 IU/ml enoxaparin (Fig. 3c).

There is only a slight correlation (r=0.262) between thrombin generation at 0.1 IU/ml heparin and thrombin generation at 0.2 IU/ml enoxaparin in individual patient plasmas (Fig. 3d), i.e. an individual patient might respond well to enoxaparin but bad to heparin as already seen in Fig. 2d.

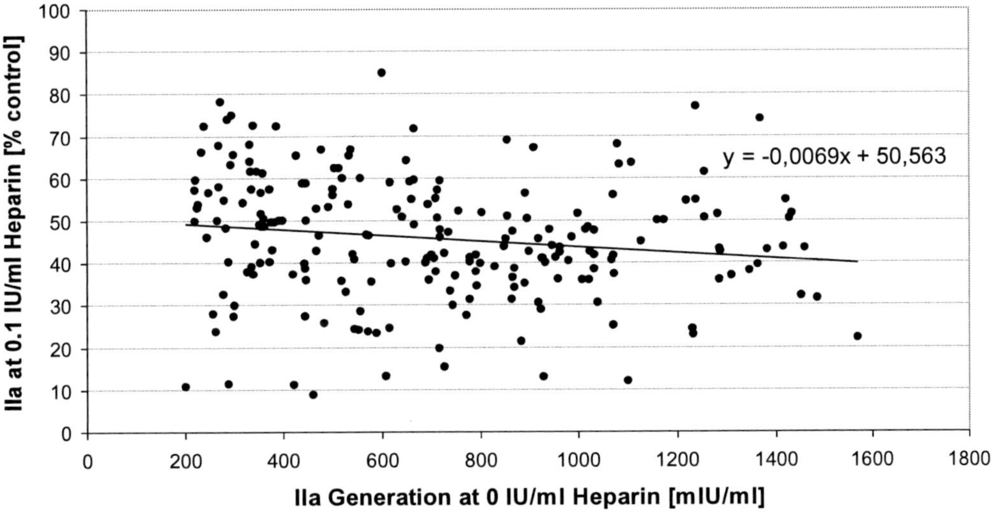

Figure 3b. IIa generation in patient plasmas with 0 IU/ml or with 0.1 IU/ml heparin. Thrombin (IIa) generation in EXCA [% unsupplemented control] was measured in the n=213 samples of patients of Fig. 3a after supplementation with 0 IU/ml (708±341 mIU/ml = 100 % IIa generation) or with 0.1 IU/ml heparin, r=- 0.163.

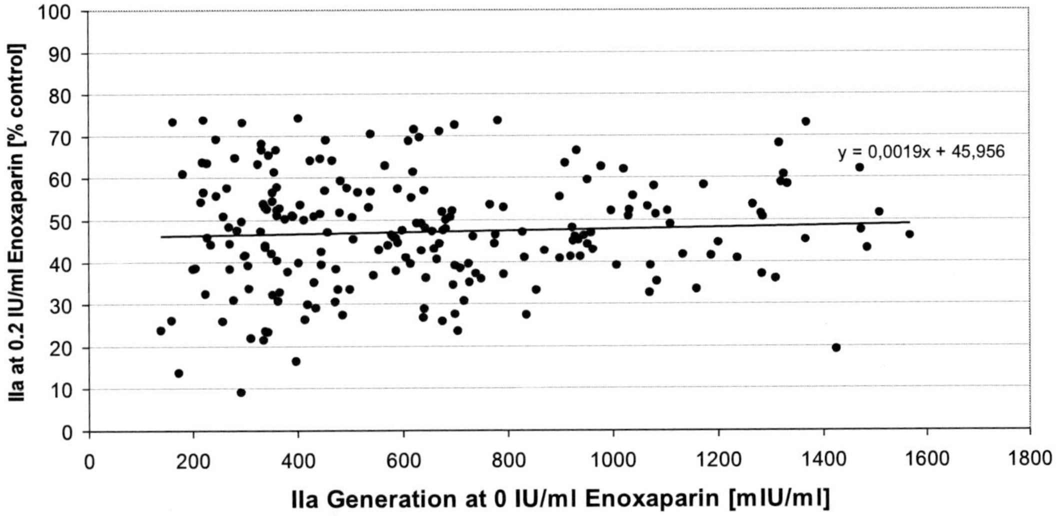

Figure 3c. IIa generation in patient plasmas with 0 IU/ml or with 0.2 IU/ml LMWH. Thrombin (IIa) generation in EXCA [% unsupplemented control] was measured in the n=213 samples of patients of Fig. 3a after supplementation with 0 IU/ml (643±340 mIU/ml = 100 % IIa generation) or with 0.2 IU/ml enoxaparin, r= 0.049.

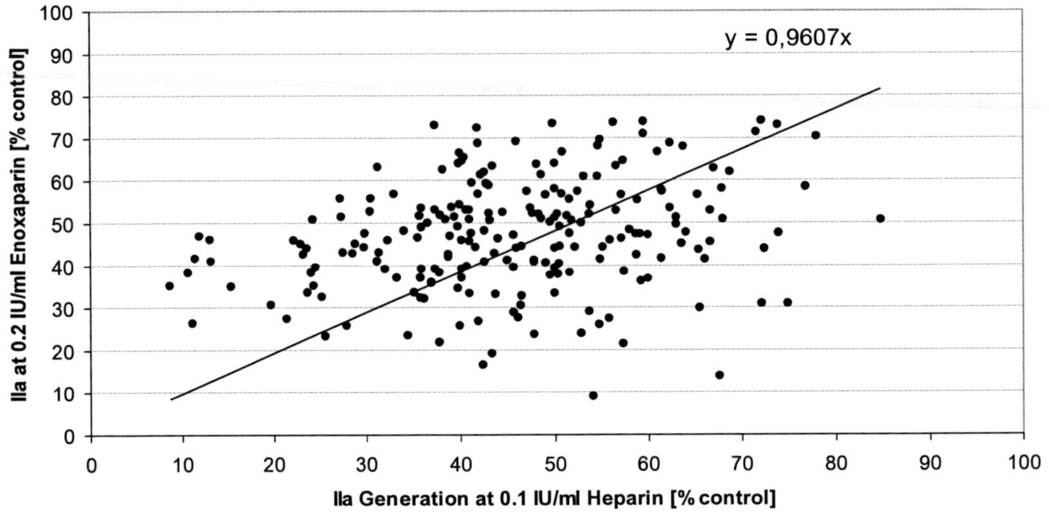

Figure 3d. IIa generation in patient plasmas with 0.1 IU/ml heparin or with 0.2 IU/ml LMWH=enoxaparin. Thrombin (IIa) generation in EXCA [% unsupplemented control] was measured in the n=213 samples of patients of Fig. 3a after supplementation with 0.1 IU/ml heparin or with 0.2 IU/ml enoxaparin, r= 0.262.

0.2 IU/ml enoxaparin results in 47±13 %, 0.5 IU/ml enoxaparin in 28±11 %, and 1 IU/ml enoxaparin in 12±9 % of IIa generation of the unsupplemented controls. The respective values for heparin are 19±9 %, 7±5 %, and 2±3 %, i.e. the results in % of thrombin generation of unsupplemented samples in these patients are very similar to that of normal donors.

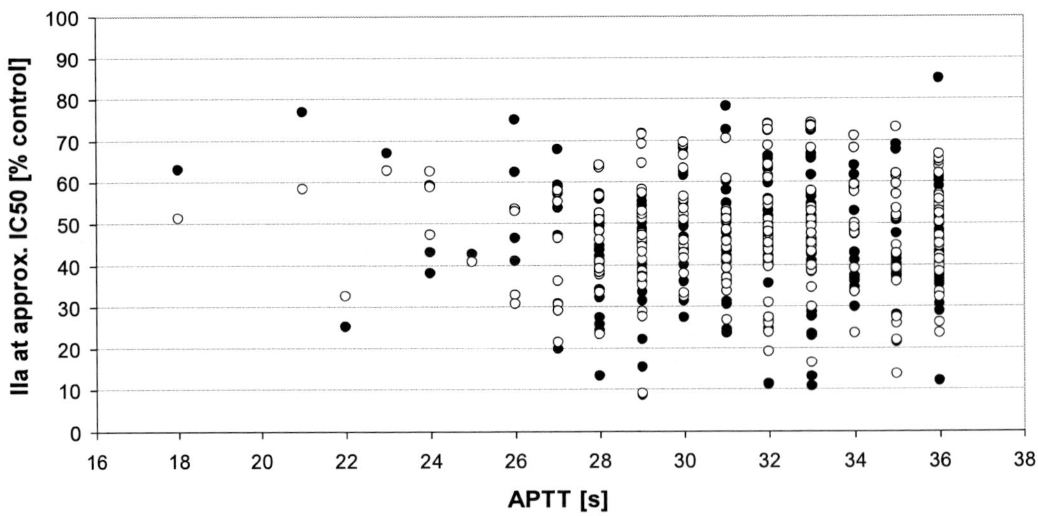

Figure 4a. APTT and IIa generation in patient plasmas. The APTT values (31.4±3.3s) were compared with the EXCA values [% of unsupplemented control] in the n=213 samples of patients of Fig. 3a after supplementation with the approximate IC50, which is 0.1 IU/ml heparin (•) or 0.2 IU/ml enoxaparin (O), r= -0.072 or r= 0.023, respectively.

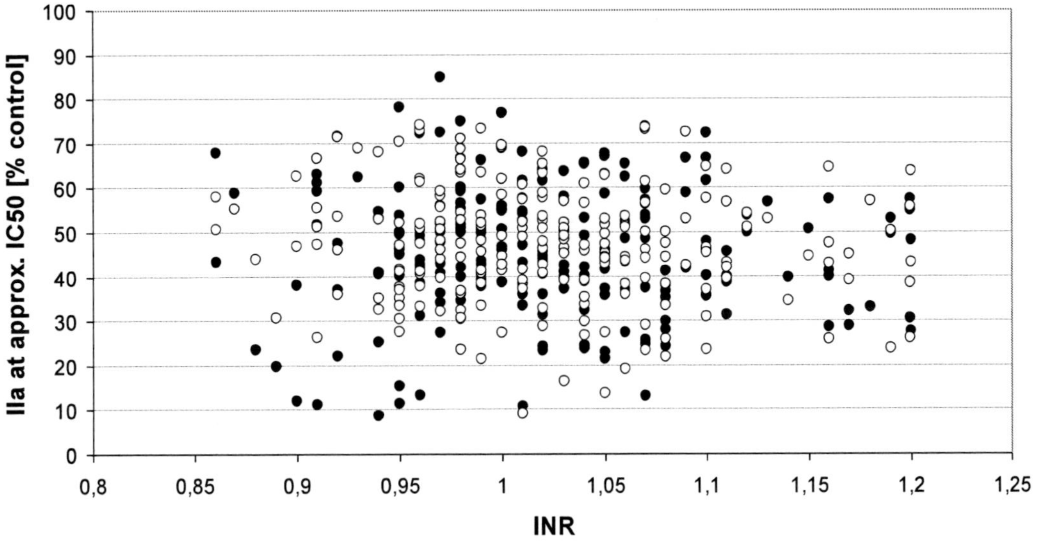

Figure 4b. INR and IIa generation in patient plasmas. The international normalized ratio (INR) values (1.02±0.07) were compared with the EXCA values [% of unsupplemented control] in the n=213 samples of patients of Fig. 3a after supplementation of plasma with the approximate IC50, which is 0.1 IU/ml heparin (●) or 0.2 IU/ml enoxaparin (O), r= -0.045 or r= – 0.101, respectively.

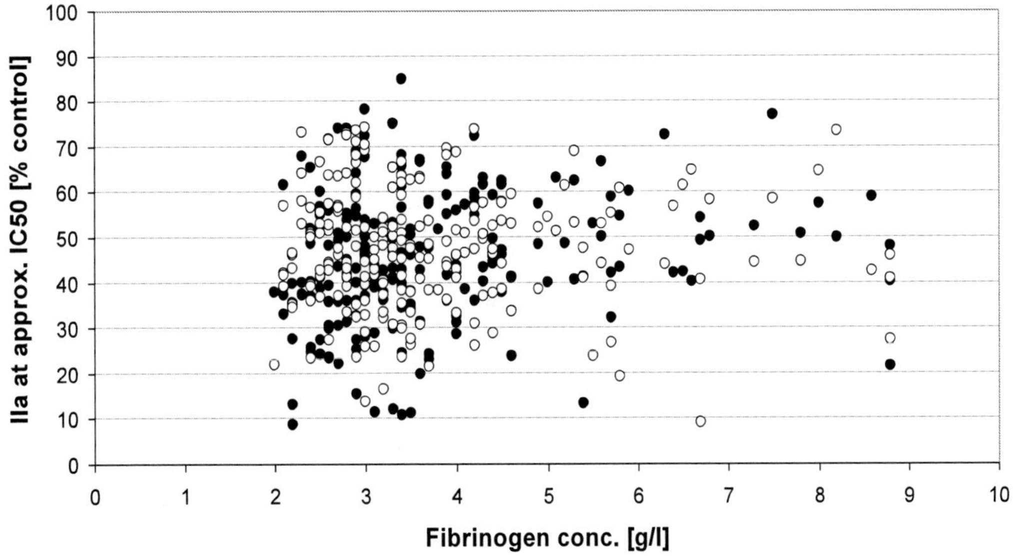

Figure 4c. Fibrinogen concentration and IIa generation in patient plasmas. The fibrinogen concentrations (3.7±1.4 g/l) were compared with the EXCA values [% of unsupplemented control] in the n=213 samples of patients of Fig. 3a after supplementation with the approximate IC50, which is 0.1 IU/ml heparin (●) or 0.2 IU/ml enoxaparin (O), r= 0.157 or r= – 0.003, respectively.

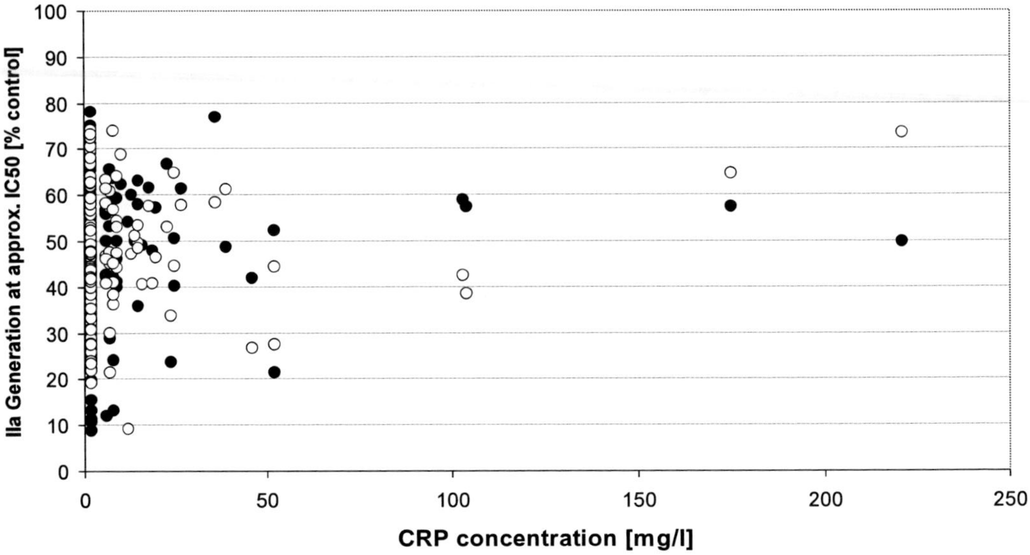

Figure 4d. CRP concentration and IIa generation in patient plasmas. The CRP concentrations (9.7±25.9 mg/l) were compared with the EXCA values [% of unsupplemented control] in the n=213 samples of patients of Fig. 3a after supplementation with the approximate IC50: 0.1 IU/ml heparin (•) or 0.2 IU/ml enoxaparin (O), r= 0.118 or r= – 0.130, respectively.

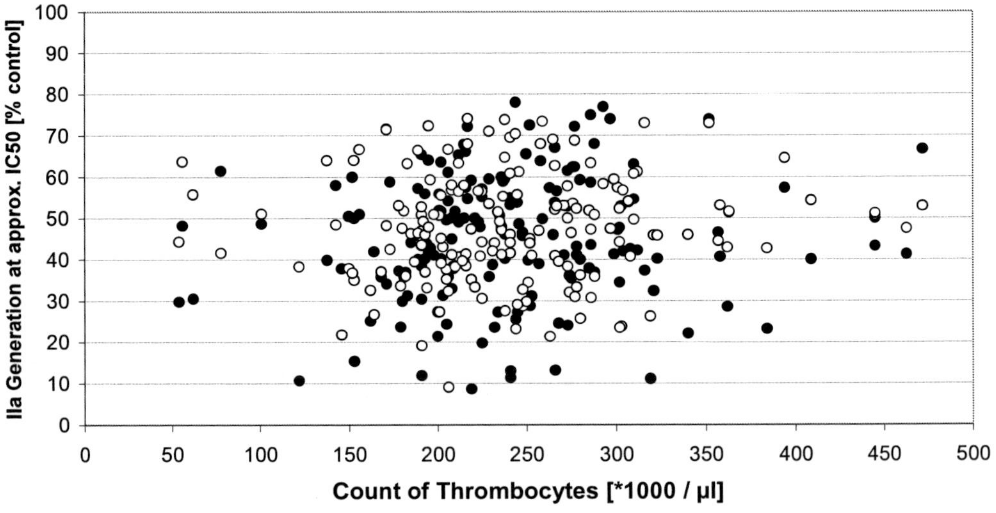

Figure 4e. Count of thrombocytes and IIa generation in patient plasmas. The platelet counts (240 000±70000/µl) were compared with the EXCA values [% unsupplemented control] in n=167 samples of patients of Fig. 3a after supplementation with the approximate IC50: 0.1 IU/ml heparin (•; 46±15 %) or 0.2 IU/ml enoxaparin (O; 47±13 %), r= 0.095 or r= 0.299, respectively.

There is no correlation between APTT, INR, CRP, or platelets with the thrombin generation in patient plasmas that were supplemented with 0.1 IU/ml heparin or with 0.2 IU/ml enoxaparin (Fig. 4).

Discussion

The present work demonstrates the sensibility of individual plasma to heparin or LMWH. The mean IC50 is about 0.08 IU/ml for heparin and 0.14 IU/ml for enoxaparin in normal donors. However, some patients might require higher doses than usual of heparin or enoxaparin, others might require less anticoagulant. In the present work the plasma was supplemented directly to the final anticoagulant concentration without further plasma dilution steps that could alter the IC50 because of higher affinity of the heparins to antithrombin at higher final concentrations of the heparins.

At anticoagulant concentrations in the range of about 10 mIU/ml enoxaparin is more effective than the potential contact activator heparin [13], at high anticoagulant concentrations (in the range of 1 IU/ml) unfractionated heparin might be potentially dangerous, since thrombin generation is inhibited by nearly 100 %.

Glycosaminoglycans as physiologic anticoagulants are superior to unphysiologic anticoagulants of the coumarin type. Life-long coumarin therapy with a target INR range of 2-3 results in about 10 % of patients in severe bleeding or in thrombo-embolic complications [14-17], i.e. an INR of 2-3 is in some patients too high and in others it is too low. This might be due to a lack of relationship between INR and the important plasmatic factors II and X [18]. Cerebral bleeding might occur in about 25 % of patients in spite of an INR $\leq$ 2.5 [19-21]. Therefore, it is suggested to replace coumarins by LMWH and to monitor their efficiency via an ultra-specific thrombin generation assay, such as the EXCA [22]. The ideal target EXCA for prophylaxis or therapy of anticoagulated patients might be about 40 % or about 10-20 % of normal thrombin generation in EXCA, respectively. For antithrombotic prophylaxis in high-risk patients (e.g. orthopaedic knee surgery) a therapeutic dosage, preferably of a LMWH heparin [23], might be used. The present data support the concept that the LMWH dosage of each individual patient should be adjusted with an ultra-specific thrombin generation assay.

Acknowledgment

This work is part of the academic thesis (MD) of Salem Ajib.

References

[1] Pollack CV Jr, Goldberg AD. The medical management of acute coronary syndromes and potential roles for new antithrombotic agents. *J Emerg Med*. 2008 Jan 26; [Epub ahead of print]

[2] Zeymer U, Gitt A, Jünger C, Bauer T, Heer T, Koeth O, Wienbergen H, Zahn R, Senges J. Efficacy and safety of enoxaparin in unselected patients with ST-segment elevation myocardial infarction. *Thromb Haemost* 2008; 99: 150-4.

[3] Gurm HS, Eagle KA. Use of Anticoagulants in ST-Segment Elevation Myocardial Infarction Patients; A Focus on Low-Molecular-Weight Heparin. *Cardiovasc Drugs Ther* 2007 Dec 29; [Epub ahead of print]

[4] Dumaine R, Borentain M, Bertel O, Bode C, Gallo R, White HD, Collet JP, Steinhubl SR, Montalescot G. Intravenous low-molecular-weight heparins compared with unfractionated heparin in percutaneous coronary intervention: quantitative review of randomized trials. *Arch Intern Med* 2007; 167: 2423-30.

[5] Dixon D, Peek B, Reeve R. Safety of enoxaparin bridge therapy in patients with mechanical heart valves. *Ann Pharmacother* 2008; 42: 143-4.

[6] De Luca G, Marino P. Adjunctive benefits from low-molecular-weight heparins as compared to unfractionated heparin among patients with ST-segment elevation myocardial infarction treated with thrombolysis. A meta-analysis of the randomized trials. *Am Heart J* 2007; 154: 1085.e1-6.

[7] Winkler AM, Sheppard CA, Fantz CR. Laboratory monitoring of heparin: challenges and opportunities. *Labmedicine* 2007; 38: 499-502.

[8] Stief TW, Wieczerzak A, Renz H. Influence of coagulation factors on extrinsic thrombin generation. *Blood Coagul Fibrinolysis* 2007; 18: 105-12.

[9] Stief TW, Otto S, Renz H. The intrinsic coagulation activity assay. *Blood Coagul Fibrinolysis* 2006; 17: 369-78.

[10] Stief TW. Inhibition of thrombin generation in recalcified plasma. *Blood Coagul Fibrinolysis* 2007; 18: 751-60.

[11] Stief TW. Specific determination of plasmatic thrombin activity. *Clin Appl Thromb Hemost* 2006; 12: 324-9.

[12] Stief TW. The fibrinogen antigenic turbidimetric assay (FIATA). The $X^2\bar{x}$ test: the corrected chi-square comparison against the control-mean. *Clin Appl Thromb/Hemost* 2007; 13: 73-100.

[13] Stief TW. The anticoagulant capacity of plasmatic unfractionated heparin decreases at 23°C. *Blood Coagul Fibrinolysis* 2007; 18: 209-12.

[14] Olsson SB, Halperin JL. Prevention of stroke in patients with atrial fibrillation. *Semin Vasc Med* 2005; 5: 285-92.

[15] Indredavik B, Rohweder G, Lydersen S. Frequency and effect of optimal anticoagulation before onset of ischaemic stroke in patients with known atrial fibrillation. *J Intern Med* 2005; 258: 133-44.

[16] Cheung CM, Tsoi TH, Huang CY. The lowest effective intensity of prophylactic anticoagulation for patients with atrial fibrillation. *Cerebrovasc Dis* 2005; 20: 114-9.

[17] Reynolds MW, Fahrbach K, Hauch O, Wygant G, Estok R, Cella C, Nalysnyk L. Warfarin anticoagulation and outcomes in patients with atrial fibrillation: a systematic review and metaanalysis. *Chest* 2004; 126: 1938-45.

[18] Sarode R, Rawal A, Lee R, Shen YM, Frenkel EP. Poor correlation of supratherapeutic international normalised ratio and vitamin K-dependent procoagulant factor levels during warfarin therapy. *Br J Haematol* 2006; 132: 604-7.

[19] Toyoda K, Okada Y, Ibayashi S, Inoue T, Yasumori K, Fukui D, Uwatoko T, Makihara N, Minematsu K. Antithrombotic therapy and predilection for cerebellar hemorrhage. *Cerebrovasc Dis* 2007; 23: 109-16.

[20] Rosand J, Eckman MH, Knudsen KA, Singer DE, Greenberg SM. The effect of warfarin and intensity of anticoagulation on outcome of intracerebral hemorrhage. *Arch Intern Med* 2004; 164: 880-4.

[21] Lee SB, Manno EM, Layton KF, Wijdicks EF. Progression of warfarin-associated intracerebral hemorrhage after INR normalization with FFP. Neurology 2006; 67:

12Lee SB, Manno EM, Layton KF, Wijdicks EF. Progression of warfarin-associated intracerebral hemorrhage after INR normalization with FFP. *Neurology* 2006; 67: 1272-4.

[22] Stief TW. Innovative tests of plasmatic hemostasis. *Laboratory Medicine* 2008; 39: 225-30.

[23] Stief TW. The efficiency of anti-activated factor X and anti-activated factor II anticoagulants. *Blood Coagul Fibrinolysis* 2007; 18: 265-9.

In: Hemostasis Laboratory Yearbook, Volume 2
Editor: Thomas W. Stief, pp. 157-160
ISBN: 978-1-60741-089-8

THE 50% INHIBITORY TIME POINT OF PLASMATIC HEPARINS

Thomas W. Stief*
Department of Clinical Chemistry
University Hospital Giessen and Marburg, Germany

ABSTRACT

Heparins (unfractionated heparin UFH or low molecular weight heparin LMWH) are among the most important physiological anticoagulants. They gain anticoagulant function in blood not until complexation with antithrombin III. What is the necessary incubation time of heparins at low dose to obtain full anticoagulant activity in plasma?

50 μl unfrozen pooled normal plasma was supplemented with 2 μl 2.6 IU/ml UFH (0.1 IU/ml final concentration) or with 2 μl 2.6 IU/ml of the LMWH enoxaparin (0.1 IU/ml final concentration) in 0.9% NaCl out of siliconized glass vials. After 1-11 min (37°C or 23°C) the extrinsic coagulation activity assay (EXCA) was performed. The EXCA is a new ultra-specific and close-to-physiological thrombin generation assay.

The approximate 50% inhibitory time point (ITP50 = 50% of the complete anticoagulant activity) was a pre-incubation time of 1 min (37°C) for low dose UFH and of 3 min (37°C) for low dose enoxaparin prior to performing the EXCA. The respective ITP50 values at 23°C were about 1.5-fold prolonged. This work demonstrates the importance of the pre-incubation time of plasmatic heparins on thrombin generation assays that analyze the sensibility of individual plasmas to heparins: after plasma supplementation with heparins there should be a minimal pre-incubation time of at least 2-fold the ITP50 to obtain nearly full function of heparins. Furthermore, these data provide evidence for an anticoagulant lack phase of some minutes that might be required in clinical heparinization (especially in low dose heparinization) of individual patients.

Keywords: heparin, low molecular weight heparin, enoxaparin, EXCA

* Correspondence to: PD Dr. Med. T. Stief, Department of Clinical Chemistry, University Hospital, D-35043 Marburg, Germany. Email: thstief@med.uni-marburg.de; Tel.+49-6421-58 64471; Fax: +49-6421-58 65594.

INTRODUCTION

Assays for thrombin generation also depend on the plasmatic content of heparins. Heparins need some minutes to associate with antithrombin III [1,2]. Therefore, an adequate preincubation time of heparin with plasma is important to obtain full activity of the heparins. The aim of the present work was to determine the necessary pre-incubation time in an ultra-specific and close-to-physiologic thrombin generation assay that is able to analyze the sensibility of plasma towards heparins at low doses.

MATERIAL AND METHODS

50 µl pooled unfrozen normal citrated plasma (1 part 106 mM sodium citrate + 9 parts of blood of 8 subjects into polypropylene (PP) blood collection tubes, Sarstedt, Nümbrecht, Germany; 10 min centrifugation at 2800g, room temperature (RT), remaining after routine analysis, stored for 4h at RT, pooled into emptied PP tubes) in U-wells polystyrol microtiter plates (NUNC, Wiesbaden, Germany; article nr. 268152, lot nr. 060385; Greiner, Frickenhausen, Germany; article nr. 650161, lot nr. 05281161) were supplemented after 1-11 min (37°C or 23°C) with 2 µl 2.6 IU/ml unfractionated heparin (ratiopharm, Ulm, Germany) or 2.6 IU/ml enoxaparin (Aventis, Frankfurt, Germany), 0.9% NaCl out of siliconized glass vials (DadeBehring, Marburg, Germany; article nr. OVKE49). For control, the plasma sample was supplemented with 2 µl 0.9% NaCl. 5 µl EXCA-trigger [3] (trigger of the extrinsic coagulation activity assay: 1 ml aliquots of once frozen/thawed 1 ng/ml human placental tissue factor without polybrene® (Thromborel S®, Behringwerke, Marburg, Germany), 250 mM $CaCl_2$, 5% human albumin (Kabi, Stockholm, Sweden) in siliconized glass vials) were added in duplicate with 0.9% NaCl-rinsed and completely emptied new polypropylene tips of Eppendorf multipettes®. After 90 s coagulation reaction time of 50 µl plasma + 2 µl heparin + 5 µl EXCA-trigger (final dilution of citrated plasma by < 13%) at 37°C in a digitally controlled water-bath, 100 µl hemostasis – stop reagent were added, that consisted in 2.5 M arginine, pH 8.6, 0.16% Triton X 100® (both from Sigma, Deisenhofen, Germany). After 3 min (RT), 25 µl 1 mM chromogenic thrombin substrate HD-CHG-Ala-Arg-pNA (Pentapharm, Basel, Switzerland) in 1.25 M arginine, pH 8.7, were added. The change in absorbance with time ΔA/t was measured by a microtiter plate photometer with a 1 mA resolution (Milenia; DPC, Los Angeles, USA); maximal ΔA= about 1050 mA, linear range of ΔA = up to about 40% of 1050 mA = 420 mA. The results were calibrated against 1 IU/ml bovine thrombin (DadeBehring) in 6.7% human albumin, that replaced the plasma sample and that resulted in a ΔA/t of about 20 mA/min (RT); 100% EXCA-control = 1.24±0.14 IU thrombin/ml (mean value ± 1 standard deviation).

The results were tested for significance ($p < 0.05$; $X^2 > 3.841$), using the non-categorical → categorical transformation of the chi-square test and 14fold determination of critical values [4]. The intra-assay coefficients of variation of the duplicate determinations were < 10%.

RESULTS AND DISCUSSION

The approximate 50% inhibitory time point (ITP50 = 50% of the whole anticoagulant activity) was obtained after pre-incubations of about 1 min at 37°C for 0.1 IU/ml heparin and of about 3 min at 37°C for 0.1 IU/ml enoxaparin prior to performing the EXCA; if the same experiment was performed at 23°C, the respective ITP50 values were about 1.5fold prolonged. The heparins need at least 2fold the ITP50 for nearly complete anticoagulant efficiency, i.e., for nearly complete association of heparins with antithrombin in plasma (Figure 1).

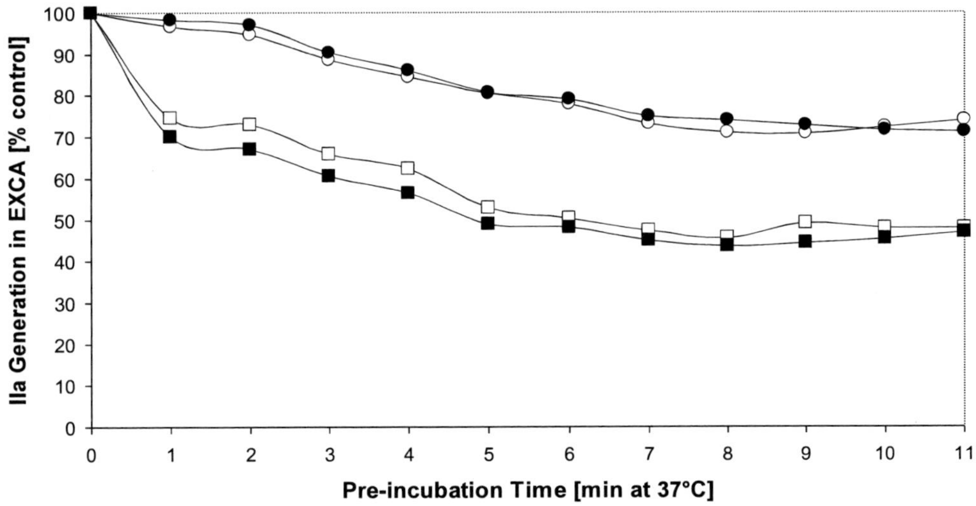

Figure 1. Influence of pre-incubation time on anticoagulant efficiency of low dose heparins. 50 µl pooled normal citrated plasma in U-wells polystyrol microtiter plates (NUNC = white symbols; Greiner = black symbols) were supplemented after 1-11 min (37°C) with 2 µl heparin (squares) or enoxaparin (circles) to obtain final plasma concentrations of 0.1 IU/ml. 5 µl EXCA-trigger (1 ng/ml tissue factor, 250 mM $CaCl_2$, 5% human albumin) were added. After 90 s (37°C), 100 µl 2.5 M arginine, pH 8.6, 0.16% Triton X 100® were added to stop hemostasis activation. After 3 min (23°C), 25 µl 1 mM HD-CHG-Ala-Arg-pNA in 1.25 M arginine, pH 8.7, were added, and $\Delta A/t$ was measured; 0 min pre-incubation time = control without anticoagulant supplementation; IIa = thrombin activity.

In the present thrombin generation experiment there was no significant difference between polystyrol U-wells from different manufacturers. However, untreated polystyrol plates should always be preferred to surface-treated or gamma-irradiated plates, that may become anticoagulant. Presently, untreated polystyrol U-microwells (Brand, Wertheim, Germany; article nr. 701300) are among the best plates for thrombin generation assays.

The used anticoagulant concentration is the approximate 50% inhibitory concentration (IC50) for plasmatic heparin and the approximate IC25 for plasmatic enoxaparin. In conclusion, after plasma supplementation with heparins there should be a minimal pre-incubation time of at least 2fold the ITP50 to obtain nearly complete function of heparins.

The interaction between the by heparin activated serpin antithrombin and thrombin or activated factor X has been described as extremely fast [5]. However the exact ITP50 of low dose heparins when added prior to ultra-specific and close-to-physiologic thrombin generation assays has not been known. The present work describes these ITP50 values for heparin and enoxaparin in plasma. It is of clinical interest to know that a heparin given to a patient needs at least about 2fold the respective ITP50 for nearly complete action. Heparin at therapeutic (high) plasma concentrations might have lower ITP50 values than heparins at prophylactic (low) plasma concentrations. Furthermore, the necessary *in vitro* pre-incubation time of heparins in plasma is important for a better understanding of thrombin generation assays that analyze the heparin sensibility of individual plasma [6].

REFERENCES

[1] Iqbal O, Mousa SA. Antiplatelet, anticoagulant, and thrombolytic drug interactions. *Methods Mol. Med.* 2004; 93: 9-20.

[2] Bick RL, Frenkel EP, Walenga J, Fareed J, Hoppensteadt DA. Unfractionated heparin, low molecular weight heparins, and pentasaccharide: basic mechanism of actions, pharmacology, and clinical use. *Hematol. Oncol. Clin. North Am.* 2005; 19: 1-51.

[3] Stief TW, Wieczerzak A, Renz H. The extrinsic coagulation activity assay. *Clin. Appl. Thromb. Hemost.* 2008; 14: 303-318.

[4] Stief TW. The fibrinogen antigenic turbidimetric assay (FIATA): the X^2x test -- the corrected chi-square comparison against the control-mean. *Clin. Appl. Thromb. Hemost.* 2007; 13: 73-100.

[5] Rau JC, Beaulieu LM, Huntington JA, Church FC. Serpins in thrombosis, hemostasis and fibrinolysis. *J. Thromb Haemost* 2007; 5 Suppl 1: 102-15.

[6] Stief TW, Ajib S, Renz H. The sensibility of individual plasma to heparins. *Hemostasis Laboratory* 2008; 1: (issue 1, in press).

In: Hemostasis Laboratory Yearbook, Volume 2
Editor: Thomas W. Stief, pp. 161-164
ISBN: 978-1-60741-089-8

FRAGMENTED ERYTHROCYTES MODULATE EXTRINSIC COAGULATION ACTIVITY

Thomas W. Stief *
Department of Clinical Chemistry
University Hospital Giessen and Marburg, Germany

ABSTRACT

When cells are fragmented, microparticles (MP) arise that are phospholipid vesicles with strange polynegative niches. MP may cause serious pro-thrombotic hemostasis problems. The ultra-specific, ultra-sensitive thrombin generation assay RECA (recalcified coagulation activity assay) detects subtle alterations of plasmatic coagulation. MP enhance thrombin generation in the RECA. The aim of the present work was to investigate a possible influence of MP without tissue factor (TF) on extrinsic coagulation. The EXCA (extrinsic coagulation activity assay) was performed with 7 individual unfrozen normal citrated plasma samples that had been supplemented with 0-1.5 g/l hemoglobin/MP, derived from hypotonic lysis of erythrocytes of the respective subject. About 1 g/l free plasmatic hemoglobin is a clinically relevant hemoglobin concentration if a patient suffers from *in vivo* hemolysis.

Plasmatic MP modulated extrinsic thrombin generation: first, thrombin generation was inhibited with a 25% inhibitory concentration (IC25) of about 0.1 g/l Hb-MP; the IC50 was approximately 0.75 g/l HB-MP; plasmatic Hb-MP concentrations > 1 g/l might enhance extrinsic IIa generation, possibly by kallikrein-thrombin-mediated activation of factor V. Thus, TF-lacking microparticles are primarily an activator of the intrinsic (and not of the extrinsic) phase of blood coagulation.

Keywords: erythrocyte fragments, microparticles, phospholipid vesicles, EXCA, RECA

INTRODUCTION

Microparticles (MP) are phospholipidic cell fragments [1] that are clinically pro-thrombotic. Especially with the ultra-specific, ultra-sensitive thrombin generation assays RECA (recalcified coagulation activity assay) and INCA (intrinsic coagulation activity assay)

* Correspondence to: PD Dr. Med. T. Stief, Department of Clinical Chemistry, University Hospital, D-35043 Marburg, Germany, Email: thstief@med.uni-marburg.de; Tel.+49-6421-58 64471; Fax +49-6421-58 65594.

the pro-thrombotic nature of MP has been shown [2,3]. The EXCA is a new ultra-specific method to test the extrinsic coagulation activity [4]. Here the influence of MP on EXCA is determined in normal citrated plasma samples.

Material and Methods

50 µl samples of n=7 normal citrated platelet-poor-plasma (1 part 106 mM sodium citrate + 9 parts of blood into polypropylene blood collection tubes, Sarstedt, Nümbrecht, Germany; 10 min centrifugation at 2800g, room temperature (RT); remaining after routine analysis, stored for 4h at 23°C) were supplemented in U-wells microtiter plates (Greiner, Frickenhausen, Germany; article nr. 650161, lot nr. 05281161) with erythrocyte microparticles (Hb-MP), generated by addition of 450 µl H_2O to 50 µl centrifuged erythrocytes (containing about 330 g/l hemoglobin) of the same donor. The final plasma concentration of Hb-MP was 0-1.5 g/l. About 1 g/l free plasmatic hemoglobin is a clinically relevant hemoglobin concentration in *in vivo* hemolysis. 5 µl trigger of EXCA (extrinsic coagulation activity assay; 1 ml aliquots of once frozen/thawed 1 ng/ml human placental tissue factor without polybrene® (Thromborel S®, Behringwerke, Marburg, Germany), 250 mM $CaCl_2$, 5 % human albumin (Kabi, Stockholm, Sweden) in siliconized 15 ml glass vials (Dade Behring; article nr. OVKE49) were added in duplicate by 0.9% NaCl - rinsed and completely emptied new polypropylene tips of Eppendorf multipettes®. After 1 min (37°C, digitally controlled water-bath), 100 µl 2.5 M arginine, pH 8.6, 0.16 % Triton X 100® (both from Sigma, Deisenhofen, Germany) were added. After 3 min (RT), 25 µl 0 or 1 mM chromogenic thrombin substrate HD-CHG-Ala-Arg-pNA (Pentapharm, Basel, Switzerland) in 1.25 M arginine, pH 8.7, were added. The change in absorbance at 405 nm with time ΔA/t was measured by a microtiter plate photometer with a 1 mA resolution (Milenia; DPC, Los Angeles, USA); maximal ΔA= about 1050 mA, linear range of ΔA = up to about 40 % of maximal ΔA = 420 mA. The results were calibrated against 1 IU/ml bovine thrombin (DadeBehring) in 6.7 % human albumin, that replaced the plasma sample and resulted in a specific ΔA of about 20 mA/min (23°C).

Results and Discussion

Figure 1 demonstrates that plasmatic MP modulated extrinsic thrombin (IIa) generation: first, IIa generation was inhibited with a 25% inhibitory concentration (IC25) of about 0.1 g/l Hb-MP; the IC50 was approximately 0.75 g/l HB-MP. Plasmatic Hb-MP concentrations > 1 g/l might enhance extrinsic IIa generation, possibly due to kallikrein – thrombin [5] mediated activation of factor V.

There appeared also a decrease in the turbidity of hemolytic plasma during the chromogenic detection phase, for which the main ΔA/t values of the thrombin generation had to be corrected: 0 g/l Hb-MP plasma had a basal absorbance of 76±14 mA, after 15 min (RT) the basal absorbance was still 76±14 mA. 1.5 g/l Hb-MP plasma had a basal absorbance of 1524±115 mA, after 15 min (RT) the basal absorbance decreased to 1492±123 mA.

The previously observed pronounced EXCA inhibition [3] might be explained by different types of polystyrol microtiterplates (sometimes they might be rather anticoagulant; U-well plates Brand®701300 are among the best).

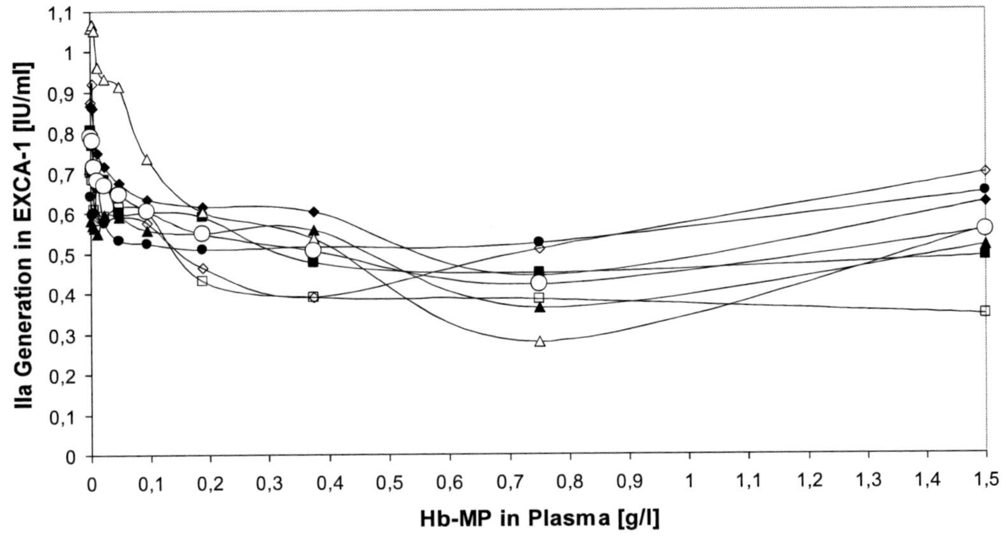

Figure 1. Modulation of extrinsic thrombin generation by erythrocyte microparticles. 50 µl samples of 7 normal plasmas were supplemented in U-wells microtiter plates with erythrocyte microparticles (Hb-MP) to 0-1.5 g/l Hb-MP in plasma. 5 µl EXCA-trigger (1 ng/ml tissue factor, 250 mM $CaCl_2$, 5 % human albumin) were added. After 1 min (37°C), 100 µl 2.5 M arginine, pH 8.6, 0.16 % Triton X 100® were added. After 3 min (23°C), 25 µl 1 mM chromogenic thrombin substrate HD-CHG-Ala-Arg-pNA in 1.25 M arginine, pH 8.7, were added and ΔA/t was measured. The results were calibrated against 1 IU/ml thrombin in 6.7 % human albumin, replacing the plasma sample; each plasma has an individual symbol; mean value of the 7 plasmas (O).

With respect to assay sensitivity for pro-coagulant changes of plasma supplemented with the intrinsic hemostasis trigger Hb-MP the order is: RECA > INCA > EXCA. Microparticles that also contain active tissue factor (e.g. when activated macrophages are destroyed), that can be more potent than intrinsic triggers of hemostasis, might primarily enhance extrinsic (and not intrinsic) coagulation [6,7].

REFERENCES

[1] Piccin A, Murphy WG, Smith OP. Ciruculating microparticles: pathophysiology and clinical implications. *Blood Rev*. 2007; 21: 157-71.

[2] Stief TW. Thrombin generation by hemolysis. *Blood Coagul. Fibrinolysis* 2007; 18: 61-6.

[3] Stief TW. Coagulation activation by lipopolysaccharides. *Clin. Appl. Thromb. Hemost.* 2007 Dec 26; [Epub ahead of print].

[4] Stief TW, Wieczerzak A, Renz H. The extrinsic coagulation activity assay. *Clin. Appl. Thromb. Hemost.* 2008; 14: 303-318.

[5] Stief TW. Kallikrein activates prothrombin. *Clin. Appl. Thromb. Hemost.* 2008 ;14: 97-8.

[6] Redman CW, Sargent IL. Circulating microparticles in normal pregnancy and pre-eclampsia. *Placenta* 2008 Jan 11; [Epub ahead of print].

[7] Saldeen T. Clotting, microembolism, and inhibition of fibrinolysis in adult respiratory distress. *Surg. Clin. North Am.* 1983; 63: 285-304.

In: Hemostasis Laboratory Yearbook, Volume 2
Editor: Thomas W. Stief, pp. 165-176

ISBN: 978-1-60741-089-8

PHOSPHOLIPIDS TRIGGER RECALCIFIED THROMBIN GENERATION

Thomas W. Stief[*]
Department of Clinical Chemistry
University Hospital Giessen and Marburg, Germany

ABSTRACT

Phospholipids are the main components of human cell membranes. With their negatively charged phosphatidyl-heads oriented towards inside or outside the cell they form polynegative bilayers. They differ with respect to the ligands at the phosphatidyl-group: there might be a choline (PC), a ethanolamine (PE), or a serine (PS). PS is slightly more negatively charged than PE or PC, which might have an effect on coagulation. The aim of the present work was to measure the thrombin generating capacity of different phospholipids in the ultra-specific, ultra-sensitive thrombin generation tests recalcified coagulation activity assay (RECA), intrinsic coagulation activity assay (INCA), and extrinsic coagulation activity assay (EXCA).

20 µl samples of individual and pooled unfrozen normal citrated plasma was supplemented with 20 µl PC, PE, or PS of different concentrations and were analyzed in the ultra-specific, ultra-sensitive thrombin generation assays RECA, INCA, and EXCA.

The approximate 200% stimulatory concentrations (SC200) for pooled normal plasma in RECA-20 were 0.5 mM PS, 1.3 mM PE, and 4.8 mM PC. When individual plasmas were tested, there were only slight differerences in the action of the PS, PE, or PC. The approximate 50% inhibitory concentrations (IC50) on the usual INCA-4 were 0.5 mM PE, 0.6 mM PS, or 1.1 mM PC. The phospholipids inhibited tissue factor - triggered thrombin generation in the EXCA at approximate IC50 values of 0.5 mM PS, PE, or PC.

It seems that the real cause of prothrombotic tendencies of some cell membranes is not the PS flop (PS translocation towards outside) but rather the membrane instability itself with generation of multiple polynegative niches within the altered membrane or within PL microparticles.

Keywords: phospholipids, phosphatidylserine, phosphatidylethanolamine, phosphatedylcholine, thrombin generation, RECA, INCA, EXCA

[*] Correspondence to: PD Dr. Med. T. Stief, Department of Clinical Chemistry, University Hospital, D-35043 Marburg, Germany. Email: thstief@med.uni-marburg.de; Tel. +49-6421-58 64471; Fax: +49-6421-58 65594.

INTRODUCTION

The main part of human cell membranes are the phospholipids (PL). Most PL consist of a glycerol backbone with two fatty acids at the first two C atoms of glycerol and a phosphate group at the third C atom. The negatively charged phosphatidyl-group is ligated to other organic compounds, as e.g. to the positively charged molecules choline (PC; lecithines) or ethanolamine (PE), and to the positively and negatively charged serine (PS). Erythrocyte membranes consist of about 60-70% PC, 20 % PE, and 6% PS [1]. The PL can move from the outer PL bilayer towards the inner one, which is called flipping and from the inner PL bilayer towards the outer one, which is called flopping. The respective flipping capacity is PC>PE>PS [2]. This transbilayer migration = flip - flop (= to inside – to outside) can be catalyzed by specific enhancers, such as the translocases [3-7]. Membranes with an increased content of phosphatidylserines (PS) are less stable; a membrane activation or membrane instability may increase the PS content and viceversa [8-11].

The slightly more negatively charged PS (when compared with other PL) is thought to play a role in hemostasis: coagulation enzymes might attach better to PS than to another PL [12]. However, PS externalization and microparticle (MP) generation seem to be coupled mechanisms in platelets [13,14]. Thus, the prothrombotic changes of PS flopping might also be primarily due to nascending strange polynegative niches: PL layers are polynegative surfaces; if pathologically folded they possess multiple niches that are often unphysiologic and activate the intrinsic system of blood hemostasis [20]. Therefore, the aim of the present study was to investigate the influence of phospholipids on coagulation using ultra-specific tests for plasmatic thrombin generation [21,22].

MATERIAL AND METHODS

Thrombin Generation in Recalcified Individual Normal Plasmas by Phospholipids (PL)

20 µl unfrozen citrated plasma (0.5 ml 106 mM sodium citrate + 4.5 ml venous blood; centrifugation at 2800g for 10 min at 23°C) from 6 individual subjects (remaining after routine analysis; remaining after routine analysis, stored for about 5h at 23°C; at the time point when the samples are usually thrown away) were pipetted into polystyrol F-well microtiter plates (Brand, Wertheim, Germany; pureGrade® article nr. 781602). 20 µl 0.9% NaCl, 20 mM phosphatidylethanolamine (PE; 1,2-dipalmitoyl-sn-glycero-3-phospho-ethanolamine; molecular weight (MW) = 692 Dalton (D); Sigma; article nr. P 1348-25MG), 20 mM phosphatidylserine (PS; 1,2-dipalmitoyl-sn-glycero-3-phospho-L-serine; MW=758 D; Sigma, Deisenhofen, Germany, article nr. P 1185-10MG), 20 mM phosphatidylcholine (PC; 1,2-dipalmitoyl-sn-glycero-3-phospho-choline; MW= 734 D; Sigma, article nr. P 4329-25MG), 10 mM PE, or 10 mM PS, all in 0.9% NaCl (37°C) were added. Afterwards, 2 µl 250 mM $CaCl_2$ were added. This reagent is the trigger for the recalcified coagulation activity assay (RECA): 1000 µl aliquots of 250 mM $CaCl_2$ in siliconized glass vials (DadeBehring; article nr. OVKE49) and stored frozen at -30°C. After 0-60 min coagulation reaction time (CRT at 37°C) 50 µl 2.5 M arginine, 0.16% Triton X 100®, pH 8.6 (Sigma) were added.

After 3 min (23°C), 25 µl 0.67 mM HD-CHG-Ala-Arg-pNA (Pentapharm, Basel, Switzerland, article nr. 081-20) in 1.25 M arginine, pH 8.7 were added and $\Delta A_{405\ nm}/t$ (23°C) was determined by a microtiter plate photometer with a 1 mA resolution (Milenia; DPC, Los Angeles, USA). The results were standardized against 1 IU/ml bovine thrombin (DadeBehring, Marburg, Germany) in 6.7% human albumin (Kabi, Stockholm, Sweden), replacing the plasma sample [21].

Thrombin Generation in Recalcified Pooled Unfrozen Normal Plasma by PL

20 µl pooled unfrozen citrated normal plasma were pipetted into polystyrol U-well microtiter plates (Brand, Wertheim, Germany; article nr. 701300). 20 µl 0.9 % NaCl, 10 mM PS or 10 mM phosphatidylcholine (L-α-phosphatidylcholine type IV; Sigma, article nr. P3644-25G) both in 0.9% NaCl were added. After 20 min (23°C) 2 µl 250 mM $CaCl_2$ (RECA-trigger) were added. After 0-11 min CRT (37°C) 50 µl 2.5 M arginine, 0.16% Triton X 100®, pH 8.6 were added. After 3 min (23°C), 25 µl 0.67 mM HD-CHG-Ala-Arg-pNA in 1.25 M arginine, pH 8.7 were added and $\Delta A_{405\ nm}/t$ (23°C) was determined. The results were standardized against 1 IU/ml bovine thrombin in 6.7% human albumin, replacing the plasma sample and resulting into a ΔA of about 10 mA/min (23°C).

Thrombin Generation in Recalcified Pooled Unfrozen Normal Plasma by PL

U-well microtiter plates were pre-filled with 20 µl 0-10 mM PS, PE, or PC. 20 µl pooled unfrozen (≤ 2h old, stored at 23°C) citrated plasma of 6 healthy donors that gave informed consent were added. Immediately thereafter, 2 µl RECA-trigger were added. After 10 min and 20 min (RECA-10 or RECA-20 = main values) or 30 min (RECA-30 = control value) (37°C) 50 µl arginine-reagent (2.5 M arginine, pH 8.6, 0.16% Triton X 100®) were added. After 3 min (23°C) 25 µl 1 mM chromogenic thrombin substrate HD-CHG-Ala-Arg-pNA in 1.25 M arginine, pH 8.7, were added and ΔA at 405 nm and ΔA at 450 nm were determined and ΔA at 405 nm minus ΔA at 450 nm was calculated. The results were standardized against 1 IU/ml thrombin in 6.7% human albumin replacing the plasma samples. All RECA-20/RECA-30 ratios were < 1, i.e. a given thrombin generation curve was at 10 or 20 min CRT in its ascending part.

Thrombin Generation in Recalcified Individual Unfrozen Normal Plasmas by PL

20 µl unfrozen (≤ 2h old, stored at 23°C) citrated plasma of n=4 healthy donors (after informed consent) were added to 20 µl 0-10 mM PS, PE, or PC in 0.9% NaCl in U-microwells. The RECA was performed with 30 min or 40 min CRT (RECA-30 = main value; RECA-40 = control value). All RECA-30/RECA-40 ratios were < 1, i.e. a given thrombin generation curve was at 30 min CRT in its ascending part.

Inhibition of Intrinsic Coagulation Activity Assay (INCA) by PL

U-well microtiter plates were pre-filled with 20 µl 0-10 mM PS, PE, or PC. 20 µl pooled unfrozen plasma of 8 healthy donors or of two individual healthy donors were added. 2 µl strong INCA-trigger (500 µl 500 mM $CaCl_2$ aliquoted in siliconized glass vials (DadeBehring; article nr. OVKE49), stored frozen at -30°C, thawed at 23°C + 500 µl Pathromtin SL® (SiO_2 based activator of the activated partial thromboplastin time; DadeBehring)) or weak INCA-trigger (500 µl 500 mM $CaCl_2$ + 400 µl H_2O + 100 µl Pathromtin SL®) were added. After 4 min (37°C) 50 µl arginine-reagent (2.5 M arginine, pH 8.6, 0.16% Triton X 100®) were added. After 3 min (23°C) 25 µl 1 mM chromogenic thrombin substrate HD-CHG-Ala-Arg-pNA in 1.25 M arginine, pH 8.7, were added and ΔA at 405 nm and ΔA at 450 nm were determined and ΔA at 405 nm minus ΔA at 450 nm was calculated. The results were standardized against 1 IU/ml thrombin in 6.7% human albumin, replacing the plasma samples [21].

Inhibition of Extrinsic Coagulation Activity Assay (EXCA) by PL

U-well microtiter plates were pre-filled with 20 µl 0-10 mM PS, PE, or PC in 0.9% NaCl. 20 µl pooled unfrozen plasma of 8 healthy donors or of two individual healthy donors were added. 2 µl EXCA-trigger (1 ng/ml human placental tissue factor (Behringwerke, Marburg, Germany), 250 mM $CaCl_2$, 5% human albumin, aliquoted in siliconized glass vials) were added. After 1 min (37°C) 50 µl arginine-reagent (2.5 M arginine, pH 8.6, 0.16% Triton X 100®) were added. After 3 min (23°C) 25 µl 1 mM chromogenic thrombin substrate HD-CHG-Ala-Arg-pNA in 1.25 M arginine, pH 8.7, were added and ΔA at 405 nm and ΔA at 450 nm were determined and ΔA at 405 nm minus ΔA at 450 nm was calculated. The results were standardized against 1 IU/ml thrombin in 6.7% human albumin, replacing the plasma samples [21].

Results and Discussion

Figure 1 demonstrates that PL enhanced thrombin generation in recalcified normal plasma. The greatest enhancer of thrombin (IIa) generation was PC, followed by PS and then by PE. At 10 min CRT the added PL increased IIa activity from 0.025 IU/ml (basal IIa value without CRT = 0.01 IU/ml) to about 0.1-1 IU/ml.

Figure 2 shows that both 4.5 mM PC and 4.5 mM PS were activators of IIa generation in RECA, especially when plasma and PL were pre-incubated for 20 min (23°C): then 3 min CRT (37°C) were sufficient to generate about 0.4 IU/ml thrombin.

Figure 3 demonstrates that PS enhanced recalcified thrombin generation more than PE or PC, especially in pooled unfrozen normal plasma (Figure 3a). The approximate 200% stimulatory concentrations (SC200 = 200% effective dose) for pooled unfrozen plasma in RECA-20 were 0.5 mM PS, 1.3 mM PE, or 4.8 mM PC. When individual plasmas were tested, there were only slight differerences in the action of the PS, PE, or PC (Figure 3b,c).

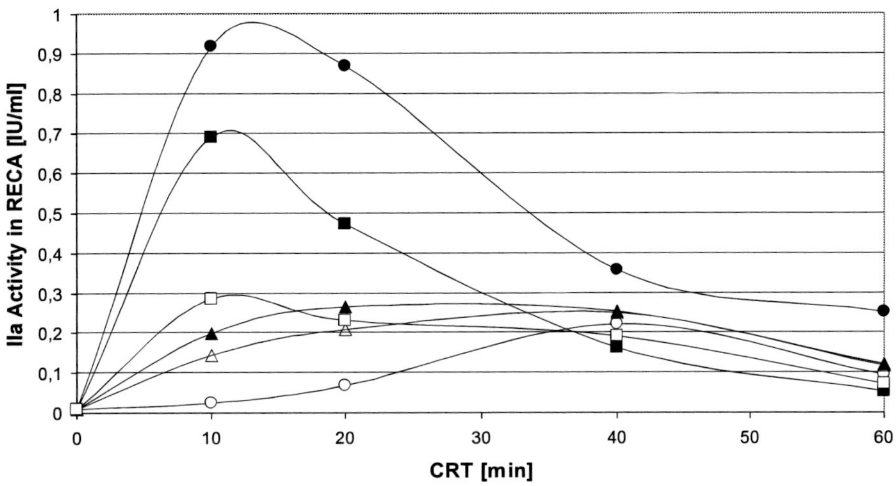

a

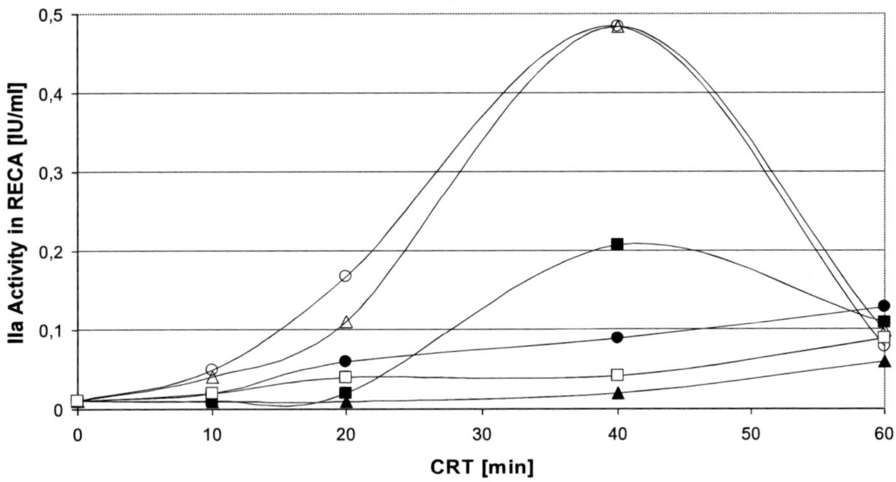

b

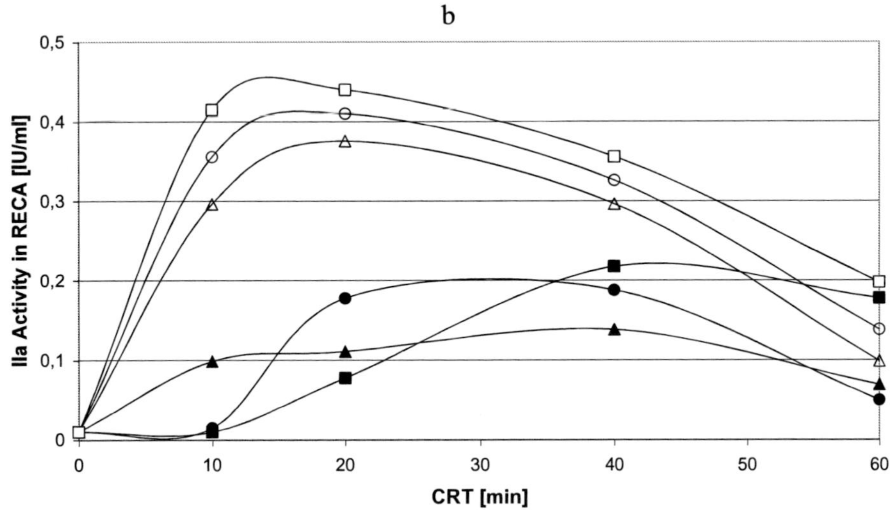

Figure 1 (continued)

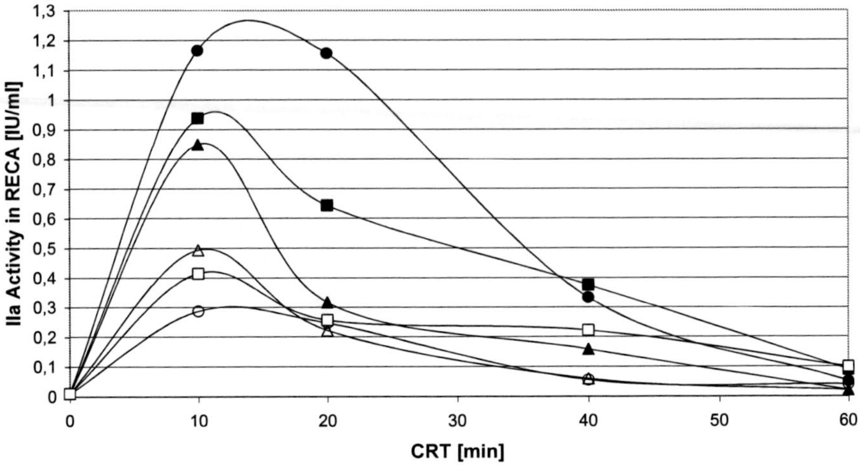

d

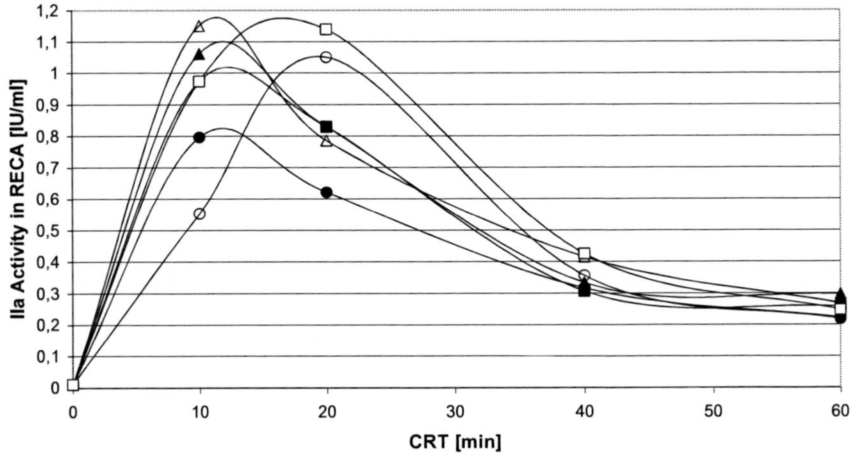

e

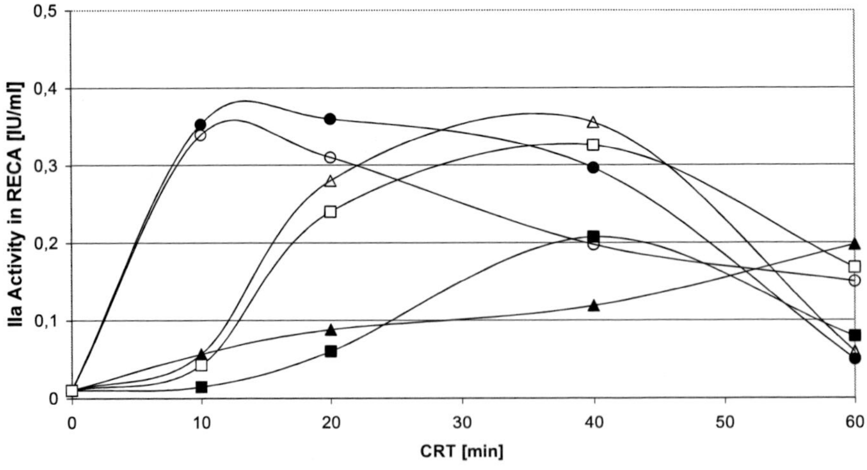

Figure 1 (continued)

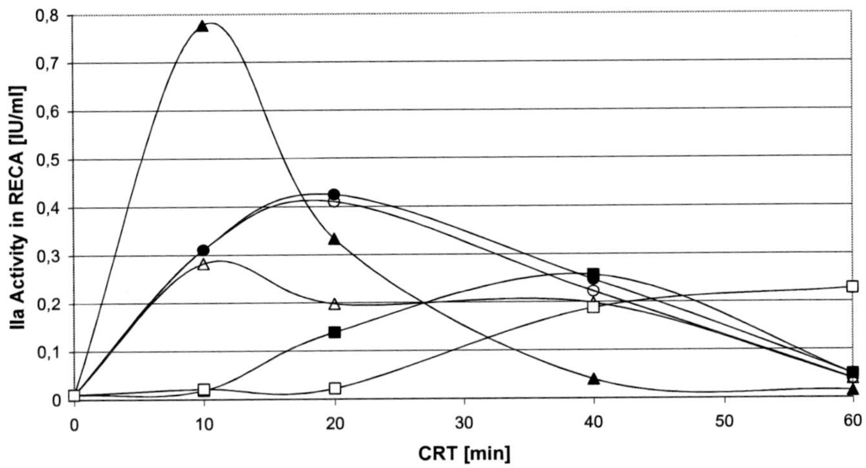

g

Figure 1. Enhanced thrombin generation in individual normal plasmas by phospholipids. 20 µl unfrozen citrated plasma from 6 individual subjects were pipetted into polystyrol F-well microwells. 20 µl 0.9% NaCl (O), 20 mM phosphatidylethanolamine (PE; ▲), 20 mM phosphatidylserine (PS; ■), 20 mM phosphatidylcholine (PC; •), 10 mM PE (Δ), or 10 mM PS (□), all in 0.9% NaCl (37°C) were added. Then 2 µl 250 mM $CaCl_2$ were added. After 0-60 min coagulation reaction time (CRT at 37°C) of this recalcified coagulation activity assay (RECA) 50 µl 2.5 M arginine, 0.16% Triton X 100, pH 8.6 were added. After 3 min (23°C), 25 µl 0.67 mM HD-CHG-Ala-Arg-pNA in 1.25 M arginine, pH 8.7 were added and ΔA/t (23°C) was determined. The results were standardized against 1 IU/ml thrombin (IIa) in 6.7 % human albumin, replacing the plasma sample. Fig. 1a: mean values of 6 individual samples. Figures 1b-1g: 6 individual plasma samples (each individual sample has an individual symbol) triggered by addition of 0.9% NaCl (zero-control; Figure 1b), 9.5 mM final PE (Figure 1c), 9.5 mM final PS (Figure 1d), 9.5 mM final PC (Figure 1e), 4.8 mM final PE (Fig. 1f), 4.8 mM final PS (Figure 1g).

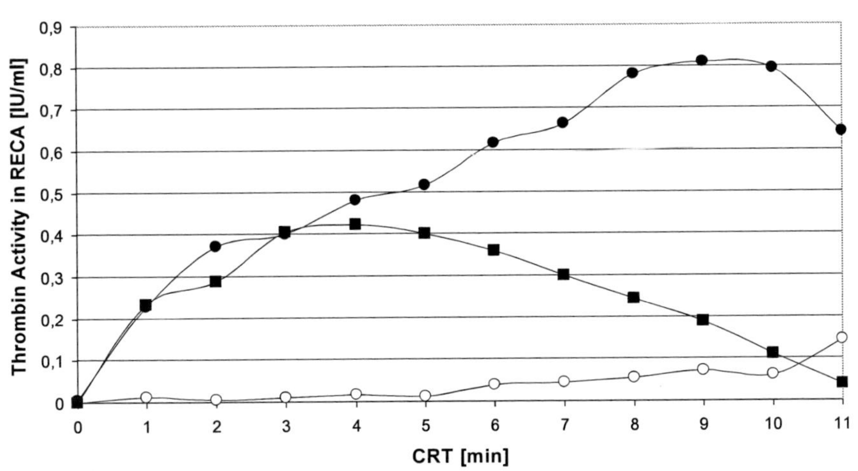

Figure 2. Enhanced IIa generation in pooled normal plasma by phospholipids. 20 µl pooled unfrozen normal citrated plasma were pipetted into polystyrol U-well microtiter plates. 20 µl 0.9% NaCl (O), 10 mM phosphatidylserine, or 10 mM phosphatidylcholine both in 0.9% NaCl were added. After 20 min (23°C) 2 µl 250 mM $CaCl_2$ were added. After 0-11 min CRT (37°C) of this RECA 50 µl 2.5 M arginine, 0.16 % Triton X 100, pH 8.6 were added. After 3 min (23°C), 25 µl 0.67 mM HD-CHG-Ala-Arg-pNA in 1.25 M arginine, pH 8.7 were added and ΔA/t (23°C) was determined.

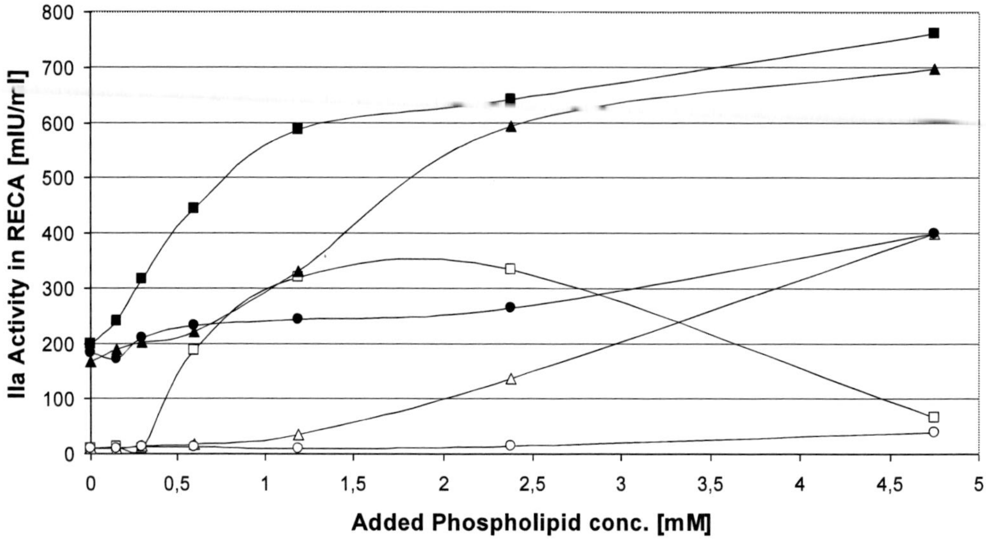

(a)

Figure 3 (a). Enhanced IIa generation in pooled normal plasma by phospholipids. U-microwells were pre-filled with 20 µl 0-10 mM PS (□,■), PE (Δ,▲), or PC (O,●). 20 µl pooled unfrozen citrated plasma of 6 healthy donors were added. Immediately thereafter, 2 µl 250 mM $CaCl_2$ were added. After 10 min (white symbols) or 20 min (black symbols) CRT (37°C) of this RECA 50 µl arginine-reagent (2.5 M arginine, pH 8.6, 0.16% Triton X 100®) were added. After 3 min (23°C) 25 µl 1 mM chromogenic thrombin substrate HD-CHG-Ala-Arg-pNA in 1.25 M arginine, pH 8.7, were added and ΔA at 405 nm and ΔA at 450 nm were determined and ΔA at 405 nm minus ΔA at 450 nm was calculated.

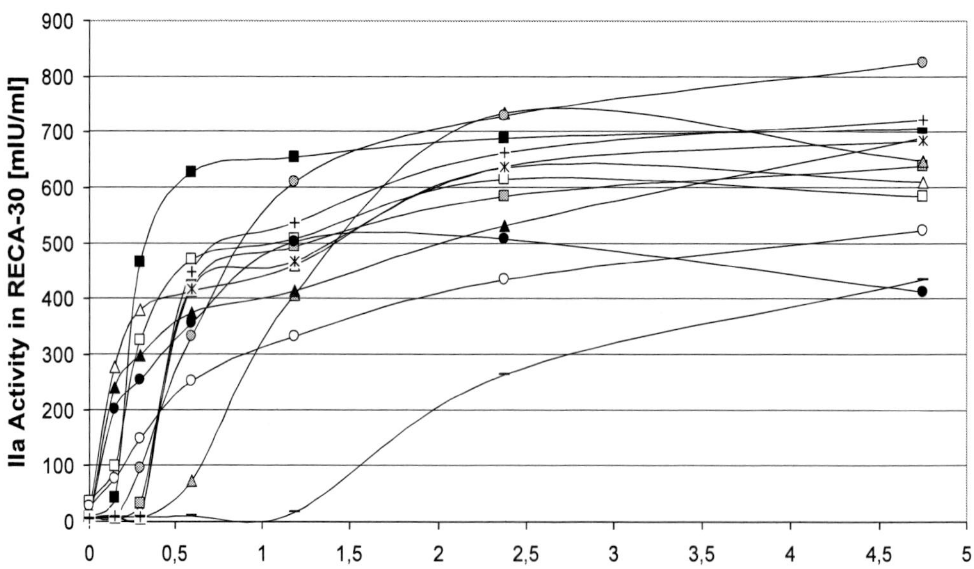

(b)

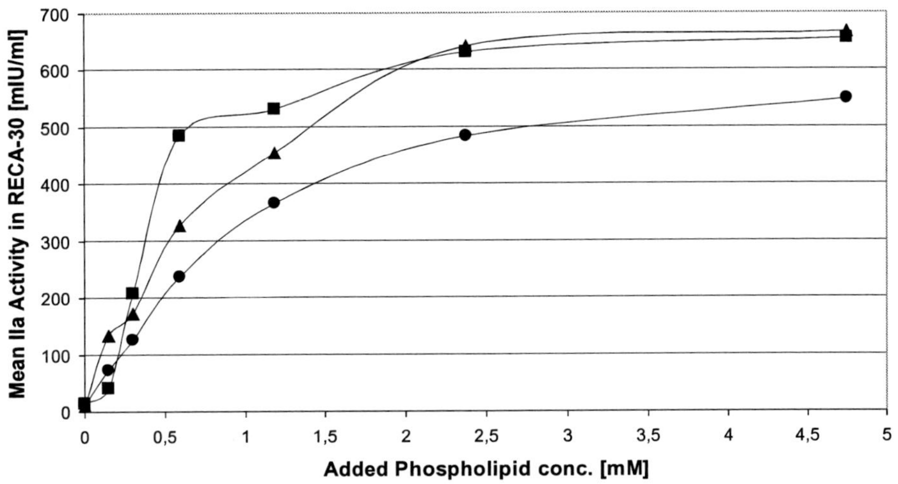

(c)

Figure 3 (b) and (c). Enhanced IIa generation in individual unfrozen plasma by phospholipids. 20 µl unfrozen citrated plasma of n=4 healthy donors (donor1=white symbols, donor2=grey symbols, donor3= black symbols, donor4= *,+,-) were added to 20 µl 0-10 mM PS (squares or *), PE (triangles or +), or PC (circles or -) in 0.9% NaCl in U-well plates were analyzed in the RECA with 30 min coagulation reaction time (RECA-30)(Figure 3b). Figure 3c represents the mean values for these 4 normal samples.

The PL seemed to have different enhancing effects especially on pooling-induced (antigen/antibody/complement mediated) pre-kallikrein to kallikrein activation [15,16].

The PL only moderately modulated thrombin generation induced by SiO_2 in a strong INCA (Figure 4a). In the usual weak INCA the approximate 50% inhibitory concentrations (IC50) were 0.5 mM PE, 0.6 mM PS, or 1.1 mM PC (Figure 4b).

The PL inhibited TF-triggered thrombin generation in the EXCA at approximate IC50 concentrations of 0.5 mM PL (PS, PE, or PC) (Figure 5).

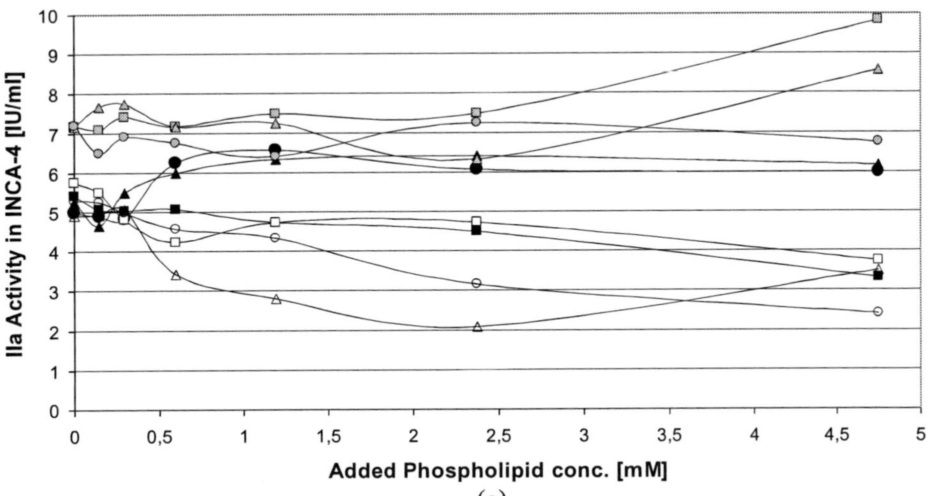

(a)

Figure 4. (Continued)

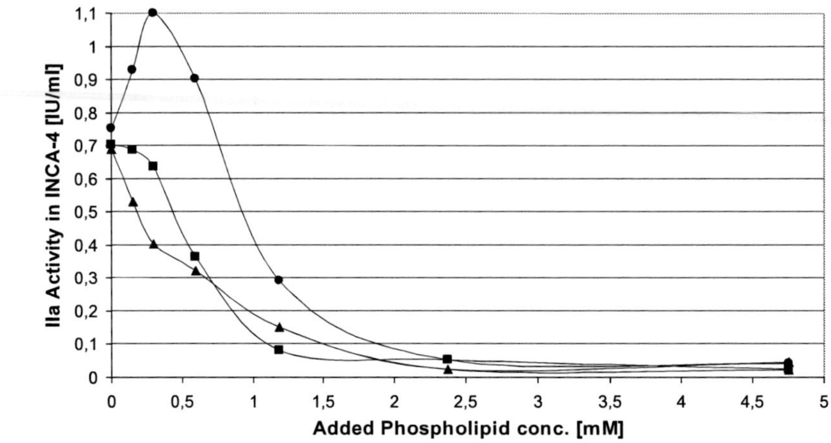

(b)

Figure 4. Inhibition of intrinsic coagulation activity assay (INCA) by phospholipids. U-microwells were pre-filled with 20 µl 0-10 mM PS (■), PE (▲), or PC (●). 20 µl pooled unfrozen citrated plasma of 8 healthy donors (black symbols) or of two individual healthy donors (donor 1: PS (□), PE (Δ), PC (O); donor 2: PS (grey□), PE (greyΔ), or PC (greyO)) were added. 2 µl strong INCA-trigger (Figure 4a: 500 µl 500 mM $CaCl_2$ + 500 µl Pathromtin SL®) or weak INCA-trigger (Figure 4b: 500 µl 500 mM $CaCl_2$ + 400 µl H_2O + 100 µl Pathromtin SL®) were added. After 4 min (37°C) 50 µl arginine-reagent (2.5 M arginine, pH 8.6, 0.16% Triton X 100®) were added. After 3 min (23°C) 25 µl 1 mM thrombin substrate HD-CHG-Ala-Arg-pNA in 1.25 M arginine, pH 8.7, were added and ΔA at 405 nm and ΔA at 450 nm were determined and ΔA at 405 nm minus ΔA at 450 nm was calculated.

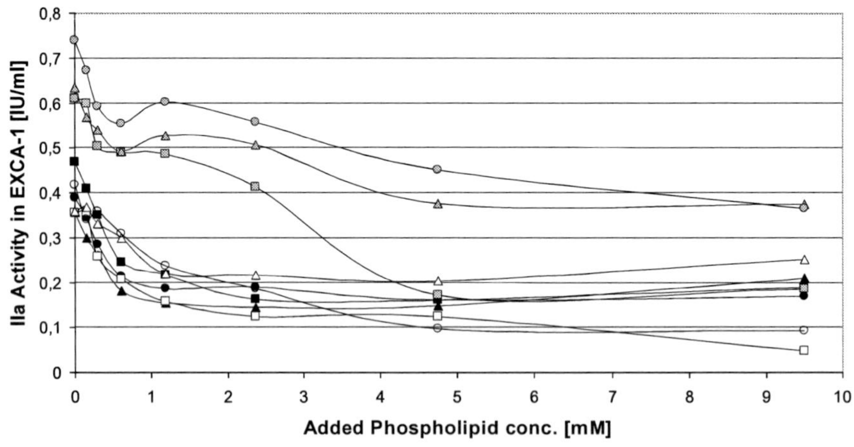

Figure 5. Inhibition of extrinsic coagulation activity assay (EXCA) by phospholipids. U-microwells were pre-filled with 20 µl 0-10 mM PS (■), PE (▲), or PC (●) in 0.9% NaCl. 20 µl pooled unfrozen citrated plasma of 8 healthy donors (black symbols) or of two individual healthy donors (donor 1: PS (□), PE (Δ), PC (O); donor 2: PS (grey□), PE (greyΔ), or PC (greyO)) were added. 2 µl EXCA-trigger (1 ng/ml human tissue factor, 250 mM $CaCl_2$, 5% human albumin) were added. After 1 min (37°C) 50 µl arginine-reagent (2.5 M arginine, pH 8.6, 0.16% Triton X 100®) were added. After 3 min (23°C) 25 µl 1 mM chromogenic thrombin substrate HD-CHG-Ala-Arg-pNA in 1.25 M arginine, pH 8.7, were added and ΔA at 405 nm and ΔA at 450 nm were determined and ΔA at 405 nm minus ΔA at 450 nm was calculated. The results were standardized against 1 IU/ml thrombin.

The present data do not support the concept that it is just the flopping of PS [3-11,17-19] that makes a cell membrane procoagulant. Instead, it seems that the real cause of prothrombotic tendencies of altered cell membranes is the membrane instability with generation of multiple polynegative niches within the modified membrane or within PL microparticles that induce a pre-kallikrein to kallikrein folding [16,20]. Phosphatidylinositol is a PL that participates in cellular signalling [23-25]; PL of the PC, PE, or PS type could also be involved in pro-thrombinic pathways of cellular signalling [26-28].

REFERENCES

[1] Boon JM, Smith BD. Chemical control of phospholipid distribution across bilayer membranes. *Med. Res. Rev.* 2002; 22: 251-81.

[2] Wu G, Hubbell WL. Phospholipid asymmetry and transmembrane diffusion in photoreceptor disc membranes. *Biochemistry* 1993; 32: 879-88.

[3] Smriti, Nemergut EC, Daleke DL. ATP-dependent transport of phosphatidylserine analogues in human erythrocytes. *Biochemistry* 2007; 46: 2249-59.

[4] Pomorski T, Menon AK. Lipid flippases and their biological functions. *Cell Mol. Life Sci.* 2006; 63: 2908-21.

[5] Gummadi SN, Kumar KS. The mystery of phospholipid flip-flop in biogenic membranes. *Cell Mol. Biol. Lett* 2005; 10: 101-21.

[6] Shukla R, Sasaki Y, Krchnák V, Smith BD. Identification of synthetic phosphatidylserine translocases from a combinatorial library prepared by directed split-and-pool synthesis. *J. Comb. Chem.* 2004; 6: 703-9.

[7] Sasaki Y, Shukla R, Smith BD. Facilitated phosphatidylserine flip-flop across vesicle and cell membranes using urea-derived synthetic translocases. *Org. Biomol. Chem.* 2004; 2: 214-9.

[8] Stebelska K, Dubielecka PM, Sikorski AF. The effect of PS content on the ability of natural membranes to fuse with positively charged liposomes and lipoplexes. *J. Membr. Biol.* 2005; 206: 203-14.

[9] Nusbaum P, Lainé C, Seveau S, Lesavre P, Halbwachs-Mecarelli L. Early membrane events in polymorphonuclear cell (PMN) apoptosis: membrane blebbing and vesicle release, CD43 and CD16 down-regulation and phosphatidylserine externalization. *Biochem. Soc. Trans* 2004; 32: 477-9.

[10] Frasch SC, Henson PM, Nagaosa K, Fessler MB, Borregaard N, Bratton DL. Phospholipid flip-flop and phospholipid scramblase 1 (PLSCR1) co-localize to uropod rafts in formylated Met-Leu-Phe-stimulated neutrophils. *J. Biol. Chem.* 2004; 279: 17625-33.

[11] Bratton DL, Fadok VA, Richter DA, Kailey JM, Guthrie LA, Henson PM. Appearance of phosphatidylserine on apoptotic cells requires calcium-mediated nonspecific flip-flop and is enhanced by loss of the aminophospholipid translocase. *J. Biol. Chem.* 1997; 272: 26159-65.

[12] Boon JM, Lambert TN, Sisson AL, Davis AP, Smith BD. Facilitated phosphatidylserine (PS) flip-flop and thrombin activation using a synthetic PS scramblase. *J. Am. Chem. Soc.* 2003; 125: 8195-201.

[13] N. Satta; F. Toti; E. Fressinaud; D. Meyer; J.-M. Freyssinet. Scott syndrome: an inherited defect of the procoagulant activity of platelets. *Platelets* 1997; 8: 117 – 124.

[14] Comfurius P, Williamson P, Smeets EF, Schlegel RA, Bevers EM, Zwaal RF. Reconstitution of phospholipid scramblase activity from human blood platelets. *Biochemistry* 1996; 35: 7631-4.

[15] Stief TW. Inhibition of thrombin generation in recalcified plasma. *Blood Coagul. Fibrinolysis* 2007; 18: 751-60.

[16] Stief TW. Kallikrein activates prothrombin. *Clin. Appl. Thromb. Hemost.* 2008; 14: 97-8.

[17] Devaux PF, Herrmann A, Ohlwein N, Kozlov MM. How lipid flippases can modulate membrane structure. *Biochim. Biophys. Acta* 2008 Apr 1. [Epub ahead of print].

[18] van Meer G, Voelker DR, Feigenson GW. Membrane lipids: where they are and how they behave. *Nat. Rev. Mol. Cell Biol.* 2008; 9: 112-24.

[19] Zhou Z. New phosphatidylserine receptors: clearance of apoptotic cells and more. *Dev. Cell* 2007; 13: 759-60.

[20] Stief TW. Coagulation activation by lipopolysaccharides. *Clin. Appl. Thromb. Hemost* 2007 Dec 26. [Epub ahead of print].

[21] Stief TW. Innovative tests of plasmatic hemostasis. *Laboratory Medicine* 2008; 39: 225-30.

[22] Stief TW. Laboratory diagnosis of the pre-phase of pathologic disseminated intravascular coagulation. *Hemostasis Laboratory* 2008; 1: (issue 1, in press).

[23] Sasaki T, Sasaki J, Sakai T, Takasuga S, Suzuki A. The physiology of phosphoinositides. *Biol. Pharm. Bull.* 2007; 30: 1599-604.

[24] Lefèvre B, Pesty A, Courtot AM, Martins CV, Broca O, Denys A, Arnault E, Poirot C, Avazeri N. The phosphoinositide-phospholipase C (PI-PLC) pathway in the mouse oocyte. *Crit. Rev. Eukaryot. Gene Expr.* 2007; 17: 259-69.

[25] Martelli AM, Cocco L, Capitani S, Miscia S, Papa S, Manzoli FA. Nuclear phosphatidylinositol 3,4,5-trisphosphate, phosphatidylinositol 3-kinase, Akt, and PTen: emerging key regulators of anti-apoptotic signaling and carcinogenesis. *Eur. J. Histochem.* 2007; 51 Suppl 1: 125-31.

[26] Lambeau G, Gelb MH. Biochemistry and physiology of mammalian secreted phospholipases A(2). *Annu. Rev. Biochem.* 2008 Apr 11. [Epub ahead of print].

[27] Yeung T, Grinstein S. Lipid signaling and the modulation of surface charge during phagocytosis. *Immunol. Rev.* 2007; 219: 17-36.

[28] Matsumoto T, Kobayashi T, Kamata K. Role of lysophosphatidylcholine (LPC) in atherosclerosis. *Curr. Med. Chem.* 2007; 14: 3209-20.

In: Hemostasis Laboratory Yearbook, Volume 2
Editor: Thomas W. Stief, pp. 177-182

ISBN: 978-1-60741-089-8

HYDROXY-ETHYL-STARCH (HES) TRIGGERS PLASMATIC THROMBIN GENERATION

Thomas W. Stief *
Department of Clinical Chemistry
University Hospital Giessen and Marburg, Germany

ABSTRACT

Severe hemorrhage or shock are clinical indications for replacement of volume. For volume replacement plasma expanders of the type of hydroxy-ethyl-starch (HES) or of the dextran type might be used or the volume is replaced by infusion of a crystalloid. Since such changes of the plasma matrix might influence normal hemostasis, the aim of this work was to measure thrombin generation in the ultra-specific, ultra-sensitive recalcified coagulation activity assay (RECA) upon recalcification of 20 µl pooled unfrozen normal citrated plasma that had been supplemented with HES of 200 kDa, HES of 70 kDa, dextran of 40 kDa, or 0.9% NaCl.

If increasing amounts of 0.9% NaCl were added to pooled normal plasma, the thrombin generation in RECA increased from < 50 mIU/ml IIa for 0-4 µl 0.9% NaCl added to 20 µl plasma to about 600 mIU/ml IIa for 6-14 µl NaCl added to 20 µl plasma, i.e. infusion of > 0.5-1 litre of volume per 3 litres of plasma can be prothrombotic. Using this volume of HES-200kDa or of HES-70kDa, the thrombin generation in RECA-30 increased about 5fold or about 8fold, respectively; with this volume of dextran the thrombin generation in RECA-30 increased about twice, when compared with the 0.9 % NaCl control.

Thus, HES may trigger the intrinsic phase of blood coagulation, especially at final plasma concentrations > 0.5%. The present data support the concept that for clinically mandatory volume replacement the plasma expanders of the HES or the dextran type might induce more hemostasis problems than just the replacement with NaCl-like solutions.

Keywords: hydroxy-ethyl-starch (HES), dextran, NaCl, volume replacement, RECA, thrombin generation.

* Correspondence to: PD Dr. Med. T. Stief, Department of Clinical Chemistry, University Hospital, D-35043 Marburg, Germany. Email: thstief@med.uni-marburg.de; Tel.: +49-6421-58 64471; Fax: +49-6421-58 65594.

INTRODUCTION

Plasma expanders are controversial drugs in intensive care medicine [1-4]. Hydroxy-ethyl-starch (HES) is a clinically important plasma expander. Since HES due to his multiple oxygen atoms is a polynegative molecule it might activate the contact (intrinsic) phase of hemostasis [5]. The aim of the present study was to investigate the influence of plasma supplemented with HES, dextran, or 0.9% NaCl on plasmatic coagulation activation, assayed by a new ultra–specific ultra-sensitive, and close-to-physiologic thrombin generation test: the recalcified coagulation activity assay (RECA) [6-8].

MATERIAL AND METHODS

Different Final Plasmatic Concentrations of Hydroxy-Ethyl-Starch (HES)

100 µl pooled normal citrated plasma (from 6 individual samples, remaining after routine analysis; citrated plasma = 0.5 ml 106 mM sodium citrate + 4.5 ml venous blood in polypropylene (PP) tubes; Sarstedt, Nümbrecht, Germany, pooling in emptied new PP tubes) in U-well microtiter plates (Brand; article nr. 701300) were supplemented with 20 µl 10% HES 200 kDa (Fresenius, Bad Homburg, Germany) or 6% HES 70 kDa (Braun, Melsungen, Germany). 60 µl of this mixture were withdrawn and diluted repetitively 1+1 on the microtiter plate with 60 µl sample (50 µl normal pool + 10 µl 0.9% NaCl). Then 5 µl RECA-trigger were added. After 20 min at 37°C (RECA-20) 100 µl arginine reagent were added. After 3 min (23°C) 25 µl 1 mM chromogenic substrate reagent were added and ΔA at 405 nm was determined. The 1 IU/ml thrombin standard resulted in a ΔA of about 20 mA/min (23°C). The maximal ΔA was about 1050 mA, the linear ΔA range was up to 40% of 1050 mA = 420 mA. The same experiment was performed with pooled normal plasma diluted 1+1 with 0.9 % NaCl in emptied new PP tubes prior to performance of the RECA.

Different Volumes Added to Pooled Normal Plasma

20 µl unfrozen pooled normal citrated plasma (from 4 individual samples; remaining after routine analysis) in polystyrol flat bottom wells (F-wells; Brand, Wertheim, Germany; pureGrade®, article nr. 781602) were supplemented in duplicate at 23°C by means of an Eppendorf-multipette® (0.9% NaCl - rinsed tips) with 0-14 µl

1. HAES-steril 10%® (HES of molecular weight (MW) = 200 kilo Dalton (kD), substitution grade 0.43-0.55 = HES-200kDa),
2. Rheohes 6%® (HES of MW = 70 kDa, substitution grade 0.58 = HES-70kDa),
3. Rheomacrodex 10% (dextran; MW= 40 kD; Pharmalink, Upplands, Vasby, Sweden),
4. 0.9% NaCl (control).

Then the recalcified coagulation activity assay (RECA) was performed: 2 µl RECA-trigger (250 mM $CaCl_2$ in siliconized glass vials) were added. After intense shaking for 5s, the plates were brought into a digitally controlled 37°C water-bath. The coagulation activation was stopped by addition of 50 µl arginine reagent (2.5 M arginine, pH 8.6, 0.16% Triton X 100®, both from Sigma, Deisenhofen, Germany) after 10 min, 30 min, or 35 min coagulation reaction time (CRT; RECA-10 and RECA-30 were the main values, RECA-35 was the control value; thrombin (IIa) generation in RECA-30 divided by thrombin generation in RECA-35 was less than 1, i.e. the thrombin generation curve was in its ascending part with nearly no fibrin (=antithrombin I) – interference [6-8]. After 3 min (23°C) 25 µl 1 mM chromogenic IIa substrate HD-CHG-Ala-Arg-pNA (Pentapharm, Basel, Switzerland) in 1.25 M arginine, pH 8.7, were added. The increase in absorbance (ΔA at 23°C) was measured at 405 nm by a microtiter plate photometer with a 1 mA resolution. The RECA was standardized with 1 IU/ml bovine thrombin (DadeBehring, Marburg, Germany) in 6.7% human albumin (Kabi, Stockholm, Sweden), replacing the 20 µl plasma sample [6-8].

Addition of 2 µl volume to 20 µl plasma imitates the infusion of 300 ml expander to 3000 ml plasma, 4 µl means 600 ml to 3000 ml plasma, 6 µl means 900 ml, to 3000 ml plasma, etc.

Results and Discussion

Figure 1a demonstrates that HES-200kDa enhanced plasmatic thrombin generation > 10fold at final plasma concentrations > 0.8%. HES-70kDa enhanced plasmatic thrombin generation > 10fold at final plasma concentrations > 0.5% (Fig. 1b). Prior to RECA performance 1+1 with 0.9% NaCl diluted pooled normal plasma generated about 20fold more thrombin even without HES when compared with undiluted pooled normal plasma. The procoagulant character of HES is better seen in undiluted plasma than in diluted plasma.

If increasing amounts of 0.9% NaCl were added to pooled normal plasma, the thrombin generation in RECA increased from < 50 mIU/ml IIa for 0-4 µl 0.9% NaCl added to 20 µl plasma to about 600 mIU/ml IIa for 6-14 µl NaCl added to 20 µl plasma (Figures 2,3). This means that infusion of > 4 µl of volume per 20 µl plasma, which approximately corresponds to > 0.5-1 litre of volume per 3 litres of plasma, can be prothrombotic. Using this volume of HES-200kDa or of HES-70kDa, the thrombin generation in RECA-30 increased about 5fold or about 8fold, respectively; with this volume of dextran the thrombin generation in RECA-30 increases about twice, when compared with the 0.9% NaCl control. Of major importance are increasing thrombin (IIa) generations, decreasing IIa activities might also be due to entrapment of IIa within the nascending fibrin [6-8]. In the present experiment a thrombin generation curve might again increase after a decrease because the reaction conditions (final volume) have changed.

The present work demonstrates, that both HES types may trigger the intrinsic phase of blood coagulation, especially at final plasma concentrations > 0.5%. It remains to be seen if the new generation HES of 130 kDa and 0.4 substitution grade is a significantly less contact activator than the here studied HES-200kDa or HES-70kDa.

The present data support the concept that for clinically mandatory volume replacement the plasma expanders of the HES or the dextran type might induce more hemostasis or nephrologic problems than just the replacement with 0.9% NaCl-like crystalloids [1,9,10]. So,

HES therapy was associated with higher rates of acute renal failure than was Ringer's lactate [11,12].

From a clinical point of view it is very difficult to judge which volume replacement therapy is the most indicated [13]. The present in vitro study on coagulation activation with the RECA helps to establish the correct solution and its dosage for fluid resuscitation.

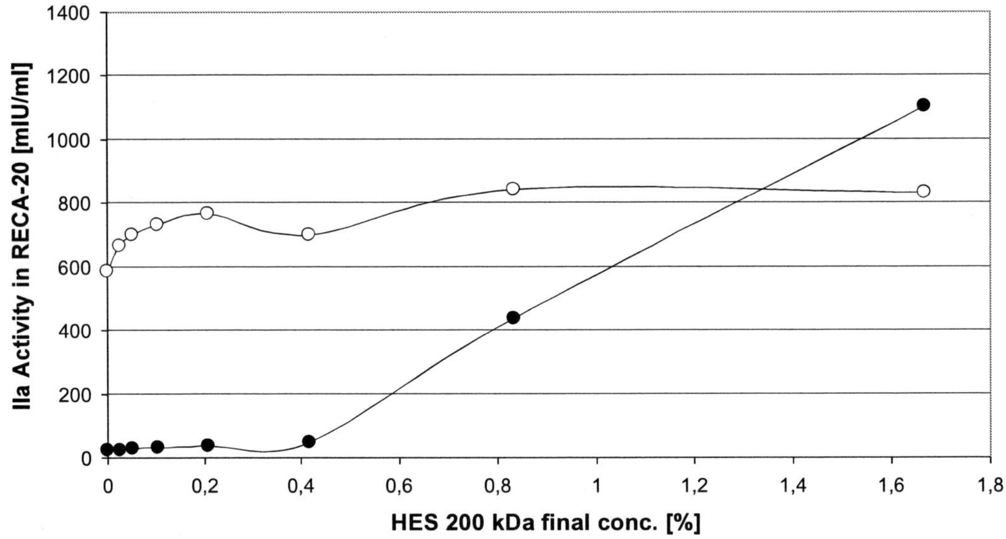

a

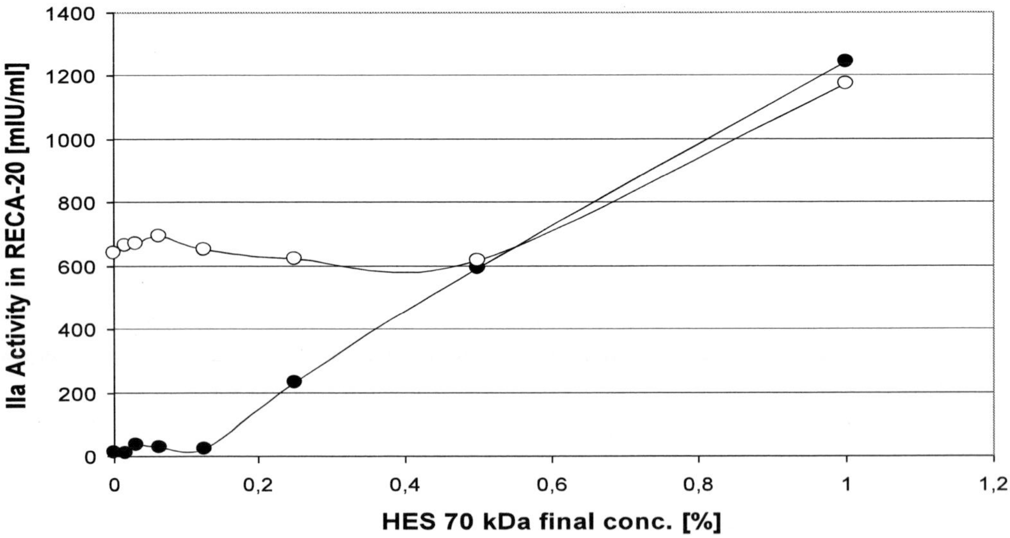

b

Figure 1. HES in RECA. 20 µl pooled unfrozen normal plasma (•) or 1+1 with 0.9 % NaCl diluted pooled normal plasma (O) in untreated polystyrol U-microwells were supplemented with HES 200 kDa (Figure 1a) and HES 70 kDa (Figure 1b). The samples were analyzed in RECA-20 (recalcified coagulation activity assay with 20 min coagulation reaction time; IIa = thrombin).

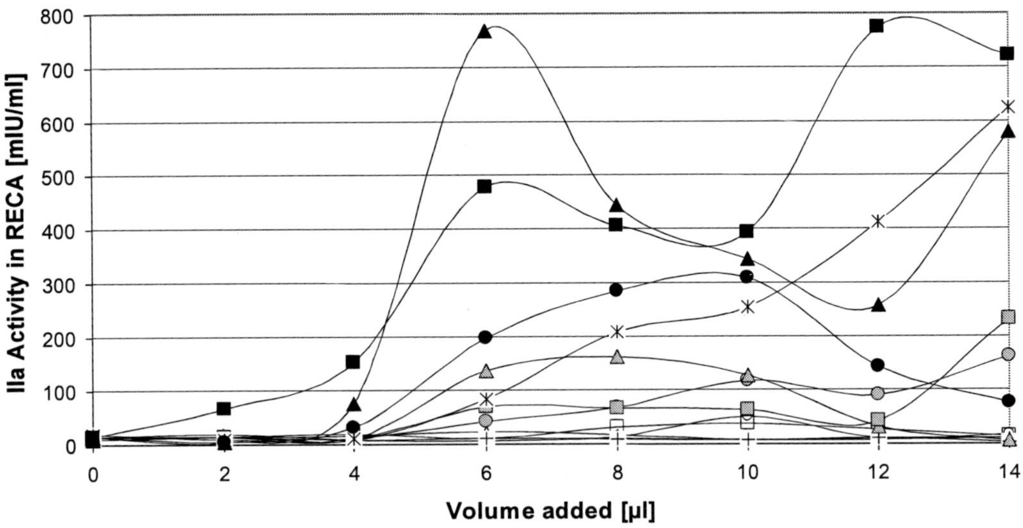

Figure 2. Thrombin (IIa) activity in RECA in dependence of added volume. 20 µl pooled unfrozen normal plasma and 0-14 µl 0.9 % NaCl (-, +, *), dextran (circles), HES-70kDa (triangles), HES-200kDa (squares) in untreated polystyrol F-wells were analyzed in RECA-5 (white symbols or -), RECA-10 (grey symbols or +), or RECA-30 (black symbols or *).

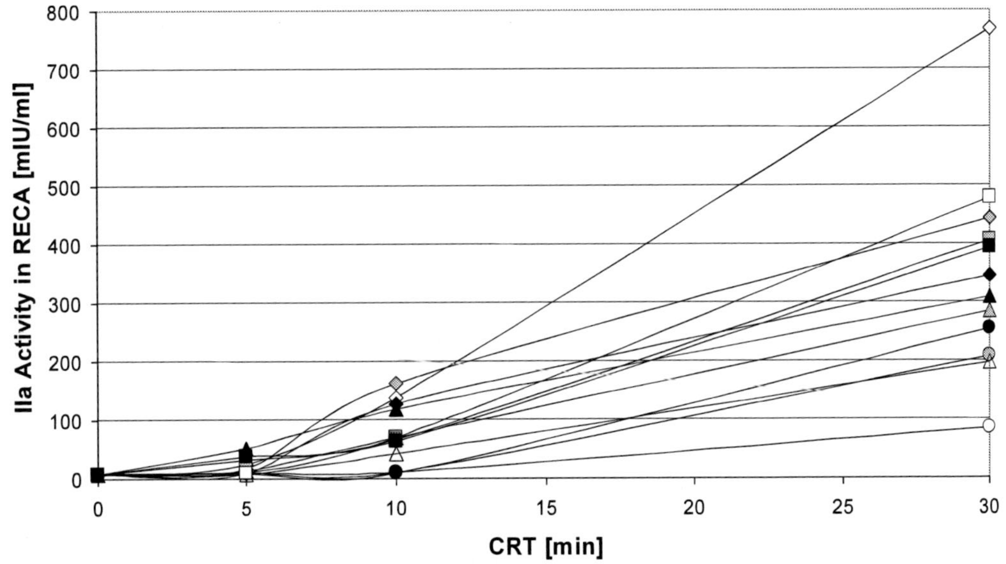

Figure 3. RECA in dependence of coagulation reaction time (CRT). 20 µl pooled unfrozen normal plasma with 6 µl (white symbols), 8 µl (grey symbols), or 10 µl 0.9 % NaCl (circles), dextran (triangles), HES-70kDa (diamonds), HES-200kDa (squares) of figure 2 were analyzed in RECA with different CRT.

REFERENCES

[1] Boldt J, Suttner S. Plasma substitutes. *Minerva Anestesiol* 2005; 71: 741-58.

[2] Vollmar B, Menger MD. Volume replacement and microhemodynamic changes in polytrauma. *Langenbecks Arch. Surg.* 2004; 389: 485-91.

[3] Dieterich HJ. Recent developments in European colloid solutions. *J. Trauma* 2003; 54(5 Suppl): S26-30.

[4] Brecher ME, Owen HG, Bandarenko N. Alternatives to albumin: starch replacement for plasma exchange. *J. Clin. Apher.* 1997; 12: 146-53.

[5] Stief TW, Ajib S, Renz H. Loss of anticoagulant action by ultra-low-dose heparin. *Hemostasis Laboratory* 2008; 1: (issue 1, in press).

[6] Stief TW. Thrombin generation by exposure of blood to endotoxin: a simple model to study disseminated intravascular coagulation. *Clin. Appl. Thromb. Hemost.* 2006; 12: 137-61.

[7] Stief TW. Innovative tests of plasmatic hemostasis. *Laboratory Medicine* 2008; 39: 225-30.

[8] Stief TW. The laboratory diagnosis of the pre-phase of pathologic disseminated intravascular coagulation. *Hemostasis Laboratroy* 2008; 1: (issue 1, in press).

[9] Boldt J. Hydroxyethylstarch as a risk factor for acute renal failure: is a change of clinical practice indicated? *Drug Saf* 2002; 25: 837-46.

[10] Strauss RG, Pennell BJ, Stump DC. A randomized, blinded trial comparing the hemostatic effects of pentastarch versus hetastarch. *Transfusion* 2002; 42: 27-36.

[11] Brunkhorst FM, Engel C, Bloos F, Meier-Hellmann A, Ragaller M, Weiler N, Moerer O, Gruendling M, Oppert M, Grond S, Olthoff D, Jaschinski U, John S, Rossaint R, Welte T, Schaefer M, Kern P, Kuhnt E, Kiehntopf M, Hartog C, Natanson C, Loeffler M, Reinhart K; German Competence Network Sepsis (SepNet). Intensive insulin therapy and pentastarch resuscitation in severe sepsis. *N .Engl. J. Med.* 2008; 358: 125-39.

[12] Brunkhorst FM, Oppert M, Leone M, Blasco V, Albanese J, Martin C. Nephrotoxicity of hydroxyethyl starch solution. *Br J Anaesth* 2008; 100: 856-857.

[13] Bunn F, Trivedi D, Ashraf S. Colloid solutions for fluid resuscitation. *Cochrane Database Syst Rev* 2008; (1): CD001319.

In: Hemostasis Laboratory Yearbook, Volume 2
Editor: Thomas W. Stief, pp. 183-190

ISBN: 978-1-60741-089-8

THERAPEUTIC HUMAN ALBUMINS TRIGGER PLASMATIC THROMBIN GENERATION

Thomas W. Stief*
Department of Clinical Chemistry
University Hospital Giessen and Marburg, Germany

ABSTRACT

Human albumin is therapeutically used for a broad range of diseases. Commercial preparations may contain activators of the intrinsic phase of hemostasis. The ultra-specific, ultra-sensitive, and close to physiologic recalcified coagulation activity assay (RECA) detects subtle prothrombotic changes of any material that comes in contact with blood. Therefore, here 3 different commercial human albumins (Behring, Baxter, Talecris) were tested for contact phase activation in the RECA with 20 min coagulation reaction time in untreated polystyrol microwells (RECA-20) and for 50% inhibitory concentration (IC50) of aprotinin against amidolysis of a chromogenic substrate.
Pooled unfrozen normal human citrated plasma supplemented with 17-33 g/l Behring-albumin had a plasmatic thrombin generation in RECA-20 of about 0.1-0.2 IU/ml; the same concentration of added albumin from Baxter or Talecris induced a plasmatic thrombin generation of about 0.2-0.6 IU/ml. The 0.9% NaCl control generated less than 0.05 IU/ml thrombin in the present RECA-20 experiment.
The approximate IC50 of aprotinin against amidolysis was 1 KIU/ml, 4 KIU/ml, or 11 KIU/ml for 5% albumin from Behring, Talecris, or Baxter, respectively, when assayed in 1+1 dilution with phosphate buffered saline. The lowest amidolytic acitivity corresponded to the lowest RECA activity.
It is suggested to test all commercial lots of human albumin before releasing them to the market with the RECA. A given industrial product should be below certain still to be defined limits of RECA, e.g., an ideal albumin lot would be one that behaves similarly as the 0.9% NaCl control. Albumin lots with elevated RECA might trigger pathologic disseminated intravascular coagulation in the patient.

Keywords: Albumin, colloid, pathologic disseminated intravascular coagulation, RECA

---

* Correspondence to: PD Dr. Med. T. Stief, Department of Clinical Chemistry, University Hospital, D-35043 Marburg, Germany. Email: thstief@med.uni-marburg.de; Tel.: +49-6421-58 64471; Fax: +49-6421-58 65594.

INTRODUCTION

Human albumin solutions are used for plasmapheresis, cardiothoracic surgery, liver cirrhosis with ascites, acute nephrotic syndromes, protein-losing gastroenterologic diseases, massive hemorrhage, or severe hypo-albuminemia [1-16]. Therapeutic human albumin might contain trace amounts of coagulation activators that especially might trigger intrinsic hemostasis similarly as other colloids such as dextran or hydroxyl-ethyl-starch (HES) [17-19]. The aim of the present study was to investigate the influence of supplemented human albumin on activation of plasmatic coagulation, assayed by a new ultra-specific, ultra-sensitive test for plasmatic thrombin generation: the recalcified coagulation activity assay (RECA) [20-24].

MATERIAL AND METHODS

Different Final Plasmatic Concentrations of Added Human Albumins

100 µl pooled unfrozen normal citrated plasma (from 6 individual samples, remaining after routine analysis; 0.5 ml 106 mM sodim citrate + 4.5 ml venous blood in polypropylene (PP) tubes; Sarstedt, Nümbrecht, Germany; pooling into emptied PP tubes) in untreated polystyrol U-microwells (Brand, Wertheim, Germany; article nr. 701300) were supplemented with 20 µl 20% human albumin from CSL Behring (Marburg, Germany), Baxter (Vienna, Austria), or Talecris (Frankfurt, Germany). 60 µl of this mixture were withdrawn and diluted repetitively 1+1 on the plate with 60 µl sample (50 µl normal pool + 10 µl 0.9% NaCl). Then the RECA was performed: 5 µl RECA-trigger (1 ml aliquots of frozen/thawed 250 mM $CaCl_2$; in siliconized 15 ml glass vials, DadeBehring, Marburg, Germany, article nr. OVKE49) were added. After 20 min at 37°C (RECA-20) 100 µl arginine reagent were added. After 3 min (23°C) 25 µl 1 mM chromogenic substrate reagent were added and ΔA at 405 nm was determined. The 1 IU/ml thrombin standard resulted in a ΔA of about 20 mA/min (23°C). The maximal ΔA was about 1050 mA, the linear ΔA range was up to 40 % of 1050 mA = 420 mA. The same experiment was performed with the same normal unfrozen pool diluted 1+1 with 0.9 % NaCl.

Different Volumes of 20% Albumin Added to Plasma

20 µl unfrozen pooled normal citrated plasma (from 4 individual samples, remaining after routine analysis) in polystyrol flat bottom wells (F-wells; Brand, Wertheim, Germany; pureGrade®, article nr. 781602) were supplemented in duplicate at 23°C by means of an Eppendorf-multipette® (0.9% NaCl - rinsed tips) with 0-14 µl

1. Human albumin 20% Behring® (salt poor, with only 125 mM Na^+; maximally 2 mM K^+, maximally 2 mM Ca^{++}, maximally 100 mM Cl^-; CSL Behring; lot nr. 58144411B),
2. Human albumin 200 g/l Baxter® (salt poor; Baxter; lot nr. VNA1FO29),

3. Plasbumin® 20 (20% human albumin, salt poor, with 145 mM Na^+, maximally 10 mM K^+, 16 mM sodium caprylate, 16 mM acetyl-tryptophane; Talecris Biotherapeutics; lot nr. 80A2433),
4. 0.9% NaCl (control).

Then the RECA was performed: 2 µl RECA-trigger (250 mM $CaCl_2$ in siliconized glass vials) were added. After intense shaking for 5s, the plates were brought into a digitally controlled 37°C water-bath. The coagulation activation was stopped by addition of 50 µl arginine reagent (2.5 M arginine, pH 8.6, 0.16% Triton X 100®, both from Sigma, Deisenhofen, Germany) after 10 min, 30 min, or 35 min coagulation reaction time (CRT; RECA-10 and RECA-30 were the main values, RECA-35 was the control value; thrombin (IIa) generation in RECA-30 divided by thrombin generation in RECA-35 was less than 1, i.e. the thrombin generation curve was in its ascending part with nearly no fibrin (=antithrombin I) – interference [20-24]. After 3 min (23°C) 25 µl 1 mM chromogenic IIa substrate HD-CHG-Ala-Arg-pNA (Pentapharm, Basel, Switzerland) in 1.25 M arginine, pH 8.7, were added. The increase in absorbance (ΔA at 23°C) was measured at 405 nm by a microtiter plate photometer with a 1 mA resolution. The RECA is standardized with 1 IU/ml bovine thrombin (DadeBehring, Marburg, Germany) in 6.7% human albumin (Kabi, Stockholm, Sweden), replacing the 20 µl plasma sample. Addition of 2 µl 20 % albumin to 20 µl plasma imitates the infusion of 300 ml 20% albumin to 3000 ml plasma and 4 µl means 600 ml 20% albumin per 3000 ml plasma, ≥ 6 µl 20% albumin per 20 µl plasma might be supra-therapeutical and might thus be of more pathophysiologic interest.

Amidolytic Activity in Human Albumins and 50% Inhibitory Concentration (IC50) of Aprotinin

50 µl 5% human albumin Behring, Baxter, Talecris, all in phosphate buffered saline (PBS; Sigma), or PBS (for control of eventual spontaneous decay of the chromogenic substrate), were incubated in duplicate for 20 min (37°C) with 50 µl 0-44.4 kallikrein inhibiting units (KIU)/ml aprotinin (Bayer, Leverkusen, Germany; 1 mg=6000 KIU; MW= about 6500 Dalton) in PBS in polystyrol microtiter plates with flat bottom (F-wells; NUNC, Wiesbaden, Germany; article nr. 446140). Then 25 µl 1 mM HD-CHG-Ala-Arg-pNA in H_2O were added and ΔA/h (37°C or 23°C) was determined.

Results and Discussion

Therapeutic human albumins in added final plasma concentrations > 15 g/l may seriously enhance thrombin generation (Figure 1): 17-33 g/l added Behring albumin induced a plasmatic thrombin generation of about 0.1-0.2 IU/ml (Fig. 1a), the same concentration of added albumin from Baxter or Talecris induced a plasmatic thrombin generation of about 0.2-0.6 IU/ml (Figures 1b,c). The 0.9% NaCl control generated less than 0.05 IU/ml thrombin in the present RECA-20 experiment. These prothrombotic changes were more pronounced in 1+1 diluted plasma at added albumin concentrations less than 2%.

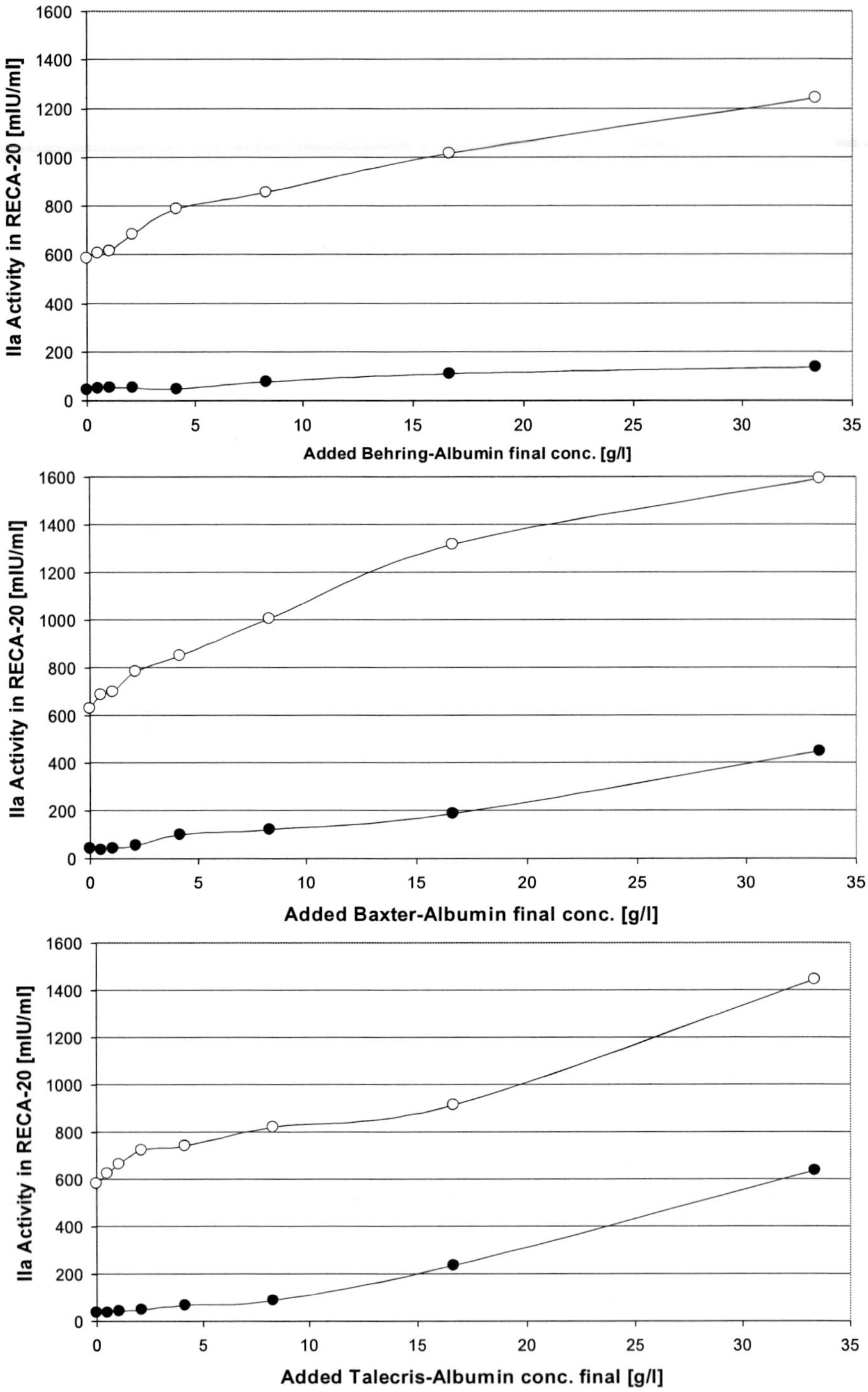

Figure 1. Different final plasmatic concentrations of added human albumins. 50 µl pooled unfrozen normal citrated plasma (●) or 1+1 with 0.9% NaCl diluted plasma pool (O) in untreated U-microwells (Brand; article nr. 701300) were supplemented with 20 % human albumin from Behring (Fig. 1a), Baxter (Fig. 1b), or Talecris (Fig. 1c). 5 µl RECA-trigger (250 mM $CaCl_2$) were added. After 20 min at 37°C (RECA-20) 100 µl 2.5 M arginine, 0.16% Triton X 100® reagent were added. After 3 min (23°C) 25 µl 1 mM chromogenic thrombin substrate were added and ΔA at 405 nm was determined.

1+1 dilution of plasma prior to the RECA enhanced thrombin generation in recalcified plasma about 10fold, even without addition of human albumin, when assayed in untreated U-wells.

With only 0-4 µl 20% human albumin added there was no increase in thrombin generation (Figures 2,3). 6 µl 20% human albumin added to 20 µl plasma means 0.9 litre albumin added to 3 litres plasma, resulting into 46 g/l additional albumin. 6 µl 20% Behring albumin generated less than 0.1 IU/ml thrombin, 6 µl 20% Baxter or Talecris albumin generated about 0.25 IU/ml thrombin in RECA-30, when assayed in F-wells.

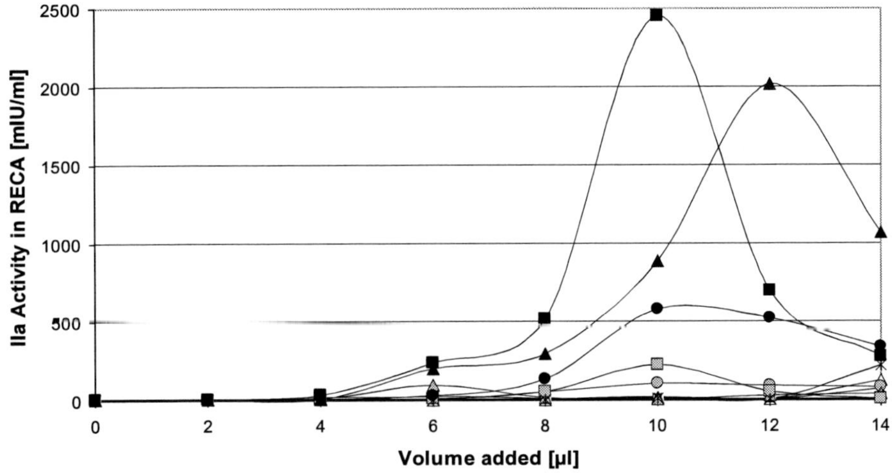

Figure 2. RECA in dependence of added volume. 0-14 µl 0.9% NaCl (-,+,*), 20 % human albumin Behring (circles), Baxter (triangles), or Talecris (squares) were analyzed in the RECA with CRT periods of 5 min (white symbols or -), 10 min (grey symbols or +), or 30 min (black symbols or *).

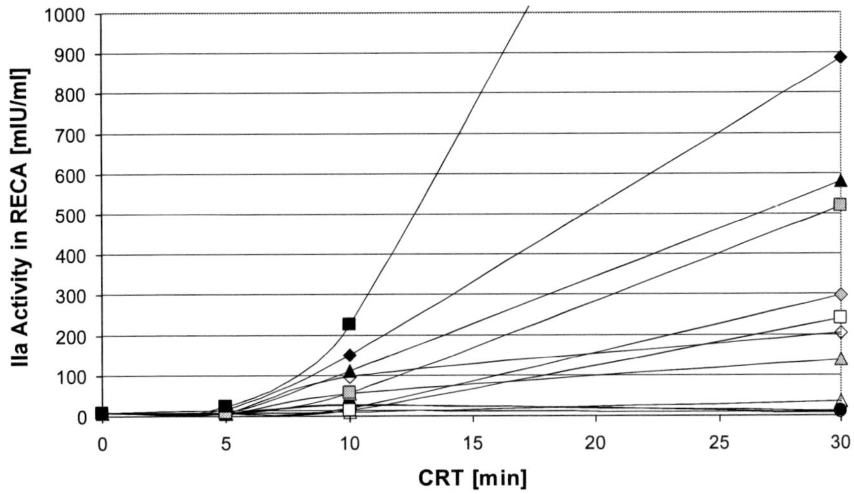

Figure 3. IIa generation in RECA in dependence of CRT. 6 µl (white symbols), 8 µl (grey symbols), or 10 µl (black symbols) 0.9% NaCl (circles), 20% human albumin Behring (triangles), Baxter (diamonds), or Talecris (squares) were analyzed in the RECA with 0-30 min CRT.

The experimental conditions with F-wells of Figs. 2,3 were more anticoagulant than that with U-wells of Figure 1. Decreasing parts of thrombin generation curves are of minor importance since thrombin may be entrapped into nascending fibrin.

Figure 4 demonstrates the presence of amidolytic activity in the investigated albumin preparations and its inhibition by aprotinin.

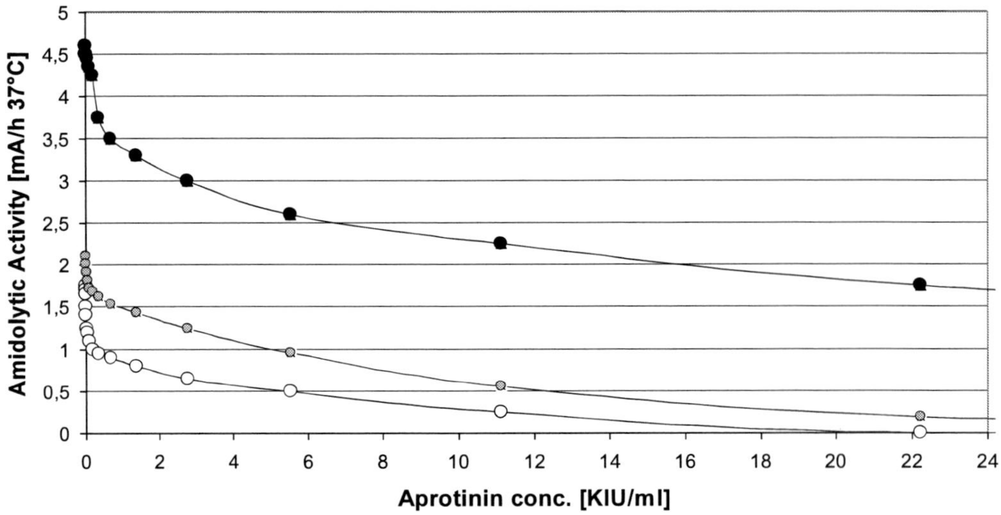

Figure 4. Amidolytic Activity of human albumins. 50 µl 5 % human albumin Behring (O), Baxter (•), or Talecris (greyO) in phosphate buffered saline (PBS) were incubated for 20 min (37°C) with 50 µl 0-44.4 KIU/ml aprotinin in PBS in F-wells. Then 25 µl 1 mM HD-CHG-Ala-Arg-pNA in H_2O were added and ΔA/h (37°C) was determined.

Without aprotinin the ΔA values at 37°C were 1.7 mA/h, 2.1 mA/h, 4.6 mA/h for 5% albumin from Behring, Talecris, or Baxter, respectively. The respective ΔA values at 23°C in absence of aprotinin were 1.0 mA/h, 1.4 mA/h, or 3.0 mA/h, i.e. the ΔA values increased about 1.5-1.7 fold when increasing the reaction temperature from 23°C to 37°C, which is typical for the contact phase of hemostasis [25]: normally, an increase of enzyme activity of about 2.5 fold would have been expected. The approximate 50 % inhibitory concentration (IC50) of aprotinin against these amidolytic activities was 1 KIU/ml, 4 KIU/ml, or 11 KIU/ml for 5% albumin from Behring, Talecris, or Baxter, respectively, when assayed in 1+1 dilution with PBS. Of interest is that the lowest amidolytic acitivity found corresponded to the lowest RECA activity.

Due to adverse hemostasis reactions of the colloids albumin or HES [1,17-19,26,27] fluid resuscitation with albumin or HES may be associated with higher mortality rates than resuscitation with saline [28,29]. Therefore, instead of using a potentially contact activating albumin for hypovolaemia in shock crystalloids may be preferable [11]. Since all colloidal plasma substitutes (HES more than albumin) interfere with the physiological mechanisms of hemostasis (platelet function, plasmatic coagulation, and fibrinolysis) [18], it is suggested to test all commercial lots of human albumin before releasing them to the market with the RECA, an industrial product should be below certain still to be defined limits of RECA, e.g. an ideal albumin lot would be one that behaves similarly as the 0.9 % NaCl control. Albumin lots with an elevated RECA value might trigger pathologic disseminated intravascular coagulation (PDIC) in the patient, similarly as PDIC is triggered by intrinsic or extrinsic coagulation activators as e.g. activated alveolar macrophages in severe lung diseases that may fragment into phospholipid-microparticles / DNA or tissue factor, respectively [30].

REFERENCES

[1] Boldt J, Suttner S. Plasma substitutes. *Minerva Anestesiol* 2005; 71: 741-58.

[2] Farrugia A, Robert P. Plasma protein therapies: current and future perspectives. *Best Pract. Res. Clin. Haematol.* 2006; 19: 243-58.

[3] Santoro A, Mancini E, Ferramosca E, Faenza S. Liver support systems. *Contrib. Nephrol.* 2007; 156: 396-404.

[4] Bosch T. Therapeutic apheresis--state of the art in the year 2005. *Ther. Apher. Dial.* 2005; 9: 459-68.

[5] Naruse K. Artificial liver support: future aspects. *J. Artif. Organs* 2005; 8: 71-6.

[6] Hughes RD. Review of methods to remove protein-bound substances in liver failure. *Int. J. Artif.Organs* 2002; 25: 911-7.

[7] Drew MJ. Plasmapheresis in the dysproteinemias. *Ther. Apher.* 2002; 6: 45-52.

[8] Siami GA, Siami FS. Plasmapheresis and paraproteinemia: cryoprotein-induced diseases, monoclonal gammopathy, Waldenström's macroglobulinemia, hyperviscosity syndrome, multiple myeloma, light chain disease, and amyloidosis. *Ther. Apher* 1999; 3: 8-19.

[9] Sternbach MS, Fawcett S, Wolsley M, Giammarco R. Plasma exchange in chronic inflammatory demyelinating polyneuropathies. *Transfus Sci.* 1996; 17: 415-22.

[10] Vermeulen LC Jr, Ratko TA, Erstad BL, Brecher ME, Matuszewski KA. A paradigm for consensus. The University Hospital Consortium guidelines for the use of albumin, nonprotein colloid, and crystalloid solutions. *Arch. Intern. Med.* 1995; 155: 373-9.

[11] Durand-Zaleski I, Bonnet F, Rochant H, Bierling P, Lemaire F. Usefulness of consensus conferences: the case of albumin. *Lancet.* 1992; 340: 1388-90.

[12] Hastings GE, Wolf PG. The therapeutic use of albumin. *Arch. Fam. Med.* 1992; 1: 281-7.

[13] Guthrie RD Jr, Hines C Jr. Use of intravenous albumin in the critically ill patient. *Am. J. Gastroenterol.* 1991; 86: 255-63.

[14] Russell JA, Navickis RJ, Wilkes MM. Albumin versus crystalloid for pump priming in cardiac surgery: meta-analysis of controlled trials. *J. Cardiothorac. Vasc. Anesth* 2004; 18: 429-37.

[15] Subcommittee of the Victorian Drug Usage Advisory Committee. Human albumin solutions: consensus statements for use in selected clinical situations. *Med. J. Aust.* 1992; 157: 340-3.

[16] Erstad BL, Gales BJ, Rappaport WD. The use of albumin in clinical practice. *Arch. Intern. Med.* 1991; 151: 901-11.

[17] de Jonge E, Levi M. Effects of different plasma substitutes on blood coagulation: a comparative review. *Crit. Care Med.* 2001; 29: 1261-7.

[18] Van der Linden P, Ickx BE. The effects of colloid solutions on hemostasis. *Can. J. Anaesth* 2006; 53 (6 Suppl): S30-9.

[19] Myllylä G. Factors determining quality of plasma. *Vox. Sang* 1998; 74 Suppl2: 507-11.

[20] Stief TW. Thrombin generation by exposure of blood to endotoxin: a simple model to study disseminated intravascular coagulation. *Clin. Appl. Thromb. Hemost.* 2006; 12: 137-61.

[21] Stief TW. The recalcified coagulation activity. *Clin. Appl. Thromb. Hemost.* 2007; Dec 26. [Epub ahead of print].

[22] Stief TW. Inhibition of thrombin generation in recalcified plasma. *Blood Coagul Fibrinolysis* 2007; 18: 751-60.

[23] Stief TW. Innovative tests of plasmatic hemostasis. *Laboratory Medicine* 2008; 39: 225-30.

[24] Stief TW. The laboratory diagnosis of the pre-phase of pathologic disseminated intravascular coagulation. *Hemostasis Laboratory* 2008; 1: (issue 1, in press).

[25] Stief TW, Otto S, Renz H. The intrinsic coagulation activity assay. Blood Coagul *Fibrinolysis* 2006; 17: 369-78.

[26] Gales BJ, Erstad BL. Adverse reactions to human serum albumin. *Ann. Pharmacother.* 1993; 27: 87-94.

[27] McClelland DB. Safety of human albumin as a constituent of biologic therapeutic products. *Transfusion* 1998; 38: 690-9.

[28] Brunkhorst FM, Engel C, Bloos F, Meier-Hellmann A, Ragaller M, Weiler N, Moerer O, Gruendling M, Oppert M, Grond S, Olthoff D, Jaschinski U, John S, Rossaint R, Welte T, Schaefer M, Kern P, Kuhnt E, Kiehntopf M, Hartog C, Natanson C, Loeffler M, Reinhart K; German Competence Network Sepsis (SepNet). Intensive insulin therapy and pentastarch resuscitation in severe sepsis. *N. Engl. J. Med.* 2008; 358: 125-39.

[29] SAFE Study Investigators; Myburgh J, Cooper DJ, Finfer S, Bellomo R, Norton R, Bishop N, Kai Lo S, Vallance S. Saline or albumin for fluid resuscitation in patients with traumatic brain injury. *N. Engl. J. Med.* 2007; 357: 874-84.

[30] Saldeen T. Clotting, microembolism, and inhibition of fibrinolysis in adult respiratory distress. *Surg. Clin. North Am.* 1983; 63: 285-304.

In: Hemostasis Laboratory Yearbook, Volume 2
Editor: Thomas W. Stief, pp. 191-198

ISBN: 978-1-60741-089-8

ARGININE LINEARIZES THE HYPERBOLIC LIMULUS KINETIC

Thomas W. Stief *

Department of Clinical Chemistry
University Hospital Giessen and Marburg, Germany

ABSTRACT

Free endotoxin in human blood can cause pathologic disseminated intravascular coagulation (PDIC). Its rapid functional determination is therefore of great clinical importance. The chromogenic Limulus test is sensitive to free lipopolysaccharide (LPS) in pg/ml quantities. Normally, the kinetic of the enzymes of the Limulus clotting system (factors C, B, G, A) is hyperbolic, as it is also typical for the human clotting system. The aim of the present study was to find out how this complicated hyperbolic kinetic can be transformed at an ideal time point into a linear kinetic.

Plasmatic LPS reactivity was determined after singlet oxygen – mediated destruction of plasmatic serine protease inhibitors. The chromogenic Limulus reagent was added in presence of different concentrations of arginine, a known competitive inhibitor of serine proteases.

The approximate 50% inhibitory concentration (IC50) of arginine against the Limulus clotting system was 50 mM. The approximate IC50 against the amidolytic activity of activated factor A was 150 mM. Since the normal range of LPS-reactivity in human plasma is 100±25% of normal (100% = about 0.8 ng/ml) and LPS-reactivities > 300% of normal may cause PDIC, the dangerous grey-zone of about 200% of normal LPS-reactivity must be determined precisely in patients at risk for PDIC. It is suggested to add 300-400 mM (final conc.) sterile arginine to a Limulus reaction, that detects pg/ml quantities of free LPS, e.g. at that reaction time point (37°C) when pooled normal plasma with about 0.8 ng/ml LPS reactivity generates an absorbance at 405 nm that is about 5-10 % of the maximal absorbance, i.e. when precise quantifications of plasmatic LPS reactivities in the critical 1-3 ng/ml range are possible.

Keywords: endotoxin, LPS, ß-glucan, limulus, arginine.

* Correspondence to: PD Dr. Med. T. Stief, Department of Clinical Chemistry, University Hospital, D-35043 Marburg, Germany. Email: thstief@med.uni-marburg.de; Tel.: +49-6421-58 64471; Fax: +49-6421-58 65594.

INTRODUCTION

Endotoxin is an old expression for certain pyrogens that are of great pathophysiologic importance in clinical hemostasis [1]. The biochemical nature of gram-negative bacterial endotoxin has been clarified as lipopolysaccharide (LPS), however there are related pyrogens from fungi that pathophysiologically [2] and clinically [3] behave like endotoxin: the ß-D-glucans. Therefore, from a pathophysiologic and clinical point of view both LPS and ß-D-glucans might be considered as endotoxins [4].

Endotoxemia is a clinically valid indicator for the pre-phase of severe sepsis [5]. The Limulus-test is an excellent tool to measure this pathophysiologic function of endotoxin (here understood as LPS or ß-D-glucan) in blood [3]: endotoxin triggers the enzyme cascade of the Limulus clotting system by interactions of LPS with factor C or of ß-D-glucan with factor G [6,7]. The serine protease activated factor A (FAa) is generated, whose activity is best monitored by means of amidolysis of a specific chromogenic substrate, such as Ile-Glu-Gly-Arg-pNA [4]. Normally, the kinetic of the Limulus-test is hyperbolic, which is typical for amplifying enzymatic cascades as e.g. also the clotting system of human blood. Many enzymes of human coagulation are serine proteases. The amino acid arginine competitively inhibits serine proteases, e.g. with 50 % inhibitory concentrations (IC50) of 10-50 mM on the thrombin generation assays recalcified coagulation activity assay (RECA), intrinsic coagulation activity assay (INCA), or extrinsic coagulation activity assay (EXCA) [8]. In the present work the IC50 of arginine on the Limulus clotting cascade is determined.

MATERIAL AND METHODS

Hyperbolic Limulus Kinetic

The present endotoxin standards were pooled citrated plasma (0.5 ml sodium citrate + 4.5 ml venous blood, centrifuged at 2800g for 10 min at 23°C, remaining after routine analysis) basally containing 1 ng/ml LPS reactivity, this pooled citrated plasma that had been supplemented with additional 2999 ng/ml purified LPS [2] (Sigma, Deisenhofen, Germany; *Escherichia coli* 0111:B4, purified by gel filtration, protein content < 1 %; Sigma, Deisenhofen, Germany; article nr. L3012-5MG) to a final super-extremely pathologic plasmatic LPS reactivity of 3000 ng/ml. This 3000 ng/ml standard had been diluted with pooled citrated plasma to final LPS-reactivities of 2 ng/ml, 4 ng/ml, 16 ng/ml, or 300 ng/ml; all citrated plasma standards had been supplemented after 15 min (23°C) with 3.2 mg/ml K_3-EDTA (ethylenediamine tetra acetic acid tripotassium salt), the approximate plasmatic K_3-EDTA concentration in EDTA-blood. An exemplary LPS reactivity of 16 ng/ml means that this plasma behaves as pooled normal plasma with 0.8 ng/ml LPS reactivity that had been supplemented with 15.2 ng/ml purified LPS; < 1 % of added LPS to plasma is active=free=unbound [11].

10 µl fresh citrated plasma of two healthy donors, fresh EDTA plasma of one healthy donor, fresh serum of the same two healthy donors, and the above frozen/thawed Limulus-reactivity plasma standards were incubated in duplicate with 10 µl 60 mM chloramine-T® (Sigma), 50 mM sodium citrate (pH 7.8) for 10 min at 37°C in half area polystyrol wells

(Corning, Schiphol-Rijk, The Netherlands; article nr. 3695). Then 10 µl antioxidant-reagent (230 mM methionine; Sigma) were added. After 3 min at 23°C, 30 µl freshly with 200 mM Tris, pH 8, reconstituted Limulus-colyophilizate-reagent Pyrochrome® (Lot Nr. 21100304C), that had been preincubated for 3 min at 23°C, were added. The lyophilized Limulus-Amebocyte-Lysate (LAL) reagent had been stored at 8°C. The specific increase in absorbance (ΔA) with time during 0-170 min (23°C) was determined as ΔA at 405 nm minus ΔA at 650 nm by a microtiter plate photometer with a 1 mA resolution (Milenia; DPC, Los Angeles, USA). The unspecific cleavage of chromogenic substrate for activated Limulus Factor A (FAa) per time (about 0.6 mA/min at 23°C for plasma and about 1 mA/min at 23°C for serum) was determined within the first 20 min of incubation and was subtracted from all ΔA values. The maximal ΔA was about 800 mA, ΔA values > 45 % of maximal ΔA (i.e. > 360 mA) were not evaluated due to exhaustion of chromogenic substrate. The specific absorbance of para-nitroaniline (pNA), when completely released out of the chromogenic substrate, decreased by about 1 mA/min (23°C).

Limulus Kinetic at 37°C Versus 23°C

Samples of pooled citrated plasma from patients containing 1.7 ng/ml LPS reactivity (remaining after routine analysis) were supplemented with 0 ng/ml or 10.3 ng/ml purified LPS (Sigma) to a LPS reactivity of 1.7 ng/ml or 12 ng/ml. After 15 min (23°C) 3.2 mg/ml K_3 - EDTA were added. 10 µl of these LPS reactivity plasma standards in sterile half well polystyrol microwells (Greiner, Frickenhausen, Germany; article nr. 675161; lot nr. 05360131) were incubated in triplicate with 10 µl 60 mM chloramine-T® in 50 mM sodium citrate, pH 7.8 for 10 min (37°C). 10 µl 230 mM methionine were added. After 3 min (23°C) 30 µl freshly reconstituted and 3 min at 23°C pre-incubated (for disappearance of turbidity) Limulus-reagent Pyrochrome® (lot nr. 20070307C) were added. The Limulus reaction was performed at 37°C (circles) or at 23°C (triangles). After 0-180 min the specific absorbance at 405 nm minus that at 450 nm was determined by a microtiter plate photometer with a 1 mA resolution (Milenia; DPC, Los Angeles, USA). The maximal ΔA was about 700 mA (45 % = 315 mA) that did not decrease. All reagents and the microtiter plates were sterile.

IC50 of Arginine on the Limulus Cascade and on FAa

Lyophilized Limulus-reagent Pyrochrome® (Cape Cod; article nr. CO120; Lot Nr. 12040104C) was reconstituted with 200 mM Tris, pH 8, frozen at -30°C and thawed at 23°C. Then 20 µl Limulus-reagent were incubated with 20 µl 0-1000 mM sterile arginine (Braun, Melsungen, Germany) in U-well microtiter plates (Greiner, Frickenhausen, Germany; article nr. 650161) for 0-180 min (37°C). The specific increase in absorbance with time (37°C) was determined as ΔA at 405 nm minus ΔA at 650 nm by a microtiter plate photometer with a 1 mA resolution (Milenia; DPC, Los Angeles, USA). The maximal ΔA was about 450 mA, ΔA values > 45 % of maximal ΔA (i.e. > 200 mA) were not evaluated due to exhaustion of chromogenic substrate.

RESULTS AND DISCUSSION

Figure 1a demonstrates the hyperbolic Limulus kinetic, when using this Pyrochrome® reagent and working at an incubation temperature of 23°C. The plasmas of the two healthy donors had LPS reactivities of about 0.9 ng/ml and about 0.6 ng/ml. 2-3 ng/ml LPS reactivity might be considered as the grey-zone of active LPS before causing pathologic disseminated coagulation activation [12]. LPS reactivities in the range of 20 ng/ml are typical for severe sepsis with PDIC [3,12]. Extreme LPS reactivities in the range of 100 ng/ml or super-extreme ones in the range of 1000 ng/ml might be found only seldomly in extremely ill patients [3,10,12].

Serum is not suitable for the Limulus-test: the maximal ΔA (at 160 min Limulus reaction time at 23°C) is only about 25 % of the maximal ΔA for plasma, i.e. FAa is destroyed by proteases of serum. Besides, since the begin of the Limulus incubation there is an unspecific ΔA of about 1 mA/min (23°C), and the Limulus kinetic with serum is completely different from the Limulus kinetic with plasma, resulting into a pseudo-LPS reactivity in the range of 10-100 ng/ml instead of one of about 1 ng/ml. Thus, for the Limulus-test instead of serum citrate-plasma or EDTA-plasma are suitable samples, the heparin of heparin-plasma artificially modulates LPS reactivity.

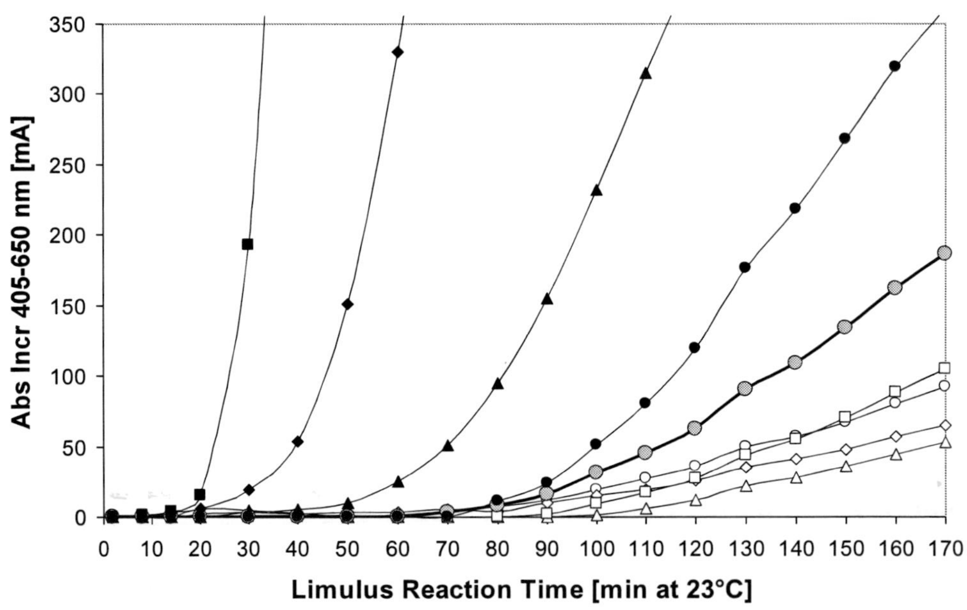

Figure 1a. Hyperbolic Limulus kinetic. 10 μl sample were incubated with 10 μl 60 mM chloramine-T® in 50 mM sodium citrate, pH 7.8, for 10 min (37°C) in half area microtiter plates. 10 μl 230 mM methionine were added and after 3 min (23°C) 30 μl Limulus-reagent Pyrochrome® were added, the reaction was incubated at 23°C, and ΔA at 405 nm minus ΔA at 650 nm was determined. The samples were: citrated plasma of healthy donor 1 (O), citrated plasma of healthy donor 2 (Δ), EDTA plasma of healthy donor 2 (◊); standards: pooled citrated/EDTA plasma with LPS reactivities of 1 ng/ml (□), 2 ng/ml (greyO), 4 ng/ml (●), 16 ng/ml (▲), 300 ng/ml (♦), 3000 ng/ml (■).

Figure 1b shows that 37°C incubation, when compared with 23°C incubation, increased the FAa activity generated by 12 ng/ml plasmatic LPS at about 100 min reaction time about

2.5 fold. In this Limulus reagent after an initial lack time the kinetic of the Limulus reaction was nearly linear instead of hyperbolic. This might be due to insufficient concentrations of the Limulus factors C, B, or A in the lyophilizate that results into exhaustion of reaction partners. With this Limulus reagent especially the low plasmatic reactivities of LPS in the critical range between 1 and 3 ng/ml were very difficult to measure precisely.

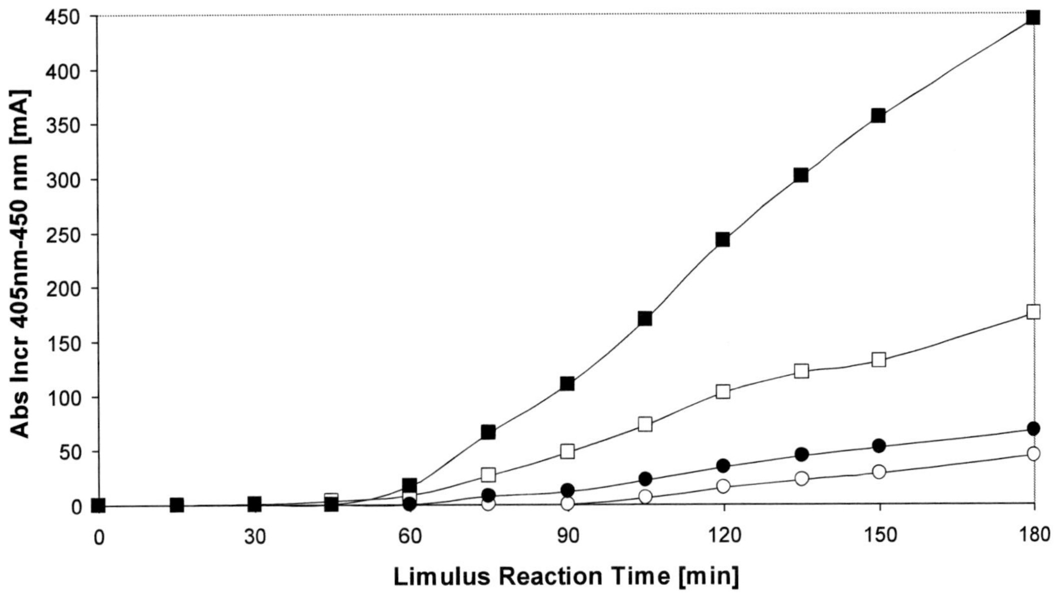

Figure 1b. Limulus reaction at 37°C versus at 23°C. 10 μl LPS reactivity standards (citrate/EDTA plasma) with 1.7 ng/ml LPS reactivity (circles) or 12 ng/ml LPS reactivity (squares) were incubated with 10 μl 60 mM chloramine-T® in 50 mM sodium citrate, pH 7.8 for 10 min (37°C) in half area wells. 10 μl 230 mM methionine were added. After 3 min (23°C) 30 μl Limulus reagent Pyrochrome® were added. The Limulus reaction was performed at 37°C (black symbols) or at 23°C (white symbols). After 0-180 min the specific absorbance at 405 nm minus that at 450 nm was determined.

The approximate IC50 of arginine on the cascade of Limulus enzymes was 50 mM; at arginine concentrations ≥ 4fold this IC50 the approximate IC50 on the amidolytic activity of FAa is 150 mM (Figure 2,3). At final arginine concentrations > 130 mM the ratio between LAL activity at 45 min and that at 15 min became the value of 3, which means that there the Limulus kinetic changed from hyperbolic to linear (Figure 4).

A linear kinetic would be easier to monitor by a clinical routine photometer. Therefore, in clinical routine analysis the complicated hyperbolic Limulus kinetic might be transformed into a linear kinetic. This linearization should be performed not until a certain reaction time that is sufficient to generate significant specific amounts of FAa even in normal plasma. Only if the normal range of plasmatic endotoxin reactivity (100±25% of normal; 100% = 0.8 ng/ml) can be measured precisely, it can be assessed if a patient is in the dangerous grey – zone of about 200% of normal, i.e. in the pre-phase of severe sepsis caused by pyrogens of gram-negative bacteria or of fungi [9].

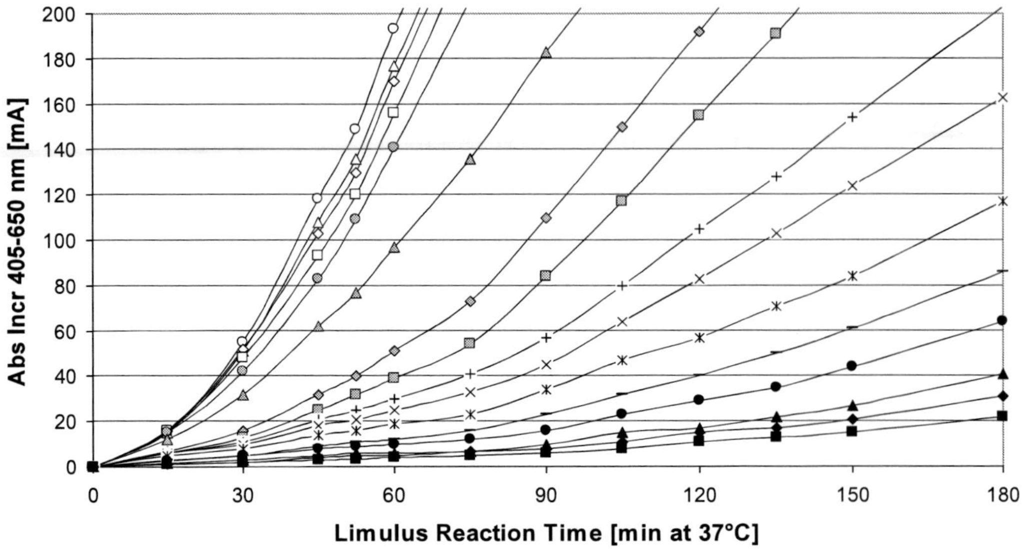

Figure 2. Limulus reaction kinetic in presence of arginine. 20 µl frozen/thawed Limulus-reagent were incubated with 20 µl 0-1000 mM sterile arginine in U-well microtiter plates at 37°C. The specific increase in absorbance (ΔA) with time was determined as ΔA at 405 nm minus ΔA at 650 nm. The final arginine concentrations were: 0 mM (O), 9 mM (Δ), 20 mM (◊), 29 mM (□), 44 mM (greyO), 54 mM (grey Δ), 67 mM (grey◊), 84 mM (grey□), 105 mM (+), 131 mM (x), 164 mM (*), 205 mM (-), 256 mM (●), 320 mM (▲), 400 mM (♦), or 500 mM (■).

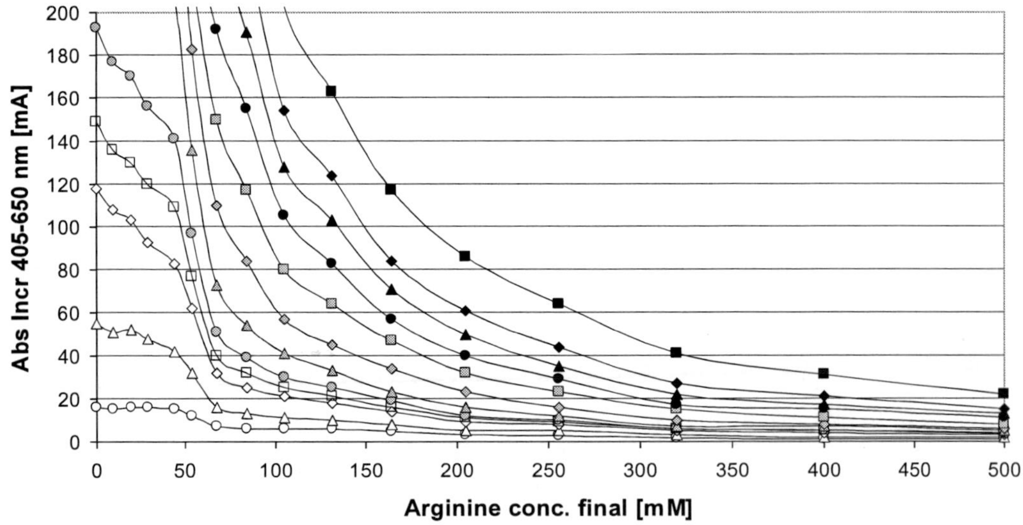

Figure 3. IC50 of arginine on the cascade of Limulus enzymes and on FAa. The Limulus reaction of figure 2 was performed with the following Limulus reaction times at 37°C: 15 min (O), 30 min (Δ), 45 min (◊), 52.5 min (□), 60 min (greyO), 75 min (greyΔ), 90 min (grey◊), 105 min (grey□), 120 min (●), 135 min (▲), 150 min (♦), 180 min (■).

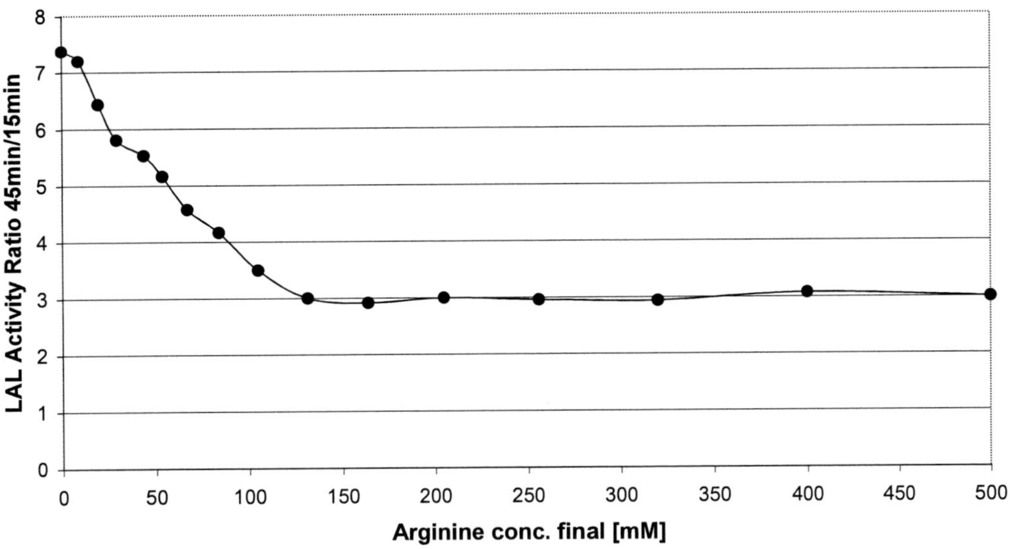

Figure 4. Ratio between ΔA within 45 min reaction time and ΔA within 15 min reaction time. The 45 min /15 min ratios of ΔA of figure 3 (symbols ◊ and O of fig. 3) were calculated. When the Limulus-Amebocyte-Lysate (LAL) kinetic is hyperbolic (without arginine) this ratio is 7.4. At final arginine concentrations > 130 mM the ratio = 3, indicating the change from hyperbolic to linear kinetic.

It is suggested to add sterile arginine at final concentrations of 300-400 mM to a Limulus reaction, that detects pg/ml quantities of free LPS, at a reaction time point (37°C) that is sufficient for precise quantification of plasmatic LPS reactivities in the critical 1-3 ng/ml range, e.g. an ideal moment might be when pooled normal plasma with about 0.8 ng/ml LPS reactivity generates an absorbance at 405 nm that is about 5-10% of the maximal absorbance.

Furthermore, arginine in concentrations of > 100 mM, preferably > 200 mM, might be a good stabilizer for the Limulus factors during the manufacturing process of the Limulus reagent to obtain a final product with a high concentration of functional Limulus factor C that is the principal binding partner of LPS and that makes the Limulus reagent so sensible to pg/ml to fg/ml quantities of free LPS.

Septic patients with severe coagulopathy have extremely high plasmatic levels of LPS; mortality increases dramatically with an increase of plasma LPS to about 100 endotoxin units/ml [10]. Effective antibiotic treatment results in a rapid decline of plasma LPS (half-life of 1-3 h), reduced coagulation activation and increased fibrinolysis capacity [10]. The endotoxin reactivity should be measured in any patient that is of risk to develop a severe sepsis. So, a patient in the grey-zone of about 200% of normal endotoxin reactivity could receive the adequate treatment in time.

REFERENCES

[1] Hurley JC. Endotoxemia: methods of detection and clinical correlates. *Clin. Microbiol. Rev.* 1995; 8: 268-92.

[2] Stief TW. Thrombin generation by exposure of blood to endotoxin: a simple model to study disseminated intravascular coagulation. *Clin. Appl. Thromb. Hemost.* 2006; 12: 137-61.

[3] Stief TW, Ijagha O, Weiste B, Herzum I, Renz H, Max M. Analysis of hemostasis alterations in sepsis. *Blood Coagul. Fibrinolysis* 2007; 18: 179-86.

[4] Stief TW. Coagulation Activation by Lipopolysaccharides. *Clin. Appl. Thromb. Hemost.* 2007 Dec 26; [Epub ahead of print].

[5] van Deventer SJ, Buller HR, ten Cate JW, Sturk A, Pauw W. Endotoxaemia: an early predictor of septicaemia in febrile patients. *Lancet* 1988; 19, 1: 605-9.

[6] Osaki T, Kawabata S. Structure and function of coagulogen, a clottable protein in horseshoe crabs. *Cell Mol. Life Sci.* 2004; 61: 1257-65.

[7] Iwanaga S. The molecular basis of innate immunity in the horseshoe crab. *Curr. Opin. Immunol.* 2002; 14: 87-95.

[8] Stief TW. Innovative tests of plasmatic hemostasis. *Laboratory Medicine* 2008; 39: 225-230.

[9] Ding JL, Ho B. A new era in pyrogen testing. *Trends Biotechnol* 2001; 19: 277-81.

[10] Brandtzaeg P, Bjerre A, Øvstebø R, Brusletto B, Joø GB, Kierulf P. Neisseria meningitidis lipopolysaccharides in human pathology. *J. Endotoxin. Res.* 2001; 7: 401-20.

[11] Stief TW. Determination of active endotoxin in plasma. *Hemostasis Laboratory* 2008; 1: (issue 1; in press).

[12] Stief TW, Max M. Active endotoxin in sepsis. *Hemostasis Laboratory* 2008; 1: (issue 1; in press).

In: Hemostasis Laboratory Yearbook, Volume 2
Editor: Thomas W. Stief, pp. 201-208 ISBN: 978-1-60741-089-8

FEIBA TRIGGERS THROMBIN GENERATION

*Thomas W. Stief**
Department of Clinical Chemistry,
University Hospital Giessen and Marburg, Germany

ABSTRACT

Background: FEIBA (factor eight inhibitor bypassing activity) is an established drug to enhance plasmatic thrombin generation in patients at risk for bleeding due to inhibitors of the intrinsic pathway of coagulation. The aim of the present work was to determine the 200 % effective dose (ED200) of FEIBA on plasmatic thrombin generation.

Material and Methods: Pools of unfrozen citrated plasma (normal or from patients on coumarin, INR=1.8) were supplemented with 0-10 U/ml FEIBA (Immuno; S-TIM4) on polystyrol U-well microtiter plates (Brand®701300) at 23°C. Immediately thereafter the ultra-specific, ultra-sensitive thrombin generation assays RECA-10 (recalcified coagulation activity assay with 10 min coagulation reaction time (CRT) at 37°C), INCA-4 (intrinsic coagulation activity assay with 4 min CRT), and EXCA-1 (extrinsic coagulation activity assay with 1 min CRT) were performed with 20 µl or 50 µl plasma samples. Thrombin generation = thrombin activity after CRT minus basal thrombin activity in citrated plasma (without CRT).

Results: The approximate ED200 of FEIBA in pooled normal plasma was about 0.02 U/ml in RECA-10, about 0.04 U/ml in INCA-4, and about 0.05 U/ml in EXCA-1. The ED200 of FEIBA added to pooled plasma from patients on coumarin was about 0.03 U/ml FEIBA in RECA-10; about 0.06 U/ml FEIBA were necessary to obtain a RECA value that is 33 % of normal.

Discussion: The RECA is a new instrument to predict and to monitor the hemostatic power of FEIBA: in patients at risk for bleeding or already in bleeding the target RECA value might be about 33-50 % of the normal one: FEIBA therapy should be individually adjusted according to the RECA value.

Keywords: FEIBA, factor eight inhibitor bypassing activity, thrombin, RECA, INCA, EXCA, ED200.

---

* Correspondence to:_PD Dr. med. T. Stief, Department of Clinical Chemistry, University Hospital, D-35043 Marburg, Germany. E-mail: thstief@med.uni-marburg.de; Tel. : +49-6421-58 64471; FAX: +49-6421-58 65594.

Introduction

Factor VIII inhibitor bypassing activity (FEIBA) is a mixture of the proenzymes of the prothrombin complex (FVII, FIX, FX, FII) and of small amounts of the respective activated calcium dependent serine proteases of the clotting system, i.e. factors VIIa, IXa, Xa, and IIa, that can bypass an intrinsic coagulation pathway that is inhibited e.g. by inhibitors against factor VIII or against factor IX; especially F Xa seems to play a critical role in the activity of FEIBA [1-6]. FEIBA dose-dependently enhances plasmatic thrombin generation [7-9]. It was the purpose of the present work to determine the 200 % effective dose (ED200) of FEIBA on new ultra-specific, ultra-sensitive, and ultra-precise thrombin generation assays.

Material and Methods

Pooled Unfrozen Normal Plasma

Unfrozen pooled normal citrated plasma (from 8 samples that remained after routine analysis; 0.5 ml 106 mM sodium citrate + 4.5 ml venous blood in polypropylene sampling tubes; Sarstedt, Nümbrecht, Germany) was supplemented with 0-16.7 U/ml FEIBA (factor VIII inhibitor bypassing activity (Immuno, Heidelberg, Germany; S-TIM4 lot nr. 05A0801B, P217928) the reconstituted solution was aliquoted in 100 µl 200 U/ml quantities, frozen at -30°C and thawed for the assay) directly in a polystyrol U-well microtiter plate (Brand, Wertheim, Germany; article nr. 701300). The repetitively 1+1 diluted plasma pool were pipetted in 20 µl aliquots by means of an Eppendorf-Multipette® with 0.9 % NaCl – rinsed new tips. After 30 min (23°C) two innovative ultra-specific, ultra-sensitive thrombin generation assays were performed: the RECA (recalcified coagulation activity assay) and the EXCA (extrinsic coagulation activity assay) [10]. The tests were standardized with 1 IU/ml bovine thrombin in 6.7 % human albumin (DadeBehring, Marburg, Germany) that replaced the plasma sample. The basal amidolytic thrombin activity in the present pools of citrated plasma was 6-10 mIU/ml. Thrombin generation = thrombin activity in the generation assay at a certain coagulation reaction time (CRT) minus basal thrombin activity in citrated plasma at 0 min CRT. If 5 % human albumin instead of plasma was supplemented in duplicate with FEIBA, 0.1 U/ml FEIBA behaved in the present assay conditions with supra-molar concentrations of arginine in the thrombin detection phase as < 3 mIU/ml thrombin.

20 µl samples of unfrozen pooled normal plasma (from 7 samples that remained after routine analysis; about 4h 23°C old) was supplemented with 0-10 U/ml FEIBA (STIM-4; Immuno, Heidelberg, Germany) on U-well plates. Immediately thereafter the thrombin generation assays RECA with 10 min CRT (RECA-10) and the extrinsic coagulation activity assay with 1 min CRT (EXCA-1) were performed in duplicate as indicated below.

Fresh Pooled Unfrozen Normal Plasma

20 µl samples of fresh unfrozen pooled normal plasma (from 7 samples; about 2h 23°C old) were supplemented with 0-0.833 U/ml FEIBA on U-well plates. Immediately thereafter

the recalcified coagulation activity assay with 10 min coagulation reaction time (RECA-10), the intrinsic coagulation activity assay with 4 min coagulation reaction time (INCA-4), and the extrinsic coagulation activity assay with 1 min coagulation reaction time (EXCA-1) were performed as follows:

RECA

2 µl RECA-trigger (250 mM $CaCl_2$ in 1 ml aliquots in siliconized glass vials, frozen at -30°C and thawed directly for the assay) were added. The plates were intensely shaken for 5s and incubated at 37°C in a digitally controlled water-bath. After 0-40 min coagulation reaction time (CRT) 50 µl arginine-reagent (2.5 M arginine, pH 8.7, 0.16 % Triton X 100® (both from Sigma, Deisenhofen, Germany) were added. 3 minutes (23°C) after the last CRT period 25 µl 1 mM chromogenic thrombin substrate HD-CHG-Ala-Arg-pNA (Pentapharm, Basel, Switzerland) in 1.25 M arginine, pH 8.7, were added. The increase in absorbance at 405 nm with time ΔA/t was determined by a microtiter plate photometer with a 1 mA resolution (Milenia; DPC, Los Angeles, USA). The maximal ΔA with these assay volumes in U-wells plates was about 1050 mA, 40 % of the maximal ΔA = about 420 mA = the upper limit of linear range of the assay without significant substrate exhaustion.

INCA

2 µl INCA-trigger were added. The present INCA trigger consisted in 500 µl 500 mM $CaCl_2$ aliquots in siliconized glass vials, frozen at -30°C and thawed for the assay were mixed with 400 µl H_2O and directly prior to the start of the assay with 100 µl SiO_2 reagent (Pathromtin SL®; DadeBehring). The plates were intensely shaken for 5s and incubated at 37°C in a digitally controlled water-bath. After 4 min coagulation reaction time (INCA-4) 50 µl arginine-reagent (2.5 M arginine, pH 8.7, 0.16 % Triton X 100® were added. After 3 minutes (23°C) 25 µl 1 mM HD-CHG-Ala-Arg-pNA in 1.25 M arginine, pH 8.7, were added. ΔA/t was determined by a microtiter plate photometer with a 1 mA resolution.

EXCA

2 µl EXCA-trigger were added. The EXCA trigger consisted in 1 ml aliquots of 1 ng/ml human placental tissue factor (Polybrene®-free Thromborel-S ®; DadeBehring) 250 mM $CaCl_2$ in siliconized glass vials, frozen at -30°C and thawed for the assay. The plates were intensely shaken for 5s and incubated at 37°C in a digitally controlled water-bath. After 1 min coagulation reaction time (EXCA-1) 50 µl arginine-reagent (2.5 M arginine, pH 8.7, 0.16 % Triton X 100® were added. After 3 minutes (23°C) 25 µl 1 mM HD-CHG-Ala-Arg-pNA in 1.25 M arginine, pH 8.7, were added. ΔA/t was determined by a microtiter plate photometer with a 1 mA resolution.

Pooled Unfrozen Plasma from Patients on Coumarin

50 µl samples of unfrozen pooled plasma (from 7 patients on coumarin, the samples remained after routine analysis, were about 4h old, stored at 23°C; INR=1.8) were supplemented with 0-3.92 U/ml FEIBA on U-well plates. Immediately thereafter the RECA-10 was performed, using 100 µl arginine-reagent and 25 µl substrate-reagent. The 1 IU/ml thrombin standard generated a ΔA at 405 nm of about 20 mA/min (23°C).

A negative control was unfrozen pooled plasma from 7 unselected patients with normal prothrombin time (PT), normal activated partial thromboplastin time (APTT), and normal fibrinogen concentration; this pool was supplemented with 1 IU/ml unfractionated heparin (ratiopharm, Ulm, Germany).

RESULTS AND DISCUSSION

Figure 1 demonstrates that the 200 % effective dose (ED200) of FEIBA in RECA-10 was about 0.03 U/ml. Of major importance are the CRT periods that belong to the ascending part of the thrombin generation curve, i.e. here CRT periods ≤ 10 min (Figure 1b), because there is still no marked negative influence of nascending fibrin (= antithrombin I [11]) on thrombin.

If a similar experiment was performed with immediate recalcification after FEIBA supplementation of plasma, the approximate ED200 was about 0.02 U/ml in RECA-10 and about 0.04 U/ml in EXCA-1 (Figure 2). With a fresh plasma-pool the approximate ED200 was about 0.02 U/ml in RECA-10, about 0.04 U/ml in INCA-4, and about 0.06 U/ml in EXCA-1 (Figure 3).

The ED200 of FEIBA added to pooled plasma from patients on coumarin (INR=1.8) was about 0.03 U/ml FEIBA in RECA-10 (Figure 4); about 0.06 U/ml FEIBA were necessary to obtain a RECA-10 value that is 33.3 % of normal (100 % = about 0.4 IU/ml thrombin). The plasma pool with 1 IU/ml unfractionated heparin did not generate additional thrombin during the RECA-10 at final FEIBA activities up to 1.96 U/ml. 3.92 U/ml FEIBA induced an additional thrombin generation of about 10 mIU/ml (thrombin activity in RECA-10 = 18 mIU/ml, basal thrombin activity in this citrated plasma-pool = 8 mIU/ml).

Thus, addition of approximately 0.02 U/ml FEIBA to unfrozen pooled normal plasma doubles the normal RECA-10 value. There might be a great lot-to-lot variation of commercial FEIBA [12]: FEIBA with high activities of factor Xa and/or thrombin might be much more active than those with low activities of these critical enzymes, factor VIIa that can also be generated by factor Xa [13] might be of secondary importance in FEIBA. Former FEIBA lots with activities in U might thus be different to actual lots with activities in IU; e.g. 0.2 U/ml FEIBA is the approximate activity that induces jugular vein thrombosis when circulating blood is locally in stasis [14]. 0.2 U FEIBA may contain approximately 1 mIU/ml thrombin that might enhance plasmatic coagulation activation by activation of the factors V and VIII [15]. In contrast, actual therapeutic doses of FEIBA are 50-100, maximally up to 200 IU/kg, which corresponds to final plasmatic FEIBA activities in the range of 1-4 IU/ml, which might be about 10fold the activities of former FEIBA preparations. Furthermore, since FEIBA is a mixture of activated serine proteases, FEIBA should be stabilized by ≥ 200 mM arginine, pH 7.4, to avoid enzyme destruction prior to infusion to the patient.

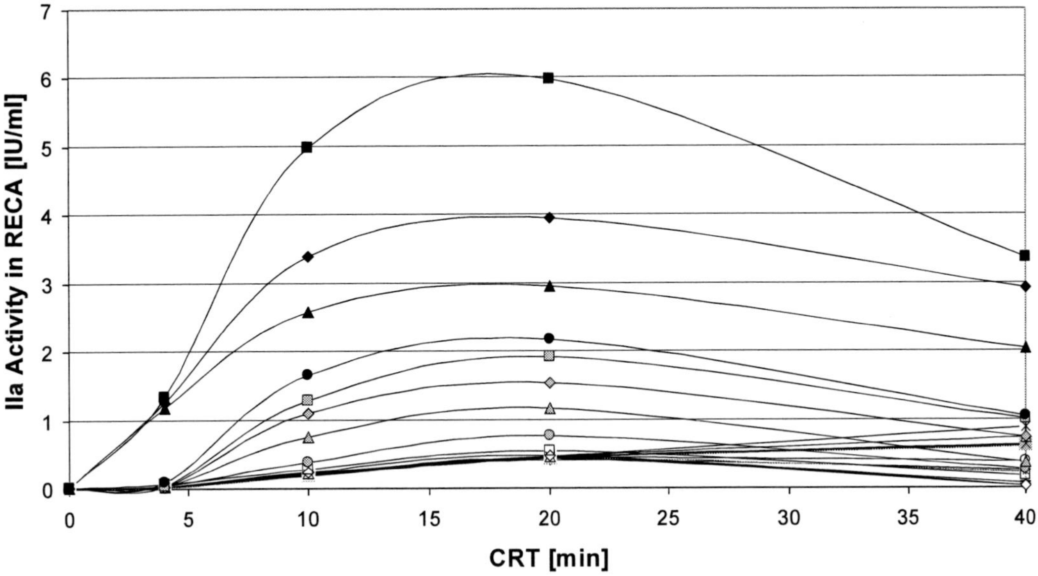

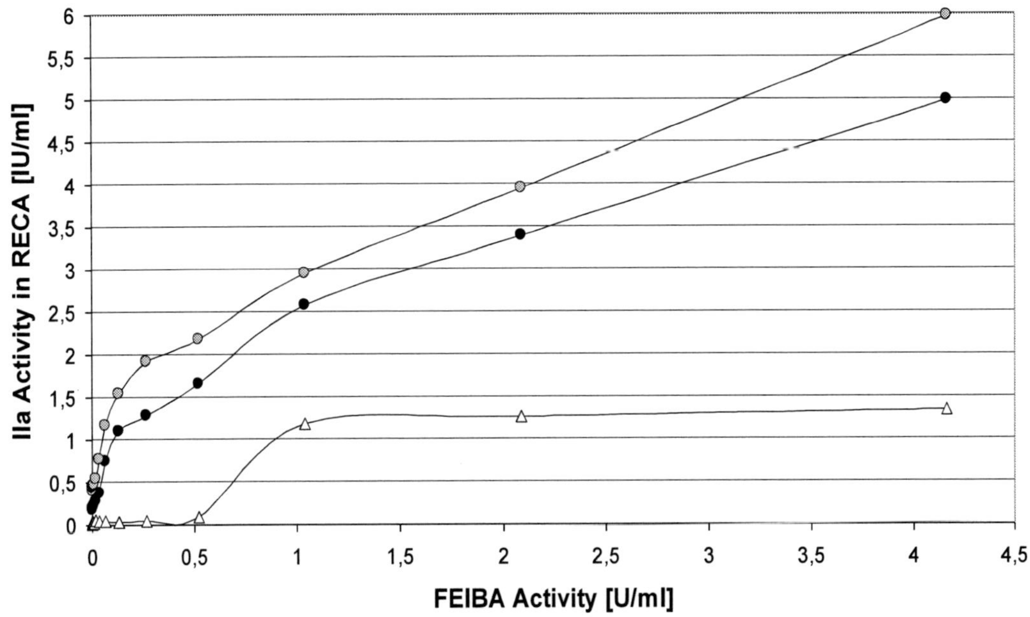

Figure 1. Thrombin generation triggered by FEIBA. Unfrozen pooled normal citrated plasma was supplemented with 0-4.17 U/ml FEIBA in a polystyrol U-well microtiter plate. After 30 min (23°C) the recalcified coagulation activity assay (RECA) was performed with a coagulation reaction time (CRT) of 0-40 min (37°C); Figure 1a: 0 IU/ml (O), 0.00003 U/ml (-), 0.00006 U/ml (+), 0.0001 U/ml (x), 0.0003 U/ml (*), 0.0005 U/ml (grey+), 0.001 U/ml (grey x), 0.002 U/ml (grey*) 0.004 U/ml (Δ), 0.008 U/ml (◊), 0.016 U/ml (□), 0.033 U/ml (greyO), 0.065 U/ml (greyΔ), 0.13 U/ml (gey◊), 0.26 U/ml (grey□), 0.52 U/ml (●), 1.04 U/ml (▲), 2.08 U/ml (♦), 4.17 U/ml (■) FEIBA. Figure 1b: CRT periods of 4 min (Δ), 10 min (●), or 20 min (greyO).

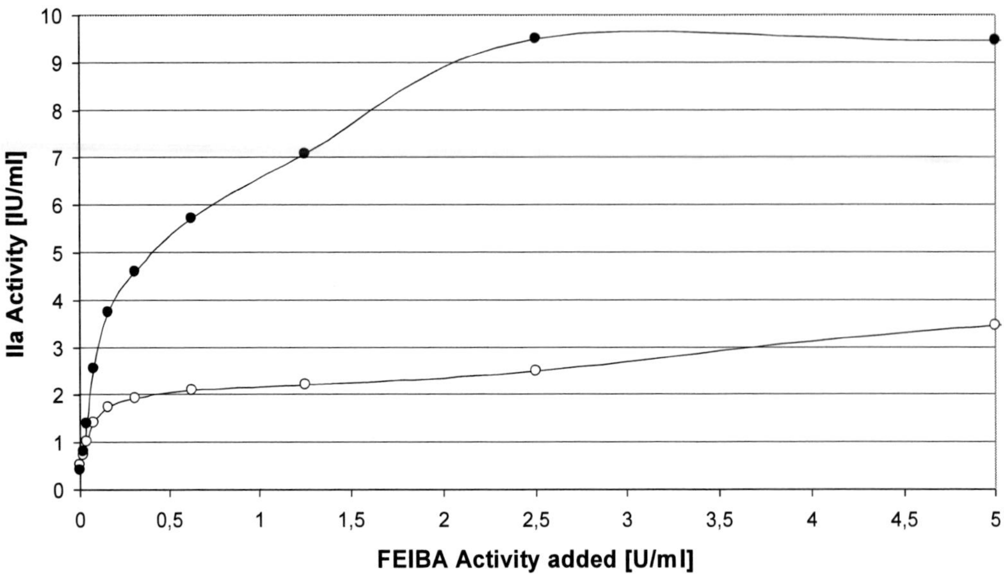

Figure 2. Thrombin generation triggered by FEIBA. Unfrozen pooled normal plasma was supplemented with 0-10 U/ml FEIBA in U-well plates. Immediately thereafter the thrombin generation assays recalcified coagulation activity assay with 10 min coagulation reaction time (RECA-10; ●) or extrinsic coagulation activity assay with 1 min coagulation reaction time (EXCA-1; O) were performed. There was no significant change between 5 U/ml and 10 U/ml FEIBA.

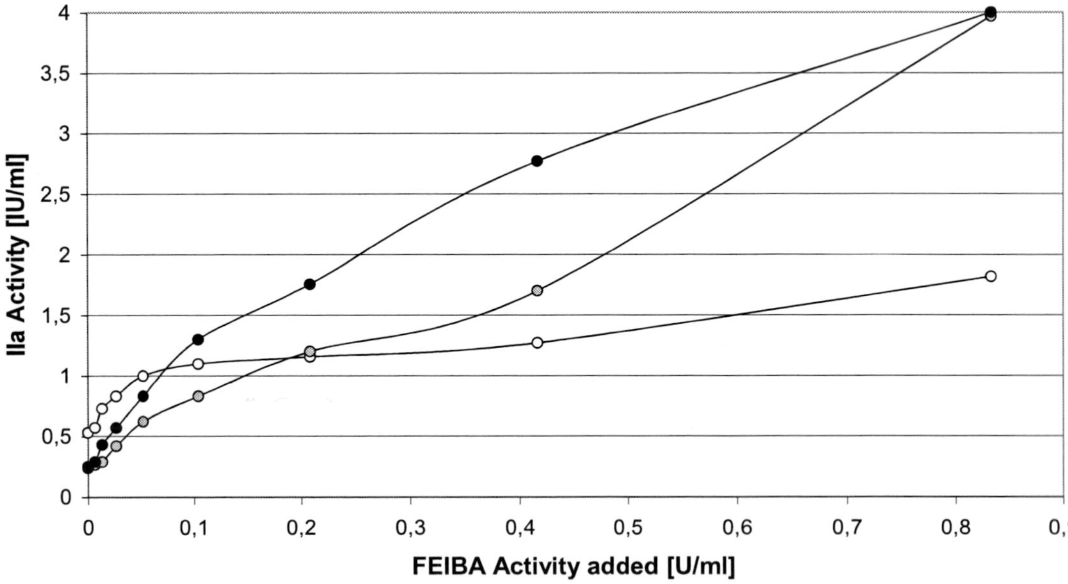

Figure 3. FEIBA triggers IIa generation. 20 µl samples of fresh unfrozen pooled normal plasma were supplemented with 0-0.833 U/ml FEIBA on U-well plates. Immediately thereafter the recalcified coagulation activity assay with 10 min coagulation reaction time (RECA-10; ●), the intrinsic coagulation activity assay with 4 min coagulation reaction time (INCA-4; greyO), or the extrinsic coagulation activity assay with 1 min coagulation reaction time (EXCA-1; O) were performed.

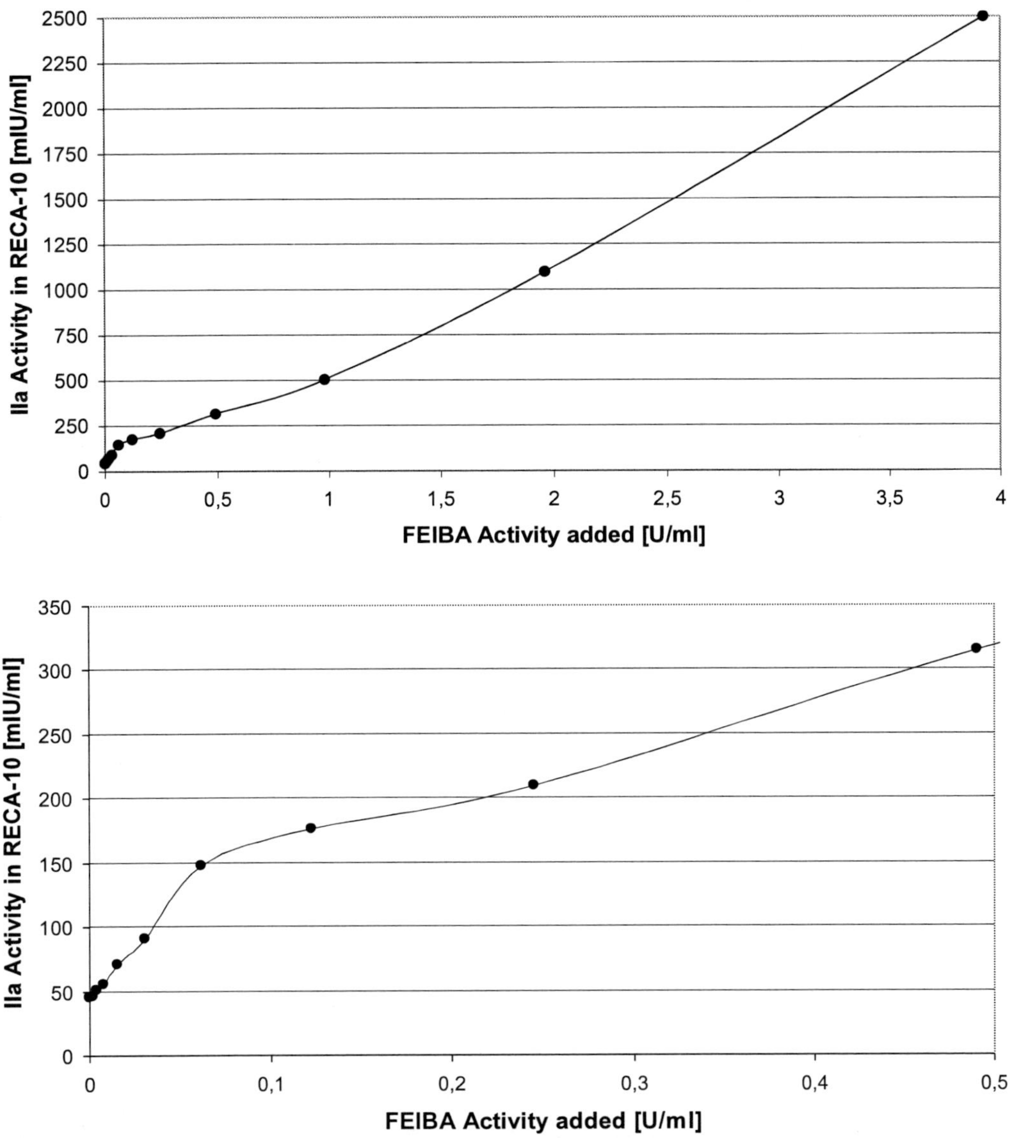

Figure 4. Pooled plasma of patients on coumarin. 50 µl samples of unfrozen pooled plasma from marcumarized patients were supplemented with 0-3.92 U/ml FEIBA on U-well plates. Immediately thereafter the RECA-10 was performed, using 100 µl arginine-reagent and 25 µl substrate-reagent.

The hemostatic efficacy of FEIBA or of recombinant factor VIIa in the individual patient can be unpredictable [1]. In some patients none of the available products are particularly effective at the usual dosages [2]. Up to now there has been a lack of standardized and validated laboratory assays that reflect the hemostatic efficacy of the bypassing agents [2]. The RECA is a new instrument to predict and to monitor the hemostatic power of FEIBA: in patients at risk for bleeding or already in bleeding the target RECA value might be about 33-50 % of the normal one: FEIBA therapy should be individually adjusted according to the RECA value.

REFERENCES

[1] Gomperts ED, Astermark J, Gringeri A, Teitel J. From theory to practice: applying current clinical knowledge and treatment strategies to the care of hemophilia A patients with inhibitors. *Blood Rev*. 2008; 22 Suppl 1: S1-11.

[2] Tjønnfjord GE, Holme PA. Factor eight inhibitor bypass activity (FEIBA) in the management of bleeds in hemophilia patients with high-titer inhibitors. Vasc Health *Risk Manag*. 2007; 3: 527-31.

[3] Turecek PL, Váradi K, Gritsch H, Schwarz HP. FEIBA: mode of action. *Haemophilia* 2004; 10 Suppl 2:3-9.

[4] Tomokiyo K, Nakatomi Y, Araki T, Teshima K, Nakano H, Nakagaki T, Miyamoto S, Funatsu A, Iwanaga S. A novel therapeutic approach combining human plasma-derived Factors VIIa and X for haemophiliacs with inhibitors: evidence of a higher thrombin generation rate in vitro and more sustained haemostatic activity in vivo than obtained with Factor VIIa alone. *Vox Sang* 2003; 85: 290-9.

[5] Gallistl S, Cvirn G, Leschnik B, Muntean W. Respective roles of factors II, VII, IX, and X in the procoagulant activity of FEIBA. *Blood Coagul Fibrinolysis* 2002; 13: 653-5.

[6] Turecek PL, Varadi K, Gritsch H, Auer W, Pichler L, Eder G, Schwarz HP. Factor Xa and prothrombin: mechanism of action of FEIBA. *Vox Sang* 1999; 77 Suppl 1:72-9.

[7] Livnat T, Martinowitz U, Zivelin A, Seligsohn U. Effects of factor VIII inhibitor bypassing activity (FEIBA), recombinant factor VIIa or both on thrombin generation in normal and haemophilia A plasma. Haemophilia 2008 Mar 25. [Epub ahead of print]

[8] Váradi K, Turecek PL, Schwarz HP. Thrombin generation assay and other universal tests for monitoring haemophilia therapy. *Haemophilia* 2004; 10 Suppl 2: 17-21.

[9] Váradi K, Negrier C, Berntorp E, Astermark J, Bordet JC, Morfini M, Linari S, Schwarz HP, Turecek PL. Monitoring the bioavailability of FEIBA with a thrombin generation assay. *J. Thromb Haemost.* 2003; 1: 2374-80.

[10] Stief TW. Innovative tests of plasmatic hemostasis. *Laboratory Medicine* 2008; 39: 225-30.

[11] Mosesson MW. Update on antithrombin I (fibrin). *Thromb Haemost* 2007; 98: 105-8.

[12] Vinazzer H. Comparison between two concentrates with factor VIII inhibitor bypassing activity. *Thromb Res.* 1982; 26: 21-9.

[13] Masys DR, Bajaj SP, Rapaport SI. Activation of human factor VII by activated factors IX and X. *Blood* 1982; 60: 1143-50.

[14] Stief TW, Fareed J. The antithrombotic factor singlet oxygen/light ($^1O_2$/hv). Clin Appl *Thromb Hemost.* 2000; 6: 22-30.

[15] Boström SL, Dagnelid E, Hansson GF, Ulvinge JC. Inhibition of thrombin-induced feedback activation of factor V: a potential pathway for inhibition of thrombin generation by melagatran. *Blood Coagul Fibrinolysis* 2004; 15: 25-30.

In: Hemostasis Laboratory Yearbook, Volume 2
Editor: Thomas W. Stief, pp. 209-220
ISBN: 978-1-60741-089-8

THROMBIN TRIGGERS ITS GENERATION

Thomas W. Stief *

Department of Clinical Chemistry,
University Hospital Giessen and Marburg, Germany

ABSTRACT

Background: The generation of plasmatic thrombin is of major importance in hemostasis regulation. The purpose of the present work was to modulate thrombin generation by addition of low activities of thrombin to citrated plasma and to quantify the resulting thrombin generation after recalcification of these plasmas.

Material and Methods: Pools of unfrozen citrated plasma (normal or from patients on coumarin) were supplemented with 0-63 mIU/ml bovine or human thrombin on polystyrol U-well microtiter plates (Brand®701300) at 23°C. Immediately thereafter the ultra-specific, ultra-sensitive thrombin generation assays RECA-10 (recalcified coagulation activity assay with 10 min coagulation reaction time (CRT) at 37°C) and EXCA-1 (extrinsic coagulation activity assay with 1 min CRT) were performed with 20 μl or 50 μl plasma samples. Thrombin generation = thrombin activity after CRT minus basal thrombin activity in citrated plasma (without CRT).

Results: The approximate 200 % effective dose (ED200) of added bovine or human thrombin on thrombin generation of pooled normal plasma in the RECA-10 was about 2-4 mIU/ml. The respective approximate ED200 in the EXCA-1 was about 5 mIU/ml added thrombin. The ED200 of thrombin added to pooled plasma from patients on coumarin (international normalized ratio = 1.8) on thrombin generation in RECA-10 was about 8 mIU/ml. To obtain in pooled coumarin-plasma a thrombin generation that is about one third of the normal RECA value about 14 mIU/ml thrombin had to be added.

Discussion: Addition of only about 2-4 mIU/ml thrombin to pooled unfrozen normal citrated plasma approximately doubles the thrombin activity generated in RECA-10 which corresponds well to the about 3 mIU/ml thrombin in pooled normal plasma that is necessary for a normal hyperbolic rate phase in the intrinsic hemostasis assay RECA. The present findings may be of importance in diagnosis and therapy of individual dysgenerations of plasmatic thrombin.

Keywords: Thrombin, factor IIa, EXCA, RECA, ED200.

---

* Correspondence to:_PD Dr. med. T. Stief, Department of Clinical Chemistry, University Hospital, D-35043 Marburg, Germany. E-mail: thstief@med.uni-marburg.de; Tel. : +49-6421-58 64471; FAX: +49-6421-58 65594

Introduction

Thrombin is the central enzyme of coagulation [1-3]. Its generation and inactivation is of major clinical importance [4-6]. The serine protease thrombin is generated by extrinsic or intrinsic triggers of coagulation that generate the extrinsic or intrinsic tenase, respectively [7,8]. Main accelerators of coagulation are the activated factors V and VIII; both are activated by thrombin. Thus, thrombin in catalytic amounts may trigger its own generation. It was the purpose of the present study to quantify the added thrombin activity that is necessary to double the normal thrombin generation [9] in innovative ultra-specific and ultra-sensitive thrombin generation assays [10].

Material and Methods

Pooled Unfrozen Normal Plasma

Unfrozen pooled normal citrated plasma (from 8 samples that remained after routine analysis; about 4h old, stored at 23°C; 0.5 ml 106 mM sodium citrate + 4.5 ml venous blood in polypropylene sampling tubes; Sarstedt, Nümbrecht, Germany; basally containing about 8 mIU/ml amidolytic thrombin activity [11]) was supplemented with 0-31.3 mIU/ml bovine thrombin (factor IIa; DadeBehring, Marburg, Germany) in 6.7 % human albumin (CSL Behring, Marburg, Germany) directly in a polystyrol U-well microtiter plate (Brand, Wertheim, Germany; article nr. 701300). The repetitively 1+1 on a microtiter plate diluted plasma pool was pipetted in 20 µl aliquots by means of an Eppendorf-Multipette® with 0.9 % NaCl – rinsed new tips. After 30 min (23°C) the ultra-specific, ultra-sensitive thrombin generation assay RECA (recalcified coagulation activity assay) was performed in duplicate. The RECA was standardized with 1 IU/ml bovine thrombin (DadeBehring) in 6.7 % human albumin (Kabi, Stockholm, Sweden) that replaced the plasma samples and resulted in a ΔA at 405 nm of about 10 mA/min (23°C) for 20 µl samples and in about 20 mA/min (23°C) for 50 µl samples; linear range = 0-40 % of maximal ΔA [10]. Thrombin generation = thrombin activity in generation assay minus basal thrombin activity in citrated plasma (about 6-10 mIU/ml).

20 µl samples of unfrozen pooled normal plasma (from 7 samples that remained after routine analysis, about 4h old, stored at 23°C) were supplemented with 0-33.25 mIU/ml bovine thrombin or human thrombin (Stago, Asnières, France) on U-well plates. Immediately thereafter the thrombin generation assays recalcified coagulation activity assay with 10 min coagulation reaction time (RECA-10), which ultra-sensitively reflects intrinsic coagulation, or the extrinsic coagulation activity assay with 1 min coagulation reaction time (EXCA-1) were performed in duplicate as follows:

RECA

2 µl RECA-trigger (250 mM $CaCl_2$ in 1 ml aliquots in siliconized glass vials (DadeBehring, article nr. OVKE49), frozen at -30°C and thawed directly for the assay) were added. The plates were intensely shaken for 5s and incubated at 37°C in a digitally controlled water-bath. After 0-40 min coagulation reaction time (CRT) 50 µl arginine-reagent (2.5 M arginine, pH 8.7, 0.16 % Triton X 100® (both from Sigma, Deisenhofen, Germany)

were added. 3 minutes (23°C) after the last CRT period 25 µl 1 mM chromogenic thrombin substrate HD-CHG-Ala-Arg-pNA (Pentapharm, Basel, Switzerland) in 1.25 M arginine, pH 8.7, were added. The increase in absorbance at 405 nm with time ΔA/t was determined by a microtiter plate photometer with a 1 mA resolution (Milenia; DPC, Los Angeles, USA). The maximal ΔA with these assay volumes in U-wells plates was about 1050 mA, 40 % of the maximal ΔA was about 420 mA (= the upper limit of linear range of the assay without significant substrate exhaustion).

EXCA

2 µl EXCA-trigger were added. The EXCA trigger consisted in 1 ml aliquots of 1 ng/ml human placental tissue factor (Polybrene®-free Thromborel-S®; DadeBehring) 250 mM $CaCl_2$ in siliconized glass vials, frozen at -30°C and thawed for the assay. The plates were intensely shaken for 5s and incubated at 37°C in a digitally controlled water-bath. After 1 min coagulation reaction time (EXCA-1) 50 µl arginine-reagent (2.5 M arginine, pH 8.7, 0.16 % Triton X 100® were added. After 3 minutes (23°C) 25 µl 1 mM HD-CHG-Ala-Arg-pNA in 1.25 M arginine, pH 8.7, were added. ΔA/t was determined by a microtiter plate photometer with a 1 mA resolution.

Fresh Pooled Unfrozen Normal Plasma

20 µl samples of fresh unfrozen pooled normal plasma (from 7 samples that remained after routine analysis, about 2h old at the moment of analysis, stored at 23°C) were supplemented with 0-16.6 mIU/ml bovine thrombin or 0-16.6 mIU/ml human thrombin on U-well plates. Immediately thereafter the thrombin generation assays RECA-10 or EXCA-1 were performed as described above.

Pooled Unfrozen Plasma from Patients on Coumarin

50 µl samples of unfrozen pooled plasma (from 7 patients on Marcumar® (phenprocoumon), the samples remained after routine analysis, were about 4h old, stored at 23°C) were supplemented with 0-19.6 mIU/ml bovine thrombin (the stock solution was 1 IU/ml bovine thrombin, 5 % human albumin in 1 ml green polypropylene tubes) on U-well plates. Immediately thereafter the RECA-10 was performed, using 100 µl arginine-reagent and 25 µl substrate-reagent. The 1 IU/ml thrombin standard generated a ΔA at 405 nm of about 20 mA/min (23°C). This coumarin-plasma-pool had an international normalized ratio (INR; trigger of Thromborel S® = placental tissue factor) of 1.8 (normal range as mean value ± 1 standard deviation = 1 ± 0.15), an activated partial thromboplastin time (APTT; trigger of Pathromtin SL® (DadeBehring) = SiO_2) of 36s (normal range: < 36s), and a fibrinogen concentration (modified Clauss-method; DadeBehring) of 4.8 g/l (normal range: 1.8-3.5 g/l). A negative control was pooled unfrozen plasma from 7 unselected patients with normal INR and normal APTT; this pool was unsupplemented or supplemented with 1 IU/ml unfractionated heparin (ratiopharm, Ulm, Germany), resulting in an APTT of 181s and an INR of 1.46 (52 % prothrombin time on the Behring Coagulation Timer®).

Further RECA Studies with Addition of Human Thrombin to Different Plasmas

Supplementation of Pooled Normal Plasma with Human Thrombin

50 µl unfrozen pooled normal plasma (4h 23°C old, remaining after routine analysis; from 11 patients not on hemostasis therapy with normal INR and APTT) were supplemented on the U-well microtiter plate with 0-15 mIU/ml human thrombin directly out of the original glass vial. Immediately thereafter the RECA-10 was performed.

Thrombin Generation in Two Plasmas of Patients on Coumarin

50 µl unfrozen plasma of two patients on Marcumar® with INR = 1.75 or INR = 2.25 (4h 23°C old, remaining after routine analysis) were assayed in the RECA with different coagulation reaction times (CRT).

Supplementation of Plasma of a Patient on Coumarin with Human Thrombin

50 µl unfrozen plasma of one patient on Marcumar® with INR = 2.25 and for control 50 µl unfrozen plasma of a patient not on hemostasis therapy with normal INR and APTT (4h 23°C old, remaining after routine analysis) were supplemented with 0-20 mIU/ml human thrombin on the plate directly out of the original glass vial and immediately thereafter assayed in the RECA-10.

Control: Normal RECA-Kinetic for Individual Unfrozen Plasmas

50 µl unfrozen citrated plasma of 8 patients not on hemostasis therapy and with normal PT, APTT, and fibrinogen and one patient not on hemostasis therapy with normal PT, APTT but with 9 g/l fibrinogen (all plasmas 4h 23°C old, remaining after routine analysis) were assayed in the RECA. The respective basal plasma turbidities at 405 nm prior to addition of the chromogenic thrombin substrate were also measured.

Control: Normal RECA-Kinetic for Pooled Unfrozen Plasma

50 µl unfrozen pooled citrated plasma from 11 patients not on hemostasis therapy and with normal INR, APTT, and fibrinogen (4h 23°C old, remaining after routine analysis) was assayed in the RECA. The respective basal plasma turbidities at 405 nm prior to addition of the chromogenic thrombin substrate were also measured.

Results and Discussion

Figure 1 demonstrates that about 4 mIU/ml bovine thrombin approximately doubled the RECA-10 value of pooled unfrozen normal plasma. Basally it was about 0.19 IU/ml thrombin, i.e. a generation of about 0.18 IU/ml thrombin additionally to the 8 mIU/ml thrombin that were basally in the pooled plasma prior to recalcification. Thus, the 200 % effective dose (ED200) of bovine thrombin on this RECA-10 of pooled plasma was about 4 mIU/ml.

Addition of 63 mIU/ml thrombin to pooled plasma clotted the plasma, entrapped thrombin [12], and resulted in a decrease of the thrombin generation curve (Figure 1b).

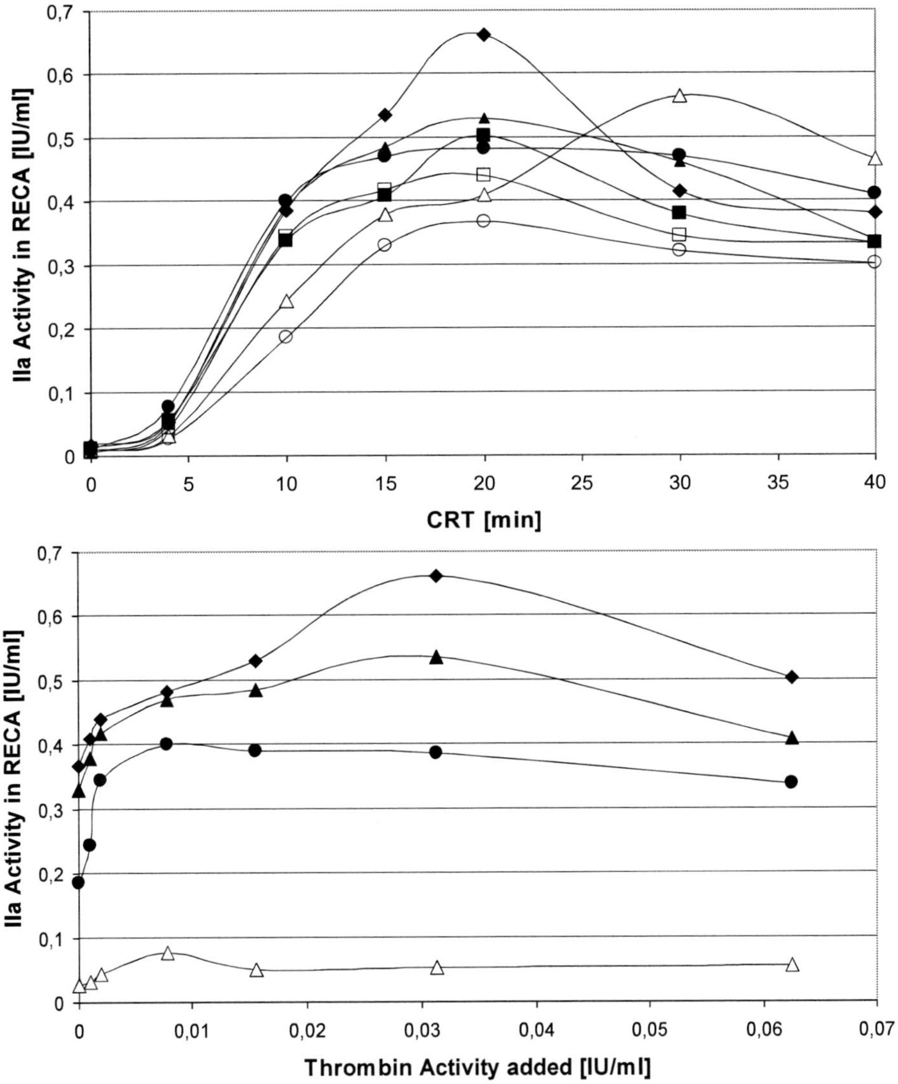

Figure 1. Thrombin generation triggered by thrombin. Unfrozen pooled normal citrated plasma was supplemented with 0-0.063 IU/ml bovine thrombin (IIa) in a polystyrol U-well microtiter plate. After 30 min (23°C) the recalcified coagulation activity assay (RECA) was performed with a coagulation reaction time (CRT) of 0-40 min (37°C); Figure 1a: 0 IU/ml (O), 2.0 mIU/ml (Δ), 3.9 mIU/ml (□), 7.8 mIU/ml (●), 15.6 mIU/ml (▲), 31.3 mIU/ml (♦), 62.5 mIU/ml (■) thrombin. Figure 1b: CRT periods of 4 min (Δ), 10 min (●), 15 min (▲), or 20 min (♦).

Only generated thrombin activities are valid that belong to the ascending part of the thrombin generation curve, because nascending fibrin might behave as antithrombin I [12]. Therefore, RECA-10 with 10 min coagulation reaction time (CRT) was here much more interesting than e.g. RECA-30 with thrombin activities in the descending part of the thrombin generation curve. If a similar experiment was performed also with human thrombin and with immediate recalcification after thrombin supplementation, the approximate ED200 was about 2 mIU/ml human or bovine thrombin in the RECA-10 (Figure 2). The approximate ED200 was about 5 mIU/ml thrombin in the EXCA-1 (Figure 2).

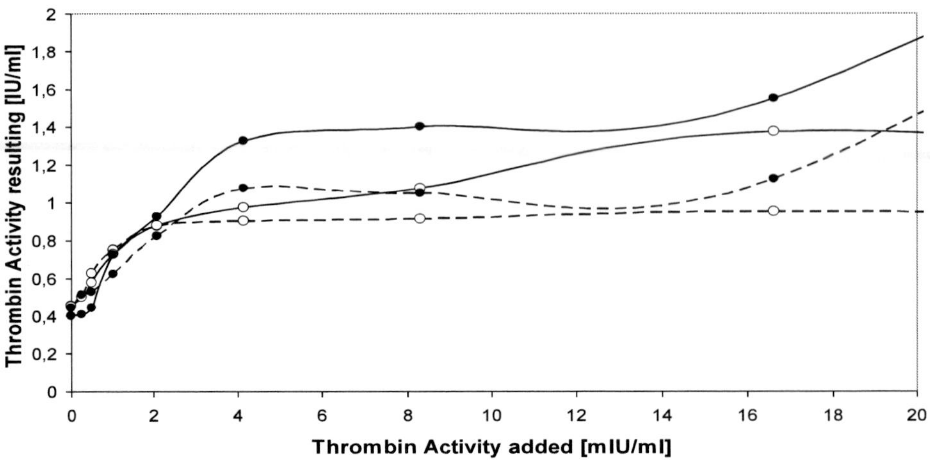

Figure 2. Thrombin triggers its own generation. Unfrozen pooled normal plasma was supplemented with bovine thrombin (slashed lines) or human thrombin (normal lines) on U-well plates. Immediately thereafter the thrombin generation assays recalcified coagulation activity assay with 10 min coagulation reaction time (RECA-10; ●) or extrinsic coagulation activity assay with 1 min coagulation reaction time (EXCA-1; O) were performed. 33 mIU/ml added thrombin in resulted in about 3 IU/ml thrombin in RECA-10.

Using a fresh plasma-pool the approximate ED200 was also about 2 mIU/ml thrombin in the RECA-10 (Figure 3); the approximate ED200 was about 13 mIU/ml thrombin in the EXCA-1 with a basal value of thrombin generation of about 0.64 IU/ml (Figure 3); the ED200 increased at higher basal thrombin generations, because the hyperbolic rate kinetic of thrombin generation is more pronounced within the initial phase of thrombin generation (up to maximally about 0.5-1 IU/ml thrombin); antithrombin I acts more efficiently at final thrombin activities that exceed the normal thrombin generation.

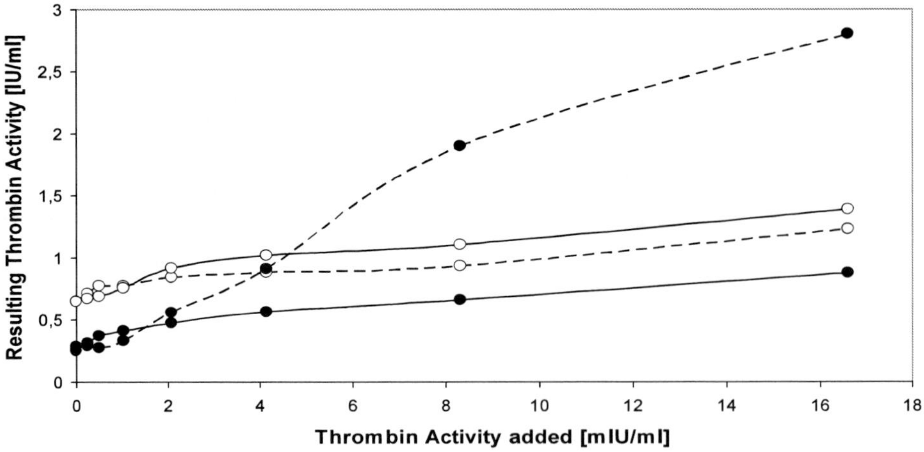

Figure 3. Thrombin triggers its own generation. 20 μl samples of fresh unfrozen pooled normal plasma were supplemented with 0-16.6 mIU/ml bovine thrombin (slashed lines) or human thrombin (normal lines) on U-well plates. Immediately thereafter the thrombin generation assays recalcified coagulation activity assay with 10 min coagulation reaction time (RECA-10; ●) or the extrinsic coagulation activity assay with 1 min coagulation reaction time (EXCA-1; O) were performed.

The ED200 of added thrombin on pooled plasma from patients on coumarin was about 8 mIU/ml (Figure 4), whereas in a control pool of normal plasma the ED200 of thrombin was about 4 mIU/ml (Figure 5), when both plasma types were tested in the 50 µl sample version in RECA-10. To obtain in pooled coumarin-plasma a thrombin generation that is about one third (33.3 %) of the normal RECA value (100 % normal RECA-10 = about 400 mA) about 14 mIU/ml thrombin had to be added (Figure 4). Due to activation of intrinsic hemostasis, pooling of plasma is pro-thrombinic (Figure 4 vs. Figure 6a).

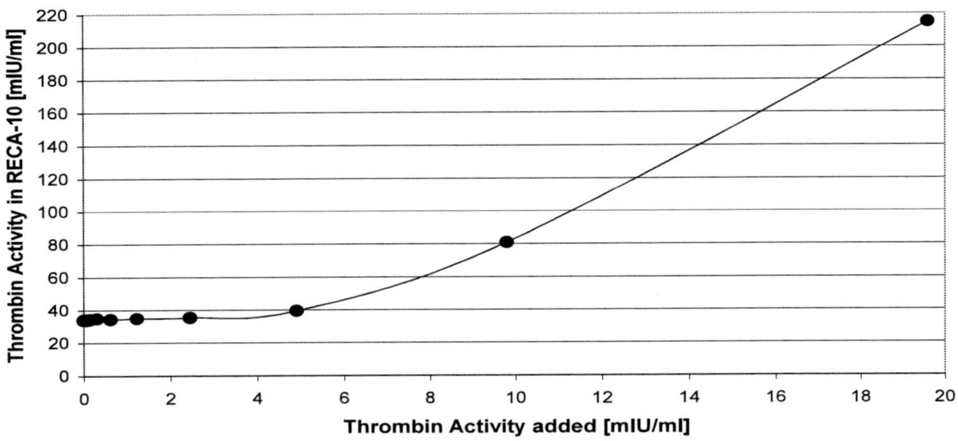

Figure 4. Pooled plasma of patients on coumarin. 50 µl samples of unfrozen pooled plasma from patients on coumarin (INR=1.8) were supplemented with 0-19.6 mIU/ml bovine thrombin on U-well plates. Immediately thereafter the RECA-10 was performed, using 100 µl arginine-reagent and 25 µl substrate-reagent. The ED200 is about 8 mIU/ml added thrombin (basal thrombin activity in this citrated pooled plasma = about 7 mIU/ml thrombin).

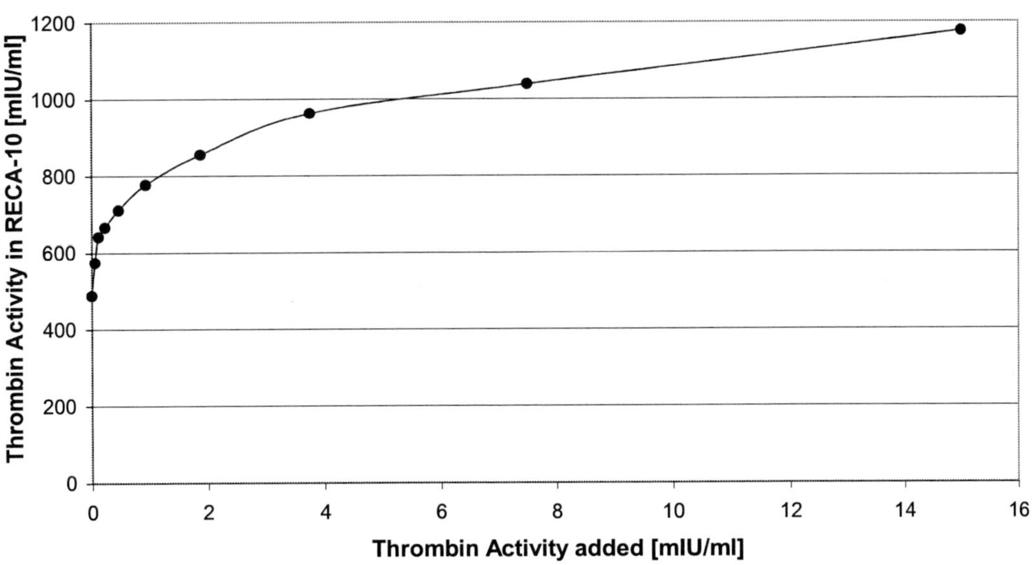

Figure 5. Human thrombin triggers thrombin generation in RECA. 50 µl unfrozen pooled normal plasma were supplemented on the U-well microtiter plate with 0-15 mIU/ml human thrombin. Immediately thereafter the RECA-10 was performed.

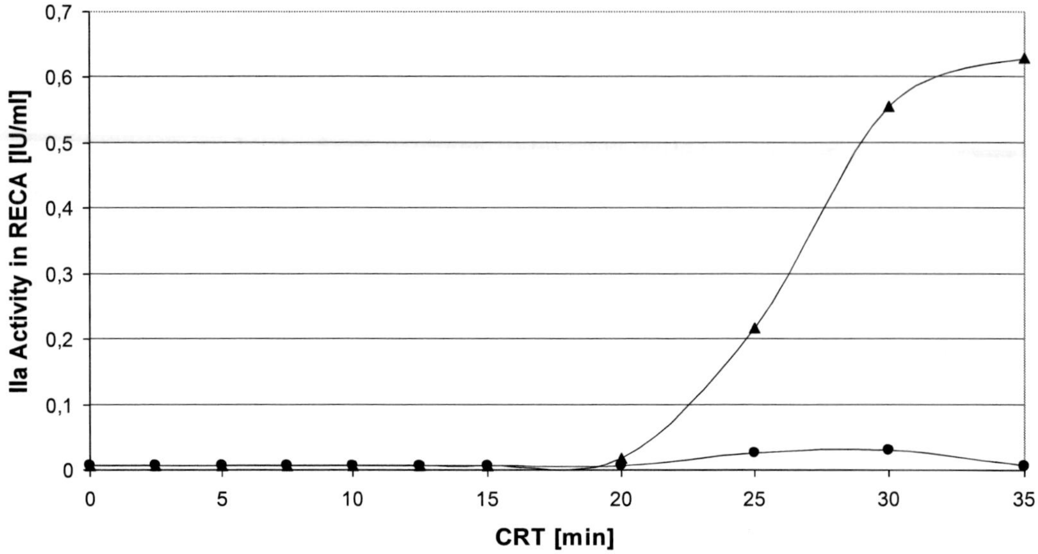

Figure 6a. Thrombin generation in two plasmas of patients on coumarin. 50 µl unfrozen plasma of two patients on coumarin with INR = 1.75 (▲) or INR = 2.25 (●) were assayed in the RECA with different coagulation reaction times (CRT).

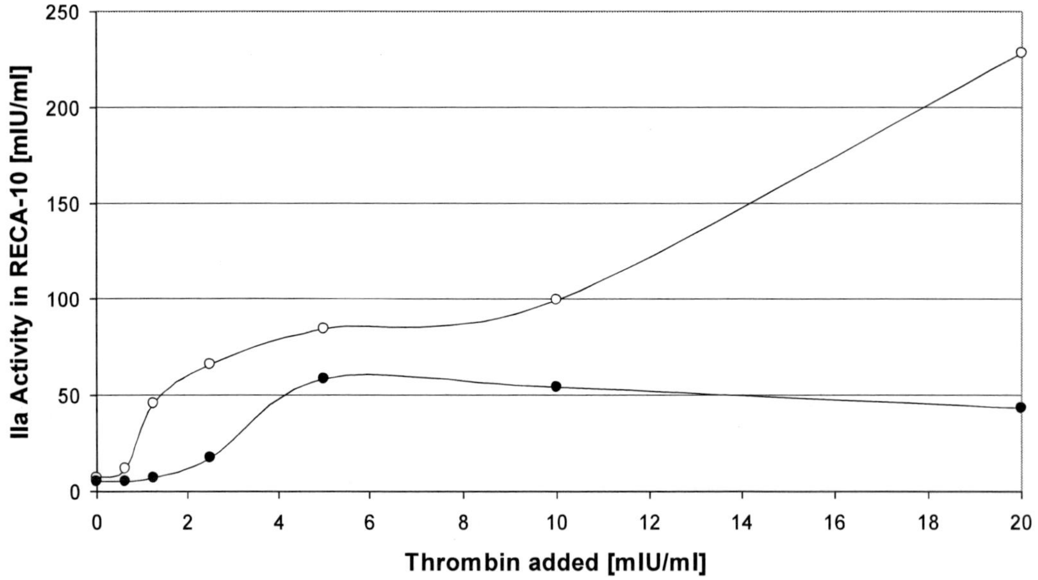

Figure 6b. Thrombin triggers its generation in plasma of a patient on coumarin. 50 µl unfrozen plasma of a patient on coumarin with INR = 2.25 (●) and for control 50 µl unfrozen plasma of a patient not on hemostasis therapy with normal PT and APTT (O) were supplemented with human thrombin on the plate and immediately thereafter assayed in the RECA-10.

The thrombin generation in RECA-10 could not be enhanced by 0-19.6 mIU/ml thrombin in a control pool that had been supplemented with 1 IU/ml unfractionated heparin (RECA-10: 0 mIU/ml additional thrombin generation).

Thrombin generation in plasma of patients on coumarin (Figure 6a) is much slower than that of normal plasma (Figure 7a): with an INR of about 2 significant thrombin generation starts at about 25 min CRT, whereas normal plasmas start at about 10-20 min CRT. Figure 6a demonstrates that it is of eminent importance to analyze the thrombin generation curves in their ascending parts, e.g. in the present experiment at 25 min CRT and not at 35 min CRT, where the thrombin generation of the INR=2.25 plasma has decreased to zero, presumably due to the action of antithrombin I, presumably a down-regulator of thrombin activities especially if they are greater than the free thrombin activity in normal blood plasma.

Figure 6b shows that the thrombin generation even in INR=2.25 plasma can be enhanced by addition of catalytic amounts of thrombin: to achieve a thrombin generation of about 50 mIU/ml in an unfrozen normal control plasma an addition of about 2 mIU/ml thrombin was necessary; for the same increase of about 50 mIU/ml in INR=2.25 plasma about 5 mIU/ml thrombin was necessary (thrombin generation = thrombin activity in generation assay minus basal thrombin activity).

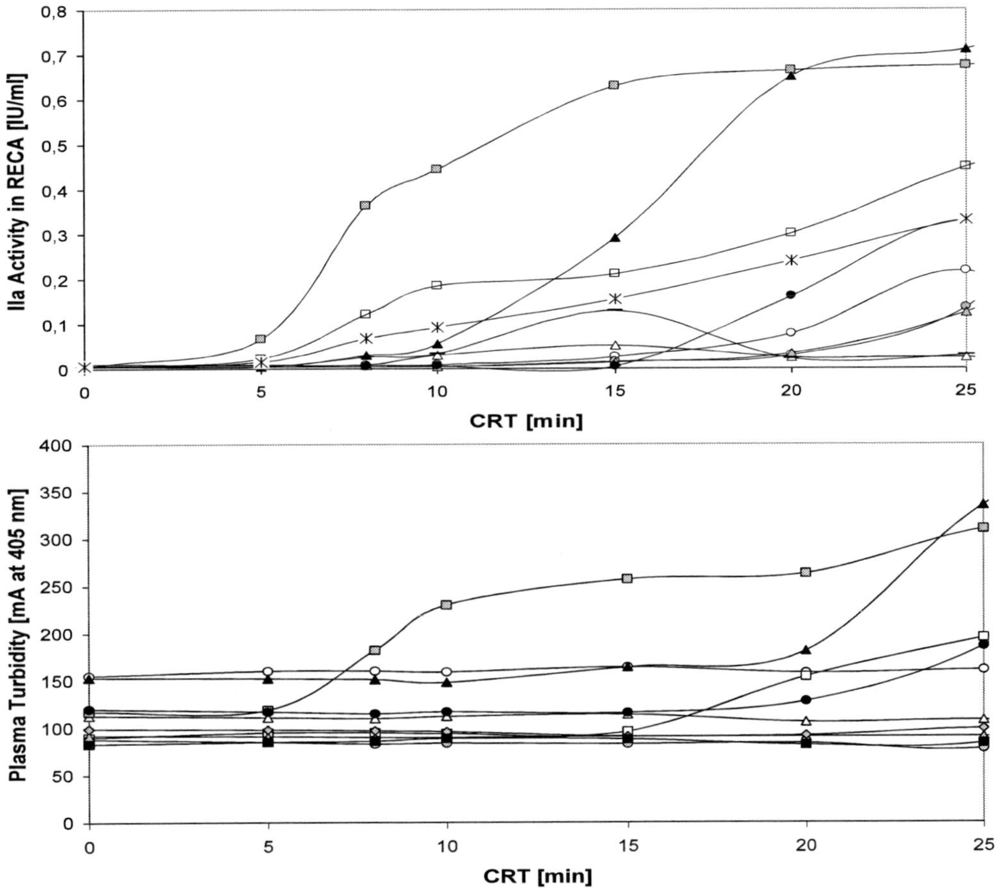

Figure 7. Normal RECA-kinetic for individual unfrozen plasmas. 50 μl unfrozen citrated plasma of 8 patients not on hemostasis therapy and with normal PT, APTT, and fibrinogen (each patient has an individual symbol; the mean value of the 9 normal plasma samples has the symbol * and one patient not on hemostasis therapy with normal PT, APTT but with 9 g/l fibrinogen (-) were assayed in the RECA (Figure 7a). The respective basal plasma turbidities prior to addition of the chromogenic thrombin substrate is shown in Figure 7b.

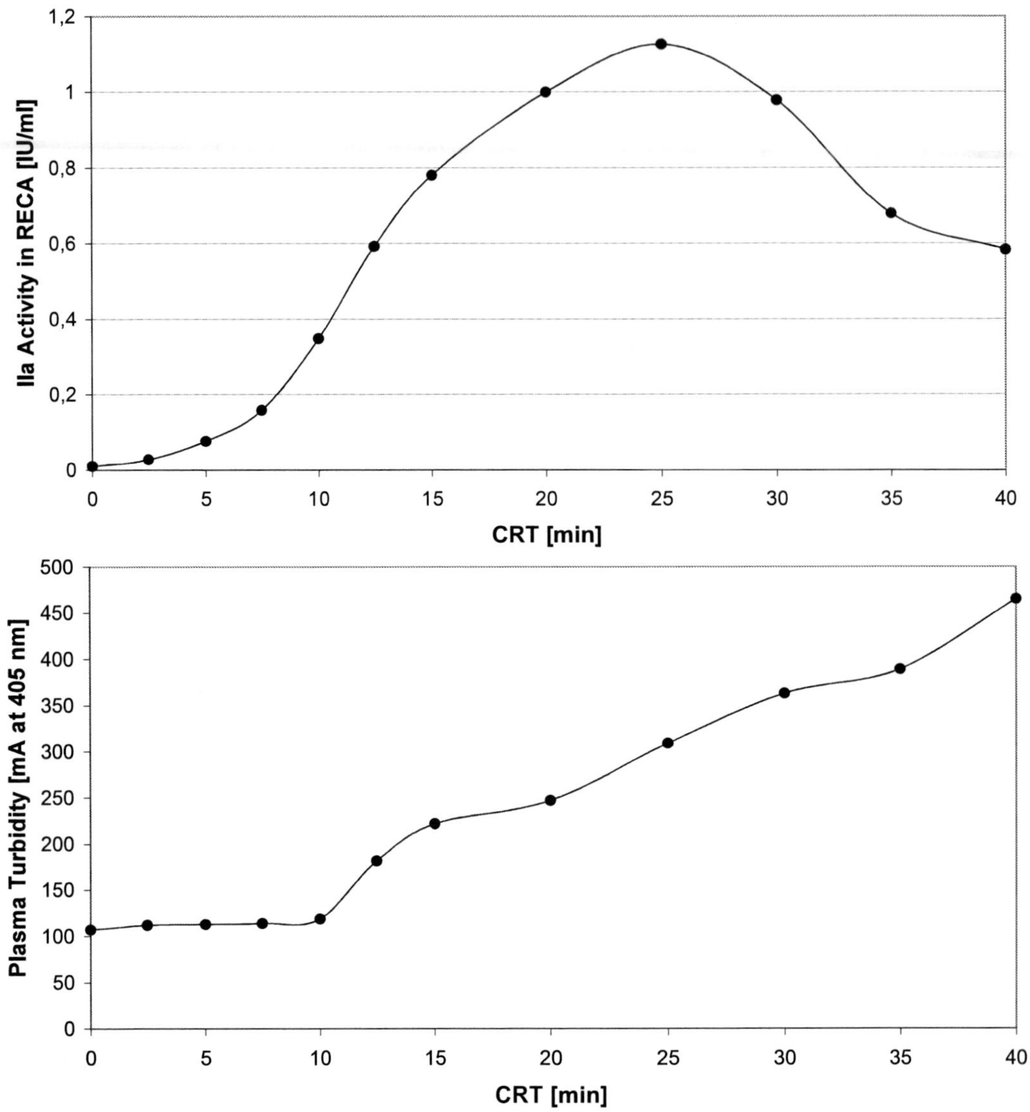

Figure 8. Normal RECA-kinetic for pooled unfrozen plasma. 50 µl unfrozen pooled citrated plasma from 11 patients not on hemostasis therapy and with normal PT, APTT, and fibrinogen was assayed in the RECA (Figure 8a). The respective basal plasma turbidities prior to addition of the chromogenic thrombin substrate is shown in Figure 8b.

The normal RECA kinetic for individual or pooled plasma is demonstrated in figure 7a or 8a, respectively. The initial kinetic of thrombin generation is hyperbolic, e.g. in pooled plasma the phase between 0 and 10 min CRT (Figure 8a). The analysis of thrombin activity should be performed preferably within this phase, never in the phase of decreasing thrombin activities due to the action of antithrombin I, which in figure 8a would be the phase with a CRT ≥ 25 min. The added arginine-reagent with final supra-molar arginine concentrations stopps hemostasis activation and completely depolymerizes uncrosslinked nascent fibrin within the initial hyperbolic phases (Figs. 7b, 8b) [10,11,13]. Factor XIIIa crosslinked and arginine resistant nascent fibrin occurred upon about 13 min CRT, thrombin activities in the phase between 10 and 20 min CRT might nevertheless be measured. With greater unspecific turbidities bichromatic detection of ΔA (ΔA at 405 nm minus ΔA at 450 nm) might be used.

The ideal RECA-CRTs of 50 µl citrated plasma on polystyrol U-well plates (Brand® 701300) are RECA-5, RECA-10, RECA-15, and RECA-20; it is of major importance to analyze the respective sample in its increasing part of the thrombin generation curve, i.e. without interference of fibrin = antithrombin I. Especially in the initial hyperbolic rate phase the thrombin generation does not depend on nascending fibrin. RECA-5 is especially indicated for strongly prothrombinic plasmas. RECA-0 might be a control value to assess the basal thrombin activity in citrated plasma prior to the addition of calcium ions.

The RECA is an excellent close-to-physiologically designed tool to measure the real prothrombinic action of any citrated plasma, however RECA for clinical routine purposes should be performed under a strongly standardized preanalytic:

- drawing of venous blood into well characterized sampling tubes
- immediate transport of the drawn blood to the laboratory (at 23±1°C)
- immediate centrifugation (at 23±1°C)
- analysis of fresh plasma within 1 h (at 23±1°C)
- usage of well characterized microtiter plates
- minimal plasma preincubation (< 10 min at 23±1°C) in the wells prior to addition of Ca^{++}.

Under these conditions the RECA quantifies the prothrombinic capacity of plasma even of critically ill patients [14-16]. Hitherto assays of hemostasis activation markers such as thrombin – antithrombin complex or prothrombin fragment 1+2 do not reflect well the clinical situation [17,18]. Plasmatic thrombin activity (the IIa Test) [10,11,18] or the RECA seem to be interesting new tests that will help the clinician to better judge any clinical situation of severe disturbance that affects primary or secondary hemostasis [19,20].

Antithrombin III (AT3) is the natural inhibitor of thrombin and low molecular weight heparins (LMWH) are nearly physiological enhancers of AT3 activity [21]. The correct dosage of LMWH and/or of AT3 should be monitored by an ultra-specific, ultra-sensitive, ultra-precise thrombin generation assay such as the EXCA or the RECA [11]. The aim should be the adequate generation of thrombin in blood: too few thrombin is dangerous because this can result in severe bleeding and too many thrombin is also dangerous because this can result in multiple thrombi that are refractory to fibrinolysis [22,23].

In conclusion, addition of about 2-4 mIU/ml thrombin to pooled unfrozen normal citrated plasma approximately doubles the thrombin activity generated in RECA-10. Interestingly, about 3 mIU/ml thrombin in pooled normal plasma is the approximate thrombin activity that is necessary for a normal hyperbolic rate phase in RECA [24]. The present findings may be of importance in diagnosis and therapy of individual dysgenerations of plasmatic thrombin.

REFERENCES

[1] Crawley JT, Zanardelli S, Chion CK, Lane DA. The central role of thrombin in hemostasis. *J. Thromb Haemost.* 2007; 5 Suppl 1: 95-101.

[2] Arnout J, Hoylaerts MF, Lijnen HR. Haemostasis. *Handb. Exp. Pharmacol.* 2006; (176 Pt 2): 1-41.

[3] Davie EW, Kulman JD. An overview of the structure and function of thrombin. *Semin. Thromb Hemost.* 2006; 32 Suppl 1:3-15.

[4] Riddel JP Jr, Aouizerat BE, Miaskowski C, Lillicrap DP. Theories of blood coagulation. J. *Pediatr. Oncol. Nurs* 2007; 24: 123-31.

[5] Harenberg J, Wehling M. Current and future prospects for anticoagulant therapy: inhibitors of factor Xa and factor IIa. *Semin. Thromb Hemost.* 2008; 34: 39-57.

[6] Tanaka KA, Levy JH. Regulation of thrombin activity--pharmacologic and structural aspects. *Hematol. Oncol. Clin. North Am.* 2007; 21: 33-50.

[7] Di Cera E. *Thrombin. Mol. Aspects Med.* 2008; 29: 203-54.

[8] Page MJ, Di Cera E. Serine peptidases: classification, structure and function. *Cell Mol. Life Sci.* 2008; 65: 1220-36.

[9] Hemker HC, Al Dieri R, De Smedt E, Béguin S. Thrombin generation, a function test of the haemostatic-thrombotic system. *Thromb Haemost.* 2006; 96: 553-61.

[10] Stief TW. Innovative tests of plasmatic hemostasis. *Laboratory Medicine* 2008; 39: 225-30.

[11] Stief TW. Specific determination of plasmatic thrombin activity. *Clin. Appl. Thromb. Hemost.* 2006; 12: 324-9.

[12] Mosesson MW. Update on antithrombin I (fibrin). *Thromb Haemost.* 2007; 98: 105-8.

[13] Masic LP. Arginine mimetic structures in biologically active antagonists and inhibitors. *Curr. Med. Chem.* 2006; 13: 3627-48.

[14] Edmunds LH Jr, Colman RW. Thrombin during cardiopulmonary bypass. *Ann. Thorac. Surg.* 2006; 82: 2315-22.

[15] Levy JH. Massive transfusion coagulopathy. *Semin. Hematol.* 2006; 43(1 Suppl 1): S59-63.

[16] Stief TW. Coagulation Activation by Lipopolysaccharides. *Clin. Appl. Thromb Hemost.* 2007 Dec 26. [Epub ahead of print].

[17] Ofosu FA. Review: Laboratory markers quantifying prothrombin activation and actions of thrombin in venous and arterial thrombosis do not accurately assess disease severity or the effectiveness of treatment. *Thromb Haemost.* 2006; 96: 568-77.

[18] Stief TW, Ijagha O, Weiste B, Herzum I, Renz H, Max M. Analysis of hemostasis alterations in sepsis. *Blood Coagul Fibrinolysis* 2007; 18: 179-86.

[19] Piccin A, Murphy WG, Smith OP. Circulating microparticles: pathophysiology and clinical implications. *Blood Rev.* 2007; 21: 157-71.

[20] Lundblad RL, White GC 2nd. The interaction of thrombin with blood platelets. *Platelets* 2005 16: 373-85.

[21] Gray E, Mulloy B, Barrowcliffe TW. Heparin and low-molecular-weight heparin. *Thromb Haemost.* 2008; 99: 807-18.

[22] Wolberg AS. Thrombin generation and fibrin clot structure. *Blood Rev.* 2007; 21: 131-42.

[23] Stief TW, Fröhlich S, Renz H. Determination of the global fibrinolytic state. Blood Coagul Fibrinolysis 2007; 18: 479-87.

[24] Stief TW. Inhibition of thrombin generation in recalcified plasma. Blood Coagul Fibrinolysis 2007; 18: 751-60.

In: Hemostasis Laboratory Yearbook, Volume 2
Editor: Thomas W. Stief, pp. 221-226
ISBN: 978-1-60741-089-8

TISSUE FACTOR TRIGGERS RECALCIFIED THROMBIN GENERATION

Thomas W. Stief*
Department of Clinical Chemistry,
University Hospital Giessen and Marburg, Germany

ABSTRACT

Background: Tissue factor (TF) as one of the main triggers of hemostasis activates factor VII (F VII) to FVIIa, a possible prothrombinic drug against severe bleeding. The purpose of the present study was to quantifiy the 200 % effective dose (ED200) of TF on thrombin generation as assayed by the new ultra-specific, ultra-sensitive thrombin generation assay RECA.

Material and Methods: Pools of unfrozen citrated plasma (normal or from patients on coumarin, INR = 1.8) were supplemented with 0-25 pg/ml human placental TF on polystyrol U-well microtiter plates (Brand®701300) at 23°C. Immediately thereafter the ultra-specific, ultra-sensitive thrombin generation assays RECA-10 (recalcified coagulation activity assay) with 10 min coagulation reaction time at 37°C (CRT) and EXCA-1 (extrinsic coagulation activity assay with 1 min CRT) were performed with 20 µl or 50 µl plasma samples. Thrombin generation = thrombin activity after CRT minus basal thrombin activity in citrated plasma (without CRT).

Results: The approximate ED200 of TF in normal RECA-10 was about 1 pg/ml. The approximate ED200 in pooled plasma of patients on coumarin (INR=1.8) was about 2.5 pg/ml; here about 12 pg/ml TF are necessary to obtain a RECA-10 value that is one third of normal.

Discussion: The present work quantifies for the first time the amount of TF that is necessary to double normal recalcified thrombin generation. This ED200 of about 1 pg/ml for pooled normal plasma and about 3fold this amount for pooled plasma of INR=1.8 is of physiological and clinical interest, e.g. in the development of TF as prothrombinic economical drug against severe bleeding. The dosis of such a prothrombinic drug amount should be individually established for each individual patient by means of an ultra-specific, ultra-sensitive thrombin generation assay, such as the RECA.

Keywords: Tissue factor, thrombin, RECA, ED200.

---

* Correspondence to:_PD Dr. med. T. Stief, Department of Clinical Chemistry, University Hospital, D-35043 Marburg, Germany. E-mail: thstief@med.uni-marburg.de; Tel. : +49-6421-58 64471; FAX: +49-6421-58 65594

Introduction

Tissue factor (TF) or contact activators (such as phospholipid microparticles) are the main triggers of hemostasis. TF is the trigger of extrinsic hemostasis [1-14]. TF activates factor VII (F VII) to F VIIa, which is currently used as a prothrombinic drug. TF might replace the expensive recombinant F VIIa if the exact TF concentration for the individual bleeding patient is known that re-establishes a nearly normal thrombin generation. There are thrombin generation data about the trigger TF [15], however measured by thrombin generation assays that are influenced artificially by kallikrein or by antithrombin I = fibrin [16]. The aim of the present study was to quantifiy for the first time the 200 % effective dose (ED200) of TF on thrombin generation as assayed by the new ultra-specific, ultra-sensitive thrombin generation assay RECA [17].

Material and Methods

Pooled Unfrozen Normal Plasma

Unfrozen pooled normal citrated plasma (from 7 remaining samples that remained after routine analysis; 0.5 ml 106 mM sodium citrate + 4.5 ml venous blood in polypropylene sampling tubes; Sarstedt, Nümbrecht, Germany) was supplemented with 0-25 pg/ml human placental tissue factor (Thromborel S®, Behringwerke, Marburg, Germany) in 5 % human albumin (CSL Behring, Marburg, Germany) aliquoted in 1 ml amounts in siliconized 20 ml glass vials (DadeBehring, article nr. OVKE49) directly in a polystyrol U-well microtiter plate (Brand, Wertheim, Germany; article nr. 701300) and repetitively 1+1 diluted. Immediately thereafter an innovative thrombin generation assays were performed: the RECA-10 (recalcified coagulation activity assay with 10 min coagulation reaction time (CRT)) [16]. The test was standardized with 1 IU/ml bovine thrombin in 6.7 % human albumin that replaced the plasma sample. The basal amidolytic thrombin activity in the present pools of citrated plasma was about 6-8 mIU/ml. Thrombin generation = thrombin activity in the generation assay at a certain coagulation reaction time (CRT) minus basal thrombin activity in citrated plasma at 0 min CRT.

Fresh Pooled Unfrozen Normal Plasma

20 µl samples of fresh unfrozen pooled normal plasma were supplemented with 0-25 pg/ml TF on U-well plates. Immediately thereafter the RECA-10 or the EXCA-1 (extrinsic coagulation activity assay with 1 min CRT) [17,18] were performed as indicated as follows:

RECA

2 µl RECA-trigger (250 mM $CaCl_2$ in 1 ml aliquots in siliconized glass vials, frozen at -30°C and thawed directly for the assay) were added. The plates were intensely shaken for 5s and incubated at 37°C in a digitally controlled water-bath. After 0-40 min coagulation

reaction time (CRT) 50 µl arginine-reagent (2.5 M arginine, pH 8.7, 0.16 % Triton X 100® (both from Sigma, Deisenhofen, Germany) were added. 3 minutes (23°C) after the last CRT period 25 µl 1 mM chromogenic thrombin substrate HD-CHG-Ala-Arg-pNA (Pentapharm, Basel, Switzerland) in 1.25 M arginine, pH 8.7, were added. The increase in absorbance at 405 nm with time ΔA/t was determined by a microtiter plate photometer with a 1 mA resolution (Milenia; DPC, Los Angeles, USA). The maximal ΔA with these assay volumes in U-wells plates was about 1050 mA, 40 % of the maximal ΔA = about 420 mA = upper limit of linear range of the assay without significant substrate exhaustion.

EXCA

2 µl EXCA-trigger were added. The EXCA trigger consisted in 1 ml aliquots of 1 ng/ml human placental tissue factor (Polybrene®-free Thromborel-S ®; DadeBehring) 250 mM $CaCl_2$ in siliconized glass vials, frozen at -30°C and thawed for the assay. The plates were intensely shaken for 5s and incubated at 37°C in a digitally controlled water-bath. After 1 min coagulation reaction time (EXCA-1) 50 µl arginine-reagent (2.5 M arginine, pH 8.7, 0.16 % Triton X 100® were added. After 3 minutes (23°C) 25 µl 1 mM HD-CHG-Ala-Arg-pNA in 1.25 M arginine, pH 8.7, were added. ΔA/t was determined by a microtiter plate photometer with a 1 mA resolution.

Pooled Citrated Plasma from Patients on Coumarin

50 µl samples of unfrozen pooled plasma (from 7 patients on Marcumar® (phenprocoumon), the samples remained after routine analysis, were about 4h old, stored at 23°C; international normalized ratio (INR) = 1.8) were supplemented with 0-19.6 pg/ml TF on U-well plates. Immediately there after the RECA-10 was performed, using 100 µl arginine-reagent and 25 µl substrate-reagent. The 1 IU/ml thrombin standard generated a ΔA at 405 nm of about 20 mA/min (23°C). A negative control was unfrozen pooled plasma from 7 unselected patients with normal prothrombin time (PT), normal activated partial thromboplastin time (APTT), and normal fibrinogen concentration; this pool was supplemented with 1 IU/ml unfractionated heparin (ratiopharm, Ulm, Germany).

RESULTS AND DISCUSSION

Figures 1 and 2 demonstrate that the approximate 200 % effective dose (ED200) of TF in normal RECA-10 was about 1 pg/ml. The approximate ED200 in pooled plasma of patients on coumarin (INR=1.8) was about 2.5 pg/ml (Figure 3); about 12 pg/ml TF are necessary to obtain a RECA-10 value that is 33 % of normal (100 % = about 0.4 IU/ml thrombin). The plasma pool with 1 IU/ml unfractionated heparin did not generate additional thrombin activity during the RECA-10 at final TF concentrations up to 19.6 pg/ml.

The present work quantifies for the first time the amount of TF that is necessary to double normal recalcified thrombin generation. This ED200 of about 1 pg/ml for pooled normal plasma and about 3fold this amount for pooled plasma of INR=1.8 is of physiological [19] and clinical interest, e.g. in the development of TF as prothrombinic economical drug for severely bleeding patients or patients at risk for severe bleeding [20]. The prothrombinic drug amount should be individually established for each patient by means of an ultra-specific, ultra-sensitive thrombin generation assay, such as the RECA.

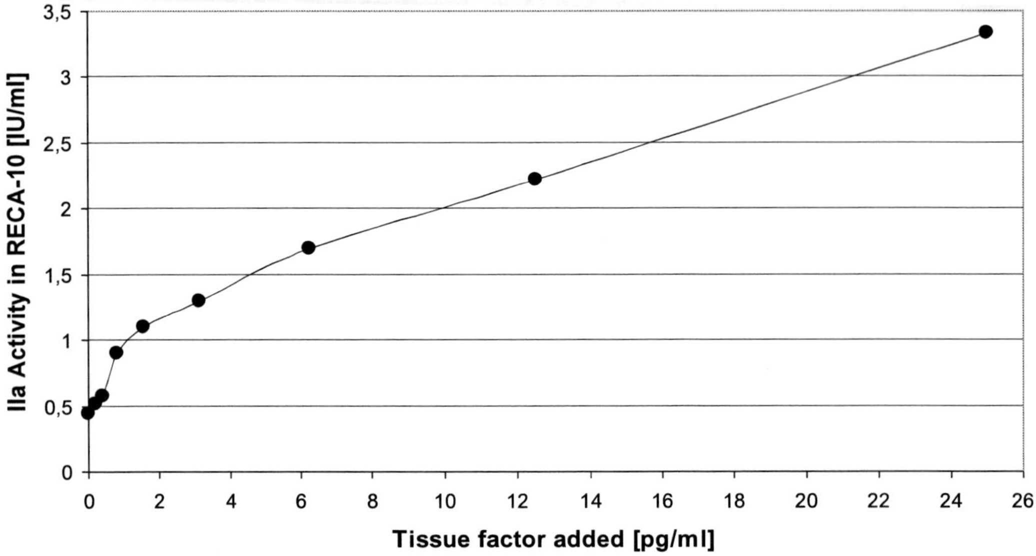

Figure 1. Thrombin generation triggered by tissue factor (TF). Unfrozen pooled normal plasma was supplemented with 0-25 pg/ml TF in U-well plates. Immediately thereafter the thrombin generation assay recalcified coagulation activity assay with 10 min coagulation reaction time (RECA-10; •) was performed.

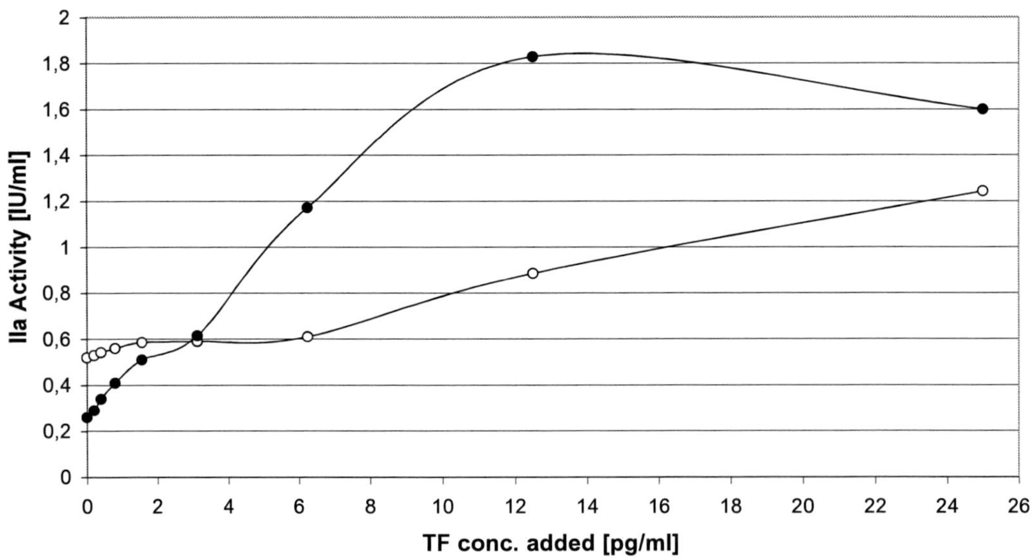

Figure 2. Quantification of IIa generation by TF. 20 µl samples of fresh unfrozen pooled normal plasma were supplemented with 0-25 pg/ml TF on U-well plates. Immediately thereafter the recalcified coagulation activity assay with 10 min coagulation reaction time (RECA-10; •) or the extrinsic coagulation activity assay with 1 min coagulation reaction time (EXCA-1; O) were performed.

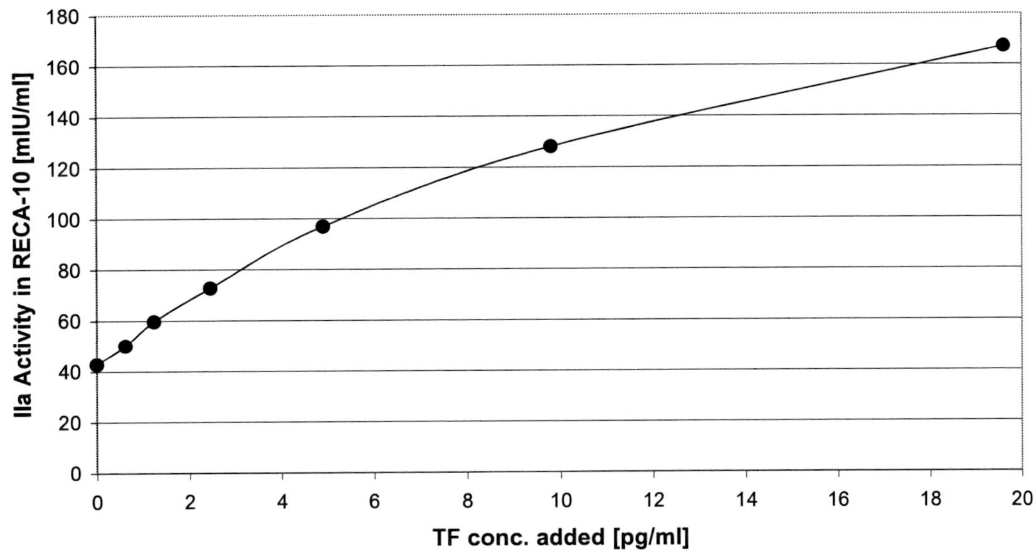

Figure 3. Pooled plasma of patients on coumarin. 50 µl samples of unfrozen pooled plasma from patients on coumarin (INR=1.8) were supplemented with 0-19.6 pg/ml TF on U-well plates. Immediately thereafter the RECA-10 was performed, using 100 µl arginine-reagent and 25 µl substrate-reagent.

REFERENCES

[1] Hedner U, Ezban M. Tissue factor and factor VIIa as therapeutic targets in disorders of hemostasis. *Annu. Rev. Med.* 2008; 59:29-41.

[2] Furie B, Furie BC. In vivo thrombus formation. *J. Thromb Haemost.* 2007; 5 Suppl 1: 12-7.

[3] Monroe DM, Key NS. The tissue factor-factor VIIa complex: procoagulant activity, regulation, and multitasking. *J. Thromb Haemost.* 2007; 5: 1097-105.

[4] Dutton RP, Stein DM. The use of factor VIIa in haemorrhagic shock and intracerebral bleeding. *Injury* 2006; 37: 1172-7.

[5] Malý MA, Tomasov P, Hájek P, Blasko P, Hrachovinová I, Salaj P, Veselka J. The role of tissue factor in thrombosis and hemostasis. *Physiol. Res.* 2007; 56: 685-95.

[6] Bosinski TJ, El Solh AA. Recombinant factor VIIa, its clinical properties, and the tissue factor pathway of coagulation. *Mini Rev. Med. Chem.* 2006; 6: 1111-7.

[7] Arnout J, Hoylaerts MF, Lijnen HR. Haemostasis. *Handb. Exp. Pharmacol.* 2006; (176 Pt 2): 1-41.

[8] Roberts HR, Hoffman M, Monroe DM. A cell-based model of thrombin generation. *Semin. Thromb Hemost.* 2006; 32 Suppl 1:32-8.

[9] Laterre PF, Wittebole X, Collienne C. Pharmacological inhibition of tissue factor. *Semin. Thromb Hemost.* 2006; 32: 71-6.

[10] Østerud B, Bjørklid E. Sources of tissue factor. *Semin. Thromb Hemost.* 2006; 32: 11-23.

[11] Furie B, Furie BC. Thrombus formation in vivo. *J. Clin. Invest* 2005; 115: 3355-62.

[12] Lösche W. Platelets and tissue factor. *Platelets* 2005; 16: 313-9.

[13] Ruf W. Emerging roles of tissue factor in viral hemorrhagic fever. *Trends Immunol.* 2004; 25: 461-4.

[14] Siddiqui FA, Desai H, Amirkhosravi A, Amaya M, Francis JL. The presence and release of tissue factor from human platelets. *Platelets* 2002; 13: 247-53.

[15] Rosenkranz A, Hiden M, Leschnik B, Weiss EC, Schlembach D, Lang U, Gallistl S, Muntean W. Calibrated automated thrombin generation in normal uncomplicated pregnancy. *Thromb Haemost.* 2008; 99: 331-7.

[16] Mosesson MW. Update on antithrombin I (fibrin). *Thromb Haemost.* 2007; 98: 105-8.

[17] Stief TW. Innovative tests of plasmatic hemostasis. *Laboratory Medicine* 2008; 39: 225-30.

[18] Stief TW, Wieczerzak A, Renz H. The extrinsic coagulation activity assay. *Clin. Appl. Thromb Hemost.* 2008; 14: 303-18.

[19] Jesty J, Beltrami E. Positive feedbacks of coagulation: their role in threshold regulation. *Arterioscler. Thromb Vasc. Biol.* 2005; 25: 2463-9.

[20] Erber WN, Perry DJ. Plasma and plasma products in the treatment of massive haemorrhage. *Best Pract. Res. Clin. Haematol.* 2006; 19: 97-112.

In: Hemostasis Laboratory Yearbook, Volume 2
Editor: Thomas W. Stief, pp. 227-235
ISBN: 978-1-60741-089-8

FACTOR VIIA TRIGGERS THROMBIN GENERATION

Thomas W. Stief*
Department of Clinical Chemistry,
University Hospital Giessen and Marburg, Germany

ABSTRACT

Background: Factor VIIa (F VIIa) is the enzyme part of the extrinsic tenase that activates factor X. F VIIa is used since about a decade to prevent or treat severe hemorrhages. Until now there has been no simple physiologic assay that quantifies the prothrombinic capacity of F VIIa in patient plasma, allowing individual adjustments of the F VIIa dosage. Here this thrombin activity is quantified with new ultra-specific, ultra-sensitive thrombin generation assays.
Material and Methods: Pools of unfrozen citrated plasma (normal or from patients on coumarin, INR=1.8) were supplemented with 0-20 µg/ml recombinant F VIIa on polystyrol U-well microtiter plates (Brand®701300) at 23°C. Immediately thereafter the thrombin generation assays RECA-10 (recalcified coagulation activity assay) with 10 min coagulation reaction time at 37°C (CRT), INCA-4 (intrinsic coagulation activity assay with 4 min CRT), and EXCA-1 (extrinsic coagulation activity assay with 1 min CRT) were performed with 20 µl or 50 µl plasma samples. Thrombin generation = thrombin activity after CRT minus basal thrombin activity in citrated plasma (without CRT).
Results: The approximate 200 % effective dose (ED200) was about 0.3 µg/ml in RECA-10 or in INCA-4, in EXCA-1 no 200% of normal thrombin generation could be reached. The ED200 of FEIBA added to pooled plasma from patients on coumarin was about 1 µg/ml FEIBA in RECA-10; about 3 µg/ml FEIBA were necessary to obtain a RECA value that is one third of normal.
Discussion: The RECA is a new instrument to predict and to monitor the hemostatic power of procoagulants, such as e.g. F VIIa: in severely bleeding patients or patients at risk for severe bleeding the target RECA value might be about 33-50 % of the normal one: therapy with prothrombinic drugs should be individually adjusted according to the RECA value.

Keywords: Factor VIIa, thrombin, RECA, ED200.

---

* Correspondence to:_PD Dr. med. T. Stief, Department of Clinical Chemistry, University Hospital, D-35043 Marburg, Germany. E-mail: thstief@med.uni-marburg.de; Tel. : +49-6421-58 64471; FAX: +49-6421-58 65594

INTRODUCTION

Tissue factor complexes with factor VII and activates it [1-4]; activated factor VII (F VIIa) is the enzyme part of this complex that then behaves as the extrinsic tenase of hemostasis that activates factor X. Recombinant F VIIa has been developed as a drug against severe bleeding [5-15]. The prothrombinic power of F VIIa as measured in 200 % effective doses (ED200) has not yet been clearly quantified. The aim of the present study was to determine the ED200 values of thrombin generation in new ultra-specific, ultra-sensitive thrombin generation assays [16].

MATERIAL AND METHODS

Pooled Unfrozen Normal Plasma

Samples of unfrozen normal citrated plasma (from 8 samples that remained after routine analysis; 0.5 ml 106 mM sodium citrate + 4.5 ml venous blood in polypropylene sampling tubes; Sarstedt, Nümbrecht, Germany; about 4h old, stored at 23°C) were pooled into completely emptied polypropylene sampling tubes (Sarstedt, Nümbrecht, Germany). The plasma pool was then supplemented with 0-10 µg/ml recombinant factor VIIa (Novo Nordisk A/S, Bagsvaerd, Denmark; lot nr. VU60276; the freshly reconstituted solution in the original glass vial contained 600 µg/ml (30 kIE/ml) recombinant factor VIIa) directly into polystyrol U-microwells (Brand, Wertheim, Germany; article nr. 701300). The repetitively 1+1 diluted plasma pool were pipetted in 20 µl aliquots by means of an Eppendorf-Multipette® with 0.9 % NaCl – rinsed new tips. After 30 min (23°C) two innovative thrombin generation assays were performed: the RECA (recalcified coagulation activity assay) and the EXCA (extrinsic coagulation activity assay). The tests were standardized with 1 IU/ml bovine thrombin in 6.7 % human albumin (DadeBehring, Marburg, Germany) that replaced the plasma sample and resulted in about 10 mA/min (23°C). The basal amidolytic thrombin activity in the present pool of citrated plasma was about 6-10 mIU/ml. If 5 % human albumin instead of plasma was supplemented in duplicate with F VIIa, 10 µg/ml F VIIa behaved in the present assay conditions with supra-molar concentrations of arginine in the thrombin detection phase as < 4 mIU/ml thrombin, underlining the ultra-specificity of thrombin generations in the presence of arginine [17-25].

20 µl samples of unfrozen pooled normal plasma (from 7 samples that remained after routine analysis, about 4h old, stored at 23°C) were supplemented with 0-20 µg/ml F VIIa directly on U-well plates by immediate repetitive 1+1 dilutions. Immediately thereafter the thrombin generation assays RECA-10 (10 min coagulation reaction time (CRT) or EXCA-1 (1 min CRT) were performed in duplicate as described below.

Fresh Pooled Unfrozen Normal Plasma

20 µl samples of fresh unfrozen pooled normal plasma (from 7 samples that remained after routine analysis, about 2h old, stored at 23°C) were supplemented with 0-20 µg/ml F VIIa on U-well plates. Immediately thereafter the thrombin generation assays RECA-10,

INCA-4 (intrinsic coagulation activity assay with 4 min CRT), or EXCA-1 were performed as described as follows:

RECA

2 µl RECA-trigger (250 mM $CaCl_2$ in 1 ml aliquots in siliconized glass vials, frozen at -30°C and thawed directly for the assay) were added. The plates were intensely shaken for 5s and incubated at 37°C in a digitally controlled water-bath. After 0-40 min coagulation reaction time (CRT) 50 µl arginine-reagent (2.5 M arginine, pH 8.7, 0.16 % Triton X 100® (both from Sigma, Deisenhofen, Germany) were added. 3 minutes (23°C) after the last CRT period 25 µl 1 mM chromogenic thrombin substrate HD-CHG-Ala-Arg-pNA (Pentapharm, Basel, Switzerland) in 1.25 M arginine, pH 8.7, were added. The increase in absorbance at 405 nm with time ΔA/t was determined by a microtiter plate photometer with a 1 mA resolution (Milenia; DPC, Los Angeles, USA). The maximal ΔA with these assay volumes in U-wells plates was about 1100 mA, 40 % of the maximal ΔA is about 440 mA, the linear range of the assay without significant substrate exhaustion.

INCA

2 µl INCA-trigger were added. The INCA trigger consisted in 500 µl 500 mM $CaCl_2$ aliquots in siliconized glass vials, frozen at -30°C and thawed for the assay were mixed with 400 µl H_2O and directly prior to the start of the assay with 100 µl SiO_2 reagent (Pathromtin SL®; DadeBehring). The plates were intensely shaken for 5s and incubated at 37°C in a digitally controlled water-bath. After 4 min coagulation reaction time (INCA-4) 50 µl arginine-reagent (2.5 M arginine, pH 8.7, 0.16 % Triton X 100® were added. After 3 minutes (23°C) 25 µl 1 mM HD-CHG-Ala-Arg-pNA in 1.25 M arginine, pH 8.7, were added. ΔA/t was determined by a microtiter plate photometer with a 1 mA resolution.

EXCA

2 µl EXCA-trigger were added. The EXCA trigger consisted in 1 ml aliquots of 1 ng/ml human placental tissue factor (Polybrene-free Thromborel-S ®; DadeBehring) 250 mM $CaCl_2$ in siliconized glass vials, frozen at -30°C and thawed for the assay. The plates were intensely shaken for 5s and incubated at 37°C in a digitally controlled water-bath. After 1 min coagulation reaction time (EXCA-1) 50 µl arginine-reagent (2.5 M arginine, pH 8.7, 0.16 % Triton X 100® were added. After 3 minutes (23°C) 25 µl 1 mM HD-CHG-Ala-Arg-pNA in 1.25 M arginine, pH 8.7, were added. ΔA/t was determined by a microtiter plate photometer with a 1 mA resolution.

Pooled Unfrozen Plasma from Patients on Coumarin

50 µl samples of unfrozen pooled plasma (from 7 patients on Marcumar® (phenprocoumon), the samples remained after routine analysis, were about 4h old, stored at 23°C; international normalized ratio (INR) = 1.8) were supplemented with 0-11.76 µg/ml FEIBA on U-well plates. Immediately thereafter the RECA-10 was performed, using 100 µl arginine-reagent and 25 µl substrate-reagent. The 1 IU/ml thrombin standard generated a ΔA at 405 nm of about 20 mA/min (23°C). A negative control was unfrozen pooled plasma from 7 unselected patients with normal prothrombin time (PT), normal activated partial

thromboplastin time (APTT), and normal fibrinogen concentration; this pool was supplemented with 1 IU/ml unfractionated heparin (ratiopharm, Ulm, Germany).

RESULTS AND DISCUSSION

Figure 1 demonstrates that the approximate ED200 of F VIIa was about 0.04-0.2 µg/ml when supplemented and 30 min preincubated pooled normal plasma was analyzed at 10-15 min CRT. Of major importance are the CRT periods that belong to the ascending part of the thrombin generation curve, i.e. here CRT periods ≤ 15 min and F VIIa concentrations < 0.6 µg/ml (Figure 1a), because there is still o marked negative influence of nascending fibrin (= antithrombin I [26]) on thrombin.

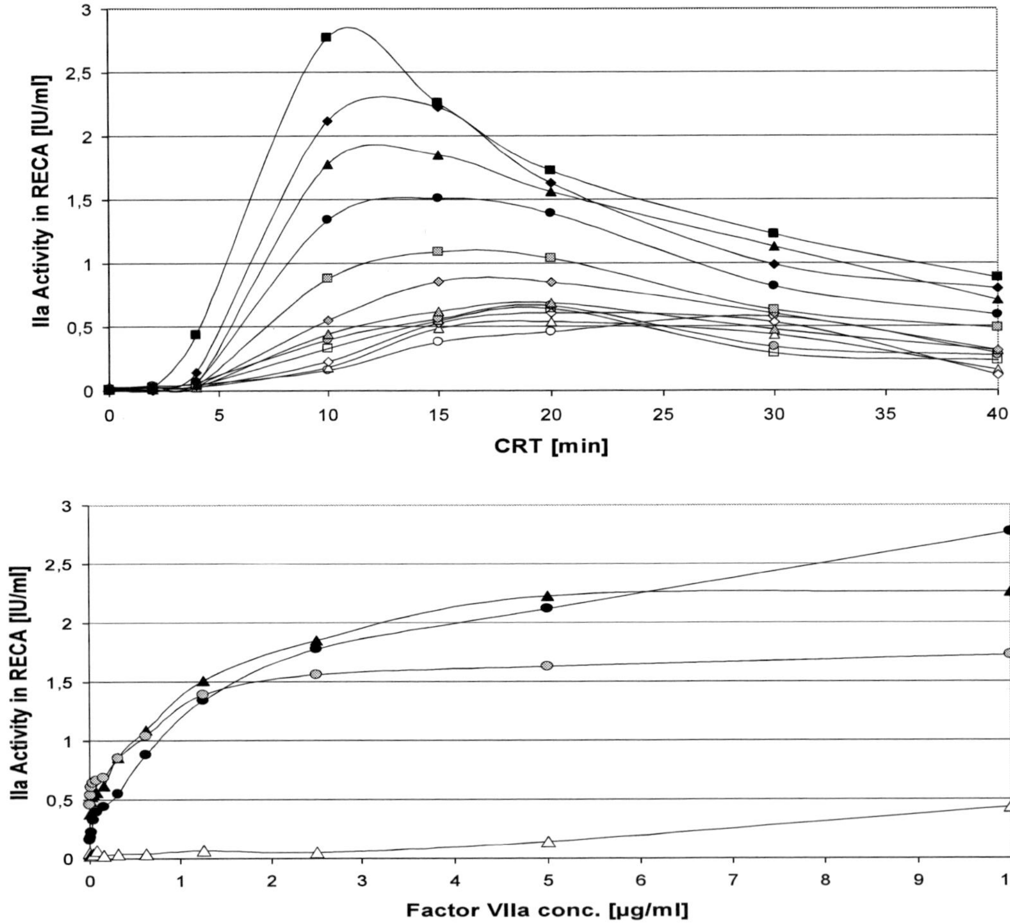

Figure 1. Thrombin generation triggered by factor VIIa. Unfrozen pooled normal citrated plasma was supplemented with 0-10 µg/ml recombinant human factor VIIa in a polystyrol U-well microtiter plate. After 30 min (23°C) the recalcified coagulation activity assay (RECA) was performed with a coagulation reaction time (CRT) of 0-40 min (37°C); Figure 1a: 0 µg/ml (O), 0.01 µg/ml (Δ), 0.02 µg/ml (◊), 0.039 µg/ml (□), 0.078 µg/ml (greyO), 0.156 µg/ml (greyΔ), 0.313 µg/ml (grey◊), 0.625 µg/ml (grey□), 1.25 µg/ml (●), 2.5 µg/ml (▲), 5 µg/ml (♦), 10 µg/ml (■) factor VIIa. Figure 1b: CRT periods of 4 min (Δ), 10 min (●), 15 min (▲), or 20 min (greyO).

If a similar experiment was performed with immediate recalcification after F VIIa supplementation of pooled normal plasma, the approximate ED200 was about 0.3 µg/ml (Figure 2); a respective ED200 in EXCA-1 could not be established because the maximal thrombin activity maximally reachable was 0.76 IU/ml at 1.25 µg/ml F VIIa with a thrombin activity of 0.47 IU/ml at 0 µg/ml F VIIa (the basal thrombin activity in this citrated plasma-pool without CRT was about 0.008 IU/ml). At final F VIIa concentrations > 2 µg/ml the added F VIIa tended to slightly inhibit thrombin generation in EXCA, 20 µg/ml F VIIa decreased the maximal thrombin activity obtained at 1.25 µg/ml F VIIa by about 20 %.

The approximate ED200 of F VIIa added to a pool of fresh plasma was about 0.3 µg/ml in RECA-10, about 0.3 µg/ml in INCA-4, no ED200 was obtainable for EXCA-1 (Figure 3). F VIIa can be given as a 4.8 mg vial (50-100 µg/kg) intravenously, which would result into a plasma concentration of about 1-2 µg/ml [27]. Sometimes much higher doses of F VIIa such as 90 µg/kg every 2-3 h might be indicated that could result into plasma concentrations of 5-10 µg/ml [28]. Especially patients that receive high amounts of F VIIa should be monitored by means of an ultra-specific thrombin generation assay to avoid prothrombotic reactions [29,30]. F VIIa should be used with caution in patients with basally enhanced thrombin generation such as in pathologic disseminated intravascular coagulation [27,31].

The approximate ED200 of F VIIa added to pooled plasma of patients on coumarin (INR=1.8) was about 1 µg/ml F VIIa (Figure 4); the F VIIa dose necessary for 1/3 (33.3 %) of normal RECA-10 (33.3 % of 0.4 IU/ml = generation of 133 mIU/ml IIa) was about 3 µg/ml F VIIa. These data are of interest to reverse a severe bleeding induced by coumarin [32]. The 100 % thrombin generation inhibiting efficiency of 1 IU/ml heparin in pooled citrated plasma was completely refractory even against 11.76 µg/ml F VIIa added to plasma.

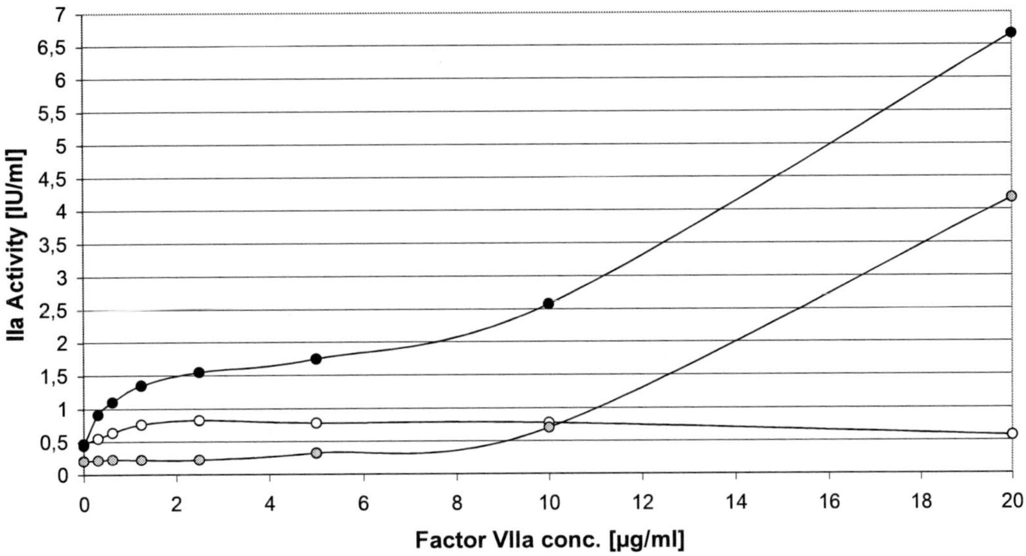

Figure 2. Thrombin generation triggered by F VIIa. Unfrozen pooled normal plasma was supplemented with 0-20 µg/ml F VIIa in U-well plates. Immediately thereafter the thrombin generation assays RECA-10 (●; recalcified coagulation activity assay with 10 min coagulation reaction time (CRT)) or EXCA-1 (O; extrinsic coagulation activity assay with 1 min CRT) were performed in duplicate.

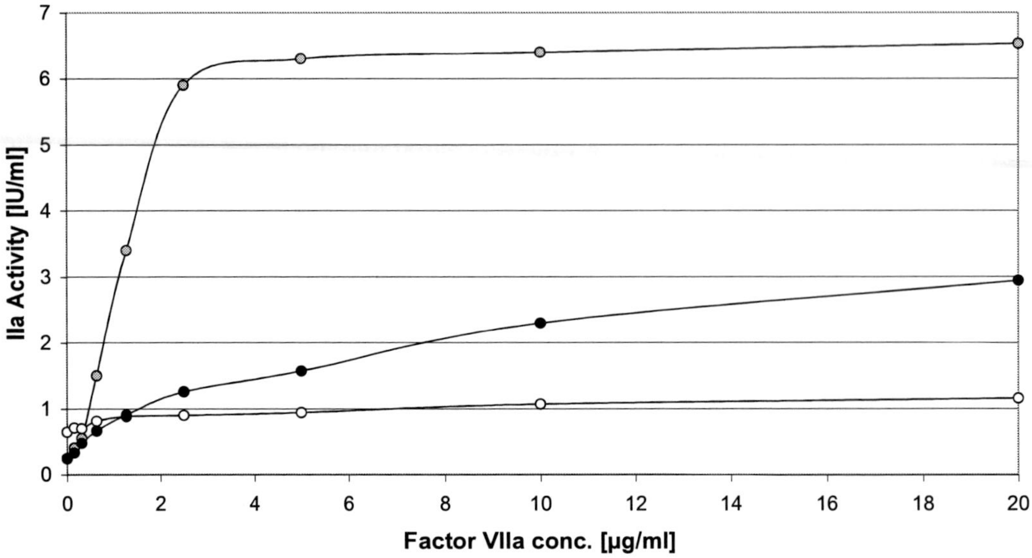

Figure 3. Quantification of IIa generation by F VIIa. 20 µl samples of fresh unfrozen pooled normal plasma were supplemented with 0-20 µg/ml recombinant F VIIa on U-well plates. Immediately thereafter the recalcified coagulation activity assay with 10 min CRT (RECA-10; ●), the intrinsic coagulation activity assay with 4 min CRT (INCA-4; greyO), or the extrinsic coagulation activity assay with 1 min CRT (EXCA-1; O) were performed in duplicate.

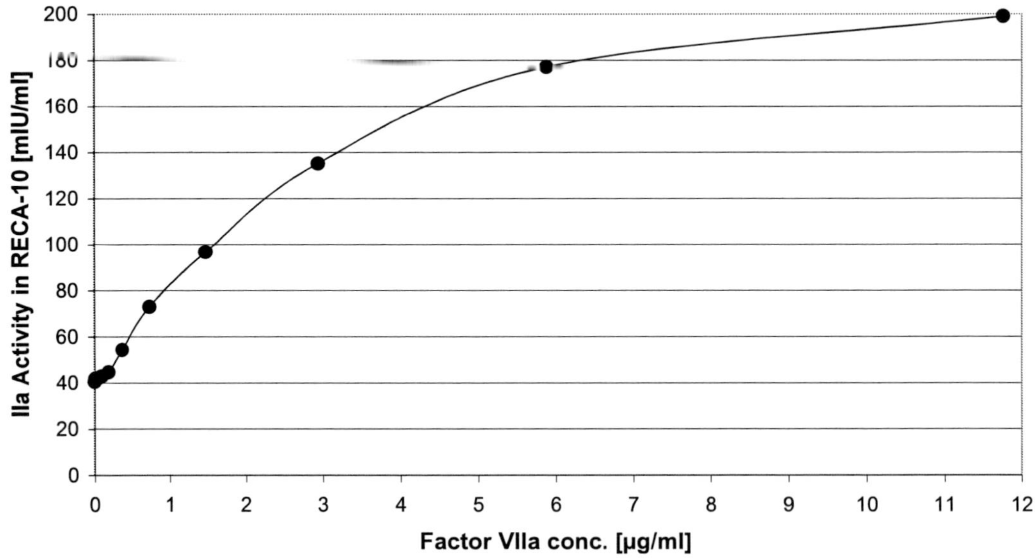

Figure 4. Pooled plasma of patients on coumarin. 50 µl samples of unfrozen pooled plasma from patients on coumarin (INR =1.8) were supplemented with 0-11.76 µg/ml recombinant factor VIIa on U-well plates. Immediately thereafter the RECA-10 was performed in duplicate, using 100 µl arginine-reagent and 25 µl substrate-reagent.

Table 1 compares the ED200 values of different prothrombinic agents [33-36]. The ED200 values for pooled plasma of patients on coumarin (PCP; INR=1.8) is about 2-3fold higher than that for pooled normal plasma (PNP). The dose of procoagulant that is necessary to obtain about one third of the normal RECA value is severalfold higher for PCP than for PNP. Of particular interest is the very low ED200 of TF (only about 1 pg/ml in PNP) that had comparable efficiency as F VIIa (about 0.3 μg/ml in PNP). This findings may be of interest to develop a very economical alternative to the rather expensive F VIIa [37-39].

The prothrombinic capacity and dosis adjustments of any new drug should be individually assessed for each individual patient by means of an ultra-specific, ultra-sensitive thrombin generation assay such as the RECA.

Table 1. Approx. ED200 values for different RECA coagulation triggers for pooled normal plasma (PNP) and for pooled plasma of patients on coumarin (PCP; INR=1.8).

	Thrombin [mIU/ml]	Factor Xa [mIU/ml]	FEIBA [U/ml]	Tissue Factor [pg/ml]	Factor VIIa [μg/ml]
ED200 for PNP	3	5	0.02	1	0.3
ED200 for PCP	8	8	0.03	2.5	1
33 % of normal dose for PCP	14	28	0.06	12	3

REFERENCES

[1] Monroe DM, Key NS. The tissue factor-factor VIIa complex: procoagulant activity, regulation, and multitasking. *J. Thromb Haemost.* 2007; 5: 1097-105.

[2] Olsen OH, Persson E. Cofactor-induced and mutational activity enhancement of coagulation factor *VIIa. Cell Mol. Life Sci.* 2008; 65: 953-63.

[3] Daubie V, Pochet R, Houard S, Philippart P. Tissue factor: a mini-review. *J. Tissue Eng. Regen Med.* 2007; 1: 161-9.

[4] Frédérick R, Pochet L, Charlier C, Masereel B. Modulators of the coagulation cascade: focus and recent advances in inhibitors of tissue factor, factor VIIa and their complex. *Curr. Med. Chem.* 2005; 12: 397-417.

[5] Bosinski TJ, El Solh AA. Recombinant factor VIIa, its clinical properties, and the tissue factor pathway of coagulation. *Mini Rev. Med. Chem.* 2006; 6: 1111-7.

[6] Hedner U, Ezban M. Tissue factor and factor VIIa as therapeutic targets in disorders of hemostasis. *Annu Rev. Med.* 2008;59:29-41.

[7] Hedner U. Mechanism of action, development and clinical experience of recombinant FVIIa. *J. Biotechnol.* 2006; 124: 747-57.

[8] Hedner U. Recombinant factor VIIa: its background, development and clinical use. *Curr. Opin. Hematol.* 2007; 14: 225-9.

[9] Gomperts ED, Astermark J, Gringeri A, Teitel J. From theory to practice: applying current clinical knowledge and treatment strategies to the care of hemophilia a patients with inhibitors. *Blood Rev.* 2008; 22 Suppl 1: S1-11.

[10] Croom KF, McCormack PL. Recombinant factor VIIa (eptacog alfa): a review of its use in congenital hemophilia with inhibitors, acquired hemophilia, and other congenital bleeding disorders. *BioDrugs* 2008; 22: 121-36.

[11] Birchall J, Stanworth SJ, Duffy MR, Doree CJ, Hyde C. Evidence for the use of recombinant factor VIIa in the prevention and treatment of bleeding in patients without hemophilia. *Transfus Med. Rev*. 2008; 22: 177-187.

[12] Gurol ME, Greenberg SM. Management of intracerebral hemorrhage. *Curr. Atheroscler Rep.* 2008; 10: 324-31.

[13] Liu-DeRyke X, Rhoney D. Hemostatic therapy for the treatment of intracranial hemorrhage. *Pharmacotherapy* 2008; 28: 485-95.

[14] Wartenberg KE, Mayer SA. Reducing the risk of ICH enlargement. *J. Neurol. Sci.* 2007 15; 261: 99-107.

[15] Bowman LJ, Uber WE, Stroud MR, Christiansen LR, Lazarchick J, Crumbley AJ 3rd, Kratz JM, Toole JM, Crawford FA Jr, Ikonomidis JS. Use of recombinant activated factor VII concentrate to control postoperative hemorrhage in complex cardiovascular surgery. *Ann. Thorac. Surg*. 2008; 85: 1669-76.

[16] Stief TW. Innovative tests of plasmatic hemostasis. *Laboratory Medicine* 2008; 39: 225-30.

[17] Stief TW. Specific determination of plasmatic thrombin activity. *Clin. Appl. Thromb Hemost.* 2006; 12: 324-9.

[18] Stief TW. Thrombin generation by exposure of blood to endotoxin: a simple model to study disseminated intravascular coagulation. *Clin. Appl. Thromb Hemost.* 2006; 12: 137-61.

[19] Stief TW. Coagulation Activation by Lipopolysaccharides. *Clin. Appl. Thromb. Hemost.* 2007 Dec 26. [Epub ahead of print].

[20] Stief TW, Otto S, Renz H. The intrinsic coagulation activity assay. *Blood Coagul Fibrinolysis* 2006; 17: 369-78.

[21] Stief TW. The Recalcified Coagulation Activity. *Clin. Appl. Thromb Hemost.* 2007 Dec 26. [Epub ahead of print].

[22] Stief TW. Kallikrein activates prothrombin.*Clin. Appl. Thromb Hemost*. 2008; 14: 97-8.

[23] Stief TW. Inhibition of thrombin generation in recalcified plasma. Blood Coagul Fibrinolysis. 2007; 18: 751-60.

[24] Stief TW. Arginine inhibits serpins. *Clin. Appl. Thromb Hemost*. 2007; 13: 213-8.

[25] Stief TW. Quantification of thrombin generation by trypsin. *Medical and Biological Sciences (*Scientific Journals International) 2007; 1/ 2: 1-8.

[26] Mosesson MW. Update on antithrombin I (fibrin). *Thromb Haemost.* 2007; 98: 105-8.

[27] Goodnough LT, Shander AS. Recombinant factor VIIa: safety and efficacy. *Curr. Opin. Hematol.* 2007; 14: 504-9.

[28] Poon MC. Clinical use of recombinant human activated factor VII (rFVIIa) in the prevention and treatment of bleeding episodes in patients with Glanzmann's thrombasthenia. *Vasc Health Risk Manag*. 2007; 3: 655-64.

[29] Fraser IS, Porte RJ, Kouides PA, Lukes AS. A benefit-risk review of systemic haemostatic agents: part 1: in major surgery. *Drug Saf.* 2008; 31: 217-30.

[30] Mahmoud A, Al-Ruzzeh S, McKeague H, Cross M. Systemic venous thrombosis after recombinant factor VIIa in the control of bleeding after cardiac surgery. *Tex. Heart Inst. J.* 2007; 34: 485-8.

[31] Stief TW. The laboratory diagnosis of the pre-phase of pathologic disseminated intravascular coagulation. *Hemostasis Laboratory* 2008; 1: (issue 1 in press)

[32] Ilyas C, Beyer GM, Dutton RP, Scalea TM, Hess JR. Recombinant factor VIIa for warfarin-associated intracranial bleeding. *J. Clin. Anesth* 2008; 20: 276-9.

[33] Stief TW. Thrombin triggers its generation. *Hemostasis Laboratory* 2008; 1: (in press).

[34] Stief TW. Factor Xa triggers thrombin generation. *Hemostasis Laboratory* 2008; 1: (in press).

[35] Stief TW. FEIBA triggers thrombin generation. *Hemostasis Laboratory* 2008; 1: (in press).

[36] Stief TW. Tissue factor triggers recalcified thrombin generation. *Hemostasis Laboratory* 2008; 1: (in press).

[37] Lyseng-Williamson KA, Plosker GL. Recombinant factor VIIa (eptacog alfa): a pharmacoeconomic review of its use in haemophilia in patients with inhibitors to clotting factors VIII or IX. *Pharmacoeconomics* 2007; 25: 1007-29.

[38] Lockwood CJ, Krikun G, Caze R, Rahman M, Buchwalder LF, Schatz F. Decidual cell-expressed tissue factor in human pregnancy and its involvement in hemostasis and preeclampsia-related angiogenesis. *Ann. N Y Acad. Sci.* 2008; 1127:67-72.

[39] Negrier C, Dargaud Y, Bordet JC. Basic aspects of bypassing agents. *Haemophilia.* 2006; 12 Suppl 6: 48-52.

In: Hemostasis Laboratory Yearbook, Volume 2
Editor: Thomas W. Stief, pp. 237-247
ISBN: 978-1-60741-089-8

TRIGGERS OF EXTRINSIC COAGULATION RESTORE THE NORMAL THROMBIN GENERATION IN FACTOR VIII OR FACTOR IX POOR PLASMA

Thomas W. Stief*
Department of Clinical Chemistry,
University Hospital Giessen and Marburg, Germany

ABSTRACT

Background: Finding the correct individual dosage of bypassing procoagulants in patients with inhibitors of factor VIII (F VIII) or IX (F IX) is a clinical challenge for every good hemostasis laboratory. The aim of the present work was to use the ultra-specific thrombin generation assay RECA (recalcified coagulation activity assay) to quantify activated thrombin generation in commercial hemophilia-like plasmas. What is the effective dose of a coagulation trigger to get a thrombin generation that is about 100 mIU/ml, which is in the range of thrombin generation in clotting normal plasma ?
Material and Methods: 20 µl plasmas completely deficient in F VIII or F IX, with 1 % F VIII or F IX, or with 10 % F VIII or F IX were supplemented in U-well plates (Brand®701300) with 0-33 mIU/ml thrombin, 0-852 mIU/ml F Xa, 0-10 U/ml FEIBA (factor eight inhibitor bypassing activity; STIM-4), 0-20 µg/ml recombinant F VII, or 0-25 pg/ml tissue factor (TF). Immediately thereafter the RECA was started with 2 µl RECA-trigger = 250 mM $CaCl_2$.
Results: The effective doses of different coagulation triggers to obtain RECA values in the range of 100 mIU/ml thrombin in commercial plasma containing 10 % F VIII or 10 % F IX were about 30-40 mIU/ml thrombin, 25-40 mIU/ml F Xa, 2.5 U/ml FEIBA, 12 µg/ml F VIIa, or 5 pg/ml TF. For 1 % F VIII plasma or 1 % F IX plasma the respective doses of F Xa or of TF are about 3-4fold higher.
Discussion: The present work might contribute to characterize the biochemistry, physiology, and pharmacology of coagulation factors VIII and IX. The ideal RECA target value for patients with deficiencies of the intrinsic pathway of blood coagulation might be about 33-50 % (about one third to one half) of normal generation of thrombin, preventing hemorrhagic and thrombotic complications.

Keywords: Factor VIII, factor IX, thrombin, RECA.

---

* Correspondence to:_PD Dr. med. T. Stief, Department of Clinical Chemistry, University Hospital, D-35043 Marburg, Germany. E-mail: thstief@med.uni-marburg.de; Tel. : +49-6421-58 64471; FAX: +49-6421-58 65594.

INTRODUCTION

A complication in hemophilia A or B is the generation of inhibitors agains factors VIII or IX [1-9]. The diagnosis of the correct individual dosage of a bypassing agent in patients with inhibitors against factors VIII or IX is a clinical challenge [10-12]. Too few of the coagulation trigger infused, and the patient will suffer from hemorrhages; too much of the coagulation trigger infused, and the patient will suffer from thromboses. Up to now there has been no simple routine assay that specifically assesses the thrombin generation in plasma of these patients. After biochemical development of the recalcified coagulation activity assay (RECA), which ultra-specifically detects normal, subnormal, or supra-normal thrombin generation in recalcified plasma [13-15], the aim of the present work was to diagnose comparable effective doses of different extrinsic coagulation enhancers on the capacity of thrombin generation of hemophilia-like commercial plasma.What is the effective dose of a coagulation trigger to get a thrombin generation that is about 100 mIU/ml, which is in the range of thrombin generation in clotting normal plasma [14] ?

MATERIAL AND METHODS

Thrombin (F IIa) Addition to F VIII or F IX Poor Plasma

Lyophilized F VIII or F IX deficient citrated plasma (DadeBehring, Marburg, Germany) or lyophilized pooled normal citrated plasma (PNP; control plasma N®, DadeBehring) were reconstituted with 1 ml H_2O. PNP was added to F VIII or F IX deficient plasma to obtain final F VIII or F IX concentrations of 0 % (= F VIII or F IX deficient plasma), 1 %, 10 %, and for control 100 % (= PNP). 20 µl of these samples were supplemented with 0-33.25 mIU/ml human thrombin (Stago, Asnières, France) or with 0-33.25 mIU/ml bovine thrombin (DadeBehring) on polystyrol U-well microtiter plates (Brand, Wertheim, Germany; article nr. 701300) by repetitive 1+1 dilution (the aliquoted 1 IU/ml thrombin stock solutions were stabilized with 5 % human albumin; CSL Behring). Immediately thereafter, 2 µl 250 mM $CaCl_2$ (trigger of the recalcified coagulation activity assay = RECA) were added. After 10 min coagulation reaction time (37°C; RECA-10) the reaction was stopped by 50 µl 2.5 M arginine, pH 8.6, 0.16 % Triton X 100® (Sigma, Deisenhofen, Germany) and after 3 min 25 µl 1 mM chromogenic thrombin substrate HD-CHG-Ala-Arg-pNA (Pentapharm, Basel, Switzerland) in 1.25 M arginine, pH 8.7 were added and the specific increase in absorbance (ΔA) at 405 nm (23°C) was determined by a microtitre plate photometer with a 1 mA resolution (Milenia; DPC, Los Angeles, USA). The results were standardized against 1 IU/ml bovine thrombin in 6.7 % human albumin (Kabi, Stockholm, Sweden) that replaced the plasma sample and resulted in a ΔA of about 10 mA/min (23°C). The linear ΔA range was up to about 420 mA = 40 % of the maximal ΔA (total cleavage of the chromogenic substrate resulting in about 1050 mA).

Factor Xa Addition to F VIII or F IX Poor Plasma

The above experiment was performed with plasmas supplemented with 0-0.852 IU/ml bovine factor Xa (Chromogenix, Mölndal, Sweden; the aliquoted 4.26 IU/ml stock solution was stabilized with 5 % human albumin).

FEIBA Addition to F VIII or F IX Poor Plasma

The above experiment was performed with plasmas supplemented with 0-10 U/ml factor eight inhibitor bypassing activity (FEIBA) (S-TIM 4; Immuno, Heidelberg, Germany; the aliquoted stock solution contained 200 U/ml).

Factor Viia Addition to F VIII or F IX Poor Plasma

The above experiment was performed with plasmas supplemented with 0-20 µg/ml recombinant human factor VIIa (Novo Nordisk, Bagsvaerd, Denmark; the aliquoted stock solution contained 600 µg/ml).

Tissue Factor Addition to FVIII or FIX Poor Plasma

The above experiment was performed with plasmas supplemented with 0-25 pg/ml human placental tissue factor (Thromborel S® without Polybrene®; Behringwerke, Marburg, Germany; the aliquoted 1 ng/ml stock solution was stabilized with 5 % human albumin).

Results and Discussion

Factor VIII

Figure 1 demonstrates that an addition of about 30 mIU/ml thrombin to reconstituted lyophilized plasma containing 0-100 % F VIII was needed to obtain a thrombin generation in RECA-10 of about 50 mIU/ml. The 0-10 % F VIII plasmas behaved as resistant to up to about 17 mIU/ml added thrombin. The commercial PNP with 100 % F VIII responded with a generation of about 10 mIU/ml or 20 mIU/ml thrombin by addition of about 4 mIU/ml bovine thrombin or human thrombin, respectively (thrombin generation = thrombin activity after CRT minus basal plasmatic thrombin activity (without CRT; here: 10-15 mIU/ml thrombin)).

A thrombin generation in lyophilized/reconstituted plasmas of about 100 mIU/ml in RECA-10 was achieved by addition of about 70 mIU/ml F Xa for 0 % or 1 % F VIII plasma or by addition of about 25 mIU/ml F Xa for 10 % F VIII plasma (Figure 2); commercial PNP with 100 % F VIII needed about 150 mIU/ml F Xa for generation of about 100 mIU/ml in RECA-10, which might be due to a different matrix (e.g. plasma stabilizers such as F Xa inhibitors) of PNP when compared with factor-deficient plasmas [16,17]. Of importance is only the ascending part of the thrombin generation curve where there is no major negative influence of nascending fibrin that entraps thrombin.

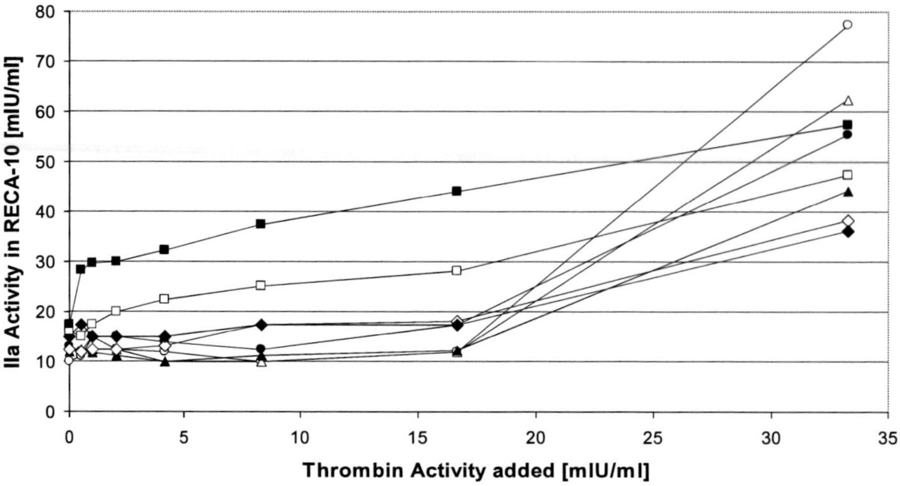

Figure 1. Thrombin addition to F VIII poor plasma. Lyophilized FVIII deficient citrated plasma or lyophilized pooled normal citrated plasma (PNP) were reconstituted with H_2O. PNP was added to FVIII deficient plasma to obtain final FVIII concentrations of 0 % (circles), 1 % (triangles), 10 % (diamonds), and for control 100 % (squares). 20 µl of these samples were supplemented with 0-33.25 mIU/ml (final added activity) human thrombin (black symbols) or bovine thrombin (white symbols) on U-well microtiter plates. Immediately thereafter, 2 µl 250 mM $CaCl_2$ (trigger of the recalcified coagulation activity assay = RECA) were added. After 10 min coagulation reaction time (37°C; RECA-10) the reaction was stopped by 50 µl 2.5 M arginine, pH 8.6, 0.16 % Triton X 100®. After 3 min (23°C) 25 µl 1 mM CHG-Ala-Arg-pNA in 1.25 M arginine, pH 8.7 were added and the ΔA at 405 nm was determined.

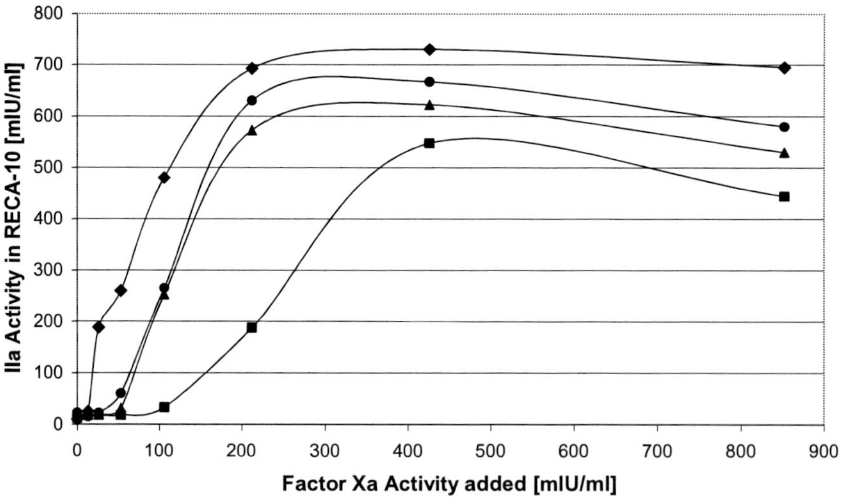

Figure 2. Factor Xa addition to F VIII poor plasma. Lyophilized FVIII deficient citrated plasma or lyophilized pooled normal citrated plasma (PNP) were reconstituted with H_2O. PNP was added to FVIII deficient plasma to obtain final FVIII concentrations of 0 % (●), 1 % (▲), 10 % (♦), and for control 100 % (■). 20 µl of these samples were supplemented with 0-852 mIU/ml (final added activity) bovine factor Xa on U-well microtiter plates. Immediately thereafter, 2 µl 250 mM $CaCl_2$ were added. After 10 min coagulation reaction time (37°C; RECA-10) the reaction was stopped by 50 µl 2.5 M arginine, pH 8.6, 0.16 % Triton X 100®. After 3 min (23°C) 25 µl 1 mM CHG-Ala-Arg-pNA in 1.25 M arginine, pH 8.7 were added and the ΔA at 405 nm was determined.

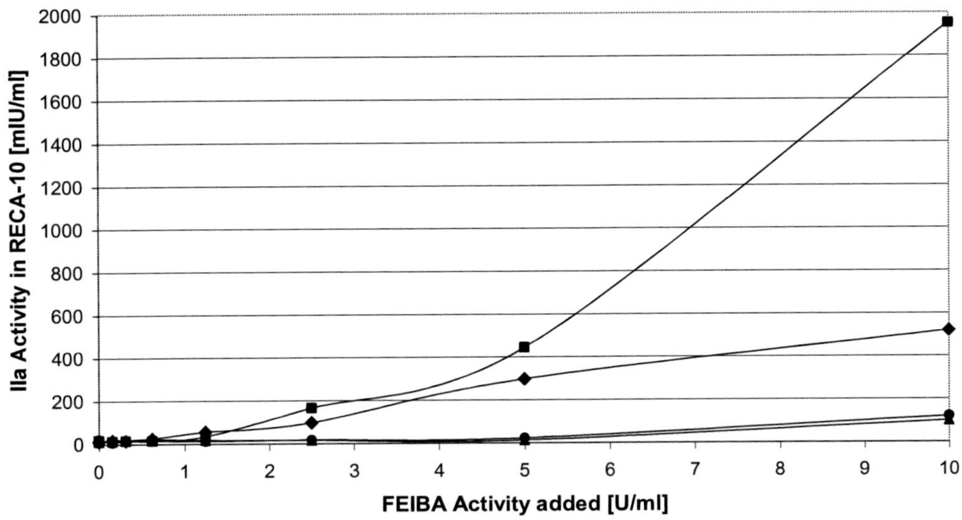

Figure 3. FEIBA addition to F VIII poor plasma. Lyophilized FVIII deficient citrated plasma or lyophilized pooled normal citrated plasma (PNP) were reconstituted with H_2O. PNP was added to FVIII deficient plasma to obtain final FVIII concentrations of 0 % (●), 1 % (▲), 10 % (♦), and for control 100 % (■). 20 µl of these samples were supplemented with 0-10 U/ml (final activity) factor eight inhibitor bypassing activity (FEIBA) on U-well microtiter plates. Immediately thereafter, 2 µl 250 mM $CaCl_2$ were added. After 10 min coagulation reaction time (37°C; RECA-10) the reaction was stopped by 50 µl 2.5 M arginine, pH 8.6, 0.16 % Triton X 100®. After 3 min (23°C) 25 µl 1 mM CHG-Ala-Arg-pNA in 1.25 M arginine, pH 8.7 were added and the ΔA at 405 nm was determined.

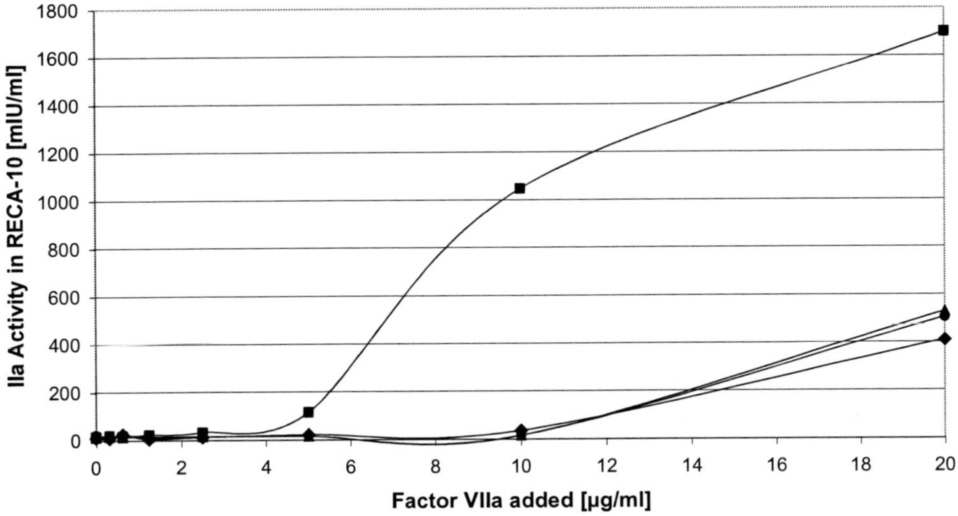

Figure 4. Factor VIIa addition to F VIII poor plasma. Lyophilized FVIII deficient citrated plasma or lyophilized pooled normal citrated plasma (PNP) were reconstituted with H_2O. PNP was added to FVIII deficient plasma to obtain final FVIII concentrations of 0 % (●), 1 % (▲), 10 % (♦), and for control 100 % (■). 20 µl of these samples were supplemented with 0-20 µg/ml (final concentration) recombinant factor VIIa on U-well microtiter plates. Immediately thereafter, 2 µl 250 mM $CaCl_2$ were added. After 10 min coagulation reaction time (37°C; RECA-10) the reaction was stopped by 50 µl 2.5 M arginine, pH 8.6, 0.16 % Triton X 100®. After 3 min (23°C) 25 µl 1 mM CHG-Ala-Arg-pNA in 1.25 M arginine, pH 8.7 were added and the ΔA at 405 nm was determined.

A thrombin generation in lyophilized/reconstituted plasmas of about 100 mIU/ml in RECA-10 was achieved by addition of about 7 pg/ml TF for 0 % or 1 % F VIII plasma, by addition of about 2 pg/ml TF for 10 % F VIII plasma, or by addition of about 6 pg/ml TF for 100 % F VIII plasma (Figure 5), which might be explained by matrix differences between these plasmas.

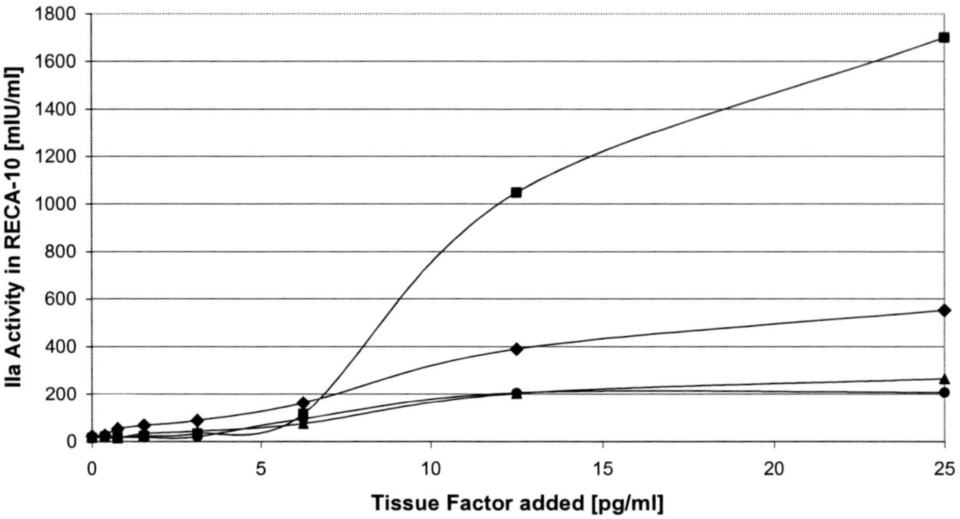

Figure 5. Tissue factor addition to F VIII poor plasma. Lyophilized FVIII deficient citrated plasma or lyophilized pooled normal citrated plasma (PNP) were reconstituted with H_2O. PNP was added to FVIII deficient plasma to obtain final FVIII concentrations of 0 % (●), 1 % (▲), 10 % (♦), and for control 100 % (■). 20 µl of these samples were supplemented with 0-25 pg/ml (final concentration) human placental tissue factor on U-well microtitre plates. Immediately thereafter, 2 µl 250 mM $CaCl_2$ were added. After 10 min coagulation reaction time (37°C; RECA-10) the reaction was stopped by 50 µl 2.5 M arginine, pH 8.6, 0.16 % Triton X 100®. After 3 min (23°C) 25 µl 1 mM CHG-Ala-Arg-pNA in 1.25 M arginine, pH 8.7 were added and the ΔA at 405 nm was determined.

Factor IX

Figure 6 demonstrates that an addition of about 30 mIU/ml thrombin to reconstituted lyophilized plasma containing 0-100 % F IX was needed to obtain a thrombin generation in RECA-10 of about 50 mIU/ml. The 0-10 % F VIII plasmas behaved as resistant to up to about15 mIU/ml added thrombin. A thrombin generation in lyophilized/reconstituted plasmas of about 100 mIU/ml in RECA-10 was achieved by addition of about 200 mIU/ml F Xa for 0 % FIX plasma, by addition of about 120 mIU/ml for 1 % F IX plasma or by addition of about 40 mIU/ml F Xa for 10 % F IX plasma (Figure 7).

A thrombin generation in lyophilized/reconstituted plasmas of about 100 mIU/ml in RECA-10 was achieved by addition of about 0.2 U/ml FEIBA for 0 % or 1 % F IX plasma, by addition of about 2.5 U/ml FEIBA for 10 % F IX plasma (Figure 8). A thrombin generation in lyophilized/reconstituted plasmas of about 100 mIU/ml in RECA-10 was achieved by addition of about 12 µg/ml F VIIa for 10 % F IX plasma (Figure 9). Lyophilized/reconstituted 0 % or 1 % F IX plasma needed > 20 µg/ml F VIIa to obtain about 100 mIU/ml in RECA-10, indicating that F IX activation is a part of the action of F VIIa.

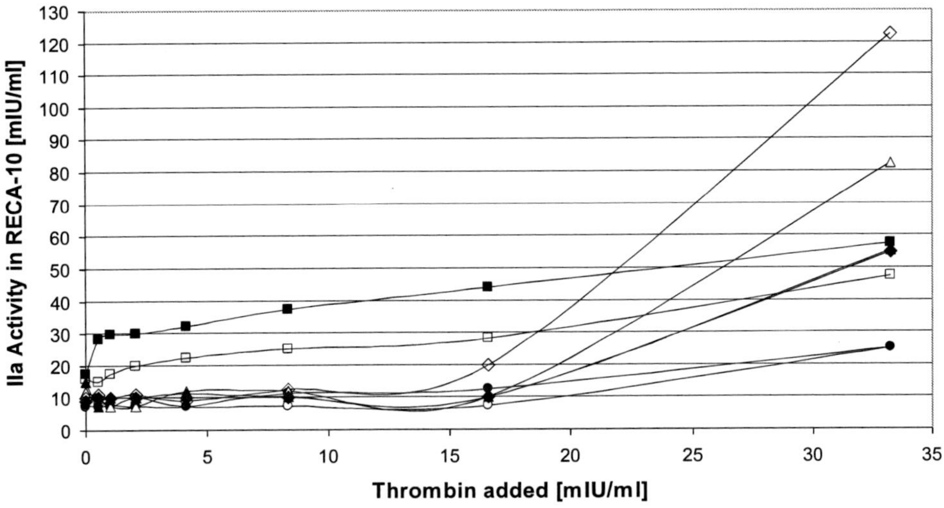

Figure 6. Thrombin addition to F IX poor plasma. Lyophilized F IX deficient citrated plasma or lyophilized pooled normal citrated plasma (PNP) were reconstituted with H_2O. PNP was added to FVIII deficient plasma to obtain final F IX concentrations of 0 % (circles), 1 % (triangles), 10 % (diamonds), and for control 100 % (squares). 20 µl of these samples were supplemented with 0-33.25 mIU/ml human thrombin (black symbols) or bovine thrombin (white symbols) on U-well microtiter plates. Immediately thereafter, 2 µl 250 mM $CaCl_2$ (trigger of the recalcified coagulation activity assay = RECA) were added. After 10 min coagulation reaction time (37°C; RECA-10) the reaction was stopped by 50 µl 2.5 M arginine, pH 8.6, 0.16 % Triton X 100®. After 3 min (23°C) 25 µl 1 mM CHG-Ala-Arg-pNA in 1.25 M arginine, pH 8.7 were added and the ΔA at 405 nm was determined.

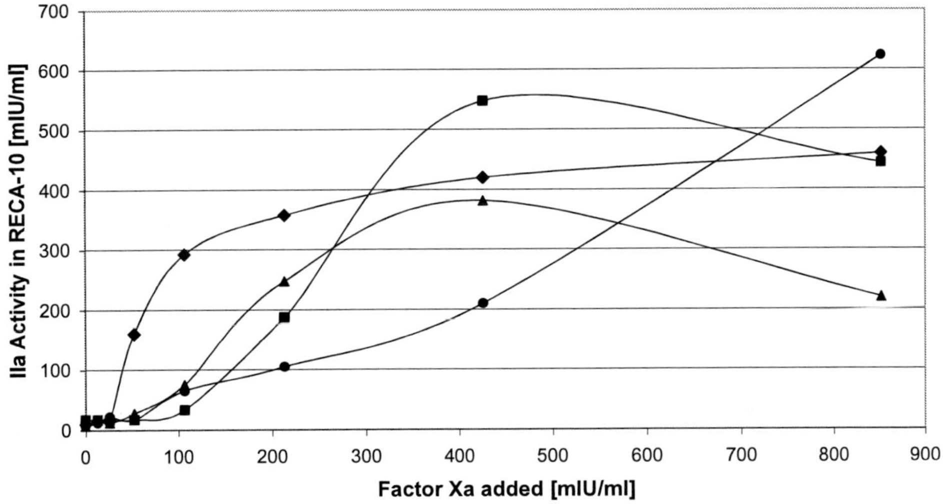

Figure 7. Factor Xa addition to F IX poor plasma. Lyophilized F IX deficient citrated plasma or lyophilized pooled normal citrated plasma (PNP) were reconstituted with H_2O. PNP was added to FVIII deficient plasma to obtain final F IX concentrations of 0 % (●), 1 % (▲), 10 % (♦), and for control 100 % (■). 20 µl of these samples were supplemented with 0-852 mIU/ml bovine factor Xa on U-well microtiter plates. Immediately thereafter, 2 µl 250 mM $CaCl_2$ were added. After 10 min coagulation reaction time (37°C; RECA-10) the reaction was stopped by 50 µl 2.5 M arginine, pH 8.6, 0.16 % Triton X 100®. After 3 min (23°C) 25 µl 1 mM CHG-Ala-Arg-pNA in 1.25 M arginine, pH 8.7 were added and the ΔA at 405 nm was determined.

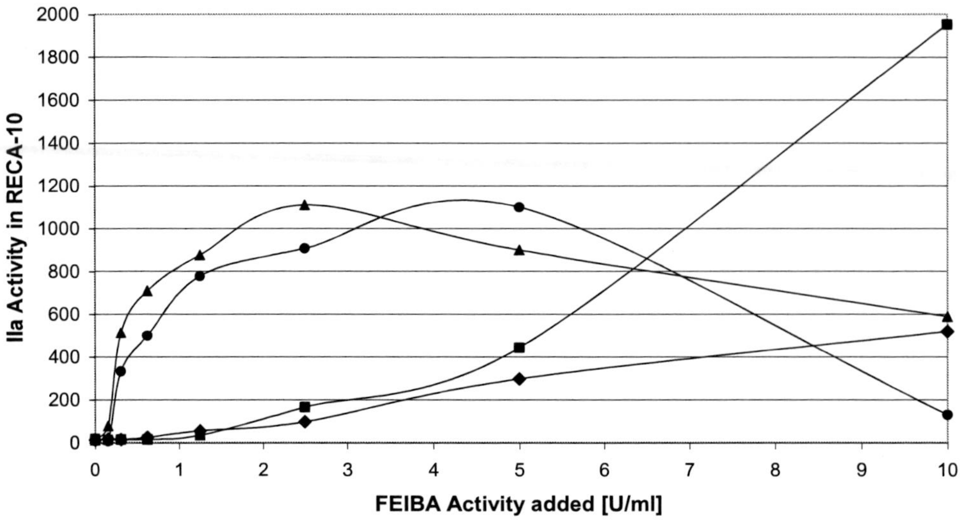

Figure 8. FEIBA addition to F IX poor plasma. Lyophilized F IX deficient citrated plasma or lyophilized pooled normal citrated plasma (PNP) were reconstituted with H_2O. PNP was added to FVIII deficient plasma to obtain final F IX concentrations of 0 % (●), 1 % (▲), 10 % (♦), and for control 100 % (■). 20 µl of these samples were supplemented with 0-10 U/ml factor eight inhibitor bypassing activity (FEIBA) on U-well microtiter plates. Immediately thereafter, 2 µl 250 mM $CaCl_2$ were added. After 10 min coagulation reaction time (37°C; RECA-10) the reaction was stopped by 50 µl 2.5 M arginine, pH 8.6, 0.16 % Triton X 100®. After 3 min (23°C) 25 µl 1 mM CHG-Ala-Arg-pNA in 1.25 M arginine, pH 8.7 were added and the ΔA at 405 nm was determined.

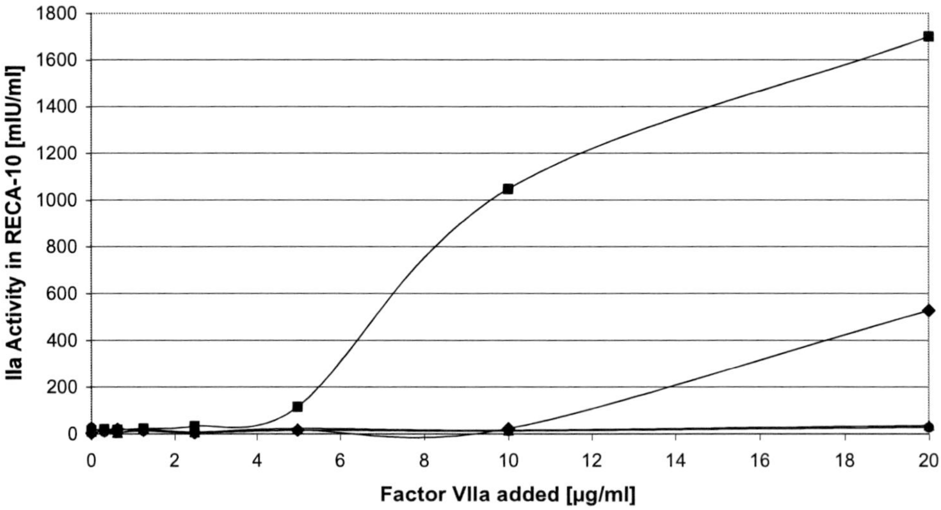

Figure 9. Factor VIIa addition to F IX poor plasma. Lyophilized F IX deficient citrated plasma or lyophilized pooled normal citrated plasma (PNP) were reconstituted with H_2O. PNP was added to F IX deficient plasma to obtain final F IX concentrations of 0 % (●), 1 % (▲), 10 % (♦), and for control 100 % (■). 20 µl of these samples were supplemented with 0-20 µg/ml recombinant factor VIIa on U-well microtiter plates. Immediately thereafter, 2 µl 250 mM $CaCl_2$ were added. After 10 min coagulation reaction time (37°C; RECA-10) the reaction was stopped by 50 µl 2.5 M arginine, pH 8.6, 0.16 % Triton X 100®. After 3 min (23°C) 25 µl 1 mM CHG-Ala-Arg-pNA in 1.25 M arginine, pH 8.7 were added and the ΔA at 405 nm was determined.

A thrombin generation in lyophilized/reconstituted plasmas of about 100 mIU/ml in RECA-10 was achieved by addition of about 13 pg/ml TF for 0 % or 1 % F IX plasm, or by addition of about 4 pg/ml TF for 10 % F IX plasma (Figure 10).

Table 1 compares the effective doses of different coagulation triggers in 10 % commercial plasma that contains only 10 % of normal F VIII or 10 % of normal F IX. When using thrombin as the coagulation trigger, added IIa activities in the range of 30-40 mIU/ml were necessary to obtain RECA-10 values in the range of 100 mIU/ml that is the approximate thrombin activity in clotting normal plasma [14].

In pooled normal plasma (lyophilized/reconstituted with a different matrix when compared with unfrozen pooled plasma) the respective trigger concentrations were 150 mIU/ml F Xa, 2 U/ml FEIBA, 5 µg/ml F VIIa, and 6 pg/ml TF. Thus, 12 µg/ml F VIIa in lyophilized/reconstitued pooled plasmas corresponded to about 25-40 mIU/ml F Xa or F IIa, to about 2.5 U/ml FEIBA, or to about 5 pg/ml TF. 1 µg F VIIa would then be approximately equivalent to about 2-3 mIU/ml F Xa or F IIa, to about 0.2 U/ml FEIBA, or to about 0.5 pg/ml TF.

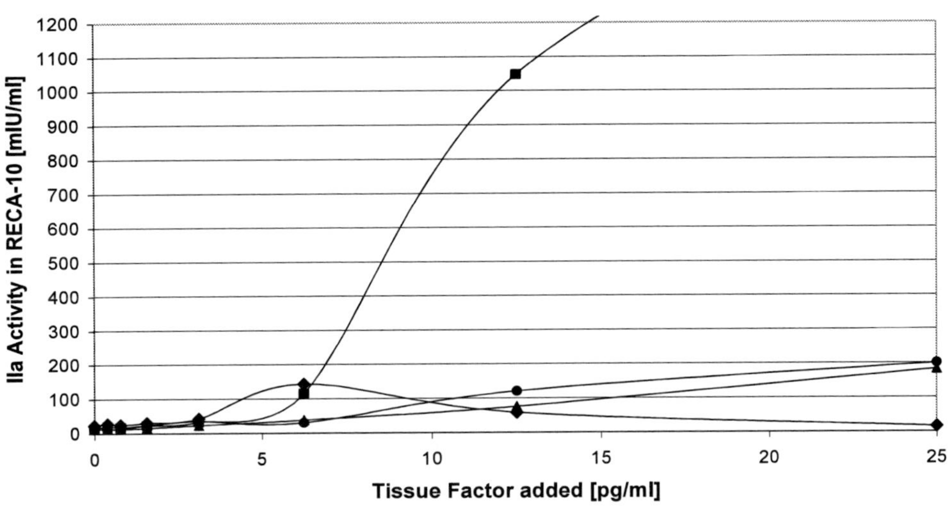

Figure 10. Tissue factor addition to F IX poor plasma. Lyophilized F IX deficient citrated plasma or lyophilized pooled normal citrated plasma (PNP) were reconstituted with H_2O. PNP was added to FVIII deficient plasma to obtain final F IX concentrations of 0 % (●), 1 % (▲), 10 % (♦), and for control 100 % (■). 20 µl of these samples were supplemented with 0-25 pg/ml human placental tissue factor on U-well microtitre plates. Immediately thereafter, 2 µl 250 mM $CaCl_2$ were added. After 10 min coagulation reaction time (37°C; RECA-10) the reaction was stopped by 50 µl 2.5 M arginine, pH 8.6, 0.16 % Triton X 100®. After 3 min (23°C) 25 µl 1 mM CHG-Ala-Arg-pNA in 1.25 M arginine, pH 8.7 were added and the ΔA at 405 nm was determined.

Table 1. Approximate trigger concentrations necessary to obtain a RECA-10 value of 100 mIU/ml.

Trigger added: *to plasma with:*	F Xa [mIU/ml]	FEIBA [U/ml]	F VIIa [µg/ml]	Tissue Factor [pg/ml]
10 % F VIII	25	2.5	12	5
10 % F IX	40	2.5	12	5

These effective doses are in a similar range as that found for unfrozen pooled plasma [15]. The respective doses of F Xa or of TF for are about 3-4fold higher both for 1 % F VIII plasma or 1 % F IX plasma.

In conclusion, the present work might contribute to characterize the biochemistry, physiology, and pharmacology of coagulation factors VIII and IX [18-20]. Triggers of extrinsic coagulation might be clinically used to bypass a dysfunctional intrinsic coagulation, e.g. in hemophilia A or B [21-24]. The correct dosage of the trigger used for each individual patient should be diagnosed by means of an ultra-specific thrombin generation assay, such as the RECA. The ideal RECA target value might be about 33-50 % (one third to one half) of normal generation of thrombin -the heart of coagulation [25]-, preventing hemorrhagic and thrombotic complications.

REFERENCES

[1] Rodriguez NI, Hoots WK. Advances in hemophilia: experimental aspects and therapy. *Pediatr. Clin. North Am.* 2008; 55: 357-76.

[2] Lyseng-Williamson KA, Plosker GL. Recombinant factor VIIa (eptacog alfa): a pharmacoeconomic review of its use in haemophilia in patients with inhibitors to clotting factors VIII or IX. *Pharmacoeconomics* 2007; 25: 1007-29.

[3] Pipe SW, Valentino LA. Optimizing outcomes for patients with severe haemophilia A. *Haemophilia* 2007; 13 Suppl 4:1-16.

[4] Khair K, Geraghty SJ. Haemophilia A: meeting the needs of individual patients. *Br. J. Nurs.* 2007; 16: 987-93.

[5] Tjønnfjord GE, Holme PA. Factor eight inhibitor bypass activity (FEIBA) in the management of bleeds in hemophilia patients with high-titer inhibitors. *Vasc. Health Risk Manag.* 2007; 3: 527-31.

[6] Dargaud Y, Negrier C. Haemophilia therapies. *Expert Opin. Biol. Ther.* 2007; 7: 651-63.

[7] Kessler CM. Advances in the treatment of hemophilia. *Clin. Adv. Hematol. Oncol.* 2008; 6: 184-7.

[8] Petrini P. Identifying and overcoming barriers to prophylaxis in the management of haemophilia. *Haemophilia* 2007; 13 Suppl 2:16-22.

[9] Berntorp E. Options for treating acute bleeds in addition to bypassing agents: extracorporeal immunoadsorption, FVIII/FIX, desmopressin and antifibrinolytics. *Haemophilia* 2006; 12 Suppl 6: 62-5.

[10] Arnout J, Hoylaerts MF, Lijnen HR. Haemostasis. *Handb Exp Pharmacol* 2006; (176 Pt 2): 1-41.

[11] DiMichele DM. Inhibitor treatment in haemophilias A and B: inhibitor diagnosis. *Haemophilia* 2006; 12 Suppl 6: 37-41.

[12] Lillicrap D, Nair SC, Srivastava A, Rodeghiero F, Pabinger I, Federici AB. Laboratory issues in bleeding disorders. *Haemophilia* 2006; 12 Suppl 3: 68-75.

[13] Stief TW. Specific determination of plasmatic thrombin activity. *Clin. Appl. Thromb. Hemost.* 2006; 12: 324-9.

[14] Stief TW. Innovative tests of plasmatic hemostasis. *Laboratory Medicine* 2008; 39: 225-30.
[15] Stief TW. Factor VIIa triggers thrombin generation. *Hemostasis Laboratory* 2008; 1: in press
[16] Stief TW, Otto S, Renz H. Influence of coagulation factors on intrinsic thrombin generation. *Blood Coagul Fibrinolysis* 2007; 18: 67-71.
[17] Stief TW, Wieczerzak A, Renz H. Influence of coagulation factors on extrinsic thrombin generation. *Blood Coagul Fibrinolysis* 2007; 18: 105-12.
[18] Fay PJ. Factor VIII structure and function. *Int. J. Hematol.* 2006; 83: 103-8.
[19] Fay PJ. Activation of factor VIII and mechanisms of cofactor action. *Blood Rev.* 2004; 18: 1-15.
[20] Howard EL, Becker KC, Rusconi CP, Becker RC. Factor IXa inhibitors as novel anticoagulants. *Arterioscler. Thromb Vasc. Biol.* 2007; 27: 722-7.
[21] Stobart K, Iorio A, Wu JK. Clotting factor concentrates given to prevent bleeding and bleeding-related complications in people with hemophilia A or B. *Cochrane Database Syst. Rev.* 2006; (2):CD003429.
[22] Dunn AL, Abshire TC. Current issues in prophylactic therapy for persons with hemophilia. *Acta Haematol.* 2006; 115: 162-71.
[23] Dunn AL. Management and prevention of recurrent hemarthrosis in patients with hemophilia. *Curr. Opin. Hematol.* 2005; 12: 390-4.
[24] Giangrande P. Haemophilia B: Christmas disease. *Expert Opin. Pharmacother* 2005; 6: 1517-24.
[25] Huntington JA. Molecular recognition mechanisms of thrombin. *J. Thromb Haemost.* 2005; 3: 1861-72.

In: Hemostasis Laboratory Yearbook, Volume 2
Editor: Thomas W. Stief, pp. 249-255
ISBN: 978-1-60741-089-8

FACTOR XA TRIGGERS THROMBIN GENERATION

Thomas W. Stief
Department of Clinical Chemistry,
University Hospital Giessen and Marburg, Germany

ABSTRACT

Background: Factor Xa (F Xa) generation and activity is important to maintain a physiologic hemostasis. F Xa is the enzyme part in the prothrombinase, that converts prothrombin into thrombin, the central enzyme of coagulation. The aim of the present work was to determine the 200 % effective dose (ED200) of F Xa on plasmatic thrombin generation.
Material and Methods: Pools of unfrozen citrated plasma (normal or from patients on coumarin, INR=1.8) were supplemented with 0-0.852 IU/ml bovine F Xa on polystyrol U-well microtiter plates (Brand®701300) at 23°C. Immediately thereafter the ultra-specific, ultra-sensitive thrombin generation assays RECA-10 (recalcified coagulation activity assay with 10 min coagulation reaction time (CRT) at 37°C) and EXCA-1 (extrinsic coagulation activity assay with 1 min CRT) were performed with 20 µl or 50 µl plasma samples. Thrombin generation = thrombin activity after CRT minus basal thrombin activity in citrated plasma (without CRT).
Results: The approximate ED200 of added F Xa on thrombin generation of pooled normal plasma in the RECA-10 was about 5 mIU/ml F Xa. The respective approximate ED200 of added F Xa in the EXCA-1 was about 80 mIU/ml F Xa. The approximate ED200 of added F Xa on thrombin generation in RECA-10 of pooled plasma of patients on coumarin (INR=1.8) was about 8 mIU/l added F Xa. To obtain in pooled coumarin-plasma a thrombin generation that is about one third of the normal RECA value about 28 mIU/ml factor Xa had to be added.
Discussion: Only about 5 mIU/ml F Xa added to pooled unfrozen normal citrated plasma approximately doubles the thrombin activity generated in RECA-10. These data may be of interest to develop new therapeutics, such as close-to-physiologic anti- F Xa anticoagulants.

Keywords: Factor Xa, thrombin, RECA, EXCA, ED200.

Introduction

Activated factor X (F Xa) is the end product of both extrinsic and intrinsic coagulation: F Xa is generated by the extrinsic tenase or by the intrinsic tenase [1-10]: F Xa together with its cofactor factor Va [11] activates prothrombin to thrombin, the central enzyme of coagulation. The adequate generation of F Xa and of thrombin is of major clinical importance: an enhanced generation may result in pathologic thrombi, a diminished generation may give rise to severe bleedings. It was the purpose of the present work to study the generation of thrombin in dependence of the activity of plasmatic F Xa.

Material and Methods

Pooled Unfrozen Normal Plasma

Unfrozen pooled normal citrated plasma (from 8 samples that remained after routine analysis; 0.5 ml 106 mM sodium citrate + 4.5 ml venous blood in polypropylene sampling tubes; Sarstedt, Nümbrecht, Germany) was supplemented with 0-1.18 nkat/ml bovine factor Xa (Chromogenix, Mölndal, Sweden; 16.67 nkat = 1 IU; the 71 nkat/ml stock solution was stabilized with 5 % human albumin (CSL Behring, Marburg, Germany) directly in a polystyrol U-well microtiter plate (Brand, Wertheim, Germany; article nr. 701300). The repetitively 1+1 diluted plasma pool were pipetted in 20 µl aliquots by means of 0.9 % NaCl - rinsed new disposable polypropylene tips of an Eppendorf-Multipette®. After 30 min (23°C) two innovative ultra-specific, ultra-sensitive thrombin generation assays [12] were performed in duplicate: the RECA-10 (recalcified coagulation activity assay with 10 min coagulation reaction time (CRT) which detects spurious alterations of intrinsic phase of coagulation) and the EXCA (extrinsic coagulation activity assay). The tests are standardized with 1 IU/ml bovine thrombin in 6.7 % human albumin (DadeBehring, Marburg, Germany) that replaced the plasma samples. Thrombin generation = thrombin activity in the generation assay at a certain CRT minus basal thrombin activity in citrated plasma at 0 min CRT (about 6-10 mIU/ml). If 5 % human albumin instead of plasma was supplemented in duplicate with F Xa, 100 mIU/ml F Xa behaved in the present assay conditions with supra-molar concentrations of arginine in the thrombin detection phase as < 9 mIU/ml thrombin.

20 µl samples of unfrozen pooled normal plasma (from 7 samples that remained after routine analysis, about 4h old, stored at 23°C) were supplemented with 0-33.25 mIU/ml bovine thrombin or human thrombin (Stago, Asnières, France) on U-well plates. Immediately thereafter the thrombin generation assays recalcified coagulation activity assay with 10 min coagulation reaction time (RECA-10), which ultra-sensitively reflects intrinsic coagulation, or the extrinsic coagulation activity assay with 1 min coagulation reaction time (EXCA-1) were performed in duplicate as follows:

RECA

2 µl RECA-trigger (250 mM $CaCl_2$ in 1 ml aliquots in siliconized glass vials, frozen at -30°C and thawed directly for the assay) were added. The plates were intensely shaken for 5s and incubated at 37°C in a digitally controlled water-bath. After 0-40 min coagulation

reaction time (CRT) 50 µl arginine-reagent (2.5 M arginine, pH 8.7, 0.16 % Triton X 100® (both from Sigma, Deisenhofen, Germany) were added. 3 minutes (23°C) after the last CRT period 25 µl 1 mM chromogenic thrombin substrate HD-CHG-Ala-Arg-pNA (Pentapharm, Basel, Switzerland) in 1.25 M arginine, pH 8.7, were added. The increase in absorbance at 405 nm with time ΔA/t was determined by a microtiter plate photometer with a 1 mA resolution (Milenia; DPC, Los Angeles, USA). The maximal ΔA with these assay volumes in U-wells plates was about 1050 mA, 40 % of the maximal ΔA = about 420 mA, that is the upper limit of linear range of the assay without significant substrate exhaustion.

EXCA

2 µl EXCA-trigger were added. The EXCA trigger consisted in 1 ml aliquots of 1 ng/ml human placental tissue factor (Polybrene®-free Thromborel-S ®; DadeBehring) 250 mM $CaCl_2$ in siliconized glass vials, frozen at -30°C and thawed for the assay. The plates were intensely shaken for 5s and incubated at 37°C in a digitally controlled water-bath. After 1 min coagulation reaction time (EXCA-1) 50 µl arginine-reagent (2.5 M arginine, pH 8.7, 0.16 % Triton X 100® were added. After 3 minutes (23°C) 25 µl 1 mM HD-CHG-Ala-Arg-pNA in 1.25 M arginine, pH 8.7, were added. ΔA/t was determined by a microtiter plate photometer with a 1 mA resolution.

Fresh Pooled Unfrozen Normal Plasma

20 µl samples of fresh unfrozen pooled normal plasma (from 7 samples that remained after routine analysis, only about 2h old at moment of analysis, stored at 23°C) were supplemented with 0-16.6 mIU/ml bovine thrombin or 0-16.6 mIU/ml human thrombin on U-well plates. Immediately thereafter the thrombin generation assays RECA-10 or EXCA-1 were performed as described above.

Pooled Unfrozen Plasma from Patients on Coumarin

50 µl samples of unfrozen pooled plasma (from 7 patients on Marcumar® (phenprocoumon), the samples remained after routine analysis, were about 4h old, stored at 23°C; INR=1.8) were supplemented with 0-53 mIU/ml bovine factor Xa on U-well plates. Immediately there after the RECA-10 was performed, using 100 µl arginine-reagent and 25 µl substrate-reagent. The 1 IU/ml thrombin standard generated a ΔA at 405 nm of about 20 mA/min (23°C). A negative control was unfrozen pooled plasma from 7 unselected patients with normal prothrombin time (PT), normal activated partial thromboplastin time (APTT), and normal fibrinogen concentration; this pool was supplemented with 1 IU/ml unfractionated heparin (ratiopharm, Ulm, Germany).

Results and Discussion

Figure 1 demonstrates that about 0.02 IU/ml bovine factor Xa approximately doubled the RECA-10 value of pooled unfrozen normal plasma, generating additional 0.2 IU/ml thrombin.

Of major importance are the CRT periods that belong to the ascending part of the thrombin generation curve, i.e. CRT periods ≤ 20 min (Figure 1b), because there is still no marked negative influence of nascending fibrin (= antithrombin I [13]) on thrombin.

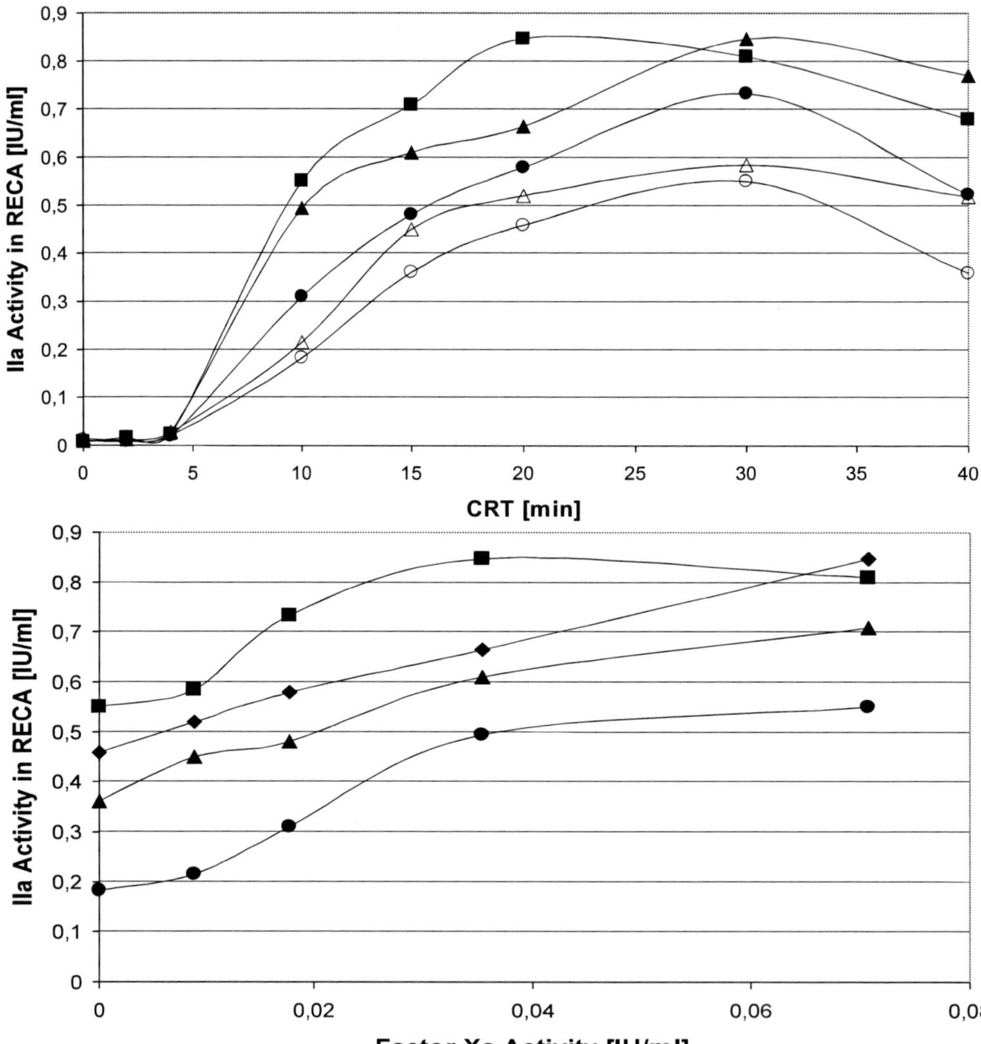

Figure 1. Thrombin generation triggered by factor Xa. Unfrozen pooled normal citrated plasma was supplemented with 0-0.071 IU/ml bovine factor Xa in a polystyrol U-well microtiter plate. After 30 min (23°C) the recalcified coagulation activity assay (RECA) was performed with a coagulation reaction time (CRT) of 0-40 min (37°C); Figure 1a: 0 IU/ml (O), 0.009 IU/ml (Δ), 0.018 IU/ml (●), 0.036 IU/ml (▲), 0.071 IU/ml (■) factor Xa. Figure 1b: CRT periods of 10 min (●), 15 min (▲), 20 min (♦), or 30 min (■).

If a similar experiment was performed with immediate recalcification after factor Xa supplementation of plasma, the approximate 200 % effective dose (ED200) was about 0.01 IU/ml F Xa in the RECA-10 (Figure 2).

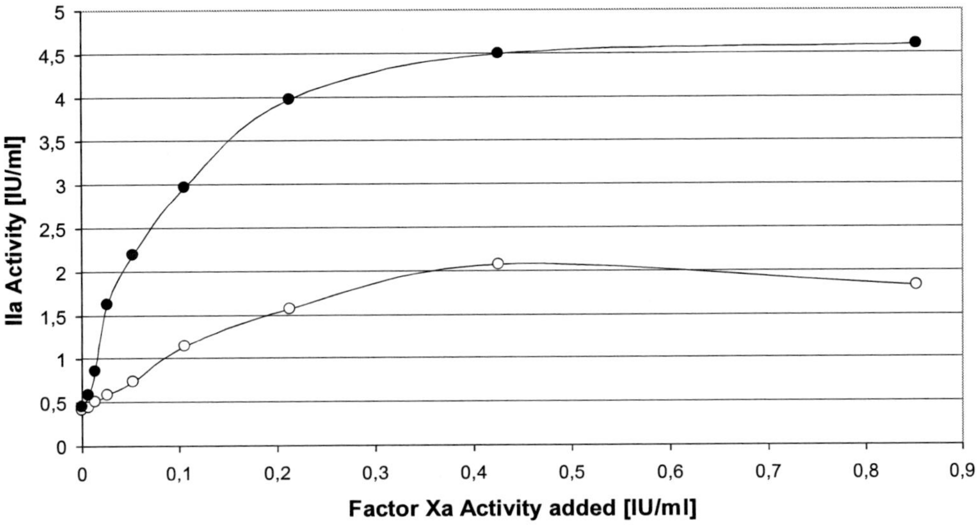

Figure 2. Thrombin generation triggered by factor Xa. Unfrozen pooled normal plasma was supplemented with 0-0.852 IU/ml bovine factor Xa on U-well plates. Immediately thereafter the thrombin generation assays recalcified coagulation activity assay with 10 min coagulation reaction time (RECA-10; •) or extrinsic coagulation activity assay with 1 min coagulation reaction time (EXCA-1; O) were performed.

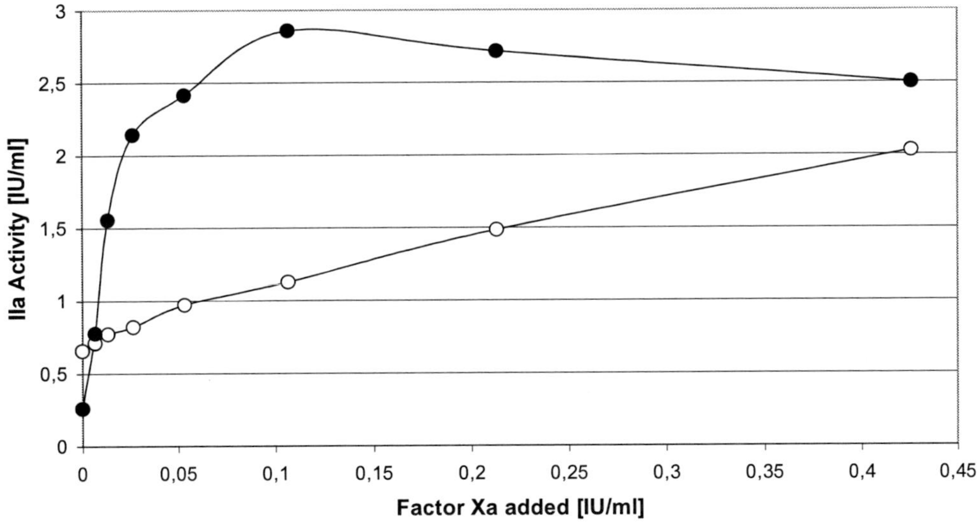

Figure 3. Thrombin generation triggered by factor Xa. 20 μl samples of fresh unfrozen pooled normal plasma were supplemented with 0-0.426 IU/ml factor Xa on U-well plates. Immediately thereafter the recalcified coagulation activity assay with 10 min coagulation reaction time (RECA-10; •) or the extrinsic coagulation activity assay with 1 min coagulation reaction time (EXCA-1; O) were performed.

The approximate ED200 was about 0.08 IU/ml F Xa in the EXCA-1 (Figure 2). With a fresh plasma-pool the approximate ED200 was about 0.005 IU/ml F Xa in the RECA-10, the approximate ED200 in the EXCA-1 was about 0.08 IU/ml (Figure 3).

The ED200 of F Xa added to pooled plasma from patients on coumarin was about 0.008 IU/ml added F Xa (Figure 4), when tested in the 50 µl sample version. To obtain in pooled coumarin-plasma a thrombin generation that is about 1/3 (33.3 %) of the normal RECA value (100 % normal RECA-10 = about 400 mA) about 0.028 IU/ml factor Xa have to be added (Figure 4). The plasma pool that had been supplemented with 1 IU/ml unfractionated heparin did not generate additional thrombin during the RECA-10.

Thus, addition of approximately 10 mIU/ml factor Xa to pooled normal plasma doubles the RECA-10 value, which means that about 10 mIU/ml F Xa induce the additional generation of about 200-400 mIU/ml thrombin in RECA-10. This is a 20-40fold augmentation of the mIU F Xa when compared with mIU thrombin. A similar 20fold augmentation could be observed for pooled plasma of patients on coumarin, when test in RECA-10. The present data support the concept to develop highly efficient and close-to physiological factor Xa inhibitors [14-18] and will augment the understanding of individual normal or pathologic generations [19] of plasmatic thrombin.

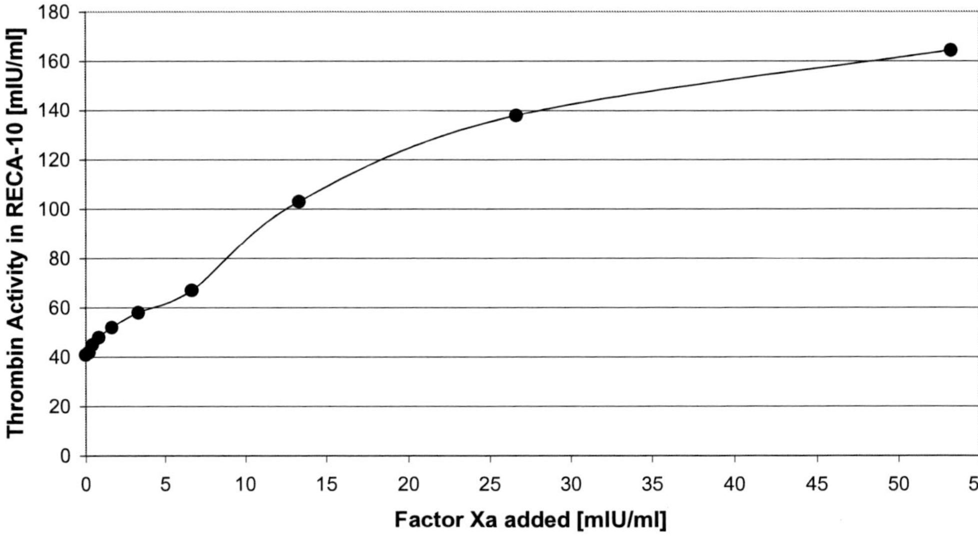

Figure 4. Pooled plasma of patients on coumarin. 50 µl samples of unfrozen pooled plasma from patients on coumarin (INR of the plasma-pool =1.8) were supplemented with bovine factor Xa on U-well plates. Immediately there after the RECA-10 was performed, using 100 µl arginine-reagent and 25 µl substrate-reagent. The approximate ED200 was about 8 mIU/ml added factor Xa (this citrated plasma pool contained basally about 7 mIU/ml thrombin).

References

[1] Arnout J, Hoylaerts MF, Lijnen HR. Haemostasis. *Handb. Exp. Pharmacol.* 2006; (176 Pt 2): 1-41.

[2] Stassen JM, Arnout J, Deckmyn H. The hemostatic system. *Curr. Med. Chem.* 2004; 11: 2245-60.

[3] Gray E, Mulloy B, Barrowcliffe TW. Heparin and low-molecular-weight heparin. *Thromb Haemost.* 2008; 99: 807-18.

[4] Jeske WP, Walenga JM, Hoppensteadt DA, Vandenberg C, Brubaker A, Adiguzel C, Bakhos M, Fareed J. Differentiating low-molecular-weight heparins based on chemical, biological, and pharmacologic properties: implications for the development of generic versions of low-molecular-weight heparins. *Semin. Thromb Hemost.* 2008; 34: 74-85.

[5] Harenberg J, Wehling M. Current and future prospects for anticoagulant therapy: inhibitors of factor Xa and factor IIa. *Semin. Thromb Hemost.* 2008; 34: 39-57.

[6] Klauss V, Spannagl M. Thrombin inhibitors and anti-factor Xa agents in the treatment of arterial occlusion. Curr Drug Targets 2006; 7: 1285-90.

[7] Wiles N, Hunt BJ. Anticoagulation via anti-Factor Xa inhibition. *Lupus* 2006; 15: 167-71.

[8] Bauer KA. New anticoagulants: anti IIa vs anti Xa -- is one better? *J. Thromb Thrombolysis* 2006; 21: 67-72.

[9] Alexander JH, Singh KP. Inhibition of factor Xa : a potential target for the development of new anticoagulants. *Am. J. Cardiovasc. Drugs* 2005; 5: 279-90.

[10] Alban S. From heparins to factor Xa inhibitors and beyond. *Eur. J. Clin. Invest* 2005; 35 Suppl 1:12-20.

[11] Steen M. Factor Va-factor Xa interactions: molecular sites involved in enzyme: cofactor assembly. *Scand. J. Clin. Lab. Invest Suppl.* 2002; 237: 5-11.

[12] Stief TW. Innovative tests of plasmatic hemostasis. *Laboratory Medicine* 2008; 39: 225-30.

[13] Mosesson MW. Update on antithrombin I (fibrin). *Thromb Haemost.* 2007; 98: 105-8.

[14] McCann CJ, Menown IB. New anticoagulant strategies in ST elevation myocardial infarction: trials and clinical implications. *Vasc Health Risk Manag.* 2008; 4: 305-13.

[15] Verheugt FW. Long-term anticoagulation in patients with coronary disease, and future developments. *Curr. Opin. Cardiol.* 2008; 23: 315-9.

[16] Walenga JM, Jeske WP, Hoppensteadt D, Fareed J. Factor Xa inhibitors. *Methods Mol. Med.* 2004; 93: 95-117.

[17] Fareed J, Hoppensteadt D, Walenga J, Iqbal O, Ma Q, Jeske W, Sheikh T. Pharmacodynamic and pharmacokinetic properties of enoxaparin: implications for clinical practice. *Clin. Pharmacokinet* 2003; 42: 1043-57.

[18] Leadley RJ Jr. Coagulation factor Xa inhibition: biological background and rationale. *Curr. Top Med. Chem.* 2001; 1: 151-9.

[19] Joseph JS, Kini RM. Snake venom prothrombin activators similar to blood coagulation factor Xa. *Curr. Drug. Targets Cardiovasc Haematol. Disord.* 2004; 4: 397-416.

In: Hemostasis Laboratory Yearbook, Volume 2
Editor: Thomas W. Stief, pp. 257-265
ISBN: 978-1-60741-089-8

FREE (ACTIVE) ENDOTOXIN PROPORTION IN SUPPLEMENTED NORMAL PLASMA

Thomas W. Stief*
Department of Clinical Chemistry,
University Hospital Giessen and Marburg, Germany

ABSTRACT

Endotoxin (here clinically understood as lipopolysaccharide (LPS) or ß-glucan) that is not neutralized by plasma proteins is of toxicologic and of pathophysiologic importance. The aim of the present study was to find out the approximate proportion of free endotoxin in relation to the total amount of endotoxin when LPS or ß-glucan are supplemented to pooled normal citrated plasma.

5 % human albumin (HA) or pooled normal citrated plasma supplemented with additional 0-95 µg/ml zymosan A (ZyA) or additional 0-1000 ng/ml LPS were incubated for 10 min at 37°C. 10 µl 60 mM chloramine-T® in 50 mM sodium citrate, pH 7.8, were added to 10 µl endotoxin-sample in half area microwells and incubated for 10 min (37°C). Then 10 µl 230 mM methionine were added. After 3 min (23°C) 30 µl *Limulus* reagent Coamatic®Chromo-LAL were added. The specific increase in absorbance (ΔA) was determined as ΔA at 405 nm minus ΔA at 450 nm after 0-210 min incubation time (37°C).

If the oxidative *Limulus* assay is performed with plasma instead of human albumin, the LPS activity in plasma is far lower than its activity in 5 % human albumin: only about 0.1 % of added LPS is active, about 99.9 % of added LPS is inactive, presumably because LPS is bound to strong plasmatic LPS inhibitors such as immunoglobulins that neutralize LPS. The reactivity of ZyA in plasma is nearly identical to that of ZyA in 5 % HA. The reactivity of LPS that enters plasma at total concentrations between 1 and 10 ng/ml is of major clinical importance. Plasmatic LPS reactivities > 200 % of normal are the threshold for PDIC. Therefore, for the purpose of clinical endotoxin analysis of patient blood with singlet oxygen treated plasmas the Pyrochrome® reagent should be used that is at least 10fold more sensitive than the Coamatic® reagent.

Keywords: Endotoxin, lipopolysaccharide, ß-glucan, zymosan A, Limulus, singlet oxygen.

---

* Correspondence to:_PD Dr. med. T. Stief, Department of Clinical Chemistry, University Hospital, D-35043 Marburg, Germany. E-mail: thstief@med.uni-marburg.de; Tel. : +49-6421-58 64471; FAX: +49-6421-58 65594

INTRODUCTION

Endotoxin is toxic for the human organism [1]. Endotoxin can be clinically understood as lipopolysaccharide (LPS) from gram-negative bacteria or as ß-glucan from fungi. That plasmatic endotoxin molecules that are not neutralized by binding to inhibitory plasma proteins such as the immunoglobulins [2-13] are the toxicologically and pathophysiologically important endotoxin molecules. This is free = unbound = active endotoxin. The aim of the present study was to find out the approximate proportion of free endotoxin in relation to the total amount of endotoxin when LPS or ß-glucan are supplemented to pooled normal citrated plasma.

MATERIAL AND METHODS

LPS was from *Escherichia coli* 055:B5 (Sigma, Deisenhofen, Germany; article nr. L2637-5MG; purified by gel filtration), 5 mg/ml were stabilized by 5 % human albumin (Kabi, Stockholm, Sweden). Zymosan A was from *Saccharomyces cerevisiae* (protein-carbohydrate complexes from yeast cell wall; Sigma; article nr. Z4250-1G).

Supplementation of Human Albumin or of Pooled Normal Citrated Plasma with Endotoxin

198 µl samples of pooled normal citrated plasma (0.5 ml 106 mM sodium citrate + 4.5 ml venous blood) from 24 normal donors that remained after routine analysis, aliquoted in 250 µl samples and stored frozen at -30°C till the experiment, 198 µl samples of unfrozen pooled normal citrated plasma, or 198 µl samples of 5 % human albumin (HA; Humalbin®; Behring, Marburg, Germany) were supplemented in 0.5 ml polypropylene tubes with 2 µl

- 0 ng/ml LPS = 5 % HA
- 100 ng/ml LPS in 5 % HA
- 1 000 ng/ml LPS in 5 % HA
- 10 000 ng/ml LPS in 5 % HA
- 100 000 ng/ml LPS in 5 % HA
- 10 µg/ml ZyA in 5 % HA
- 100 µg/ml ZyA in 5 % HA
- 1 000 µg/ml ZyA in 5 % HA

or with 10 µl 2 000 µg/ml ZyA in 5 % HA resulting in respective final additional concentrations of

- 0 ng/ml LPS
- 1 ng/ml LPS
- 10 ng/ml LPS
- 100 ng/ml LPS
- 1000 ng/ml LPS

- 0.1 µg/ml ZyA
- 1 µg/ml ZyA
- 10 µg/ml ZyA
- 95 µg/ml ZyA

either in pooled normal plasma or in 5 % HA. The samples were incubated for 10 min at 37°C. Then the nonradicalic oxidative *Limulus* assay was performed that in contrast to heat mediated denaturation of plasmatic serine protease inhibitors [14] works with relatively gentle singlet oxygen treatment of the plasma samples at physiological pH that does not result in a loss of free LPS and that does not liberate neutralized LPS [15]: 10 µl of these supplemented samples were incubated in triplicate with 10 µl 60 mM chloramine-T® (Sigma) in 50 mM sodium citrate, pH 7.8, in glue-film-covered polystyrol half area microwells (Greiner, Frickenhausen, Germany; article nr. 675161) for 10 min at 37°C in a sterile incubator. Then 10 µl 230 mM methionine (Sigma) were added. After 3 min (23°C) 30 µl *Limulus*-reagent COAMATIC® Chromo-LAL (Cape Cod, Falmouth, USA; Chromogenix article nr. 82 28 90; kit nr. CX03020; lot nr. 337028) were added; the co-lyophilizate between the Limulus factors C, B, G, A and the chromogenic substrate S-2834 (Ac-Ile-Glu-Gly-Lys-pNA) at pH 7 had been freshly reconstituted with 3.2 ml H_2O. The covered microtiter plate was incubated at 37°C (sterile incubator) and the specific increase in absorbance (ΔA) was determined as ΔA at 405 nm minus ΔA at 450 nm after 0-210 min incubation time. Of particular interest might be the time needed to increase the absorbance of the reaction mixture by 200 mA, that is specific for the respective added endotoxin. 5 % HA supplemented with 0.1 ng/ml or 0.01 ng/ml LPS was additionly assayed to determine this time point at nearly no substrate exhaustion. The present 5 % HA preparation contained basally about 0.1 µg/ml ZyA.

Different Concentrations of the *Limulus* Reagent

198 µl pooled normal citrated plasma (once frozen/thawed) were supplemented with 2 µl 0, 1000, or 10000 ng/ml LPS in 5 % HA, resulting in final additional plasmatic LPS concentrations of 0, 10, or 100 ng/ml. 198 µl 5 % HA were supplemented with 2 µl 100 ng/ml LPS in 5 % HA that was repetitively diluted 1:10 with 5 % HA to obtain final additional LPS concentrations of 0, 1, 10, 100, 1000 pg/ml in 5 % HA. The samples were incubated for 10 min (37°C; sterile incubator).

10 µl of these samples were incubated in triplicate for 10 min (37°C; sterile incubator) with 10 µl 60 mM chloramine-T®, 50 mM sodium citrate pH 7.8 in half area microwells. Then 10 µl 230 mM methionine were added. After 3 min (23°C) 30 µl *Limulus* reagent (Coamatic®-Chromo LAL) 3fold concentrated, 2fold concentrated, or 1fold concentrated were added (therefore the lyophilized *Limulus* reagent had been reconstituted with 1067 µl H_2O instead of the usual 3200 µl, resulting in a 3fold concentrated *Limulus* reagent; this 3fold concentrated *Limulus* reagent was diluted with H_2O to obtain a 2fold and a 1fold concentrated *Limulus* reagent directly prior to the addition of the *Limulus* reagent to the microwells). The microwells were incubated at 37°C (sterile incubator) and ΔA at 405 nm minus ΔA at 450 nm was determined.

The maximal ΔA values for 1fold concentrated *Limulus* reagent were about 1100 mA (45 % = 495 mA), for 2fold concentrated *Limulus* reagent about 2200 mA (45 % = 990 mA), and for 3fold concentrated *Limulus* reagent about 3300 mA (45 % = 1485 mA). At 3h (37°C) *Limulus* reaction time the ΔA values for unsupplemented plasma were for all types of *Limulus* reagent about 40 mA; for unsupplemented 5 % human albumin the ΔA values were about 200 mA for 1fold concentrated *Limulus* reagent and about 100 mA for 2fold or 3fold concentrated *Limulus* reagent.

Results and Discussion

Figure 1a demonstrates the *Limulus* reaction kinetic of pure LPS or pure ß-glucan in 5 % human albumin. The strongly hyperbolic nature of this kinetic is typical for LPS, the *Limulus* kinetic of ß-glucan is only slightly hyperbolic. This is due to the complex enzymatic cascade of the *Limulus* factors C, B, and A for LPS and due to the relatively simple enzymatic cascade consisting only of *Limulus* factors G and A for ß-glucan. Figures 1b and 1c are log-log plots that compare the concentration of endotoxin in 5 % HA with the time needed to increase the absorbance of the reaction mixture by 200 mA. 200 mA is far below the critical value of 45 % of the maximal ΔA, which is 560 mA: only ΔA values < 560 mA are valid, because up to this value there is nearly no substrate exhaustion. Lin-lin plots (LPS concentration versus ΔA, e.g. with Pyrochrome® reagent [15,18]) are more sensible to lowest reactivities of LPS (free LPS at about 0.1-1 pg/ml) than log-log plots (LPS concentration versus time of reaction onset, e.g. with Coamatic® reagent).

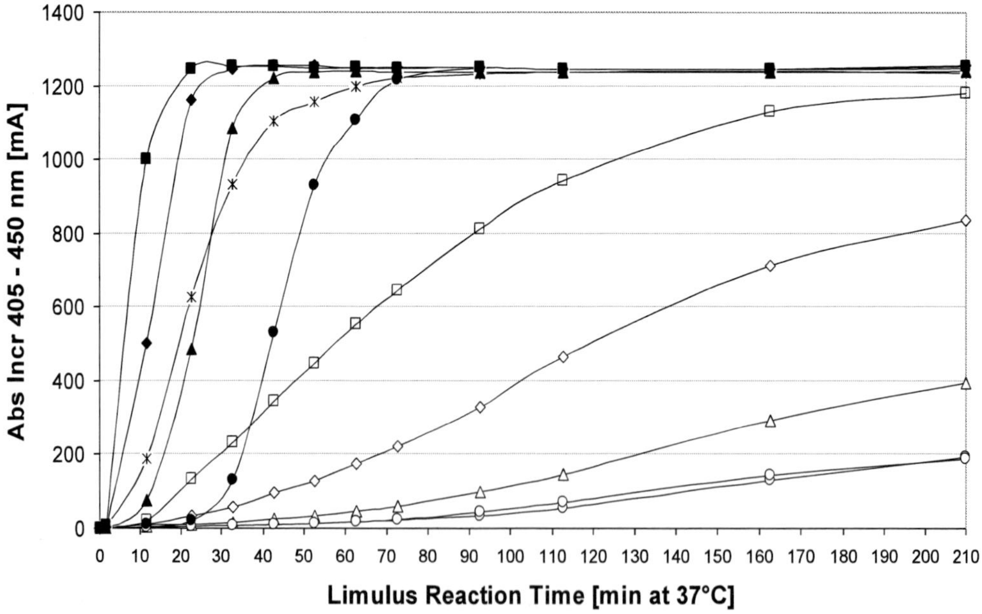

Figure 1. (Continued)

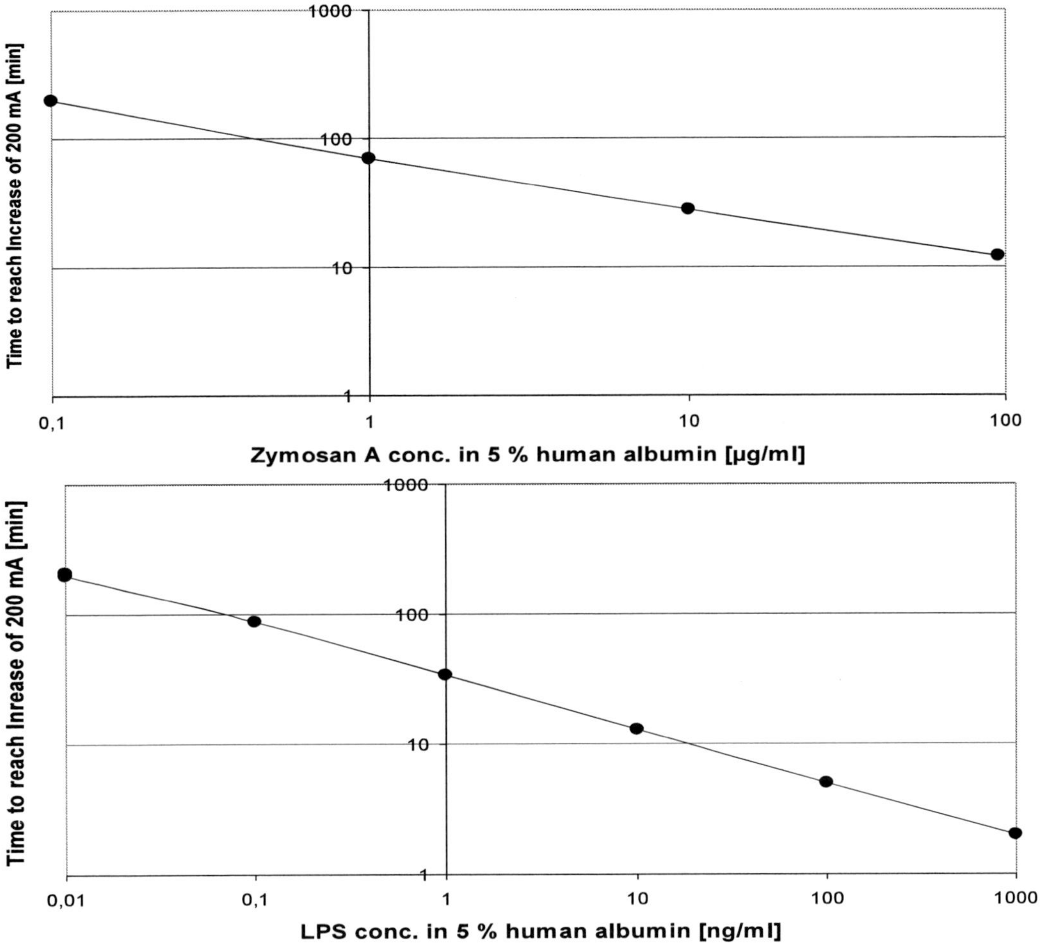

Figure 1. Endotoxin activity in supplemented 5 % human albumin. 5 % human albumin (HA) supplemented with additional 0.1 µg/ml (Δ), 1 µg/ml (◊), 10 µg/ml (Q), 95 µg/ml (*) zymosan A, 1 ng/ml (●), 10 ng/ml (▲), 100 ng/ml (♦), 1000 ng/ml (■) lipopolysaccharide (LPS), or not additionally supplemented (O) were incubated for 10 min at 37°C. 10 µl 60 mM chloramine-T® in 50 mM sodium citrate, pH 7.8, were added to 10 µl endotoxin-sample in half area microwells and incubated for 10 min (37°C). Then 10 µl 230 mM methionine were added. After 3 min (23°C) 30 µl Limulus-reagent Coamatic® Chromo-LAL were added. The specific increase in absorbance (ΔA) was determined as ΔA at 405 nm minus ΔA at 450 nm after 0-210 min incubation time (37°C) (Figure 1a). Figs. 1b,c demonstrate the time needed to increase the absorbance of the reaction mixture by 200 mA, that is specific for the respective added endotoxin.

If the oxidative *Limulus* assay is performed with plasma (Figure 2) instead of human albumin (Figure 1a), the activity of LPS in plasma is far lower than its activity in 5 % human albumin: only about 0.1 % of added 100 ng/ml or 1000 ng/ml LPS are active, about 99.9 % of added LPS are inactive, presumably because LPS is bound to strong plasmatic LPS inhibitors such as immunoglobulins that neutralize LPS. The present *Limulus* reagent Coamatic® is not sensitive to total plasmatic LPS concentrations below 10-100 ng/ml, which would be in the very low pg/ml range of free LPS. Especially this reactivity range is of major importance since pooled normal human plasma contains about 1 ng/ml LPS in total (100 % of normal = 0.8 ng/ml LPS reactivity, 1 standard deviation = 25 % of normal).

Plasmatic LPS reactivities > 200 % of normal are the threshold for PDIC. Therefore, for the purpose of clinical analysis of patient plasmas the Pyrochrome® reagent should be used because its sensitivity is at least 10fold better [16-18].

When compared with LPS, the ß-glucan zymosan A is only minimally inhibited in plasma: the reactivity of zymosan A in plasma is nearly identical to that in 5 % HA (Figure 2).

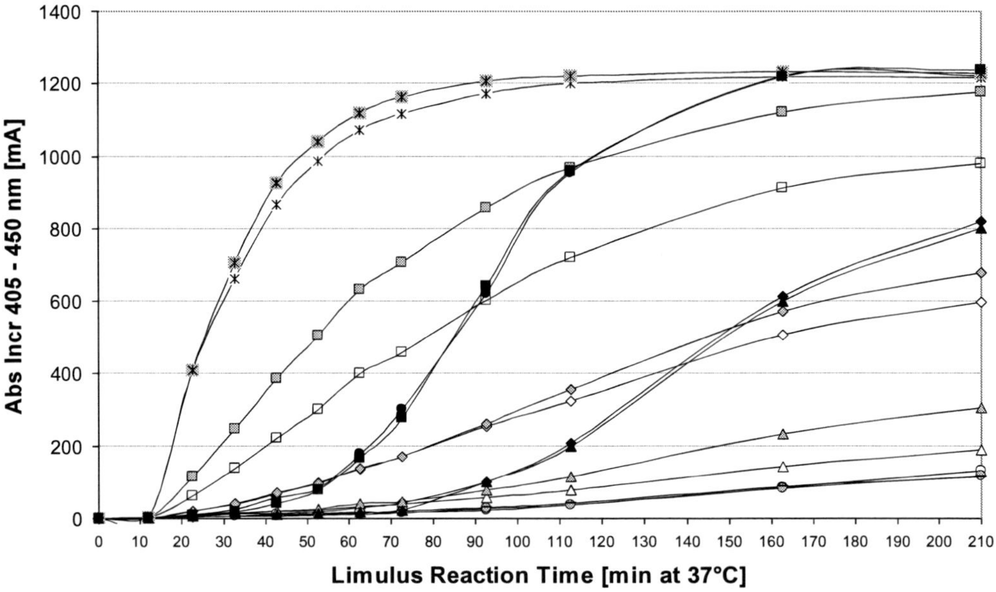

Figure 2. Endotoxin activity in supplemented pooled normal citrated plasma. Pooled normal citrated plasma that was unfrozen (white symbols or * for zymosan A; -, ▲, or ● for LPS) or that was once frozen/thawed (grey symbols or grey * for zymosan A; _, ♦, or ■ for LPS) was supplemented with additional 0 µg/ml (circels), 0.1 µg/ml (triangles), 1 µg/ml (diamonds), 10 µg/ml (squares), 95 µg/ml asteriscs) zymosan A, with additional 0 ng/ml (-,_) 100 ng/ml (▲, ♦), or 1000 ng/ml (●, ■) LPS were incubated for 10 min at 37°C. Then 10 µl of these endotoxin-samples were assayed for endotoxin activity as described in Figure 1.

It should be noted that the *Limulus* reaction depends not only on the type of *Limulus* reagent but also on the final assay concentration of proteins, e.g. albumin can inhibit or stabilize the *Limulus* reaction for endotoxin: up to about 1 % human albumin in the sample may inhibit the *Limulus* cascade reaction up to about 80 %, human albumin concentrations ≥ 2 % in the sample may stabilize the *Limulus* cascade resulting into a generation of activated *Limulus* factor A that is similar to samples without protein.

The sensitivity of the Coamatic® reagent can be increased about 10fold, if the lyophilized reagent is reconstituted with 1.6 ml H_2O instead of the usual 3.2 ml H_2O, i.e. if it is 2fold concentrated (Figure 3a,b); then the reactivity of 10 ng/ml LPS added to normal plasma can be measured: it behaves as about 5 pg/ml LPS (about 0.05 % of 10 ng/ml) in 5 % albumin. 100 ng/ml LPS in plasma behave as about 50 pg/ml LPS (about 0.05 % of 100 ng/ml) in 5 % albumin, when specifically analyzed at a reaction time of 120 min at 37°C (Figure 3b).

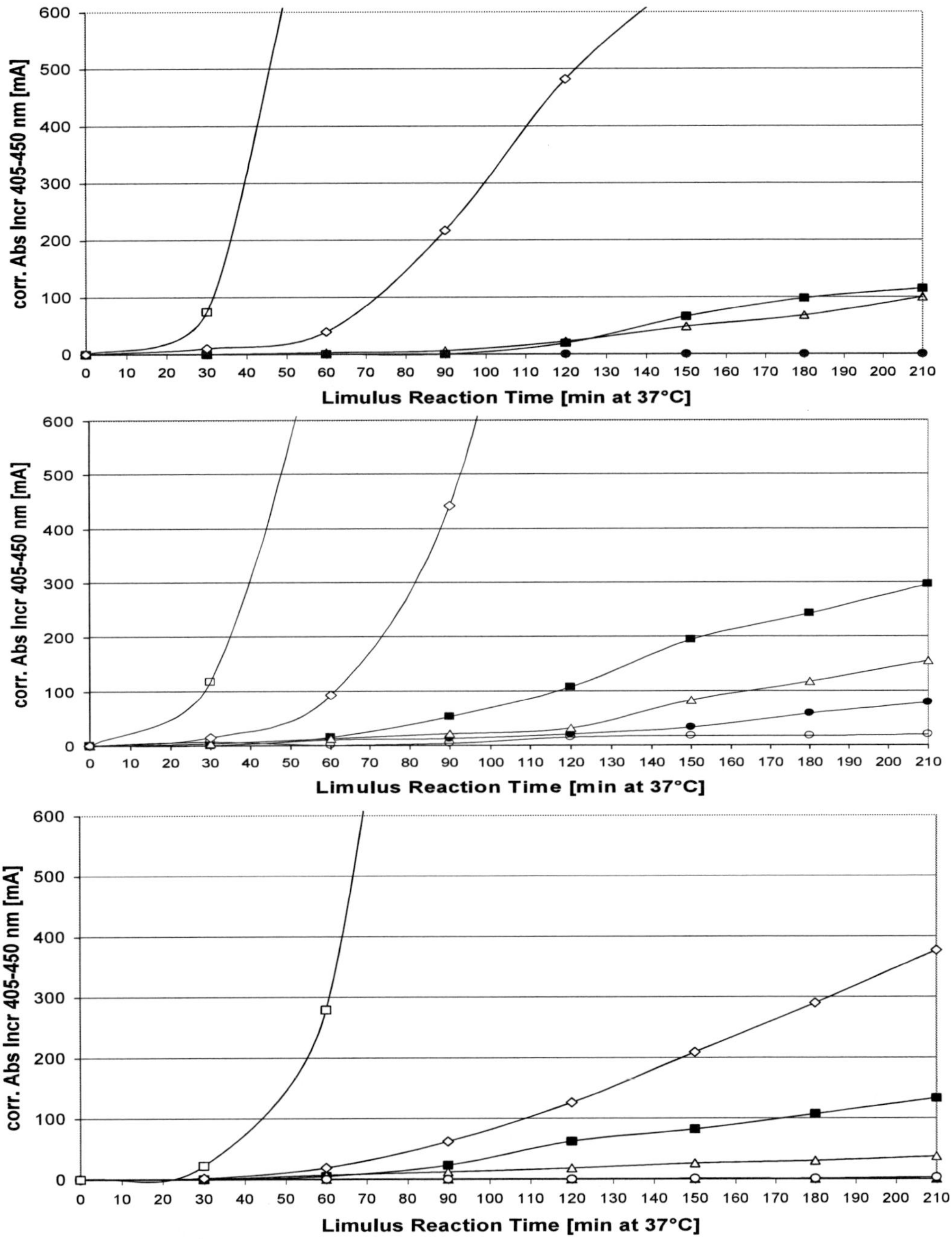

Figure 3. Different concentrations of the *Limulus* reagent. Pooled normal citrated plasma (once frozen/thawed) was supplemented with 0, 10 (●), or 100 (■) ng/ml LPS. 5 % human albumin was supplemented with 0, 1 (○), 10 (Δ), 100 (◊), 1000 (□) pg/ml LPS. After incubation for 10 min at 37°C 10 μl of these samples were incubated for 10 min (37°C) with 10 μl 60 mM chloramine-T®, 50 mM sodium citrate pH 7.8 in half area microwells. Then 10 μl 230 mM methionine were added. After 3 min (23°C) 30 μl *Limulus* reagent Coamatic® 1fold concentrated (Figure 3a), 2fold concentrated (Figure 3b), or 3fold concentrated (Figure 3c) were added. The microwells were incubated at 37°C and the corrected (corr.) values for ΔA at 405 nm minus ΔA at 450 nm were determined by subtracting ΔA of the unsupplemented plasma sample or of the 5 % albumin sample from the respective ΔA values of the supplemented samples.

If a 3fold concentrated *Limulus* reagent is used, the kinetic of the assay is slowed down (Figure 3c), presumably due to high final concentrations of Mg^{++} (the usual 1fold concentrated *Limulus* reagent contains about 50 mM Mg^{++} ions). Mg^{++} at final assay concentrations > 50 mM inhibits cascades of serine proteases [19].

In conclusion, the *Limulus* test for singlet-oxygen oxidated plasma is a powerful tool to determine the reactivity of endotoxins in human plasma. However, the *Limulus* reagent should contain sufficient concentrations of the factors C, B, G, A that allow reactivity determinations with a detection limit of about 0.1 ng/ml LPS in plasma which corresponds to free LPS in the range of about 0.1 pg/ml.

REFERENCES

[1] Stief TW. Coagulation Activation by Lipopolysaccharides. *Clin. Appl. Thromb Hemost.* 2007 Dec 26 [Epub ahead of print]

[2] Teng NN, Kaplan HS, Hebert JM, Moore C, Douglas H, Wunderlich A, Braude AI. Protection against gram-negative bacteremia and endotoxemia with human monoclonal IgM antibodies. *Proc. Natl. Acad. Sci. USA* 1985; 82: 1790-4.

[3] Bennett-Guerrero E, Barclay GR, Weng PL, Bodian CA, Feierman DE, Vela-Cantos F, Mythen MG. Endotoxin-neutralizing capacity of serum from cardiac surgical patients. *J. Cardiothorac. Vasc. Anesth.* 2001; 15: 451-4.

[4] Hellman J, Warren HS. Antiendotoxin strategies. *Infect Dis. Clin. North Am.* 1999; 13: 371-86.

[5] Peterson EM, de la Maza LM, Brade L, Brade H. Characterization of a neutralizing monoclonal antibody directed at the lipopolysaccharide of Chlamydia pneumoniae. *Infect. Immun.* 1998; 66: 3848-55.

[6] Wisniewski MA, Kazemi M, Fang IS, Knight LS, Huntenburg CC, Bubbers JE, Schneidkraut MJ. Comparison of binding specificity and the function of two human IgM anti-lipid A monoclonal antibodies. *Circ. Shock* 1994; 44: 230-7.

[7] Fang IS, Wisniewski MA, Huntenburg CC, Knight LS, Bubbers JE, Schneidkraut MJ. Inhibition of lipopolysaccharide-associated endotoxin activities in vitro and in vivo by the human anti-lipid A monoclonal antibody SdJ5-1.17.15. *Infect Immun.* 1993; 61: 3873-8.

[8] Di Padova FE, Brade H, Barclay GR, Poxton IR, Liehl E, Schuetze E, Kocher HP, Ramsay G, Schreier MH, McClelland DB, et al. A broadly cross-protective monoclonal antibody binding to Escherichia coli and Salmonella lipopolysaccharides. *Infect Immun.* 1993; 61: 3863-72.

[9] Corriveau CC, Danner RL. Antiendotoxin therapies for septic shock. *Infect Agents Dis.* 1993 ; 2: 44-52.

[10] Warren HS, Amato SF, Fitting C, Black KM, Loiselle PM, Pasternack MS, Cavaillon JM. Assessment of ability of murine and human anti-lipid A monoclonal antibodies to bind and neutralize lipopolysaccharide. *J. Exp. Med.* 1993; 177: 89-97.

[11] Mashimo J, Mizutani T, Mita A, Kasai N. Neutralization of Shwartzman-inducing activity by antibodies recognizing the Re core or lipid A structures of

lipopolysaccharide from Salmonella minnesota R595 and Pseudomonas vesicularis JCM1477. *Microbiol. Immunol.* 1991; 35: 423-34.

[12] Ward DC, Michalek SM, McGhee JR. Monoclonal antibodies to salmonella lipopolysaccharide: functional analysis of anti-lipid A antibodies. *Clin. Exp. Immunol.* 1988 ; 72: 157-63.

[13] Warren HS, Novitsky TJ, Bucklin A, Kania SA, Siber GR. Endotoxin neutralization with rabbit antisera to Escherichia coli J5 and other gram-negative bacteria. *Infect Immun.* 1987 ; 55: 1668-73.

[14] Obata T, Nomura M, Kase Y, Sasaki H, Shirasawa Y. Early detection of the Limulus amebocyte lysate reaction evoked by endotoxins. *Anal. Biochem.* 2008; 373: 281-6.

[15] Stief TW. Determination of active endotoxin in plasma. *Hemostasis Laboratory* 2008; 1: (issue 1 in press).

[16] Stief TW, Ijagha O, Weiste B, Herzum I, Renz H, Max M. Analysis of hemostasis alterations in sepsis. *Blood Coagul Fibrinolysis* 2007 ; 18: 179-86.

[17] Stief TW, Max M. Active endotoxin in sepsis. *Hemostasis Laboratory* 2008; 1: (issue 1 in press).

[18] Stief TW. Arginine linearizes the hyperbolic Limulus kinetic. *Hemostasis Laboratory* 2008; 1: (issue 2 in press).

[19] Stief TW, Richter A, Bünder R, Maisch B, Renz H. Functional determination of plasminogen activator in arginine-stabilized plasma. *Clin. Appl. Thromb. Hemost.* 2005; 11: 311-23.

In: Hemostasis Laboratory Yearbook, Volume 2
Editor: Thomas W. Stief, pp. 267-287
ISBN: 978-1-60741-089-8

NEUTROPHIL GRANULOCYTES IN HEMOSTASIS

Thomas W. Stief[*]
Institute of Clinical Chemistry,
University Hospital Giessen and Marburg,
D-35043 Marburg, Germany

ABSTRACT

This review focuses on the antithrombotic action of activated polymorphonuclear neutrophil granulocytes (PMN). PMN with about 4000 cells/µl are the main leukocyte type in normal human blood. They are the first line of defence against invading bacteria or fungi. About 50 % of all blood PMN are always slightly activated and express adhesion molecules (e.g. CD11b/CD18) that bind endothelial surface proteins (e.g. ICAM-1). PMN roll over the endothelium to patrol for the existence of any pathogen that may stick to the endothelium and that may threaten vessel patency. In this sense also fibrin might be considered as a special type of pathogen. CD11b/CD18 receptors of PMN bind to fibrin and activate the cell. Activated PMN via membrane assembly of NADPH-oxidase (Nox2) generate high concentrations of H_2O_2 that reacts via catalysis of released myeloperoxidase to HOCl. The hypochlorite reacts with amino groups to chloramines, an important biological source of the excited nonradical oxidant singlet molecular oxygen ($^1O_2^*$). $^1O_2^*$ is an inter- and intra- cellular communication signal and a destructive bullet. Light quants (hν, especially those at about 425 nm) may enhance PMN patrolling and may direct and recruit PMN to a pathologic focus, such as a pathologic thrombus. CD11b/CD18 binding induces H_2O_2 generation and viceversa.

$^1O_2^*$ is a selective oxidant. Due to its nonradical nature, $^1O_2^*$ is relatively inoffensive to normal mammalian cells but highly destructive against pathogens. $^1O_2^*$ inactivates important components of hemostasis, such as thrombocytes, fibrinogen, factors V, VIII, X, α2-antiplasmin, and PAI-1 with 50 % inhibitory concentrations of 1-2 mM in blood or plasma. It is suggested to imitate the physiologic PMN mediated thrombolysis by intravascular injection of blue photons or of sub-millimolar concentrations of chloramines.

Keywords: Neutrophils, polymorphonuclear granulocytes (PMN), hemostasis, fibrinolysis.

---

[*] Correspondence to: PD Dr. med. T. Stief, Department of Clinical Chemistry, University Hospital, D-35043 Marburg, Germany. email: thstief@med.uni-marburg.de; Tel. : +49-6421-58 64471; FAX: +49-6421-58 65594

INTRODUCTION

Polymorphonuclear neutrophil granulocytes (PMN) with a diameter of about 12-15 µm have a poly-segmented lengthy nucleus, many cytoplasmic granules, large glycogen stores, and a highly convoluted surface [1]. PMN as cells of the innate immune response guarantee the sterility of blood or of alveoli [2-8]. PMN are with about 4000 ± 2000 cells / µl the main leukocyte type in flowing blood. These flowing cells are about 50 % of all blood PMN, the other 50 % of all blood PMN are rolling over the endothelium, i.e. normally 50 % roll and 50 % flow [9]. Flowing PMN are inactive, rolling PMN are slightly activated. Rolling PMN patrol for invading pathogens (e.g. bacteria or fungi) that are attached to the endothelium. Pathogens strongly activate PMN, activated PMN fight against these pathogens [10], the PMN release pro-inflammatory cytokins such as interferon-gamma (IFN-γ) [11], interleukin-1 (IL-1), tumor necrosis factor–alpha (TNF-α), or granulocyte-colony stimulating factor (G-CSF) [1,12-14]. Pathological deposits of fibrin on endothelial cells threatens vessel patency; thus, a pathological thrombus might also be considered as a type of pathogen. The present review focuses on the interaction of PMN with fibrin.

PMN ROLLING AND DIAPEDESIS

The half-life of PMN in the blood circulation is only about 9h [1]. The physiologic PMN rolling over the endothelium is mediated by reversible binding of PMN CD11b/CD18 to endothelial intercellular adhesion molecule (ICAM) - 1 [15,16] or by selectin/selectin receptor interactions, e.g. binding of endothelial selectins to PMN selectin receptors [17-19].

CD11b/CD18 of slightly activated (primed [20]) PMN not only bind ICAM-1 but also fibrin [21,22]. Enhanced CD11b/CD18 binding results in increased cell activation and viceversa [23,24,195,196].

PMN respond to cell activators such as plasmatic lipopolysaccharide (LPS) at about 3-10 ng/ml with enhanced adhesion [1,23]. LPS concentrations > 10-100 ng/ml are toxic for PMN [1,24,25] resulting in defective oxidant production [23]. Thus, there is great clinical need to examine more closely the plasmatic reactivity of endotoxin (free endotoxin) in relation to pathophysiology [23]. The monocytes/macrophages seem to play a much greater role in the pathophysiology of sepsis and pathologic disseminated intravascular coagulation (PDIC) than the PMN [26,153,154]: only about 5 ng/ml LPS added to normal citrated blood induced a destruction of about 20 % of blood monocytes within 60 min (37°C), the monocytes decreased linearly as a function of LPS incubation time; the PMN were resistant to up to 100 ng/ml LPS in blood [154]. Monocyte derived microparticles trigger intrinsic hemostasis.

Glucocorticoids reduce the adhesion of PMN to the endothelial surface [27,35], possibly by downregulation of the expression of CD11b, CD18, or L-selectin (CD62L) [28-31] by decreasing chemotaxis [32,33], or by proteolytic cleavage and release of L-selectin (CD62L) or of CD18 from the surface of the PMN [34]. 1h after injection of 200 IU ACTH there appeared an about 10fold increase in plasmatic corticoid concentration (basal conc. =3 ng/ml); 2h after injection of ACTH the blood PMN (not other blood leukocytes) began to increase, 4h after ACTH injection the PMN count approximately doubled [1].

The nucleus of the PMN is multi-segmented and lengthy. So it allows the PMN to line up its nucleus in a straight line, which is a prerequisite for rapid migration through the endothelium [1]. To reach a pathogenic focus in the interstitium, blood PMN traverse the endothelium [36] without proteolytic destruction; the PMN traverse the basal lamina possibly by proteolysis [37-39]. *In vivo*, PMN mostly penetrate endothelial cells through small openings called "fenestrae" of the cell membrane [36,37,40,41]. These pores of about 50 nm in diameter, whose normal function might be to enable plasma contact with the subendothelial tissue, can widen up to a size of 3-5 µm, if a PMN penetrates the endothelium [36,42]. PMN look for thin regions of the endothelium, which could be opened fenestrae, or zones where the upper and the lower membrane of the endothelial cell are in close contact [36]. During penetration there appears a rearrangement of the cellular cytoskeleton [43]. *In vitro*, PMN might penetrate the endothelium preferably by paracellular lysis of tight junctions [36].

PMN GRANULES

Neutrophils possess four different types of granules that were classified according to the moment they occur in the maturing cell [4]:

1. primary granules
2. secondary granules
3. tertiary granules
4. secretory vesicles.

The primary granules contain myeloperoxidase, proteases (e.g. urokinase, elastase, cathepsins), phospholipases (PLA_2) [44], and polycationic peptides/proteins (e.g. defensins). Myeloperoxidase generates the powerful oxidant HOCl out of H_2O_2 and Cl^-. The proteases degrade peri-cellular proteins. The polycations are toxic for germs, enhance the activity of the proteases [45,46] and activate PMN [4].

The secondary granules are also known as the specific granules; they contain the cytochrome b558 components gp91phox and p22phox, alkaline phosphatase, lactoferrin and gelatinase B (= matrix metalloprotease 9 = MMP9) [4]. Tertiary granules are similar as secondary granules, but they are bigger than primary or secondary ones and contain especially lactoferrin and polycations [1]. The secretory vesicles contain cytochrome b558, alkaline phosphatase, CD16, decay accelerating factor, and albumin as stabilizing protein [47].

The granules are translocated to the plasma membrane (or to the membrane of a phagosome) after assembly of microtubules and remodelling of the actin cytoskeleton [4,48]. In the translocation machinery with a possible GTP-ase switch actin is first polymerized to "mini-steel-ropes" (flexible cytoskeleton [180]), along them the granules are then transported to the plasma membrane, and myosin may act as "mini-motor" [4,47]. Secretory vesicles are first released, followed by the tertiary / secondary granules. The myeloperoxidase containing primary granules are the last ones to be released, i.e. myeloperoxidase is released not until H_2O_2 production has started. The degranulation is regulated by phospholipid mediators (e.g. phosphatidyl-inositol-4,5-diphosphate (PIP_2) [4].

Oxidant Metabolism

PMN generate high concentrations of reactive oxygen species (ROS) by a combined action of membranous NADPH-oxidase and released myeloperoxidase. The main reactive ROS are hydrogen peroxide (H_2O_2), hydroxyl radical (·OH), and excited singlet molecular oxygen ($^1O_2$*). First, the NADPH-oxidase generates H_2O_2 that may break to 2 ·OH, or that may react to HOCl by myeloperoxidase catalysis. HOCl reacts with amino groups to chloramines. Chloramines or HOCl can generate $^1O_2$* by reaction with H_2O_2; $^1O_2$* reacts with C=C bonds to yield excited carbonyls (R-C=O*) that emit at about 425 nm or it reacts with sulphur atoms in methionine or cysteine [85]. The ROS type might be modulated by certain cellular enzymes, cofactors, or reaction conditions [165-167]. ROS at high concentrations act as bullets, at low concentrations they may also act as cell signals. Especially $^1O_2$* might play an important role in inter- and intra- cellular communication. PMN might possess membraneous (opsin-like or chromophore-like [92,207,208]) receptors for singlet oxygen and/or photons, e.g. the chemotactic IL-8 receptor belongs to the rhodopsin-like serpentines that are receptors with 7 transmembrane helices and that are coupled to G-proteins [155]. Retinoids (vitamin A and its derivatives) are involved in a broad range of events of cell maturation, differentiation, and signalling that are up to now not completely understood [157,158,159,161]. Interestingly, all-trans retinoic acid (ATRA) is an important regulator of granulocyte differentiation [49,160]: ATRA up-regulates the expression of CD 11b, CD 11c, CD 15, CD 65, CD 54, CD 38. ATRA establishes complete remissions in acute promyelocytic leukaemia (M_3), a feared hyper-acute form of leukaemia. Especially the pathologic disseminated intravascular coagulation or the primary hyperfibrinolysis, which are frequent complications of M_3, can be avoided by oral ATRA prior to definitive chemotherapy [156,161].

NADPH-Oxidase

Reduced nicotine amide adenine dinucleotide phosphate (NADPH) is the intracellular cofactor of an important PMN weapon: the NADPH-oxidase. NADPH is generated by cellular uptake of glucose [52,53], degradation of cellular glycogen stores, phosphorylation of glucose, and action of the glucose-6-phosphat-dehydrogenase. The NADPH-oxidase is a complex of proteins that are membrane bound or that originally belong to the cytosol of the cell. The cytosolic subunits of the NADPH-oxidase are p67phox, that with its NADPH binding site is of importance for normal oxidase function [54], p47phox [55], the phosphoinositide-binding protein p40phox [47,212], and the regulatory cytoplasmic G-protein Rac (Rac1 or Rac2) [56]. For activation of NADPH-oxidase, p40phox has to be separated from p67phox, p40phox regulates the activity of NADPH-oxidase [57,212].

The membranous subunits of the NADPH-oxidase are gp91phox and p22phox that are the ß-chain and the α-chain, respectively, of cytochrome b558. The abbreviation phox stands for phagocytic oxidase (= NAPH-oxidase 2 = Nox2). 1 molecule of cytochrome b558 binds also 1 molecule of Rap1a, a 22kDa guanosine 5`-triphospate (GTP) – binding protein that is also present in the specific granules [58]. Active phospholipase C mediates Rap1a activation. Rap1a and Rac might be switches of the NADPH-oxidase [59,60].

About 85 % of the cytochrom b558 molecules are within the specific granules or secretory vesicles of an inactive (resting) cell, about 15 % of the flavocytochrome b558 molecules are already located in the plasma membrane [58]. Upon cell activation the active NADPH-oxidase is assembled at the cell membrane by translocation of the membranous NADPH-oxidase subunits and of the cytosolic NADPH-oxidase subunits to the cell membrane (or to the membrane of a phagosome). In inactive (resting) PMN the cytochrome b558 containing granules are randomly distributed all over the interior of the cell (see e.g. Figure 1A of [47]). Upon activation, actin "mini-steel-ropes" are formed by focal polymerization that enable the transport to the plasma membrane (see e.g. Figure 1B of [47]). Finally, the complete NADPH-oxidase is assembled at the plasma membrane, the PMN looks like a "mini-tank" with multiple "mini-guns" directed towards all sites (see e.g. Figure 1D of [47]). High concentrations of H_2O_2 are generated pericellularly: 1 million activated PMN generate about 100 nmol H_2O_2 [61], i.e. considering areas of PMN infiltration with about 1 million activated PMN/µl, these PMN might generate an ambience of H_2O_2 in the range of 100 mM. The PMN myeloperoxidase transforms the rather radicalic H_2O_2 into slightly radicalic HOCl [62] that e.g. reacts with H_2O_2 to nonradicalic chloramines, mainly taurine-chloramine. Chloramines are anti-bacterial, anti-fungal, anti-viral, anti-parasitic, anti-tumoral, and anti-thrombotic [63-82,85,92]: chloramines act against all pathogen-types. PMN might generate ambiences of about 1-10 mM chloramine [10,83]. H_2O_2 and HOCl/chloramines might act synergistically [84]. Chloramines are important physiologic sources of the nonradical excited oxidant singlet oxygen ($^1O_2^*$) [85] that at neutral-physiologic pH selectively reacts with sulphur atoms (in methionine or cysteine) or with C=C bonds [86,87]. The latter reaction yields excited carbonyls (R-C=O*), that emit photons of about 425 nm (in the blue spectrum of light), which might be of physiologic importance for specific and aimed cell signalling within the dark blood stream that is partially filled with red cells [88]. $^1O_2^*$ is anticoagulant, profibrinolytic, and complement activating [89-94]. These nonradical oxidants are well tolerable to normal mammalian cells [95,96]. gp91phox is the most important part of the NADPH-oxidase: intracellularly it binds the NADPH binding protein p67phox, intramembranously it contains FAD (flavin adenine dinucleotide) and 2 hemes, extracellularly it contains a binding site for molecular oxygen (O_2) [56]. So, gp91phox is the main transporter of electrons from inside to outside the cell, i.e. the gp91phox part of the NADPH-oxidase is responsible for the electrons – flop (Figure 1).

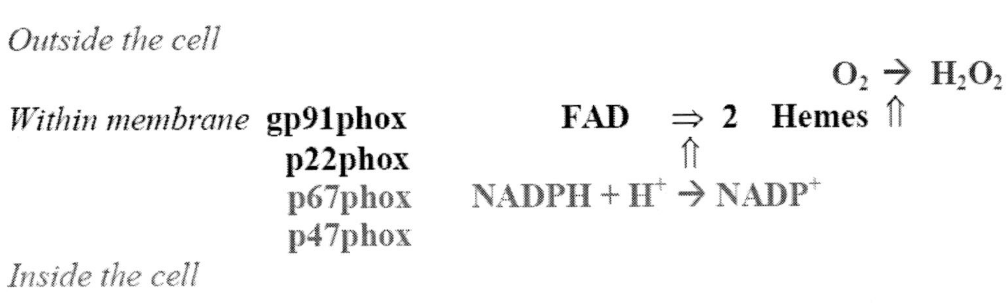

Figure 1. Main parts of assembled NADPH-oxidase of activated PMN. H atoms/electrons from inside the cell (in blue), bound in NADPH, are transported via p67phox to the nearby gp91phox with its FAD and its hemes (gp91phox = main intramembraneous part, p67phox = main intracellular part of the NADPH-oxidase [8,27]). The electrons are then transferred to O_2 and H_2O_2 is formed outside the cell or inside a phagosome (in red). The flux of H atoms or of electrons is indicated by the symbol ⇑.

The activity of the NADPH-oxidase is regulated by protein phosphorylation [50,58], e.g. by protein kinase C, furthermore alkaline phosphatase for phosphorylation of membrane proteins [97] is associated with gp91phox and p22phox within the same cell granules [47].

Three isoforms of NADPH-oxidase are expressed in the vascular wall: endothelial cells and adventitial fibroblasts have a NADPH-oxidase similar to that of PMN with gp91phox = Nox2 as the main component [98]; the NADPH-oxidase of vascular smooth muscle cells is different to gp91phox, these isoforms are named Nox1 and Nox4 [99,100].

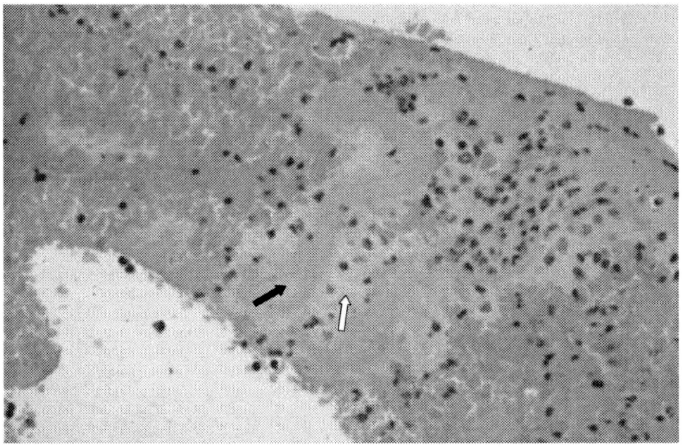

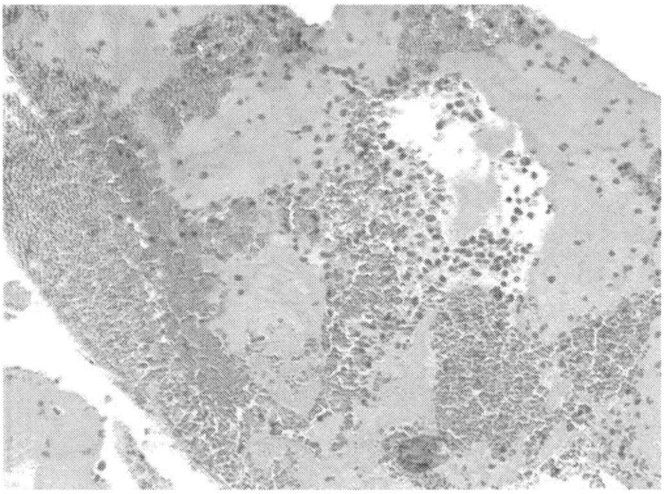

Figure 2. Thrombolysis *in vivo* by PMN. A thrombus was generated in the left jugular vein of rabbits by injection of 0.2 U factor eight inhibitor bypassing activity (FEIBA) per ml plasma and 15 min stasis of blood stream in this vein segment [92]. The generator of excited singlet oxygen ($^1O_2^*$) chloramine-T® in 0.9 % NaCl or 0.9 % NaCl (control) was infused over 30 min to reach final blood concentrations of 0.5 mM or 0 mM (control). 60 min after the end of the drug-infusion the left jugular vein was excised. The minimal rest-thrombi (<5% of control) of the treated animals were histologically (hematoxylin-eosin stained) compared with the full control thrombi (100% control). PMN massively infiltrated the thrombus, if the circulating blood of the respective animal was treated with $^1O_2^*$, the PMN/erythrocytes ratio in animals without $^1O_2^*$ therapy of about 1/2000 could increase more than about 1000fold in favour of the PMN [92]. Areas of destroyed erythrocytes are coloured in dark-pink (→), areas of pericellular fibrinolysis around single PMN with less erythrocytes, that were fibrinolytically released from the thrombus, are coloured in white to light-pink (⇒).

SINGLET OXYGEN ($^1\Delta O_2$*) AND HEMOSTASIS

The nonradical excited reactive oxygen species (ROS) $^1O_2^*$ is a molecule of both cellular signalling and destruction. At low doses ROS behave as cell signals: they regulate cell cycle, protein kinases, and gene expression [99,101,102]. At high doses $^1O_2^*$ is pathogen-destructive and signalling: blue light quants of about 425 nm derived from the $^1\Delta O_2$* reaction product excited carbonyl (R-C=O*) are emitted, when PMN are strongly activated. In the dark blood stream they may act as inter- or intra- cellular signals. This signalling side effect can be compared to the gun fire of soldiers against invading bandits at night: nearby other soldiers see the exact location of the battle, are recruited to this crime scene, and amplify the gun fire against the invasive bandits.

The expression of gp91phox mRNA in the artery wall is upregulated during atherogenesis [99]. Hydroxyl radicals (·OH) may also be formed, especially if transition metal catalysts (Fe^{3+}/ Fe^{2+}) are interacting (Fenton reaction) [58,99]. For normal mammalian cells ·OH is rather bad, because ·OH unspecifically breaks protein chains or forms tyrosine dimers that might crosslink proteins [103,104], $^1O_2$ or inhibitors of ·OH [105] are rather good. Whereas it seems to be clear that the genesis of ·OH promotes atherogenesis, the generation of subtoxic levels of the nonradical $^1O_2$ by gp91phox (=Nox2), Nox1, and Nox4 might well be anti-thrombotic or anti-atheroscerotic [106]: patients with chronic granulomatous disease (CGD), an illness of dysfunctional NADPH-oxidase (defective gp91phox, p22phox, p67phox, p47phox (the main components of Nox-2; defective p40phox has not been reported) [56]), often suffer from severe atherosclerosis [58,107,108].

PMN-NADPH-oxidase deficient mice can develop atherosclerosis [109]. In the pre-phase of atherosclerosis, that might be called thrombo-atherosclerosis, there appears a pathological fibrin clot. This clot can be lysed by recruited PMN that have become activated by $^1O_2^*$ generating endothelium, that were activated by bound fibrin [110], by activated platelets, or by other activated PMN [102,111-120]. PMN via CD11b/CD18 bind to the C-gamma-terminus of D-domains in fibrin [115] and become activated. Consequently, a $^1O_2$* and R-C=0* (excited singlet oxygen or excited carbonyl) - mediated decrease of the count of flowing blood PMN in favour of PMN that chemotactically adhere to and infiltrate the pathologic clot on the endothelium might be physiological [121-123,162,163,164] In contrast, in the late phases of atherosclerosis, infiltration of tissue factor (TF) expressing macrophages (M∅) [124-128] but also of PMN [129] that via ROS might enhance TF production or PLA_2 activity of M∅ [130] might be pathological. Patients with dysfunctional PMN, e.g. patients positive for anti-cytoplasmic antibodies (ANCA) often suffer from thrombosis [131,132,178].

Also fibroblasts bind fibrin via ICAM-1 [133]. Activated fibroblasts transform the immature fibrin clot into mature fibrotic tissue, i.e. thrombosis could be a pre-form of fibrosis [134].

CELLULAR FIBRINOLYSIS

Fibrinolysis consists of a plasmatic part and a cellular one [135,136]. The plasmatic part is the plasmatic fibrinolysis system with plasmin as the central enzyme. The cellular part are the PMN with their urokinase, elastase, and singlet oxygen [51,138-140]. If pathologic amounts of fibrin are deposited over endothelium, that are beginning to obstruct the vessel lumen, the blood PMN are activated. If the PMN system is insufficient, e.g. because there is too much fibrin as e.g. in PDIC, this cellular fibrinolysis is frustrane [141]. D-dimer degradation by PMN elastase makes the D-dimer result difficult to interprete, since the plasmatic D-dimer concentration would then depend on at least 4 totally different hemostasis enzymes: thrombin, factor XIIIa, plasmin, and elastase. Circulating plasmatic thrombin seems to be a superior parameter for diagnosis of coagulation activation, e.g. in sepsis [142,211].

Corticoids suppress PMN adhesion to the endothelium and result into thrombosis [143-146]. Physiologic PMN activators such as singlet oxygen or G-CSF induce enhanced adhesion to endothelial cells via CD11b/CD18 – ICAM-1 interaction and subsequently into thrombolysis [83,147-150]. PMN recruitment to a pathologic thrombus is a prerequisite for efficient thrombolysis, mediated by singlet oxygen, urokinase, plasmin, and elastase [151,152].

Imitation of the physiologic PMN mediated thrombolysis is of major clinical interest to avoid severe bleeding complications. PMN can be activated e.g. by about 2 µg/ml G-CSF [83,179], by about 0.5 mM chloramines [92,147], or by usual therapeutic doses of vancomycine that precipitates fibrinogen [89,92] to a possible CD11b/CD18 activator (about 0.25 mmol/l of vancomycine activates blood PMN comparably efficiently as about 0.5 mmol/l of chloramine). Blood concentrations of about 0.5 mM chloramine do not significantly alter the normal blood coagulation because the 50 % inhibitory concentration of chloramine against susceptible coagulation components is $\geq$ 1 mM [92].

CONCLUSIONS

For several decades there has been a controversial if leukocytes are the cause or the consequence of pathologic coagulation activation. Now it seems to be clear that MØ with their TF and their phospholipase A_2, that are potent activators of extrinsic and intrinsic coagulation, respectively, can be rather pathologic [197-205], and PMN with their $^1O_2$* + urokinase, that mediate peri-cellular fibrinolysis (see e.g. the PMN in the right upper corner of figure 4B of [172]), are rather physiologic [169-171,175-177]. If it is difficult to selectively lyse a pathologic thrombus via individually adjusted therapeutic activation of plasmatic fibrinolysis [173] (with about 0.1-0.2 U/ml plasmatic plasmin [174]), the PMN- mediated selective fibrinolysis might be stimulated: PMN with their CD11b/CD18 receptors adhere selectively to and destroy pathologic deposits of fibrin [206]; CD11b/CD18 binding enhances the generation of reactive oxygen species, and CD11b/CD18 is activated via redox reactions [181-196]. So, the intravascular release of $^1O_2$* or of photons might be an innovative therapy, e.g. to selectively activate anti-thrombotic PMN without major hemostasis complications [92,147,168,208-211].

REFERENCES

[1] Paape MJ, Bannerman DD, Zhao X, Lee JW. The bovine neutrophil: Structure and function in blood and milk. *Vet. Res.* 2003; 34: 597-627.

[2] Tate MD, Brooks AG, Reading PC. The role of neutrophils in the the upper and lower respiratory tract during influenza virus infection of mice. *Respir. Res.* 2008 Aug 1; 9: 57. [Epub ahead of print].

[3] Sugui JA, Kim HS, Zarember KA, Chang YC, Gallin JI, Nierman WC, Kwon-Chung KJ. Genes differentially expressed in conidia and hyphae of Aspergillus fumigatus upon exposure to human neutrophils. *PLoS ONE* 2008; 3: e2655.

[4] Lacy P, Eitzen G. Control of granule exocytosis in neutrophils. *Front Biosci.* 2008; 1; 13: 5559-70.

[5] Hogg JC. The traffic of polymorphonuclear leukocytes through pulmonary microvessels in health and disease. *Am. J. Respir.* 1994; 163: 769-778.

[6] Dinauer MC. Disorders of neutrophil function: an overview. *Methods Mol. Biol.* 2007; 412: 489-504.

[7] Malech HL. The role of neutrophils in the immune system: an overview. *Methods Mol.* Biol 2007; 412: 3-11.

[8] Sawyer DW, Donowitz GR, Mandell GL.Polymorphonuclear neutrophils: an effective antimicrobial force. *Rev. Infect. Dis.* 1989; 11 Suppl 7: S1532-44.

[9] Harlan JM. Leukocyte-endothelial interactions. *Blood* 1985; 65: 513-25.

[10] Weiss SJ. Tissue destruction by neutrophils. *N. Engl. J. Med.* 1989; 320: 365-76.

[11] Ellis TN, Beaman BL. Murine polymorphonuclear neutrophils produce interferon-gamma in response to pulmonary infection with Nocardia asteroids. *J. Leukocyte Biol.* 2002; 72: 373-81.

[12] Ellis TN, Beaman BL. Interferon-gamma activation of polymorphonuclear neutrophil function. *Immunology* 2004; 112: 2-12.

[13] Sohn EJ, Paape MJ, Connor EE, Bannerman DD, Fetterer RH, Peters RR. Bacterial lipopolysaccharide stimulates bovine neutrophil production of TNF-alpha, IL-1beta, IL-12 and IFN-gamma. *Vet. Res.* 2007; 38: 809-18.

[14] Djeu JY. Cytokines and anti-fungal immunity. *Adv. Exp. Med. Biol.* 1992; 319: 217-23.

[15] Sigal A, Bleijs DA, Grabovsky V, Vliet SJ, Dwir O, Figdor CG, van Kooyk Y, Alon R. The LFA-1 integrin supports rolling adhesions on ICAM-1 under physiological shear flow in a permissive cellular environment. *J. Immunol.* 2000; 165: 442-52.

[16] Gaboury JP, Kubes P. Reductions in physiologic shear rates lead to CD11/CD18-dependent, selectin-independent leukocyte rolling in vivo. *Blood* 1994; 83: 345-50.

[17] McEver RP. Adhesive interactions of leukocytes, platelets, and the vessel wall during hemostasis and inflammation. *Thromb. Haemost.* 2001; 86: 746-56.

[18] Etzioni A, Tonetti M. Leukocyte adhesion deficiency II- from A to almost Z. *Immunological Reviews* 2000; 178: 138-47.

[19] Davenpeck KL, Berens KL, Dixon RAF, Dupre B, Bochner BS. Inhibition of adhesion of human neutrophils and eosinophils to P-selectin by the sialyl Lewis^{x} antagonist TBC1269: preferential activity against neutrophil adhesion in vitro. *J. Allergy Clin. Immunol.* 2000; 105: 769-75.

[20] Stie J, Jesaitis AJ. Reorganization of the human neutrophil plasma membrane is associated with functional priming: implications for neutrophil preparations. *J. Leukoc. Biol.* 2007; 81: 672-85.

[21] Sakamoto S, Okanoue T, Itoh Y, Sakamoto K, Nishioji K, Nakagawa Y, Yoshida N, Yoshikawa T, Kashima K. Intercellular adhesion molecule-1 and CD18 are involved in neutrophil adhesion and its cytotoxicity to cultured sinusoidal endothelial cells in rats. *Hepatology* 1997; 26: 658-63.

[22] Loike JD, Silverstein R, Wright SD, Weitz JI, Huang AJ, Silverstein SC. The role of protected extracellular compartments in interactions between leukocytes, and platelets, and fibrin/fibrinogen matrices. *Ann. N Y Acad. Sci.* 1992; 667: 163-72.

[23] Wagner JG, Roth RA. Neutrophil migration during endotoxemia. *J. Leukoc. Biol.* 1999; 66: 10-24.

[24] Stief TW. Coagulation Activation by Lipopolysaccharides. *Clin. Appl. Thromb. Hemost.* 2007 Dec 26.

[25] Arditi M, Zhou J, Dorio R, Rong GW, Goyert SM, Kim KS. Endotoxin-mediated endothelial cell injury and activation: role of soluble CD14. *Infect. Immun.* 1993; 61: 3149-56.

[26] Charavaryamath C, Janardhan KS, Caldwell S, Singh B. Pulmonary intravascular monocytes/macrophages in a rat model of sepsis. *Anat. Rec. A Discov. Mol. Cell Evo*l. *Biol.* 2006; 288: 1259-71.

[27] Farsky SP, Sannomiya P, Garcia-Leme J. Secreted glucocorticoids regulate leukocyte-endothelial interactions in inflammation. A direct vital microscopic study. *J. Leukoc. Biol.* 1995; 57: 379-86.

[28] Filep JG, Delalandre A, Payette Y, Földes-Filep E. Glucocorticoid receptor regulates expression of L-selectin and CD11/CD18 on human neutrophils. *Circulation* 1997; 96: 295-301.

[29] Hill GE, Alonso A, Thiele GM, Robbins RA. Glucocorticoids blunt neutrophil CD11b surface glycoprotein upregulation during cardiopulmonary bypass in humans. *Anesth Analg*. 1994; 79: 23-7.

[30] Brandt MM, Lynam E, Sklar LA. Methylprednisolone inhibits three classes of neutrophil receptors in human blood in vitro. *J. Surg. Res.* 1993; 55: 632-9.

[31] Gilbert RO, Kim CA, Yen A. Modulation, in vivo and in vitro, of surface expression of CD18 by bovine neutrophils. *Am. J. Vet Res*. 1992; 53: 1675-8.

[32] Schramm R, Liu Q, Thorlacius H. Expression and function of MIP-2 are reduced by dexamethasone treatment in vivo. *Br. J. Pharmacol.* 2000; 131: 328-34.

[33] Barton AE, Bayley DL, Mikami M, Llewellyn-Jones CG, Stockley RA. Phenotypic changes in neutrophils related to anti-inflammatory therapy. *Biochim. Biophys. Acta* 2000; 1500: 108-18.

[34] Burton JL, Kehrli ME Jr, Kapil S, Horst RL. Regulation of L-selectin and CD18 on bovine neutrophils by glucocorticoids: effects of cortisol and dexamethasone. *J. Leukoc. Biol.* 1995; 57: 317-25.

[35] Ballabh P, Simm M, Kumari J, Krauss AN, Jain A, Califano C, Lesser ML, Cunningham-Rundles S. Neutrophil and monocyte adhesion molecules in bronchopulmonary dysplasia, and effects of corticosteroids. *Arch. Dis. Child Fetal Neonatal. Ed* 2004; 89: F76-83.

[36] Kvietys PR, Sandig M. Neutrophil diapedesis: paracellular or transcellular? News *Physiol. Sci.* 2001; 16:15-9.
[37] Hoshi O, Ushiki T. Neutrophil extravasation in rat mesenteric venules induced by the chemotactic peptide N-formyl-methionyl-luecylphenylalanine (fMLP), with special attention to a barrier function of the vascular basal lamina for neutrophil migration. *Arch. Histol Cytol.* 2004; 67: 107-14.
[38] Lin M, Jackson P, Tester AM, Diaconu E, Overall CM, Blalock JE, Pearlman E. Matrix metalloproteinase-8 facilitates neutrophil migration through the corneal stromal matrix by collagen degradation and production of the chemotactic peptide Pro-Gly-Pro. *Am. J. Pathol.* 2008; 173: 144-53.
[39] Tschesche H, Bakowski B, Schettler A, Knäuper V, Reinke H, Krämer S. Leukodiapedesis, compartmentalisation and secretion of PMN leukocyte proteinases, and activation of PMN leukocyte procollagenase. *Adv. Exp. Med. Biol.* 1991; 297: 39-53.
[40] Faustmann PM, Dermietzel R. Extravasation of polymorphonuclear leukocytes from the cerebral microvasculature. Inflammatory response induced by alpha-bungarotoxin. *Cell Tissue Res*. 1985; 242: 399-407.
[41] Hoshi O, Ushiki T. Scanning electron microscopic studies on the route of neutrophil extravasation in the mouse after exposure to the chemotactic peptide N-formyl-methionyl-leucyl-phenylalaninphenylalanine (fMLP). *Arch. Histol. Cytol.* 1999; 62: 253-60.
[42] Michel CC, Neal CR. Openings through endothelial cells associated with increased microvascular permeability. *Microcirculation* 1999; 6: 45-54.
[43] Wolosewick JJ. Distribution of actin in migrating leukocytes in vivo. *Cell Tissue Res.* 1984; 236: 517-25.
[44] Solodkin-Szaingurten I, Levy R, Hadad N. Differential behavior of sPLA2-V and sPLA2-X in human neutrophils. *Biochim. Biophys. Acta* 2007; 1771: 155-63.
[45] Gabay JE, Scott RW, Campanelli D, Griffith J, Wilde C, Marra MN, Seeger M, Nathan CF. Antibiotic proteins of human polymorphonuclear leukocytes. *Proc. Natl. Acad. Sci. USA* 1989; 86: 5610-4.
[46] Stief TW. Polycations neutralize PAI-1. *Hemostasis Laboratory* 2008; 1: 109-118.
[47] Seguchi H, Kobayashi T. Study of NADPH oxidase-activated sites in human neutrophils. *J. Electron. Microsc.* 2002; 51: 87-91.
[48] Burgoyne RD, Morgan A. Secretory granule exocytosis. *Physol. Rev.* 2003; 83: 581-632.
[49] Di Noto R, Lo Pardo C, Schiavone EM, Ferrara F, Manzo C, Vacca C, Del Vecchio L. All-trans retinoic acid (ATRA) and the regulation of adhesion molecules in acute myeloid leukemia. *Leuk. Lymphoma* 1996; 21: 207-9.
[50] El-Benna J, Dang PM, Gougerot-Pocidalo MA. Priming of the neutrophil NADPH oxidase activation: role of p47phox phosphorylation and NOX2 mobilization to the plasma membrane. *Semin. Immunopathol.* 2008; 30: 279-89.
[51] Stief TW. Singlet oxygen potentiates thrombolysis. *Clin. Appl. Thromb. Hemost.* 2007; 13: 259-78.
[52] Schuster DP, Brody SL, Zhou Z, Bernstein M, Arch R, Link D, Mueckler M. Regulation of lipopolysaccharide-induced increases in neutrophil glucose uptake. *Am. J. Physiol. Lung Cell Mol. Physiol.* 2007; 292: L845-51.

[53] Ha H, Lee HB. Reactive oxygen species as glucose signaling molecules in mesangial cells cultured under high glucose. *Kidney Int.* 2000; 58: 19-25.

[54] Han CH, Lee MH. Activation domain in p67phox regulates the steady state reduction of FAD in gp91phox. *J. Vet. Sci.* 2000; 1: 27-31.

[55] Shen K, Sergeant S, Hantgan RR, McPhail LC, Horita DA. Mutations in the PX-SH3A Linker of p47(phox) Decouple PI(3,4)P2 Binding from NADPH Oxidase Activation. *Biochemistry.* 2008 Aug 2. [Epub ahead of print].

[56] Babior BM. NADPH oxidase. *Curr. Opin. Immunol.* 2004; 16: 42-7.

[57] Vergnaud S, Paclet MH, El Benna J, Pocidalo MA, Morel F. Complementation of NADPH oxidase in p67-phox-deficient CGD patients: p67-phox/-40-phox interaction. *Eur. J. Biochem.* 2000; 267: 1059-67.

[58] Sheppard FR, Kelher MR, Moore EE, McLaughlin NJ, Banerjee A, Silliman CC. Structural organization of the neutrophil NADPH oxidase: phosphorylation and translocation during priming and activation. *J. Leukoc. Biol.* 2005; 78: 1025-42.

[59] Gabig TG, Crean CD, Mantel PL, Rosli R. Function of wild-type or mutant Rac2 and Rap1a GTPases in differentiated HL60 cell NADPH oxidase activation. *Blood* 1995; 85: 804-11.

[60] Yan J, Li F, Ingram DA, Quilliam LA. Rap1a is a key regulator of FGF2-induced angiogenesis and together with Rap1b controls human endothelial cell functions. *Mol. Cell Biol.* 2008 Jul 14. [Epub ahead of print].

[61] Nathan CF. Respiratory burst in adherent human neutrophils: triggering by colony-stimulating factors CSF-GM and CSF-G. *Blood* 1989; 73: 301-6.

[62] Stief TW. Oxidized fibrin stimulates the activation of pro-urokinase and is the preferential substrate of human plasmin. *Blood Coagul Fibrinolysis* 1993; 4: 117-21.

[63] Thomas EL. Myeloperoxidase-hydrogen peroxide-chloride antimicrobial system: effect of exogenous amines on antibacterial action against Escherichia coli. *Infect. Immun.* 1979; 25: 110-6.

[64] Weiss SJ, Lampert MB, Test ST. Long-lived oxidants generated by human neutrophils: characterization and bioactivity. *Science* 1983; 222: 625-8.

[65] Weiss SJ, Klein R, Slivka A, Wei M. Chlorination of taurine by human neutrophils. Evidence for hypochlorous acid generation. *J. Clin. Invest* 1982; 70: 598-607.

[66] Schuller-Levis GB, Park E. Taurine and its chloramine: modulators of immunity. *Neurochem. Res.* 2004; 29: 117-26.

[67] Stief TW. Singlet oxygen ($^1O_2$)-oxidizable lipids in the HIV membrane, new targets for AIDS therapy? *Med. Hypotheses* 2003; 60: 575-7.

[68] Stief TW. The physiology and pharmacology of singlet oxygen. *Med. Hypotheses* 2003; 60: 567-72.

[69] Dudani AK, Martyres A, Fliss H. Short communication: rapid preparation of preventive and therapeutic whole-killed retroviral vaccines using the microbicide taurine chloramine. *AIDS Res. Hum. Retroviruses* 2008; 24: 635-42.

[70] Fürnkranz U, Nagl M, Gottardi W, Köhsler M, Aspöck H, Walochnik J. Cytotoxic activity of N-chlorotaurine on Acanthamoeba spp. *Antimicrob Agents Chemother* 2008; 52: 470-6.

[71] Gottardi W, Arnitz R, Nagl M. N-Chlorotaurine and ammonium chloride: an antiseptic preparation with strong bactericidal activity. *Int. J. Pharm.* 2007; 335: 32-40.

[72] Reeves EP, Nagl M, O'Keeffe J, Kelly J, Kavanagh K. Effect of N-chlorotaurine on Aspergillus, with particular reference to destruction of secreted gliotoxin. *J. Med. Microbiol.* 2006; 55: 913-8.

[73] Romanowski EG, Yates KA, Teuchner B, Nagl M, Irschick EU, Gordon YJ. N-chlorotaurine is an effective antiviral agent against adenovirus in vitro and in the Ad5/NZW rabbit ocular model. *Invest Ophthalmol. Vis. Sci.* 2006; 47: 2021-6.

[74] Klamt F, Shacter E. Taurine chloramine, an oxidant derived from neutrophils, induces apoptosis in human B lymphoma cells through mitochondrial damage. *J. Biol. Chem.* 2005; 280: 21346-52.

[75] Gottardi W, Nagl M. Chemical properties of N-chlorotaurine sodium, a key compound in the human defence system. *Arch. Pharm.* 2002; 335: 411-21.

[76] Gottardi W, Hagleitner M, Nagl M. The influence of plasma on the disinfecting activity of the new antimicrobial agent N-chlorotaurine-sodium in comparison with chloramine T. *J. Pharm. Pharmacol.* 2001; 53: 689-97.

[77] Nagl M, Teuchner B, Pöttinger E, Ulmer H, Gottardi W. Tolerance of N-chlorotaurine, a new antimicrobial agent, in infectious conjunctivitis - a phase II pilot study. *Ophthalmologica* 2000; 214: 111-4.

[78] Nagl M, Gottardi W. Rapid killing of Mycobacterium terrae by N-chlorotaurine in the presence of ammonium is caused by the reaction product monochloramine. *J. Pharm. Pharmacol.* 1998; 50: 1317-20.

[79] Nagl M, Pfausler B, Schmutzhard E, Fille M, Gottardi W. Tolerance and bactericidal action of N-chlorotaurine in a urinary tract infection by an omniresistant Pseudomonas aeruginosa. *Zentralbl Bakteriol.* 1998; 288: 217-23.

[80] Nagl M, Larcher C, Gottardi W. Activity of N-chlorotaurine against herpes simplex- and adenoviruses. *Antiviral Res.* 1998; 38: 25-30.

[81] Nagl M, Nguyen VA, Gottardi W, Ulmer H, Höpfl R. Tolerability and efficacy of N-chlorotaurine in comparison with chloramine T for the treatment of chronic leg ulcers with a purulent coating: a randomized phase II study. *Br. J. Dermatol.* 2003; 149: 590-7.

[82] Yazdanbakhsh M, Eckmann CM, Roos D. Killing of schistosomula by taurine chloramine and taurine bromamine. *Am. J. Trop Med. Hyg.* 1987; 37: 106-10.

[83] Stief TW. Modulation of granulocytc mediated thrombolysis. *Hemostasis Laboratory* 2008; 1: 77-102.

[84] Mashino T, Fridovich I. NADPH mediates the inactivation of bovine liver catalase by monochloroamine. *Arch. Biochem. Biophys.* 1988; 265: 279-85.

[85] Stief TW. Regulation of hemostasis by singlet-oxygen ($^1\Delta O_2$*). *Curr. Vasc. Pharmacol.* 2004; 2: 357-62.

[86] Shechter Y, Burstein Y, Patchornik A. Selective oxidation of methionine residues in proteins. *Biochemistry* 1975; 14: 4497-503.

[87] Peskin AV, Winterbourn CC. Kinetics of the reactions of hypochlorous acid and amino acid chloramines with thiols, methionine, and ascorbate. *Free Radic Biol. Med.* 2001; 30: 572-9.

[88] Stief TW. The blood fibrinolysis/deep-sea analogy: a hypothesis on the cell signals singlet oxygen/photons as natural antithrombotics. *Thromb. Res.* 2000; 99: 1-20.

[89] Stief TW. The fibrinogen antigenic turbidimetric assay (FIATA): the X^2x test -- the corrected chi-square comparison against the control-mean. *Clin. Appl. Thromb. Hemost* 2007; 13: 73-100.

[90] Fujimoto Y, Ikeda M, Sakuma S. Monochloramine potently inhibits arachidonic acid metabolism in rat platelets. *Biochem. Biophys. Res. Commun.* 2006; 344: 140-5.

[91] Stief TW, Jeske WP, Walenga J, Schultz C, Kretschmer V, Fareed J. Singlet oxygen inhibits agonist-induced P-selectin expression and formation of platelet aggregates. *Clin. Appl. Thromb. Hemost.* 2001; 7: 219-24.

[92] Stief TW, Fareed J. The antithrombotic factor singlet oxygen/light ($^1O_2/h\nu$). *Clin. Appl. Thromb. Hemost.* 2000; 6: 22-30.

[93] Stief TW, Kurz J, Doss MO, Fareed J. Singlet oxygen inactivates fibrinogen, factor V, factor VIII, factor X, and platelet aggregation of human blood. *Thromb. Res.* 2000; 97: 473-80.

[94] Vogt W. Complement activation by myeloperoxidase products released from stimulated human polymorphonuclear leukocytes. *Immunobiology* 1996; 195: 334-46.

[95] Neher A, Nagl M, Schrott-Fischer A, Ichiki H, Gottardi W, Gunkel AR, Stephan K. N-chlorotaurine, a novel endogenous antimicrobial agent: tolerability testing in a mouse model. *Arch. Otolaryngol. Head Neck Surg.* 2001; 127: 530-3.

[96] Nagl M, Miller B, Daxecker F, Ulmer H, Gottardi W. Tolerance of N-chlorotaurine, an endogenous antimicrobial agent, in the rabbit and human eye--a phase I clinical study. *J. Ocul. Pharmacol. Ther.* 1998; 14: 283-90.

[97] Shanmugham LN, Petrarca C, Castellani ML, Symeonidou I, Frydas S, Vecchiet J, Falasca K, Tetè S, Conti P, Salini V. IL-1beta induces alkaline phosphatase in human phagocytes. *Arch. Med. Res.* 2007; 38: 39-44.

[98] Rada B, Hably C, Meczner A, Timár C, Lakatos G, Enyedi P, Ligeti E. Role of Nox2 in elimination of microorganisms. *Semin. Immunopathol.* 2008; 30: 237-53.

[99] Bengtsson SH, Gulluyan LM, Dusting GJ, Drummond GR. Novel isoforms of NADPH oxidase in vascular physiology and pathophysiology. *Clin. Exp. Pharmacol. Physiol.* 2003; 30-54.

[100] Rada B, Leto TL. Oxidative innate immune defenses by Nox/Duox family NADPH oxidases. *Contrib. Microbiol.* 2008; 15: 164-87.

[101] Schäppi MG, Jaquet V, Belli DC, Krause KH. Hyperinflammation in chronic granulomatous disease and anti-inflammatory role of the phagocyte NADPH oxidase. *Semin. Immunopathol.* 2008; 30: 255-71.

[102] Miyoshi T, Matsumoto AH, Shi W. Paradoxical increase in LDL oxidation by endothelial cells from an atherosclerosis-resistant mouse strain. *Atherosclerosis* 2007; 192: 259-65.

[103] Calingasan NY, Gibson GE. Vascular endothelium is a site of free radical production and inflammation in areas of neuronal loss in thiamine-deficient brain. *Ann. N Y Acad. Sci.* 2000; 903: 353-6.

[104] Tak PP, Zvaifler NJ, Green DR, Firestein GS. Rheumatoid arthritis and p53: how oxidative stress might alter the course of inflammatory diseases. *Immunology Today* 2000; 21: 78-82.

[105] O'Brien NC, Charlton B, Cowden WB, Willenborg DO. Nitric oxide plays a critical role in the recovery of Lewis rats from experimental autoimmune encephalomyelitis and the maintenance of resistance to reinduction. *J. Immunol.* 1999; 163: 6841-7.

[106] Matheny HE, Deem TL, Cook-Mills JM. Lymphocyte migration through monolayers of endothelial cell lines involves VCAM-1 signaling via endothelial cell NADPH Oxidase. *J. Immunol.* 2000; 164: 6550-9.

[107] Wyche KE, Wang SS, Griendling KK, Dikalov SI, Austin H, Rao S, Fink B, Harrison DG, Zafari AM. C242T CYBA polymorphism of the NADPH oxidase is associated with reduced respiratory burst in human neutrophils. *Hypertension* 2004; 43: 1246-51.

[108] Stasia MJ, Li XJ. Genetics and immunopathology of chronic granulomatous disease. *Semin. Immunopathol.* 2008; 30: 209-35.

[109] Kirk EA, Dinauer MC, Rosen H, Chait A, Heinecke JW, LeBoeuf RC. Impaired superoxide production due to a deficiency in phagocyte NADPH oxidase fails to inhibit atherosclerosis in mice. *Arterioscler. Thromb. Vasc. Biol.* 2000; 20: 1529-35.

[110] Bach TL, Barsigian C, Yaen CH, Martinez J. Endothelial cell VE-cadherin functions as a receptor for the ß15-42 sequence of fibrin. *J. Biol. Chem.* 1998; 273: 30719-28.

[111] Cockwell P, Tse WY, Savage CO. Activation of endothelial cells in thrombosis and vasculitis. *Scand. J. Rheumatol.* 1997; 26: 145-50.

[112] Ruf A, Schlenk RF, Maras A, Morgenstern E, Patscheke H. Contact-induced neutrophil activation by platelets in human cell suspensions and whole blood. *Blood* 1992; 80: 1238-46.

[113] Vercellotti GM, Severson SP, Duane P, Moldow CF. Hydrogen peroxide alters signal transduction in human endothelial cells. *J. Lab. Clin. Med.* 1991; 117: 15-24.

[114] Kirton CM, Nash GB. Activated platelets adherent to an intact endothelial cell monolayer bind flowing neutrophils and enable them to transfer to the endothelial surface. *J. Lab. Clin. Med.* 2000; 136: 303-13.

[115] Trezzini C, Schalch L, Jungi TW. The triggering of fibrinogen receptors on mononuclear phagocytes of healthy subjects and of a thrombasthenia Glanzmann patient promotes the generation of reactive oxygen species. *Blood Coagul. Fibrinolysis* 1990; 1: 363-73.

[116] Jungi TW, Spycher MO, Nydegger UE, Barandum S. Platelet-leukocyte interaction: selective binding of thrombin-stimulated platelets to human monocytes, polymorphonuclear leukocytes and related cell lines. *Blood* 1986; 67: 629-36.

[117] Sherman LA, Lee J. Specific binding of soluble fibrin to macrophages. *J. Exp. Med.* 1977; 145: 76-85.

[118] Colvin RB. Fibrinogen-fibrin interactions with fibroblasts and macrophages. *Ann. NY Acad. Sci.* 1983; 408: 621-633.

[119] Neelamegham S, Taylor AD, Shankaran H, Smith CW, Simon SI. Shear and time-dependent changes in Mac-1, LFA-1, and ICAM-3 binding regulate neutrophil homotypic adhesion. *J. Immunol.* 2000; 164: 3798-805.

[120] Rubel C, Fernandez GC, Dran G, Bompadre MB, Isturiz MA, Palermo MS. Fibrinogen promotes neutrophil activation and delays apoptosis. *J. Immunol.* 2001; 166: 2002-10.

[121] Brennan ML, Anderson MM, Shih DM, Qu XD, Wang X, Mehta AC, Lim LL, Shi W, Hazen SL, Jacob JS, Crowley JR, Heinecke JW, Lusis AJ. Increased atherosclerosis in myeloperoxidase-deficient mice. *J. Clin. Invest.* 2001; 107: 419-30.

[122] Almekhlafi MA, Hu WY, Hill MD, Auer RN. Calcification and endothelialization of thrombi in acute stroke. *Ann. Neurol.* 2008 Jun 20. [Epub ahead of print].

[123] Järemo P, Nilsson O. Interleukin-6 and neutrophils are associated with long-term survival after acute myocardial infarction. *Eur. J. Intern. Med.* 2008; 19: 330-3. Epub 2008 Feb 20.

[124] Shepherd J, Hilderbrand SA, Waterman P, Heinecke JW, Weissleder R, Libby P. A fluorescent probe for the detection of myeloperoxidase activity in atherosclerosis-associated macrophages. *Chem. Biol.* 2007; 14: 1221-31.

[125] McMillen TS, Heinecke JW, LeBoeuf RC. Expression of human myeloperoxidase by macrophages promotes atherosclerosis in mice. *Circulation* 2005; 111: 2798-804.

[126] Aviram M, Rosenblat M. Paraoxonases 1, 2, and 3, oxidative stress, and macrophage foam cell formation during atherosclerosis development. *Free Radic. Biol. Med.* 2004; 37: 1304-16.

[127] Nakayama K, Nitto T, Inoue T, Node K. Expression of the cytochrome P450 epoxygenase CYP2J2 in human monocytic leukocytes. *Life Sci.* 2008 Jul 12. [Epub ahead of print].

[128] Lambert JM, Lopez EF, Lindsey ML. Macrophage roles following myocardial infarction. *Int. J. Cardiol.* 2008 Jul 23. [Epub ahead of print].

[129] van Leeuwen M, Gijbels MJ, Duijvestijn A, Smook M, van de Gaar MJ, Heeringa P, de Winther MP, Tervaert JW. Accumulation of myeloperoxidase-positive neutrophils in atherosclerotic lesions in LDLR-/- mice. *Arterioscler. Thromb. Vasc. Biol.* 2008; 28: 84-9.

[130] Cadroy Y, Dupouy D, Boneu B, Plaisancie H. Polymorphonuclear leukocytes modulate tissue factor production by mononuclear cells: role of reactive oxygen species. *J. Immunol.* 2000; 164: 3822-8.

[131] Mitarai T. Anti-neutrophil cytoplasmic autoantibodies associated renal diseases and thrombotic microangiopathy. *Intern. Med.* 1998; 37: 207-10.

[132] Tervaert JW, Stegeman CA, Kallenberg CG. Novel therapies for anti-neutrophil cytoplasmic antibody-associated vasculitis. *Curr. Opin. Nephrol. Hypertens* 2001; 10: 211-7.

[133] Liu X, Piela-Smith TH. Fibrin(ogen)-induced expression of ICAM-1 and chemokines in human synovial fibroblasts. *J. Immunol.* 2000; 165: 5255-61.

[134] Anstee QM, Goldin RD, Wright M, Martinelli A, Cox R, Thursz MR. Coagulation status modulates murine hepatic fibrogenesis: implications for the development of novel therapies. *J. Thromb. Haemost.* 2008; 6: 1336-43.

[135] Van Giezen JJJ, Chung-A-Hing JE, Vegter CB, Bouma BN, Jansen JWCM. Fibrinolytic activity in blood is distributed over a cellular and the plasma fraction which can be modulated separately. *Thromb. Haemost.* 1994; 72: 887-92.

[136] Moir E, Robbie LA, Bennett B, Booth NA. *Polymorphonuclear leucocyte mediate spontaneous thrombus lysis via urokinase*. ISTH 1999 Washington.

[137] Stief TW, Fröhlich S, Renz H. Determination of the global fibrinolytic state. *Blood Coagul. Fibrinolysis* 2007; 18: 479-87.

[138] Stief TW. Singlet oxygen enhances intrinsic thrombolysis: the intrinsic oxidative clot lysis assay (INOXCLA). *Clin. Appl. Thromb. Hemost.* 2007; 13: 369-83.

[139] Haj MA, Neilly IJ, Robbie LA; Adey GD, Bennett B. Influence of white blood cells on the fibrinolytic response to sepsis: studies of septic patients with or without severe leucopenia. *Br. J. Haematol.* 1995; 90: 541-7.

[140] Bach-Gansmo ET, Halvorsen S, Godal HC, Skjönsberg OH. D-Dimers are degraded by human neutrophil elastase. *Thromb. Res.* 1996; 82: 177-86.
[141] Brown KA, Brain SD, Pearson JD, Edgeworth JD, Lewis SM, Treacher DF. Neutrophils in development of multiple organ failure in sepsis. *Lancet* 2006; 368: 157-69.
[142] Stief TW, Ijagha O, Weiste B, Herzum I, Renz H, Max M. Analysis of hemostasis alterations in sepsis. *Blood Coagul. Fibrinolysis* 2007; 18: 179-86.
[143] Andrade J, Al Ali A, Saw J, Wong GC. Acute stent thrombosis in a patient with giant cell arteritis. *Can. J. Cardiol.* 2008; 24: e25-6.
[144] Menon SP, Rajkumar SV, Lacy M, Falco P, Palumbo A. Thromboembolic events with lenalidomide-based therapy for multiple myeloma. *Cancer* 2008; 112: 1522-8.
[145] Jilma B, Cvitko T, Winter-Fabry A, Petroczi K, Quehenberger P, Blann AD. High dose dexamethasone increases circulating P-selectin and von Willebrand factor levels in healthy men. *Thromb. Haemost.* 2005; 94: 797-801.
[146] Frank RD, Altenwerth B, Brandenburg VM, Nolden-Koch M, Block F. Effect of intravenous high-dose methylprednisolone on coagulation and fibrinolysis markers. *Thromb. Haemost* 2005; 94: 467-8.
[147] Stief TW. Nonradical excited oxygen species induce selective thrombolysis in vivo. *Thromb. Res.* 1991; 62: 147-63.
[148] Falanga A, Marchetti M, Evangelista V, Manarini S, Oldani E, Giovanelli S, Galbusera M, Cerletti C, Barbui T. Neutrophil Activation and hemostatic changes in healthy donors receiving granulocyte colony-stimulating factor. *Blood* 1999; 93: 2506-14.
[149] Stief T. G-CSF enhances cellular fibrinolysis. *Clin. Appl. Thromb. Hemost.* 2006 ; 12: 122.
[150] Kleemann R, Zadelaar S, Kooistra T. Cytokines and atherosclerosis: a comprehensive review of studies in mice. *Cardiovasc. Res.* 2008; 79: 360-76.
[151] Gyetko MR, Sud S, Kendall T, Fuller JA, Newstead MW, Standiford TJ. Urokinase receptor-deficient mice have impaired neutrophil recruitment in response to pulmonary pseudomonas aeruginose infection. *J. Immunol.* 2000; 165: 1513-9.
[152] Plow EF, Felez J, Miles LA. Cellular regulation of fibrinolysis. *Thromb. Haemost.* 1991; 66: 32-6.
[153] Vinazzer HA. Antithrombin III in shock and disseminated intravascular coagulation. *Clin. Appl. Thromb. Hemost.* 1995; 1: 62-65.
[154] Stief TW. Thrombin generation by exposure of blood to endotoxin: a simple model to study disseminated intravascular coagulation. *Clin. Appl. Thromb. Hemost.* 2006; 12: 137-61.
[155] Kelvin DJ, Michiel DF, Johnston JA, Lloyd AR, Sprenger H, Oppenheim JJ, Wang JM. Chemokines and serpentines: the molecular biology of chemokine receptors. *J. Leukoc. Biol.* 1993; 54: 604-12.
[156] Wang ZY, Chen Z. Acute promyelocytic leukemia: from highly fatal to highly curable. *Blood* 2008; 111: 2505-15.
[157] Clagett-Dame M, McNeill EM, Muley PD. Role of all-trans retinoic acid in neurite outgrowth and axonal elongation. *J. Neurobiol.* 2006; 66: 739-56.
[158] Lane MA, Bailey SJ. Role of retinoid signalling in the adult brain. *Prog. Neurobiol.* 2005; 75: 275-93.

[159] Salih HR, Kiener PA. Alterations in Fas (CD 95/Apo-1) and Fas ligand (CD178) expression in acute promyelocytic leukemia during treatment with ATRA. *Leuk. Lymphoma* 2004; 45: 55-9.
[160] Capitani S, Marchisio M, Neri LM, Brugnoli F, Gonelli A, Bertagnolo V. Phosphoinositide 3-kinase is associated to the nucleus of HL-60 cells and is involved in their ATRA-induced granulocytic differentiation. *Eur. J. Histochem.* 2000; 44: 61-5.
[161] Hofmann SL. Retinoids--"differentiation agents" for cancer treatment and prevention. *Am. J. Med. Sci.* 1992; 304: 202-13.
[162] Warso MA, Lands WE. Presence of lipid hydroperoxide in human plasma. *J. Clin. Invest.* 1985; 75: 667-71.
[163] Petrone WF, English DK, Wong K, McCord JM. Free radicals and inflammation: superoxide-dependent activation of a neutrophil chemotactic factor in plasma. *Proc. Natl. Acad. Sci. USA* 1980; 77: 1159-63.
[164] McCord JM. A superoxide-activated chemotactic factor and its role in the inflammatory process. *Agents Actions* 1980; 10: 522-7.
[165] McCord JM.Superoxide radical: controversies, contradictions, and paradoxes. *Proc. Soc. Exp. Biol. Med.* 1995; 209: 112-7.
[166] Khan AU, Kasha M. Singlet molecular oxygen in the Haber-Weiss reaction. *Proc. Natl. Acad. Sci. USA* 1994; 91: 12365-7.
[167] McCord JM, Day ED Jr. Superoxide-dependent production of hydroxyl radical catalyzed by iron-EDTA complex. *FEBS Lett.* 1978; 86: 139-42.
[168] Salin ML, McCord JM. Superoxide dismutases in polymorphonuclear leukocytes. *J. Clin. Invest* 1974; 54: 1005-9.
[169] Sluiter W, de Vree WJ, Pietersma A, Koster JF. Prevention of late lumen loss after coronary angioplasty by photodynamic therapy: role of activated neutrophils. *Mol. Cell Biochem.* 1996; 157: 233-8.
[170] Klebanoff SJ, Locksley RM, Jong EC, Rosen H. Oxidative response of phagocytes to parasite invasion. *Ciba Found Symp.* 1983; 99: 92-112.
[171] Rosen H, Klebanoff SJ. Bactericidal activity of a superoxide anion-generating system. A model for the polymorphonuclear leukocyte. *J. Exp. Med.* 1979; 149: 27-39.
[172] Rosen H, Klebanoff SJ. Formation of singlet oxygen by the myeloperoxidase-mediated antimicrobial system. *J. Biol. Chem.* 1977; 252: 4803-10.
[173] Merhi Y, King M, Guidoin R. Acute thrombogenicity of intact and injured natural blood conduits versus synthetic conduits: neutrophil, platelet, and fibrin(ogen) adsorption under various shear-rate conditions. *J. Biomed. Mater. Res.* 1997; 34: 477-85.
[174] Collen D, Lijnen HR. The fibrinolytic system in man. *Crit. Rev. Oncol. Hematol.* 1986; 4: 249-301.
[175] Stief TW, Richter A, Bünder R, Maisch B, Renz H. Monitoring of plasmin and plasminogen activator activity in blood of patients under fibrinolytic treatment by reteplase. *Clin. Appl. Thromb. Hemost.* 2006; 12: 213-8.
[176] Kwaan HC, Astrup T. Demonstration of cellular fibrinolytic activity by the histochemical fibrin slide technique. *Lab. Invest.* 1967; 17: 140-5.
[177] Langleben D, Moroz LA. Interspecies variation in the cellular phase of blood fibrinolytic activity. *Proc. Soc. Exp. Biol. Med.* 1991; 196: 270-2.

[178] Humphries JE, Vasudevan J, Gonias SL. Fibrinogenolytic and fibrinolytic activity of cell-associated plasmin. *Arterioscler. Thromb.* 1993; 13: 48-55.

[179] Calderwood JW, Williams JM, Morgan MD, Nash GB, Savage CO. ANCA induces beta2 integrin and CXC chemokine-dependent neutrophil-endothelial cell interactions that mimic those of highly cytokine-activated endothelium. *J. Leukoc. Biol.* 2005; 77: 33-43.

[180] Broudy VC, Kaushansky K, Harlan JM, Adamson JW. Interleukin 1 stimulates human endothelial cells to produce granulocyte-macrophage colony-stimulating factor and granulocyte colony-stimulating factor. J. *Immunol.* 1987; 139: 464-8.

[181] Kitagawa Y, Van Eeden SF, Redenbach DM, Daya M, Walker BA, Klut ME, Wiggs BR, Hogg JC. Effect of mechanical deformation on structure and function of polymorphonuclear leukocytes. *J. Appl. Physiol.* 1997; 82: 1397-405.

[182] Ramamoorthy C, Kovarik WD, Winn RK, Harlan JM, Sharar SR. Neutrophil adhesion molecule expression is comparable in perinatal rabbits and humans. *Anesthesiology* 1997; 86: 420-7.

[183] Schwartz BR, Harlan JM. Sulfhydryl reducing agents promote neutrophil adherence without increasing surface expression of CD11b/CD18 (Mac-1, Mo1). *Biochem. Biophys. Res. Commun.* 1989; 165: 51-7.

[184] Vedder NB, Harlan JM. Increased surface expression of CD11b/CD18 (Mac-1) is not required for stimulated neutrophil adherence to cultured endothelium. *J. Clin. Invest* 1988; 81: 676-82.

[185] Rochon YP, Kavanagh TJ, Harlan JM. Analysis of integrin (CD11b/CD18) movement during neutrophil adhesion and migration on endothelial cells. *J. Microsc.* 2000; 197: 15-24.

[186] Nagata M, Yamamoto H, Shibasaki M, Sakamoto Y, Matsuo H. Hydrogen peroxide augments eosinophil adhesion via beta2 integrin. *Immunology* 2000; 101: 412-8.

[187] Lu H, Ballantyne C, Smith CW. LFA-1 (CD11a/CD18) triggers hydrogen peroxide production by canine neutrophils. *J. Leukoc. Biol.* 2000; 68: 73-80.

[188] Lu H, Youker K, Ballantyne C, Entman M, Smith CW. Hydrogen peroxide induces LFA-1-dependent neutrophil adherence to cardiac myocytes. *Am. J. Physiol. Heart Circ. Physiol.* 2000; 278: H835-42.

[189] Blouin E, Halbwachs-Mecarelli L, Rieu P. Redox regulation of beta2-integrin CD11b/CD18 activation. *Eur. J. Immunol.* 1999; 29: 3419-31.

[190] Repo H, Rochon YP, Schwartz BR, Sharar SR, Winn RK, Harlan JM. Binding of human peripheral blood polymorphonuclear leukocytes to E-selectin (CD62E) does not promote their activation. *J. Immunol.* 1997; 159: 943-51.

[191] Fraticelli A, Serrano CV Jr, Bochner BS, Capogrossi MC, Zweier JL. Hydrogen peroxide and superoxide modulate leukocyte adhesion molecule expression and leukocyte endothelial adhesion. *Biochim. Biophys Acta* 1996; 1310: 251-9.

[192] Wikman A, Lundahl J, Fernvik E, Shanwell A. Altered expression of adhesion molecules (L-selectin and Mac-1) on granulocytes during storage. *Transfusion* 1994 ; 34: 167-71.

[193] Vaporciyan AA, Ward PA. Enhanced generation of $\cdot O_2^-$ by human neutrophils via a complement iC3b/Mac-1 interaction. *Biol. Signals* 1993; 2: 126-35.

[194] Shappell SB, Toman C, Anderson DC, Taylor AA, Entman ML, Smith CW. Mac-1 (CD11b/CD18) mediates adherence-dependent hydrogen peroxide production by human and canine neutrophils. *J. Immunol.* 1990; 144: 2702-11.

[195] Skoglund G, Cotgreave I, Rincon J, Patarroyo M, Ingelman-Sundberg M. H_2O_2 activates CD11b/CD18-dependent cell adhesion. *Biochem. Biophys. Res. Commun.* 1988; 157: 443-9.

[196] Berton G, Lowell CA. Integrin signalling in neutrophils and macrophages. *Cell Signal* 1999; 11: 621-35.

[197] Wang Q, Doerschuk CM. Neutrophil-induced changes in the biomechanical properties of endothelial cells: roles of ICAM-1 and reactive oxygen species. *J. Immunol.* 2000; 164: 6487-94.

[198] Darley-Usmar VM, Lelchuk R, O'Leary VJ, Knowles M, Rogers MV, Severn A. Oxidation of low-density lipoprotein and macrophage derived foam cells. *Biochem. Soc. Trans* 1990; 18: 1064-6.

[199] Aleksandrowicz P, Wolf K, Falzarano D, Feldmann H, Seebach J, Schnittler H. Viral haemorrhagic fever and vascular alterations. *Hamostaseologie* 2008; 28: 77-84.

[200] Naito M. Macrophage differentiation and function in health and disease. *Pathol. Int.* 2008; 58: 143-55.

[201] Wynn TA. Cellular and molecular mechanisms of fibrosis. *J. Pathol.* 2008; 214: 199-210.

[202] Allavena P, Sica A, Solinas G, Porta C, Mantovani A. The inflammatory micro-environment in tumor progression: the role of tumor-associated macrophages. *Crit. Rev. Oncol. Hematol.* 2008; 66: 1-9.

[203] Papatheodorou L, Weiss N. Vascular oxidant stress and inflammation in hyperhomocysteinemia. *Antioxid. Redox. Signal* 2007; 9: 1941-58.

[204] Meerarani P, Moreno PR, Cimmino G, Badimon JJ. Atherothrombosis: role of tissue factor; link between diabetes, obesity and inflammation. *Indian J. Exp. Biol.* 2007; 45: 103-10.

[205] Croce K, Libby P. Intertwining of thrombosis and inflammation in atherosclerosis. *Curr. Opin. Hematol.* 2007; 14: 55-61.

[206] Serruys PW, García-García HM, Buszman P, Erne P, Verheye S, Aschermann M, Duckers H, Bleie O, Dudek D, Bøtker HE, von Birgelen C, D'Amico D, Hutchinson T, Zambanini A, Mastik F, van Es GA, van der Steen AF, Vince DG, Ganz P, Hamm CW, Wijns W, Zalewski A; for the Integrated Biomarker and Imaging Study-2 Investigators. Effects of the Direct Lipoprotein-Associated Phospholipase A2 Inhibitor Darapladib on Human Coronary Atherosclerotic Plaque. *Circulation* 2008 Sep 1. [Epub ahead of print]

[207] Witting PK, Zeng B, Wong M, McMahon AC, Rayner BS, Sapir AJ, Lowe HC, Freedman SB, Brieger DB. Polymorphonuclear leukocyte phagocytic function increases in plasminogen knockout mice. *Thromb. Res.* 2008; 122: 674-82.

[208] Bouly JP, Schleicher E, Dionisio-Sese M, Vandenbussche F, Van Der Straeten D, Bakrim N, Meier S, Batschauer A, Galland P, Bittl R, Ahmad M. Cryptochrome blue light photoreceptors are activated through interconversion of flavin redox states. *J. Biol. Chem.* 2007; 282: 9383-91.

[209] Hoang N, Schleicher E, Kacprzak S, Bouly JP, Picot M, Wu W, Berndt A, Wolf E, Bittl R, Ahmad M. Human and Drosophila cryptochromes are light activated by flavin photoreduction in living cells. *PLoS Biol.* 2008; 6: e160.

[210] Stief TW. Hemostasis tolerable singlet oxygen as a perspective in AIDS therapy. *Hemostasis Laboratory* 2008; 1: 21-40.

[211] Stief TW. The laboratory diagnosis of the pre-phase of pathologic disseminated intravascular coagulation. *Hemostasis Laboratory* 2008; 1: 2-20.

[212] Tian W, Li XJ, Stull ND, Ming W, Suh CI, Bissonnette SA, Yaffe MB, Grinstein S, Atkinson SJ, Dinauer MC. FcγR-stimulated activation of the NADPH oxidase: phosphoinositide-binding protein $p40^{phox}$ regulates NADPH oxidase activity after enzyme assembly on the phagosome. *Blood* 2008; 112: 3867-77.

In: Hemostasis Laboratory Yearbook, Volume 2
Editor: Thomas W. Stief, pp. 289-294
ISBN: 978-1-60741-089-8

PRE-ANALYTIC COAGULATION ACTIVATION BY DIFFERENT BLOOD SAMPLING TUBES

Thomas W. Stief *

Department of Clinical Chemistry,
University Hospital Giessen and Marburg, Germany

ABSTRACT

Background: Plastic tubes or siliconized glass tubes are currently used for diagnostic blood sampling. In the present work thrombin generation of pooled normal plasma stored in different tubes was studied in the ultra-specific, ultra-sensitive thrombin generation assay RECA (recalcified coagulation activity assay).

Material and Methods: 600 µl unfrozen pooled normal citrated plasma was incubated for 30 min at 23°C in emptied polypropylene (PP) tubes from Sarstedt, or emptied polyethylene (PE) tubes, emptied siliconized glass tubes, unsiliconized glass tubes from Becton Dickinson. Then the recalcified coagulation activity assay (RECA) was performed with 50 µl pooled normal plasma in U-polystyrol-microwells (Brand®701300), 5 µl RECA-trigger (250 mM $CaCl_2$), 0-35 min coagulation reaction time at 37°C (CRT), 100 µl arginine-reagent (2.5 M arginine, pH 8.6, 0.16 % Triton X 100®), 3 min incubation, addition of 25 µl 1 mM chromogenic thrombin substrate HD-CHG-Ala-Arg-pNA in 1.25 M arginine, pH 8.7, and determination of ΔA at 405 nm.

Results: The plastic tubes (either made of PP or of PE) generated much less thrombin in RECA than glass tubes. PE tubes behaved very similarly as PP tubes: at 20 min CRT (=RECA-20) the plastic tubes generated 0.04-0.05 IU/ml thrombin. Siliconized glass tubes generated about 10fold more thrombin at RECA-20 and unsiliconized glass tubes generated about 10fold more thrombin than siliconized glass tubes, when analyzed at RECA-10 or RECA-15.

Discussion: Pre-analytic alteration of plasma should be minimized. For ultra-specific, ultra-sensitive thrombin generation assays there should be neither blood-collection-tube-induced increased thrombin generation nor blood-collection-tube-induced decreased thrombin generation of the recalcified plasma sample. For this purpose plastic tubes of the type of polypropylene or of polyethylene are preferable to procoagulant siliconized glass tubes.

Keywords: Thrombin, RECA, polypropylene, polyethylene, siliconized glass, pre-analytic.

---

* Correspondence to: PD Dr. med. T. Stief, Department of Clinical Chemistry, University Hospital, D-35043 Marburg, Germany. email: thstief@med.uni-marburg.de; Tel. : +49-6421-58 64471; FAX: +49-6421-58 65594.

INTRODUCTION

Thrombin generation is of great clinical and of great analytical interest. To diagnose normal or pathological thrombin generation in recalcified citrated plasma, the pre-analytic conditions are of primary importance [1]. The blood collection tube should be made of such a material that there is neither false in-vitro activation nor false in-vitro inhibition of the recalcified plasma [2]. Currently, siliconized glass tubes or plastic tubes are clinically used. The aim of the present work was to compare thrombin generation of plasmas stored in different tubes by means of the ultra- specific, -sensitive, and -precise thrombin generation assay RECA (recalcified coagulation activity assay) [3-6].

MATERIAL AND METHODS

Pre-Incubation of Pooled Normal Plasma in Different Tubes

600 µl unfrozen pooled normal citrated plasma (from 6 individual samples that remained after routine analysis; 4.5 ml venous blood drawn into polypropylene (PP) tubes that contained 0.5 ml 106 mM sodium citrate; Sarstedt, Nümbrecht, Germany; the blood was centrifuged at 2800g for 10 min; the analyzed plasma samples remained after routine analysis, were 4±1 h old, were stored at 23°C, and were then pooled into emptied PP tubes for the present quality assurance of routine analysis of thrombin activity of patient plasma) was given in duplicate into emptied 2.7 ml polyethylene (PE) tubes from Becton Dickinson (BD; Plymouth, UK, article nr. 363048, lot nr. 8190145, valid thru 03-2009, containing 0.27 ml 105 mM sodium citrate), 5 ml emptied BD-glass tubes (article nr. 367714, lot nr. 8176993, valid thru 12-2009, containing 0.5 ml 105 mM sodium citrate), 5 ml BD-glass tubes (article nr. 367614, lot nr. 8157482, valid thru 11-2009), or 5 ml emptied PP tubes from Sarstedt (article nr. 05.1071, lot nr. 8092002, valid thru 08-2009). After 30 min pre-incubation time at 23°C or at 37°C 50 µl samples were added to polystyrol U-well microtiter plates (Brand, Wertheim, Germany, article nr. 701300). 5 µl 250 mM $CaCl_2$ (trigger of the recalcified coagulation activity assay = RECA) were added and the RECA was performed with coagulation reaction times (CRT) of 0-35 min. Thrombin generation = thrombin activity after a certain CRT minus basal thrombin activity (0 min CRT).

The pre-incubation experiment at 23°C was repeated with another pool of unfrozen citrated normal plasma.

Influence of Repetitive Addition of Pooled Normal Citrated Plasma to Emptied PP Tubes

4 ml unfrozen normal citrated plasma from 6 individual samples were pooled into an emptied PP tube, 1000 µl pooled plasma were withdrawn and were added to a second PP tube, 500 µl pooled plasma were withdrawn and added to a third PP tube. The following reaction conditions were as described above.

Coagulation Activation by Siliconized Glass Vials

4 ml unfrozen normal citrated plasma from 6 individual samples were pooled into an emptied Sarstedt-PP tube, 500 µl pooled normal plasma were withdrawn and added to a DadeBehring siliconized glass vial (article nr. OVKE49®) or to an inverted white polystyrol top of this glass vial. The reaction conditions were as indicated above.

RESULTS AND DISCUSSION

Figure 1 demonstrates that the plastic tubes (either made of PP or of PE) generated much less thrombin in RECA than glass tubes. PE tubes behaved very similarly as PP tubes: at 20 min CRT (=RECA-20) the plastic tubes generated 0.04-0.05 IU/ml thrombin. Siliconized glass tubes generated about 10fold more thrombin at RECA-20 and unsiliconized glass tubes generated about 10fold more thrombin than siliconized glass tube, when analyzed at RECA-10 or RECA-15. For comparison of both glass types here RECA-10 or RECA-15 is superior to RECA-20, because only thrombin activities that belong to the ascending part of the thrombin generation curve are valid, decreasing or near-maximal thrombin activities might be difficult to interprete due nascending fibrin = antithrombin I, that entraps thrombin.

If the pre-incubation is performed at 37°C instead of the usual pre-analytic temperature of about 23°C, thrombin generation in the unsiliconized glass tubes did not change when compared with 23°C (Figure 2).

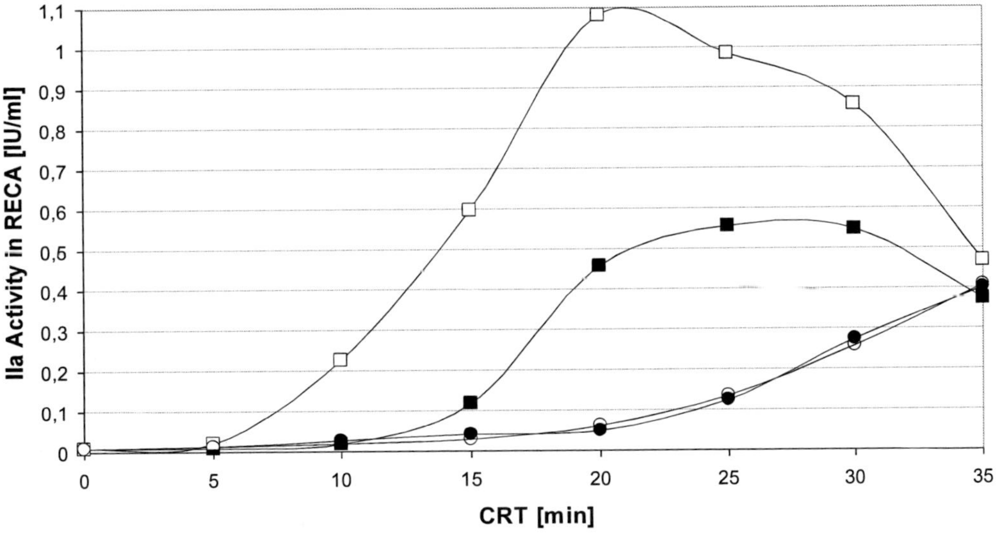

Figure 1. Pre-incubation of pooled normal plasma in different tubes for 30 min at 23°C. 600 µl unfrozen pooled normal citrated plasma was given into emptied 2.7 ml polyethylene tubes from Becton Dickinson (BD) (●), emptied 5 ml BD-glass tubes (■), 5 ml BD-glass tubes (□), or emptied 5 ml PP tubes from Sarstedt (O). After 30 min pre-incubation time at 23°C 50 µl samples were added to U-well microtiter plates (Brand®701300). 5 µl 250 mM $CaCl_2$ (trigger of the recalcified coagulation activity assay = RECA) were added and the RECA was performed with coagulation reaction times (CRT) of 0-35 min. Thrombin (IIa) generation = IIa activity minus basal IIa (at 0 min CRT).

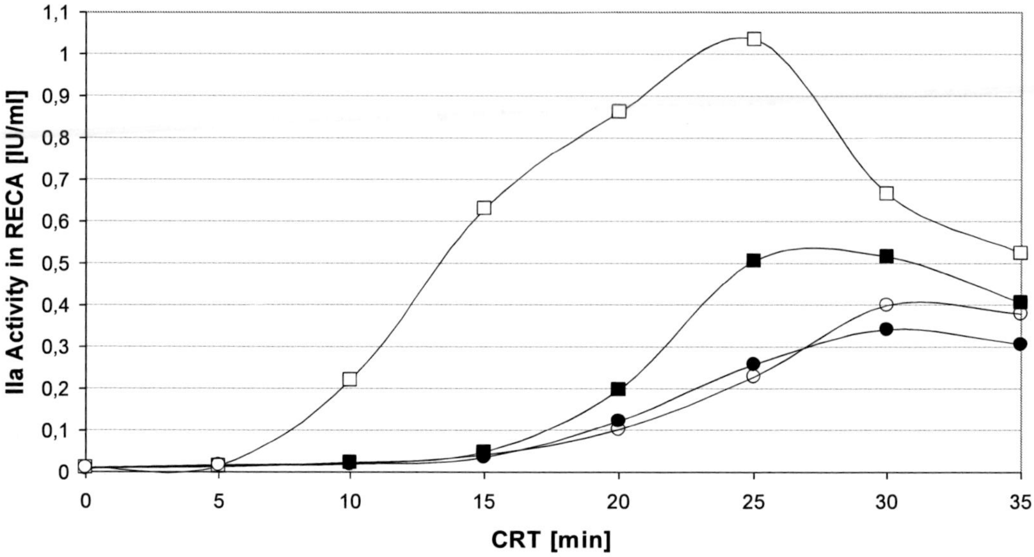

Figure 2. Pre-incubation of pooled normal plasma in different tubes for 30 min at 37°C. The experiment of figure 1 was performed with a pre-incubation period of 30 min at 37°C (water-bath) with emptied BD-polyethylene tubes (●), emptied BD-glass tubes (■), BD-glass tubes (□), or emptied PP tubes from Sarstedt (O).

The siliconized glass tubes generated at 37°C about halve the amount of thrombin when compared with 23°C incubation. PP and PE generated at 37°C about twice the amount of thrombin when compared with 23°C incubation. Thus, 37°C incubation of plasma in PP or PE was slightly procoagulant. The PP tubes seemed to contain a substance that favours thrombin generation: repetitive addition of pooled normal plasma to several PP tubes increased about 3fold thrombin generation at RECA-15, if the pooled plasma in the first PP tube was withdrawn, added to a second PP tube, withdrawn from this second one and given to a third PP tube (Figure 3). For thrombin activity comparisons the lowest CRT that generates significant thrombin activities is best; thrombin generations at high CRTs might be artificially altered by antithrombin I (descending part of the IIa generation curve).

The similar thrombin generation in both plastic types (PP or PE) could again be observed, when the experiment of figure 1 was repeated with another pool of normal citrated plasma (Figure 4).

Another type of siliconized glass are the 15 ml OVKE-49® vials of DadeBehring. These vials can be used for 1 ml aliquots of triggers of RECA, INCA (intrinsic coagulation activity assay), or EXCA (extrinsic coagulation activity assay). Therefore, thrombin generation was studied with pooled plasma pre-incubated in this type of siliconized glass. At RECA-10 OVKE-49® vials generated about twice the amount of thrombin when compared with PP tubes (Figure 5). At higher CRTs the thrombin generation in PP tubes was slightly higher than in OVKE-49® vials, i.e. this siliconized glass is slightly procoagulant at more important lower CRTs and becomes slightly anticoagulant at less important higher CRTs.

SiO_2 with its polynegative niches is a known activator of the contact phase of coagulation. Plastic also might possess polynegative niches that might fold pre-kallikrein into kallikrein but these polynegative structures also might behave like heparinoids.

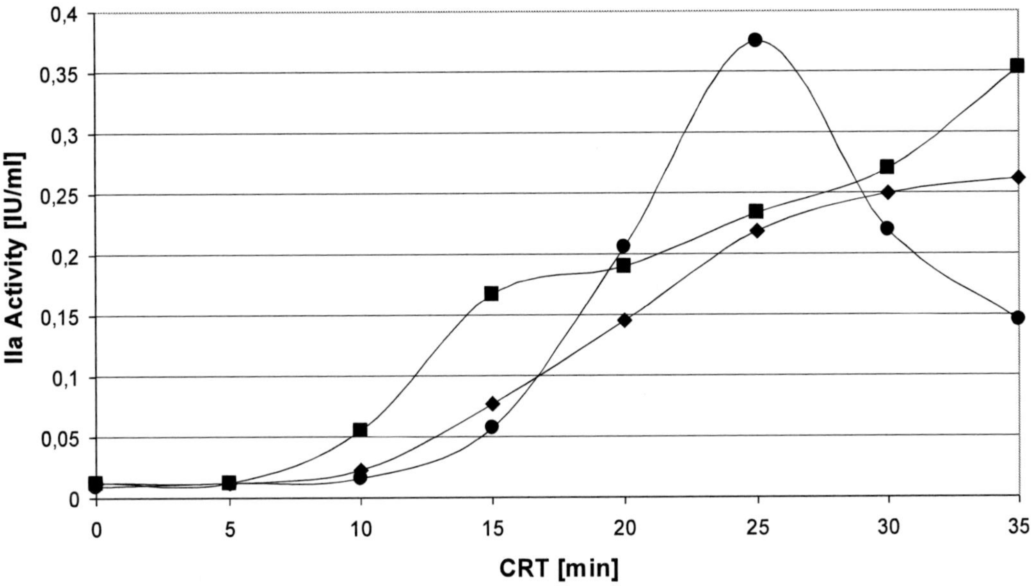

Figure 3. Influence of repetitive addition of pooled normal plasma to emptied PP tubes. 4 ml unfrozen normal citrated plasma of 6 individual samples were pooled into an emptied polypropylene (PP) tube (●), 1000 µl pooled normal plasma were withdrawn and added to a second PP tube (♦), 500 µl pooled normal plasma were withdrawn and added to a third PP tube (■). The reaction conditions were as indicated in figure 1.

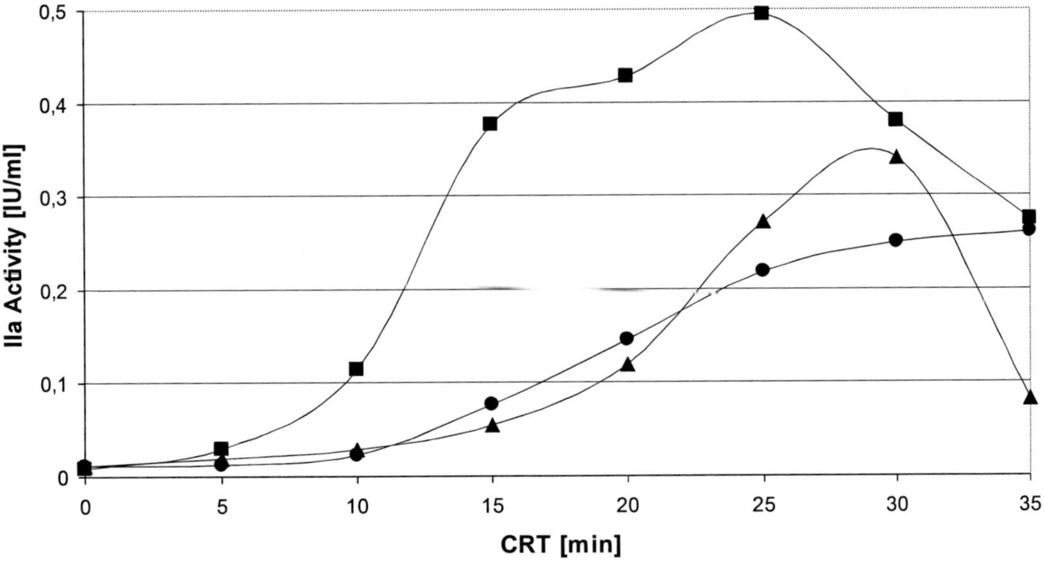

Figure 4. Pre-incubation of another pool of normal plasma in different tubes for 30 min at 23°C. The experiment of figure 1 was repeated with another poold of citrated normal plasma, using emptied BD-glass (■), BD-poly-ethylene (▲), or Sarstedt-polypropylene (●) tubes. The reaction conditions were as indicated in figure 1.

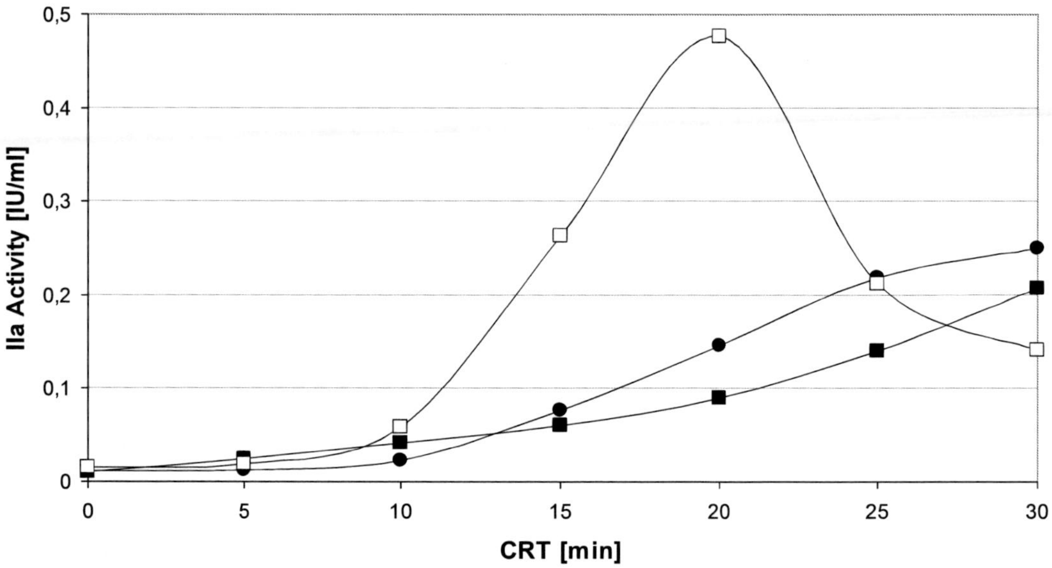

Figure 5. Coagulation activation by siliconized glass vials. 4 ml normal citrated plasma were pooled into an emptied PP tube (●), 500 µl were withdrawn and added to a siliconized glass vial (DadeBehring; OVKE49®) (■) or to an inverted white polystyrol top of this glass vial (□). The reaction conditions were as indicated in figure 1.

Pre-analytic alteration of plasma should be minimized. For ultra-specific, ultra-sensitive thrombin generation assays there should be neither blood-collection-tube-induced increased thrombin generation nor blood-collection-tube-induced decreased thrombin generation of the recalcified plasma sample. For this purpose plastic tubes of the nature of polypropylene or of polyethylene are preferable to procoagulant siliconized glass tubes.

REFERENCES

[1] Schleicher E. The clinical chemistry laboratory: current status, problems and diagnostic prospects. *Anal. Bioanal. Chem*. 2006; 384: 124-31.

[2] Stief TW. Influence of the surface on thrombin generation. *Int. J. Lab. Hematol*. 2008; 30: 269-77.

[3] Stief TW. Inhibition of thrombin generation in recalcified plasma. *Blood Coagul. Fibrinolysis* 2007; 18: 751-60.

[4] Stief TW. Specific determination of plasmatic thrombin activity. *Clin. Appl. Thromb. Hemost*. 2006; 12: 324-9.

[5] Stief TW. Thrombin generation by exposure of blood to endotoxin: a simple model to study disseminated intravascular coagulation. *Clin. Appl. Thromb. Hemost*. 2006; 12: 137-61.

[6] Stief TW. Innovative tests of plasmatic hemostasis. *Laboratory Medicine* 2008; 39: 225-230.

In: Hemostasis Laboratory Yearbook, Volume 2
Editor: Thomas W. Stief, pp. 295-299

ISBN: 978-1-60741-089-8

CONVERSION OF A MEASURED ΔA WITHIN THE NON-LINEAR PART OF A SUBSTRATE CLEAVAGE KINETIC INTO THE TRUE ΔA

Thomas W. Stief*
Department of Clinical Chemistry,
University Hospital Giessen and Marburg, Germany

ABSTRACT

Background: Enzyme reactions often are coupled with the generation of coloured substances. If the enzyme kinetic is still in its linear part, it is easy to convert the respective concentration of a coloured substance into the correct enzyme activity. The aim of the present work was to convert ΔA-values in the non-linear part of an enzyme kinetic into the true ones.

Material and Methods: As exemplary enzyme the hemostasis enzyme thrombin was used. As exemplary substrate HD-CHG-Ala-Arg-pNA at 0.14 mM final concentration, which here is approximately 0.5fold the Km value, was used. 50 µl 0-1 IU/ml bovine thrombin in 6.7 % human albumin were incubated in polystyrol U-well microtiter plates with 100 µl 2.5 M arginine, pH 8.6, 0.16 % Triton X 100®, 5 µl 0.9 % NaCl and 25 µl 1 mM chromogenic pNA-substrate in 1.25 M arginine, pH 8.7 were added and ΔA at 405 nm was determined after 40 min or after 105 min at 23°C.

Results and Discussion: The enzyme kinetic leaves the linear part of the curve at about 40 % of the maximal ΔA. ΔA-values in the non-linear part of the enzyme kinetic can be converted into true ΔA-values by usage of one of the following transformation formulas: $y = 111.09e^{0.0033x}$ or $y = 0.0032x^2 - 0.9853x + 331.81$ with "x" being the ΔA value measured and "y" being the true ΔA-value. These conversion formulas may help to diagnose a pathological enzyme activity within short time periods, avoiding repetition of measurements.

Keywords: Absorbance increase, ΔA, linear kinetic, non-linear kinetic, transformation, chromogenic substrate.

* Correspondence to: PD Dr. med. T. Stief, Department of Clinical Chemistry, University Hospital, D-35043 Marburg, Germany. email: thstief@med.uni-marburg.de; Tel. : +49-6421-58 64471; FAX: +49-6421-58 65594.

Introduction

Chromogenic assays are increasingly used in applied enzymology, e.g. many hemostasis tests base on chromogenic detection of serine proteases such as kallikrein, thrombin, or plasmin [1-3]. The typical chromogenic substrate used is a tripeptide coupled to a para-nitroaniline (pNA) group. To obtain high enzyme specificity the final test concentration is typically approximately in the range of 0.5 fold the Km value (Michaelis-constant) [4-6]. The enzyme that shall be measured cleaves the colourless pNA-bound chromogenic substrate and releases the now yellow – coloured free pNA. Up to a certain concentration of free pNA there appears a linear relationship between enzyme activity and free pNA concentration. From increases of absorbance (ΔA) within this linear part of the enzyme kinetic the enzyme activity can easily be calculated. In clinical-chemical analysis high activities of enzymes might occur in pathologic samples, the enzyme kinetic might leave the linear part and might enter the non-linear part of substrate cleavage, i.e. the part of the enzyme kinetic where substrate exhaustion begins. The purpose of the present work was to mathematically convert such measured free chromophore concentrations into the true free chromophore concentration that would have occurred without substrate exhaustion.

Material and Methods

Substrate Cleavage in Dependence of Thrombin Activity

50 µl 0-1 IU/ml (in repetitive 2+1 dilutions or in repetitive 1+1 dilutions) bovine thrombin (DadeBehring, Marburg, Germany) in 6.7 % human albumin (Kabi, Stockholm, Sweden) were added to polystyrol U-well microtiter plates (Brand, Wertheim, Germany, article nr. 701300). 100 µl 2.5 M arginine, pH 8.6, 0.16 % Triton X 100® (Sigma, Deisenhofen, Germany), 5 µl 0.9 % NaCl (for compensation of trigger volume in ultra-specific thrombin generation assays [3]), and 25 µl 1 mM chromogenic thrombin substrate HD-CHG-Ala-Arg-pNA (Pentapharm, Basel, Switzerland) in 1.25 M arginine, pH 8.7 were added and ΔA at 405 nm was determined after 40 min or after 105 min at 23°C by a microtiter plate photometer with a 1 mA resolution (Mileania; DPC, Los Angeles, USA).

Results and Discussion

The final test concentration of chromogenic substrate in the present experiments was 0.14 mM. The respective Km value of thrombin against this chromogenic substrate under the present assay conditions is approximately 0.25-0.4 mM [4], higher pNA-substrate concentrations may result in artificially enhanced kallikrein activities [5,6], possibly by polynegative (-pNA) activation of kallikrein.

Figure 1 demonstrates that the linear part of the enzyme kinetic is up to about 40 % of the maximal absorbance increase (ΔA) which is approximately 1050 mA (40 % = 420 mA). ΔA values > 420 mA belong to the non-linear part of the enzyme kinetic, i.e. such a ΔA value cannot be simply linearly converted into the correspondent enzyme activity. However, the ΔA values measured in Figure 1 (x-axis) can be plotted against the theoretical true ΔA values (y-axis) that would have occurred, if the whole kinetic would have been in its initial linear phase. Then, an approximation function is: $y = 111.09\ e^{0.0033x}$.

The same procedure applied for figure 2 gives an approximation function of: $y = 0.0032x^2 - 0.9853x + 331.81$.

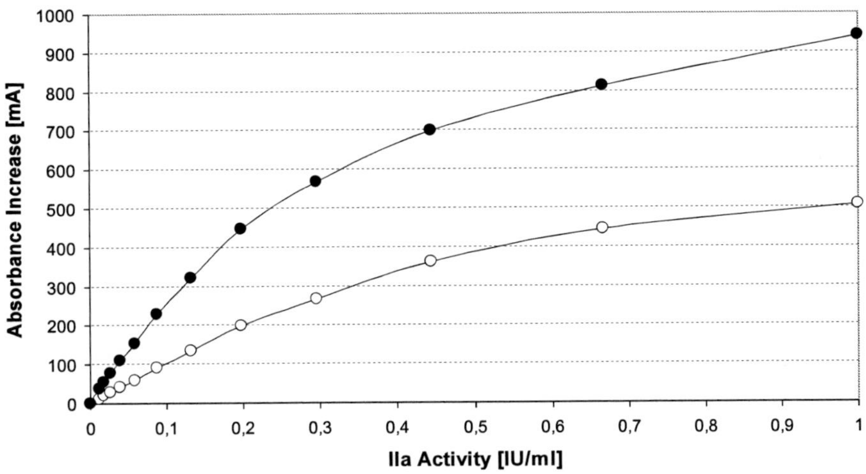

Figure 1. Substrate cleavage in dependence of thrombin activity. 50 µl 0-1 IU/ml (repetitive 2+1 dilutions) thrombin (IIa) in 6.7 % human albumin were added to U-well microtiter plates. 100 µl 2.5 M arginine, pH 8.6, 0.16 % Triton X 100®, 5 µl 0.9 % NaCl, and 25 µl 1 mM HD-CHG-Ala-Arg-pNA in 1.25 M arginine, pH 8.7 were added and ΔA at 405 nm was determined after 40 min (○) or 105 min (●) at 23°C.

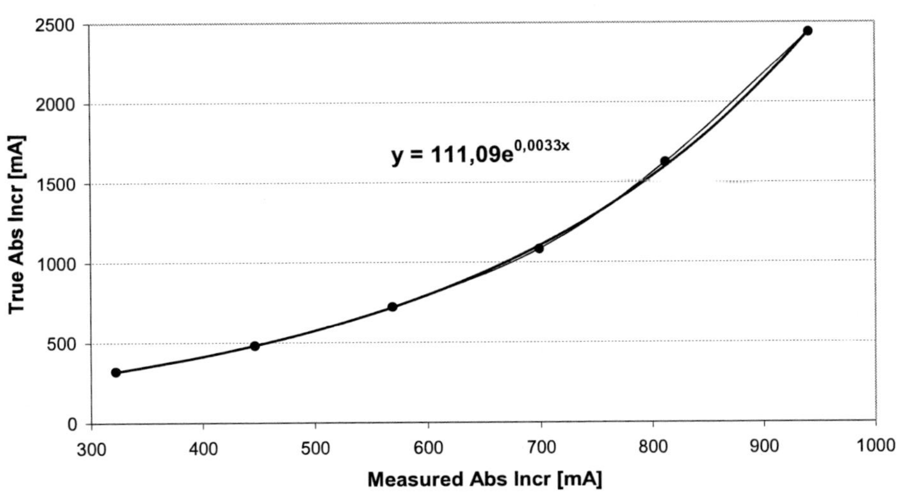

Figure 2. Approximation formula 1. The absorbance-increase (ΔA)- values measured in Figure 1 (x-axis) were plotted against the theoretical true ΔA - values (y-axis) that would have occurred if the whole kinetic would have been in its initial linear phase. An approximation function is: $y = 111.09\ e^{0.0033x}$.

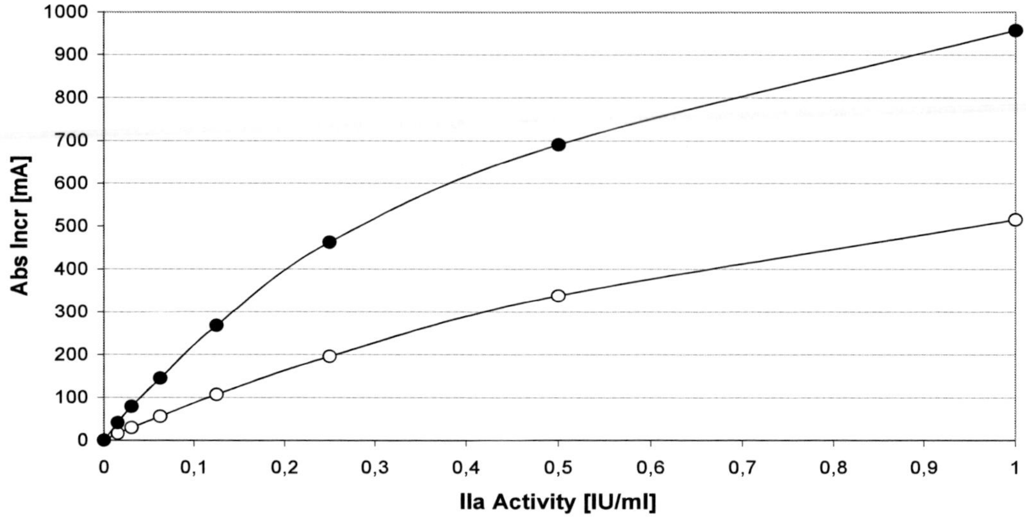

Figure 3. Substrate cleavage in dependence of thrombin activity. 50 µl 0-1 IU/ml (repetitive 1+1 dilutions) thrombin (IIa) in 6.7 % human albumin were added to U-well microtiter plates. 100 µl 2.5 M arginine, pH 8.6, 0.16 % Triton X 100®, 5 µl 0.9 % NaCl, and 25 µl 1 mM HD-CHG-Ala-Arg-pNA in 1.25 M arginine, pH 8.7 were added and ΔA at 405 nm was determined after 40 min (○) or 105 min (●) at 23°C.

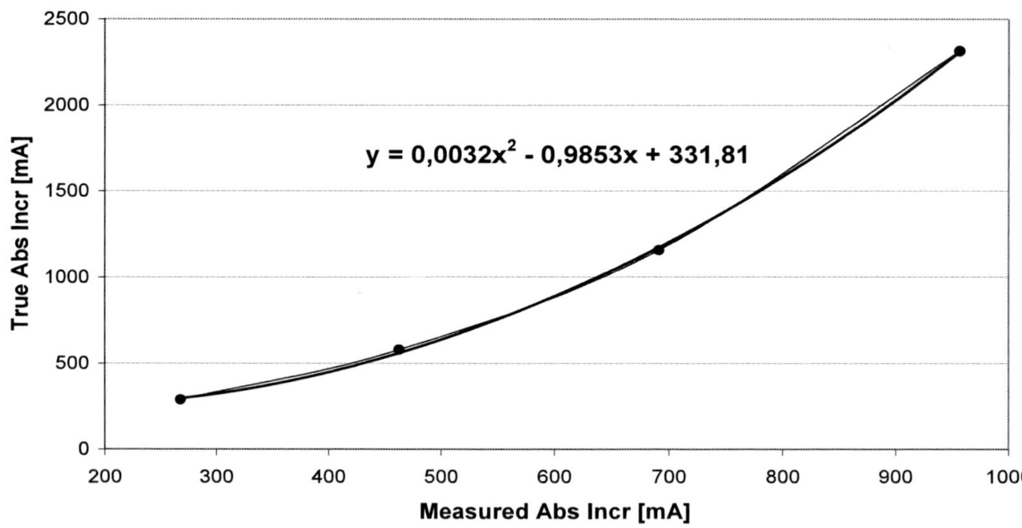

Figure 4. Approximation formula 2. The absorbance-increase (ΔA)- values measured in Fig. 3 (x-axis) were plotted against the theoretical true ΔA - values (y-axis) that would have occurred, if the whole kinetic would have been in its initial linear phase. An approximation function is: $y = 0.0032x^2 - 0.9853x + 331.81$.

Both conversion formulas give similar results. Thus, by using formula 1 or 2 a ΔA value within the non-linear part of an enzyme kinetic with substrate concentrations in the approximate 0.5 fold Km range can be converted into the true ΔA value in the linear part of the respective enzyme kinetic. This procedure facilitates the routine- or the research-diagnostic of pathologic activities of a broad range of different enzymes [7,8].

REFERENCES

[1] Gast A, Tschopp TB. Inhibition of extrinsic and intrinsic thrombin generation by a novel synthetic thrombin inhibitor (Ro 46-6240), recombinant hirudin and heparin in human plasma. *Blood Coagul. Fibrinolysis* 1995; 6: 553-60.

[2] Memari N, Jiang W, Diamandis EP, Luo LY. Enzymatic properties of human kallikrein-related peptidase 12 (KLK12). *Biol. Chem.* 2007; 388: 427-35.

[3] Stief TW. Innovative tests of plasmatic hemostasis. *Laboratory Medicine* 2008; 39: 225-230.

[4] Stief TW. Specific determination of plasmatic thrombin activity. *Clin. Appl. Thromb. Hemost.* 2006; 12: 324-9.

[5] Oliveira L, Araujo-Viel MS, Juliano L, Prado ES. Substrate activation of porcine pancreatic kallikrein by N alpha derivatives of arginine 4-nitroanilides. *Biochemistry* 1987; 26: 5032-5.

[6] Sousa MO, Miranda TL, Maia CN, Bittar ER, Santoro MM, Figueiredo AF. Kinetic peculiarities of human tissue kallikrein: 1--substrate activation in the catalyzed hydrolysis of H-D-valyl-L-leucyl-L-arginine 4-nitroanilide and H-D-valyl-L-leucyl-L-lysine 4-nitroanilide; 2--substrate inhibition in the catalyzed hydrolysis of N-alpha-p-tosyl-L-arginine methyl ester. *Arch. Biochem. Biophys.* 2002; 400: 7-14.

[7] Zabłotna E, Dysasz H, Lesner A, Jaśkiewicz A, Kaźmierczak K, Miecznikowska H, Rolka K. A simple method for selection of trypsin chromogenic substrates using combinatorial chemistry approach. *Biochem. Biophys. Res. Commun.* 2004; 319: 185-8.

[8] Wysocka M, Kwiatkowska B, Rzadkiewicz M, Lesner A, Rolka K. Selection of new chromogenic substrates of serine proteinases using combinatorial chemistry methods. *Comb. Chem. High Throughput Screen* 2007; 10: 171-80.

In: Hemostasis Laboratory Yearbook, Volume 2
Editor: Thomas W. Stief, pp. 301-364

ISBN: 978-1-60741-089-8

Asparaginase Modulates Thrombin Generation

Thomas W. Stief **and Danuta Chalkitis***
Department of Clinical Chemistry,
University Hospital Giessen and Marburg, Germany

Abstract

Background: The bacterial enzyme asparaginase that attacks asparagines or glutamines is clinically used as part of the therapy of acute lymphoblastic leukaemia (ALL). Asparaginase is known to be pro-thrombotic in some patients. It was the aim of the present work to identify such problematic plasmas by means of in-vitro addition of asparaginase immediately followed by performance of a new ultra-specific and -sensitive thrombin generation assay: the recalcified coagulation activity assay (RECA).

Material and Methods: 50 μl samples of n=57 individual unfrozen citrated normal plasmas and of n=7 pools of 7±1 individual unfrozen citrated normal plasmas were supplemented by repetitive 1+1 dilution in polystyrol U-microwells (Brand®701300) with 0-100 U/ml *Escherichia coli* - asparaginase. Immediately thereafter the RECA was performed with coagulation reaction times (CRT) of 0-20 min (37°C). The approximate 200 % stimulatory concentrations (SC200) or the approximate 50 % inhibitory concentrations (IC50) of plasmatic asparaginase were determined using the respective most sensible CRT.

Results: For 29 plasma samples (51 %) there appeared only a SC200 (approx. SC200-mean = 10 U/ml asparaginase). 12 samples (21 %) had only an IC50 (approx. IC50-mean = 10 U/ml asparaginase). 14 samples (24.5 %) had both a SC200 and an IC50 (approx. SC200-mean = 40 U/ml and approx. IC50-mean = 4 U/ml asparaginase). 2 plasma samples (3.5 %) had neither a SC200 nor an IC50. Of the n=29 individual plasma samples with only a SC200 for asparaginase about one third (10/29) had a SC200 < 3 U/ml, about one third (10/29) had a SC200 of 3-20 U/ml, and about one third (9/29) had a SC200 > 20 U/ml.

Discussion: The present asparaginase preparation might pathologically activate or pathologically inactivate intrinsic coagulation. The present work demonstrates that the coagulation - altering capacity of any drug (e.g. asparaginase) in individual plasma samples can be measured prior to the administration of this drug to the patient. With the RECA, the patient´s individual coagulation response to any drug can be pre-viewed, allowing individual dosage adjustments.

Keywords: Asparaginase, thrombin, RECA, SC200, IC50.

---

* Correspondence to: PD Dr. med. T. Stief, Department of Clinical Chemistry, University Hospital, D-35043 Marburg, Germany. email: thstief@med.uni-marburg.de; Tel. : +49-6421-58 64471; FAX: +49-6421-58 65594

INTRODUCTION

Asparaginase is a bacterial enzyme that transforms asparagine or glutamine to NH_3 and aspartic acid or glutamic acid, respectively [1]. L-Asparaginase is clinically used in combination with cytostatics and glucocortidoids to treat acute lymphoblastic leukaemia (ALL) or Non-Hodgkin´s Lymphoma (NHL) because lymphoblasts are much more susceptible to asparaginase than mature lymphocytes [2,3]. At plasma concentrations > 0.4 IU/ml about 90 % of all free asparagines or of all free glutamines and about 40 % of all free arginines are deaminated [1,4]. An important side reaction of plasmatic asparaginase is the enhancement of thrombin generation [5], probably via triggering the intrinsic phase of hemostasis. Therefore up to about one third of the patients treated with asparaginase + glucocorticoids develop severe thromboses, mainly of the upper venous system [23].

Recently, new ultra-specific, ultra-sensitive, ultra-precise thrombin generation assays have been developed [6-8]. It was the aim of the present work to quantify plasmatic thrombin generation by means of the recalcified coagulation activity assay (RECA) in unfrozen normal citrated plasma that has been supplemented with asparaginase.

MATERIAL AND METHODS

Thrombin (IIa) Generation in Dependence of Plasmatic Asparaginase Activity

50 µl samples of n=57 individual unfrozen citrated normal plasmas, of n=7 pools of 7±1 individual unfrozen citrated normal plasma, and of one healthy donor (4.5 ml venous blood drawn into polypropylene tubes that contained 0.5 ml 106 mM sodium citrate; Sarstedt, Nümbrecht, Germany; blood was centrifuged at 2800g for 10 min; the analyzed plasma samples remained after routine analysis, were 4±1 h old, and were stored at 23°C for the present quality assurance of thrombin activity analysis of patient plasma) were supplemented by repetitive 1+1 dilution in polystyrol U-microwells (Brand, Wertheim, Germany, article Nr. 701300) with 0-100 U/ml *Escherichia coli* - asparaginase (medac, Hamburg, Germany; 10000 U/ original vial, lot nr. M80125AE, valid thru 07-2010; aliquoted; freshly reconstituted asparaginase and aliquoted frozen/thawed asparaginase of the same lot nr. resulted in similar thrombin generation curves).

The recalcified coagulation activity assay (RECA) was performed. The RECA was started with 5 µl 250 mM $CaCl_2$ in 1 ml frozen/thawed aliquots in 20 ml siliconized glass vials (DadeBehring, Marburg, Germany; article nr. OVKE49) using 0.9 % NaCl – rinsed new disposable polypropylene tips for the Eppendorf-Multipette®. After coagulation reaction times (CRT) of 0-20 min (exceptionally 0-30 min) at 37°C (in a digitally controlled water-bath) 100 µl arginine reagent were added to stop hemostasis activation. This stop reagent consisted in 2.5 M arginine, pH 8.6, 0.16 % Triton X 100® (Sigma, Deisenhofen, Germany). 25 µl 1 mM chromogenic thrombin substrate HD-CHG-Ala-Arg-pNA (Pentapharm, Basel, Switzerland) in 1.25 M arginine, pH 8.7 were added. After 3 min (23°C) the increase of absorbance at 405 nm with time (ΔA/t) at 23°C was measured by a microtiter plate photometer with a 1 mA resolution (Milenia; DPC, Los Angeles, USA). The RECA was standardized with 1 IU/ml bovine thrombin (DadeBehring) in 6.7 % human albumin (Kabi, Stockholm, Sweden) that replaced the plasma sample. The maximal ΔA was about 1050 mA; 40 % of the maximal ΔA = upper limit of linearity = 420 mA. The intra-assay coefficients of variation (CV) were < 10 %.

The approximate 50 % inhibitory concentration (IC50) and the approximate 200 % stimulatory concentration (SC200) of the added asparaginase was determined by Lin-Lin plots of the plasmatic asparaginase activity (concentration = conc.) versus the thrombin activity measured for RECA-5, RECA-10, RECA-15, or RECA-20, i.e. RECA with CRTs of 5, 10, 15, or 20 min, respectively. Thrombin generation = thrombin activity at a certain CRT minus basal thrombin activity (at 0 min CRT). Since all plasmas basally contain a thrombin activity prior to recalcification (thrombin entrapped in α2-macroglobulin) the thrombin generation in RECA is calculated as thrombin activity after CRT minus basal thrombin activity (0 min CRT = plasma + arginine-reagent + calcium-reagent + substrate-reagent). The normal basal thrombin activity in EDTA-plasma is 5.5 ± 1.1 mIU/ml (mean value ±1 standard deviation) [9]. In citrated plasma, that has been stored for about 4h at 23°C, the normal basal thrombin activity is usually higher (about 10 ± 2 mIU/ml) due to in vitro activation of hemostasis (EDTA and/or arginine stabilize plasma much better than citrate).

For determination of the approx. IC50 or of the approx. SC200, that RECA curve is considered that is the most sensible (with the lowest values for IC50 or SC200). Thrombin activities are only considered that belong to the ascending part of the thrombin generation curve, i.e. where the thrombin activity at a certain time point is lower than the thrombin activity at a following time point: thrombin activities in the descending part of the thrombin generation curve also depend on the action of antithrombin I = fibrin [10]. If there is no increase in plasma turbidity within a certain CRT, then the respective generated IIa activity might also be valid.

RESULTS

It was the purpose of the present study to follow thrombin generation after asparaginase supplementation of many normal plasma samples. So it becomes possible to judge the pro–thrombinic or anti-thrombinic power of the present lot of asparaginase. Furthermore, with this exemplary work the analytic power of the RECA assay system itself is proven. Therefore, a high number of exemplary curves of *a) coagulation reaction time (CRT)* and of *b) asparaginase dose response* have been included in the present work: for *a)* the CRT is plotted on the x-axis and the resulting thrombin (IIa) activity is plotted on the y-axis; for *b)* the added asparaginase activity is plotted on the x-axis and the resulting thrombin activity is plotted on the y-axis.

Normal thrombin generation - curves without addition of asparaginase (symbol "O" in all CRT - figures) are hyperbolic up to the moment, where sufficient thrombin is generated to form antithrombin I = fibrin, usually detectable as a significant increase in plasmatic turbidity.

Figures 1-20 demonstrate 20 typical thrombin activity curves for plasma samples that have an asparaginase-SC200. The range of approximate SC200 is between < 1 U/ml (Figure 1) and up to 100 U/ml (Figure 20).

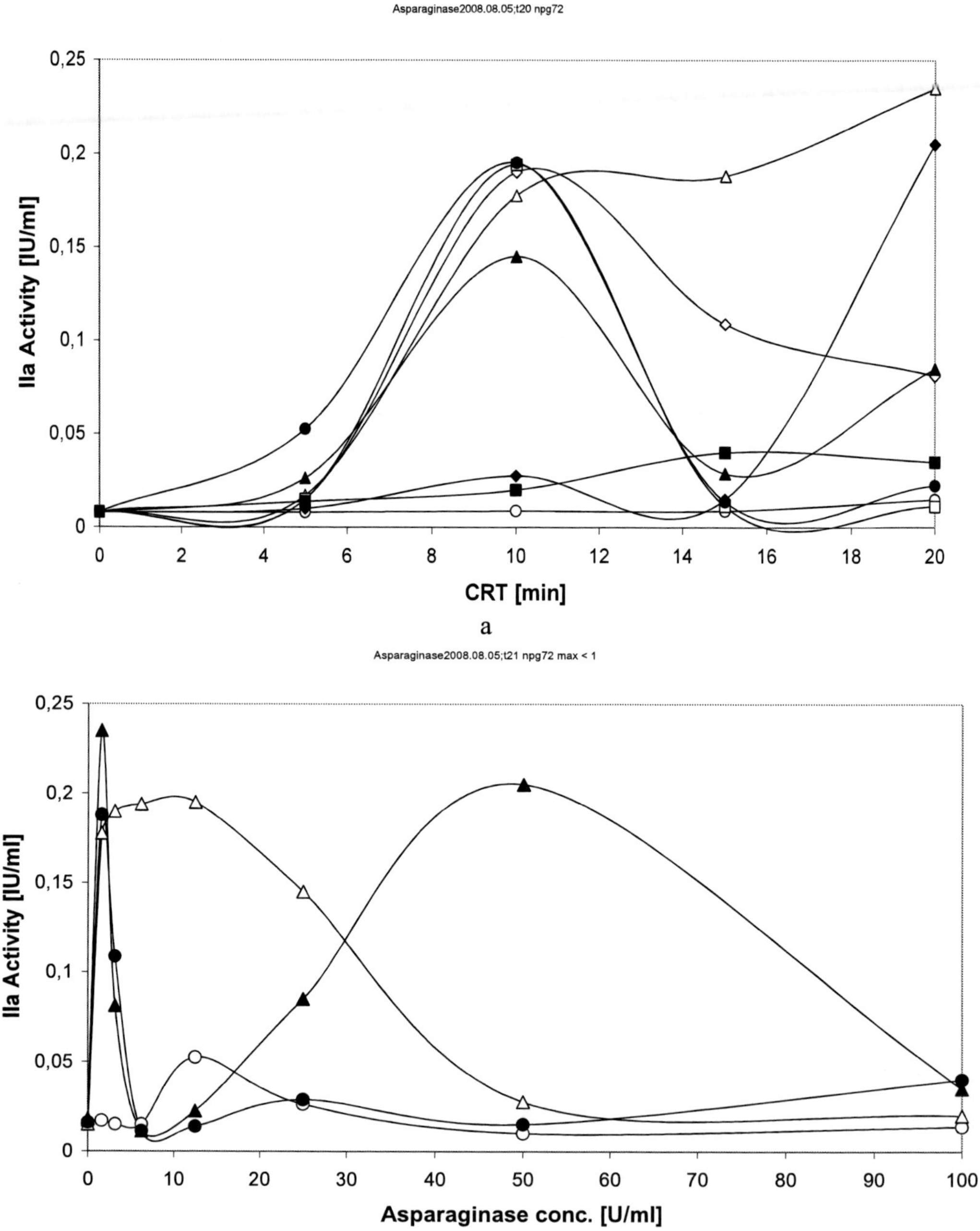

Figure 1. IIa generation in dependence of asparaginase concentration in sample 1. 50 µl unfrozen citrated normal plasma (sample 1) were supplemented in U-microwells (Brand®701300) with 0-100 U/ml asparaginase by repetitive 1+1 dilution. The RECA was performed. Figure 1a: 0 (O), 1.6 (Δ), 3.1 (◊), 6.3 (□), 12.5 (●), 25 (▲), 50 (♦), or 100 (■) U/ml asparaginase. Figure 1b: coagulation reaction times (CRT) of 5 min (O), 10 min (Δ), 15 min (●), or 20 min (▲). The approx. SC200 was less than 1 U/ml asparaginase. Thrombin generation = thrombin activity generated minus basal thrombin activity.

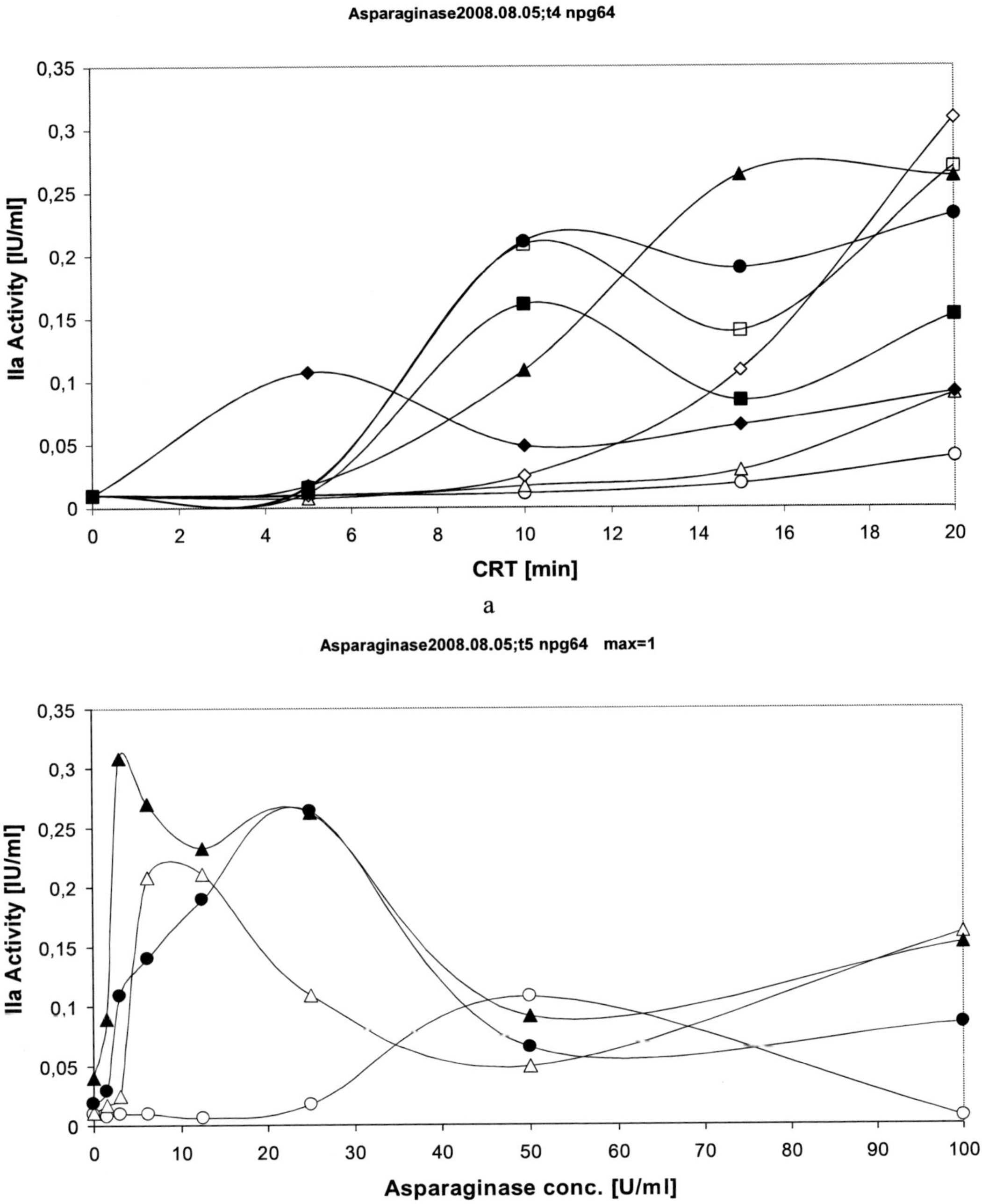

Figure 2. IIa generation in dependence of asparaginase concentration in sample 2. 50 µl unfrozen citrated normal plasma (sample 2) were supplemented in the U-microwells (Brand®701300) with 0-100 U/ml asparaginase by repetitive 1+1 dilution. The RECA was performed. Figure 2a: 0 (O), 1.6 (Δ), 3.1 (◊), 6.3 (□), 12.5 (●), 25 (▲), 50 (♦), or 100 (■) U/ml asparaginase. Figure 2b: coagulation reaction times (CRT) of 5 min (O), 10 min (Δ), 15 min (●), or 20 min (▲); approx. SC200 = 1 U/ml asparaginase.

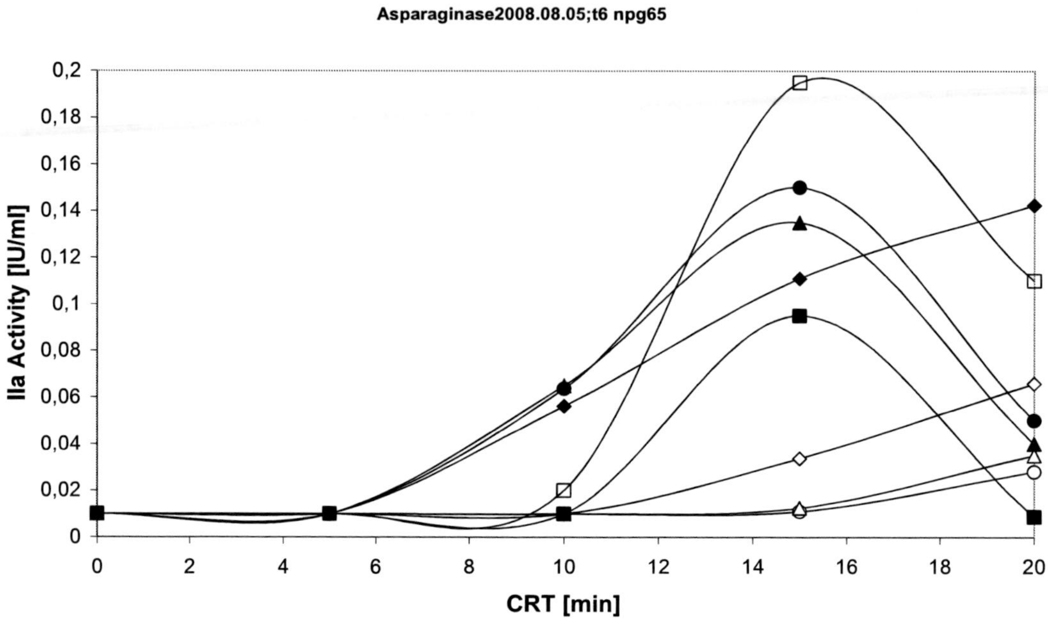

a

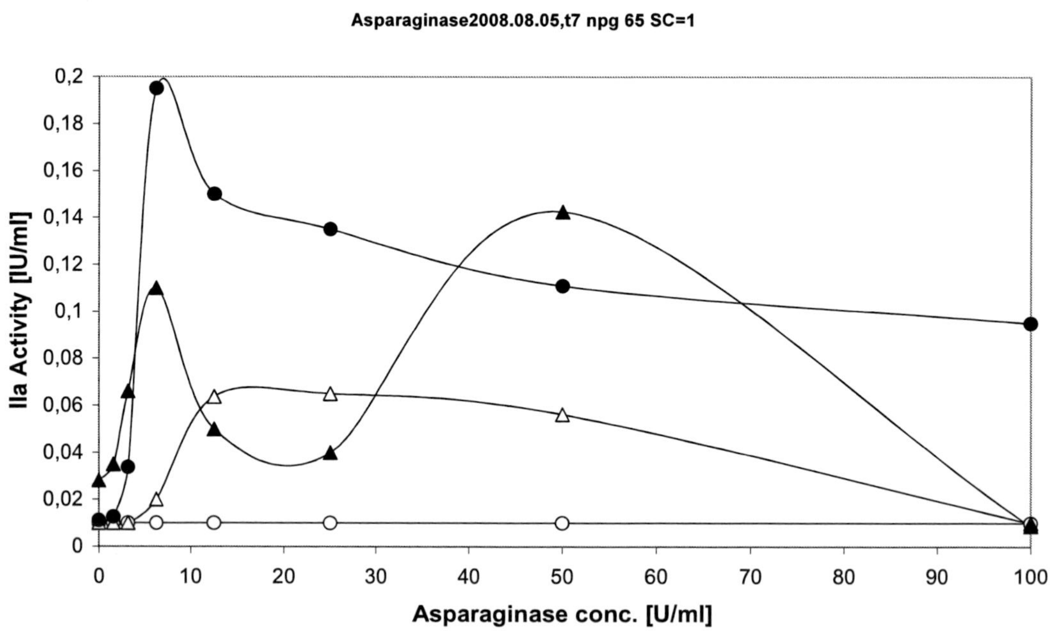

b

Figure 3. IIa generation in dependence of asparaginase concentration in sample 3. 50 µl unfrozen citrated normal plasma (sample 3) were supplemented in the U-microwells (Brand®701300) with 0-100 U/ml asparaginase by repetitive 1+1 dilution. The RECA was performed. Figure 3a: 0 (O), 1.6 (Δ), 3.1 (◊), 6.3 (□), 12.5 (●), 25 (▲), 50 (♦), or 100 (■) U/ml asparaginase. Figure 3b: coagulation reaction times (CRT) of 5 min (O), 10 min (Δ), 15 min (●), or 20 min (▲); approx. SC200 = 1 U/ml asparaginase.

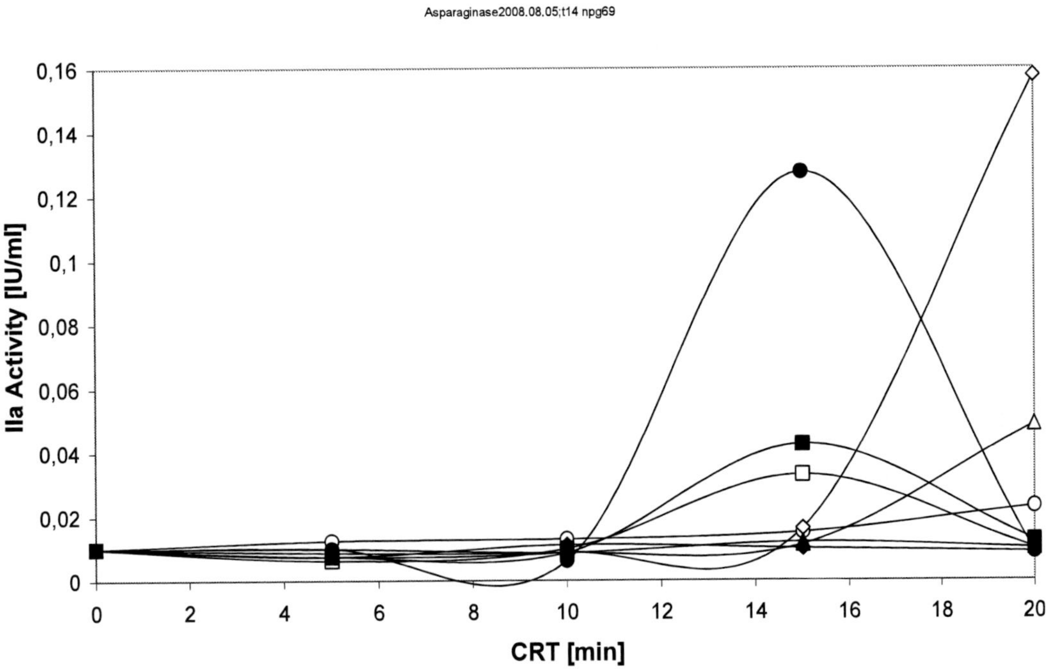

a

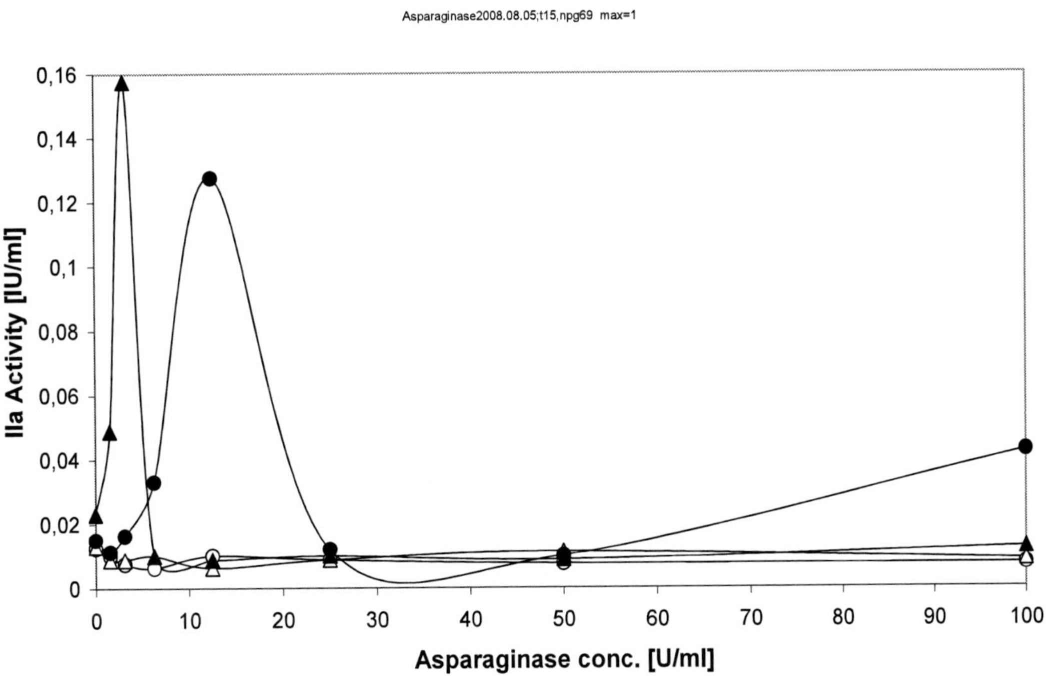

Figure 4. IIa generation in dependence of asparaginase concentration in sample 4. 50 µl unfrozen citrated normal plasma (sample 4) were supplemented in the U-microwells (Brand®701300) with 0-100 U/ml asparaginase by repetitive 1+1 dilution. The RECA was performed. Figure 4a: 0 (O), 1.6 (Δ), 3.1 (◊), 6.3 (□), 12.5 (●), 25 (▲), 50 (♦), or 100 (■) U/ml asparaginase. Figure 4b: coagulation reaction times (CRT) of 5 min (O), 10 min (Δ), 15 min (●), or 20 min (▲). Approx. SC200 = 1 U/ml asparaginase.

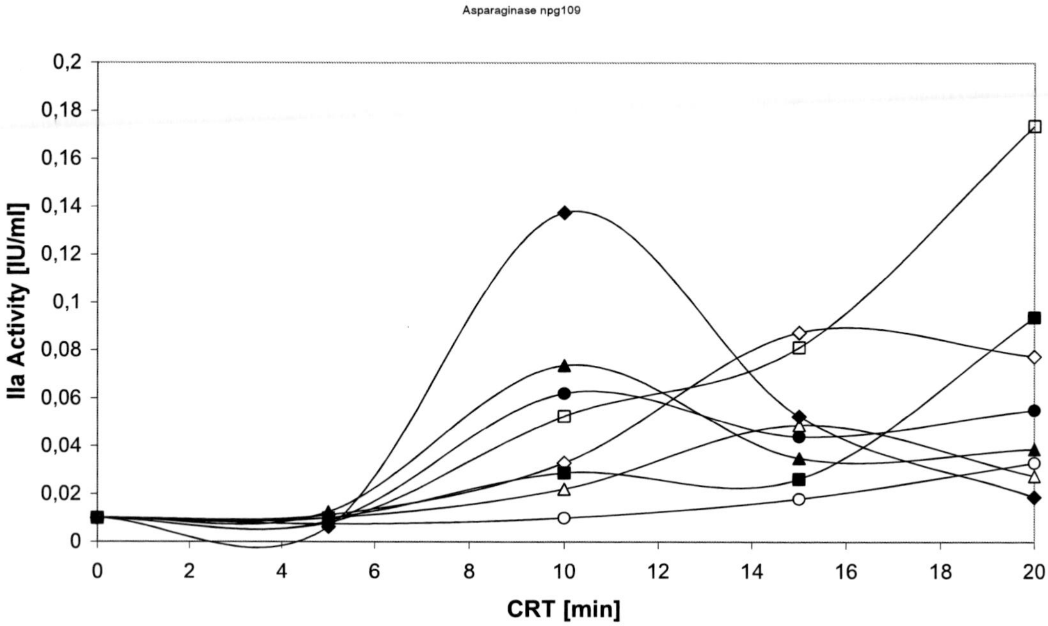

a

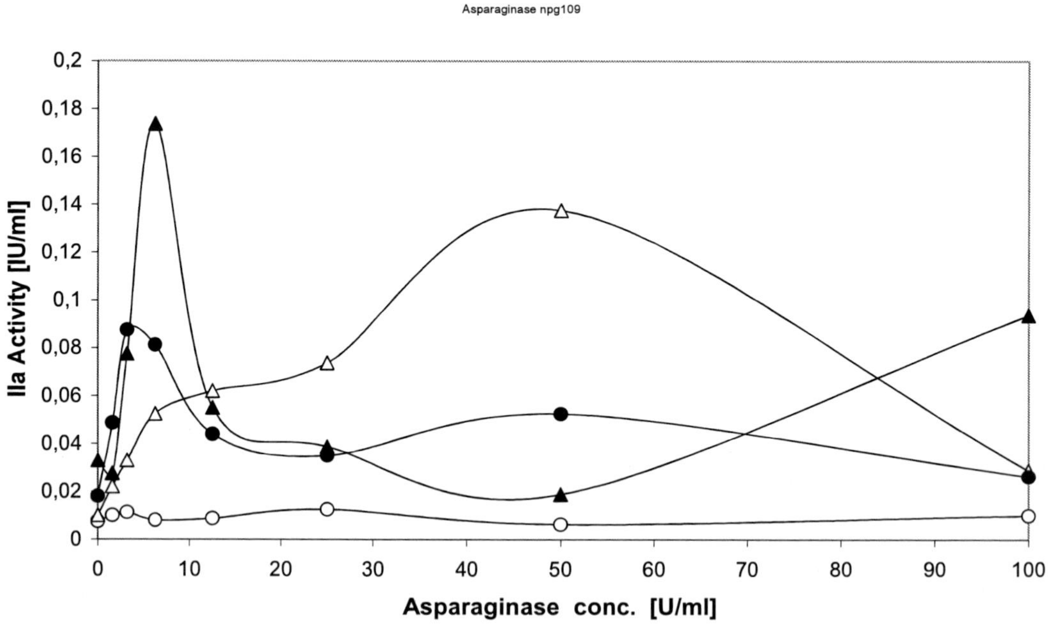

b

Figure 5. IIa generation in dependence of asparaginase concentration in sample 5. 50 µl unfrozen citrated normal plasma (sample 5) were supplemented in U-microwells (Brand®701300) with 0-100 U/ml asparaginase by repetitive 1+1 dilution. The RECA was performed. Figure 5a: 0 (O), 1.6 (Δ), 3.1 (◊), 6.3 (□), 12.5 (●), 25 (▲), 50 (♦), or 100 (■) U/ml asparaginase. Figure 5b: coagulation reaction times (CRT) of 5 min (O), 10 min (Δ), 15 min (●), or 20 min (▲). Approx. SC200 = 1 U/ml asparaginase.

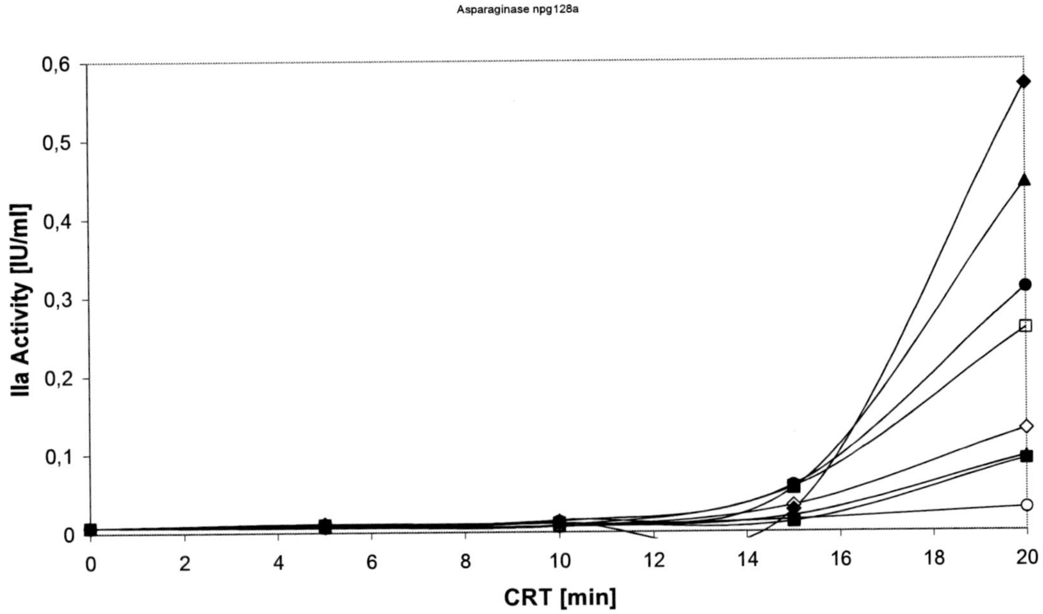

a

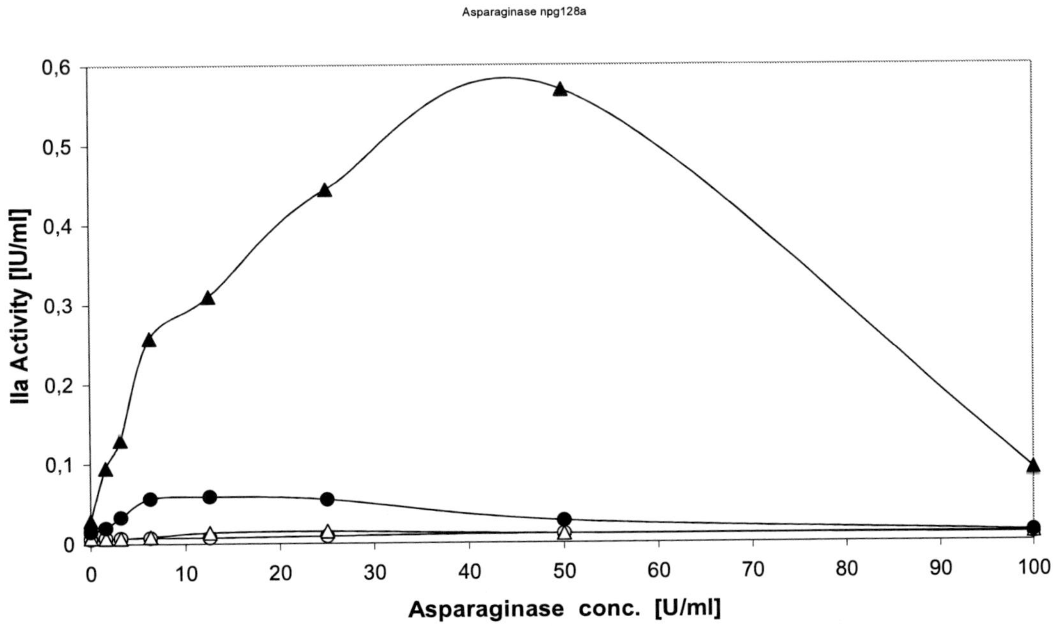

b

Figure 6. IIa generation in dependence of asparaginase concentration in sample 6. 50 µl unfrozen citrated normal plasma (sample 6) were supplemented in the U-microwells (Brand®701300) with 0-100 U/ml asparaginase by repetitive 1+1 dilution. The RECA was performed. Figure 6a: 0 (O), 1.6 (Δ), 3.1 (◊), 6.3 (□), 12.5 (●), 25 (▲), 50 (♦), or 100 (■) U/ml asparaginase. Figure 6b: coagulation reaction times (CRT) of 5 min (O), 10 min (Δ), 15 min (●), or 20 min (▲). Approx. SC200 = 1 U/ml asparaginase.

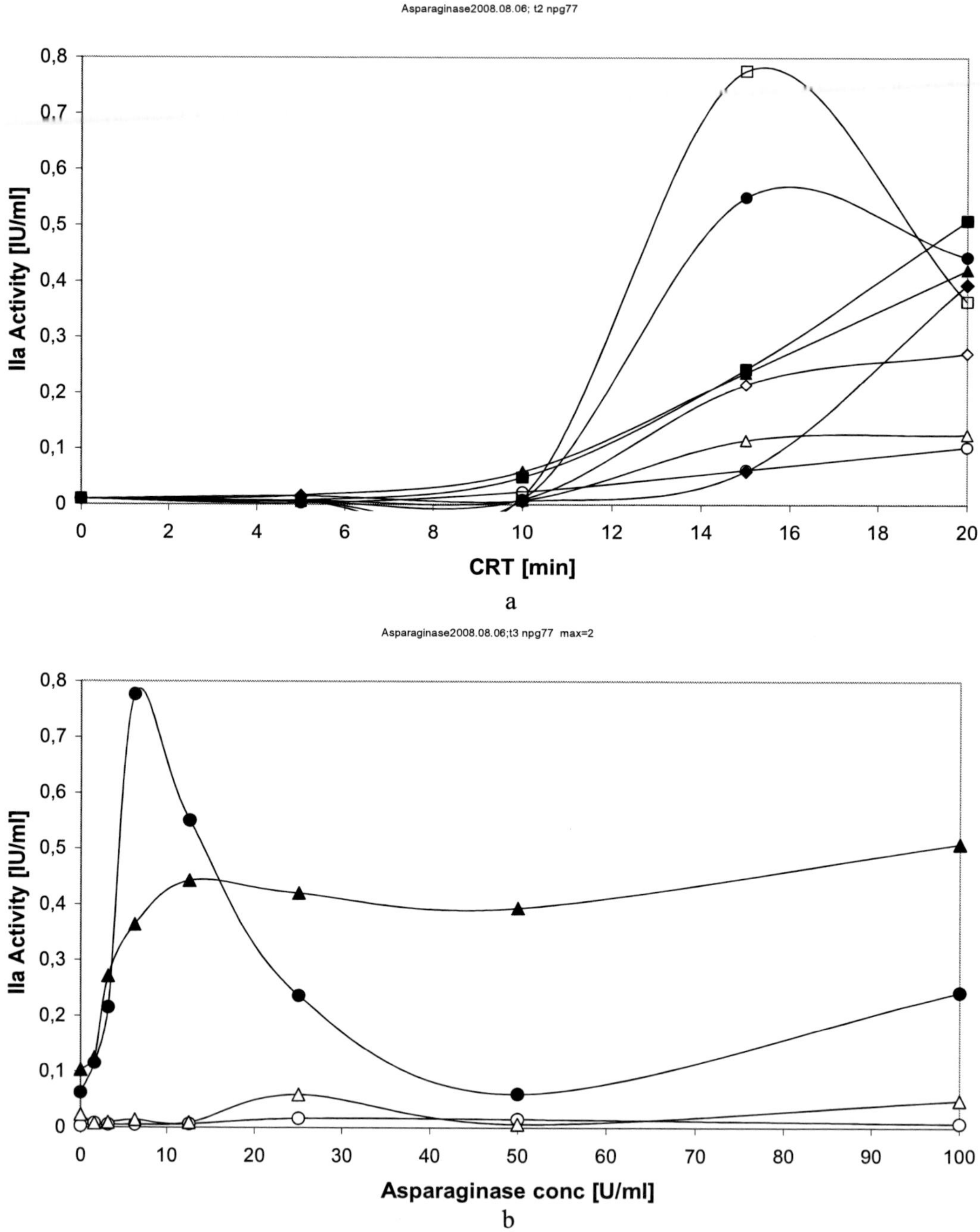

Figure 7. IIa generation in dependence of asparaginase concentration in sample 7. 50 µl unfrozen citrated normal plasma (sample 7) were supplemented in the U-microwells (Brand®701300) with 0-100 U/ml asparaginase by repetitive 1+1 dilution. The RECA was performed. Figure 7a: 0 (O), 1.6 (Δ), 3.1 (◊), 6.3 (□), 12.5 (●), 25 (▲), 50 (♦), or 100 (■) U/ml asparaginase. Figure 7b: coagulation reaction times (CRT) of 5 min (O), 10 min (Δ), 15 min (●), or 20 min (▲). The approx. SC200 was about 2 U/ml asparaginase.

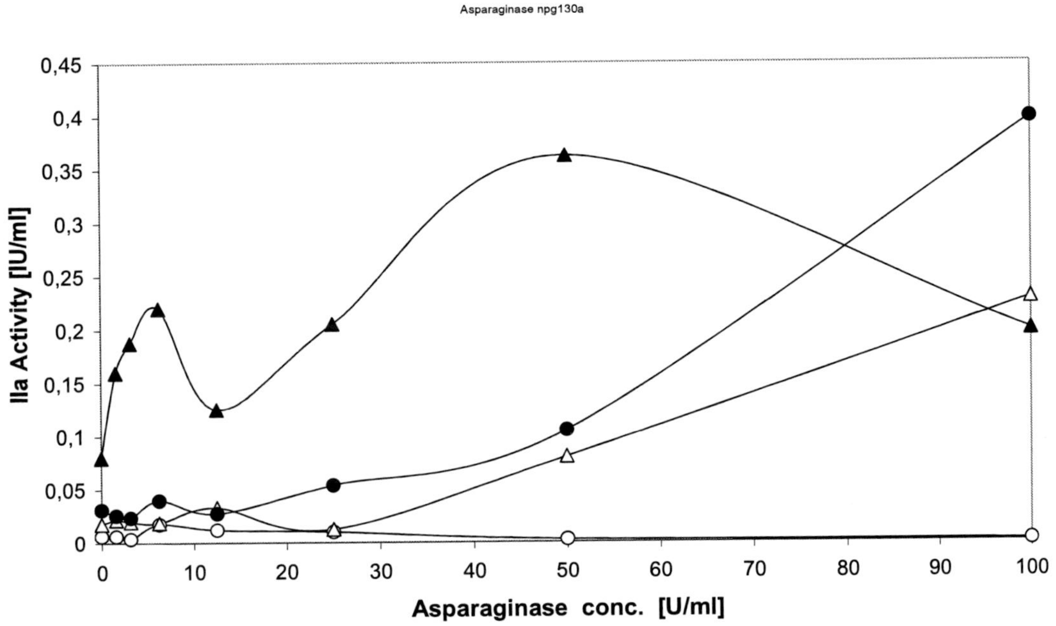

a

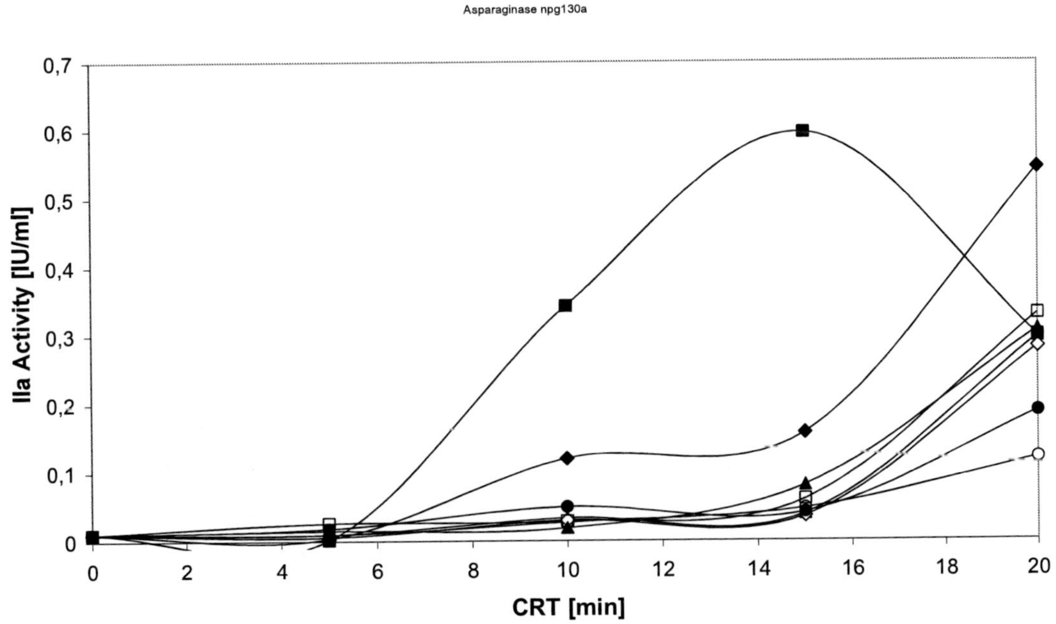

b

Figure 8. IIa generation in dependence of asparaginase concentration in sample 8. 50 µl unfrozen citrated normal plasma were supplemented in the U-microwells (Brand®701300) with 0-100 U/ml asparaginase by repetitive 1+1 dilution. The RECA was performed. Figure 8a: 0 (O), 1.6 (Δ), 3.1 (◊), 6.3 (□), 12.5 (•), 25 (▲), 50 (♦), or 100 (■) U/ml asparaginase. Figure 8b: coagulation reaction times (CRT) of 5 min (O), 10 min (Δ), 15 min (•), or 20 min (▲). The approx. SC200 was about 2 U/ml asparaginase.

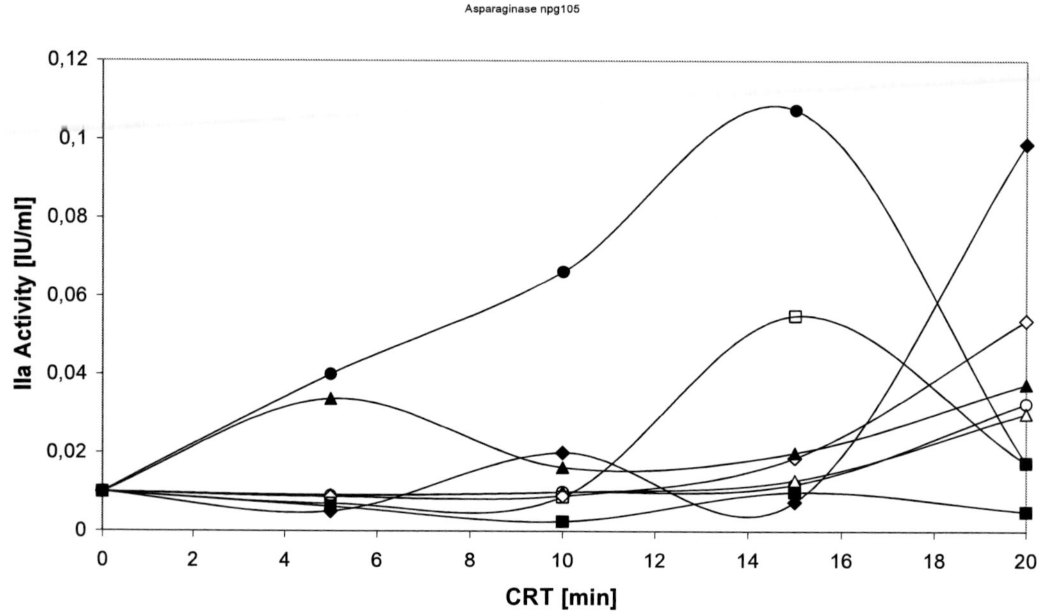

a

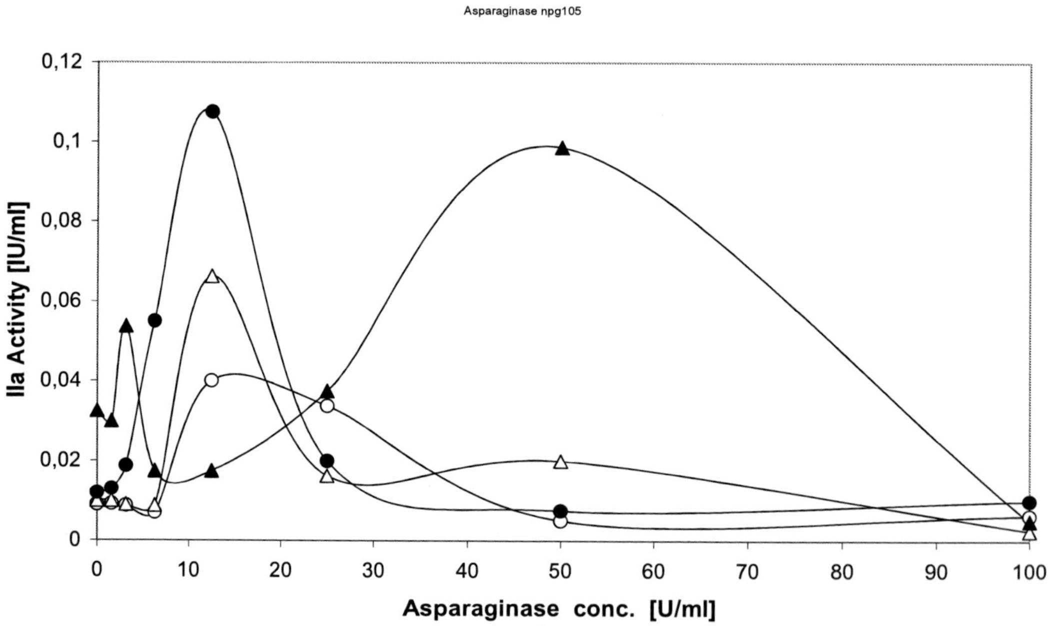

b

Figure 9. IIa generation in dependence of asparaginase concentration in sample 9. 50 µl unfrozen citrated normal plasma (sample 9) were supplemented in the U-microwells (Brand®701300) with 0-100 U/ml asparaginase by repetitive 1+1 dilution. The RECA was performed. Figure 9a: 0 (O), 1.6 (Δ), 3.1 (◊), 6.3 (□), 12.5 (●), 25 (▲), 50 (♦), or 100 (■) U/ml asparaginase. Figure 9b: coagulation reaction times (CRT) of 5 min (O), 10 min (Δ), 15 min (●), or 20 min (▲). The approx. SC200 was about 2 U/ml asparaginase.

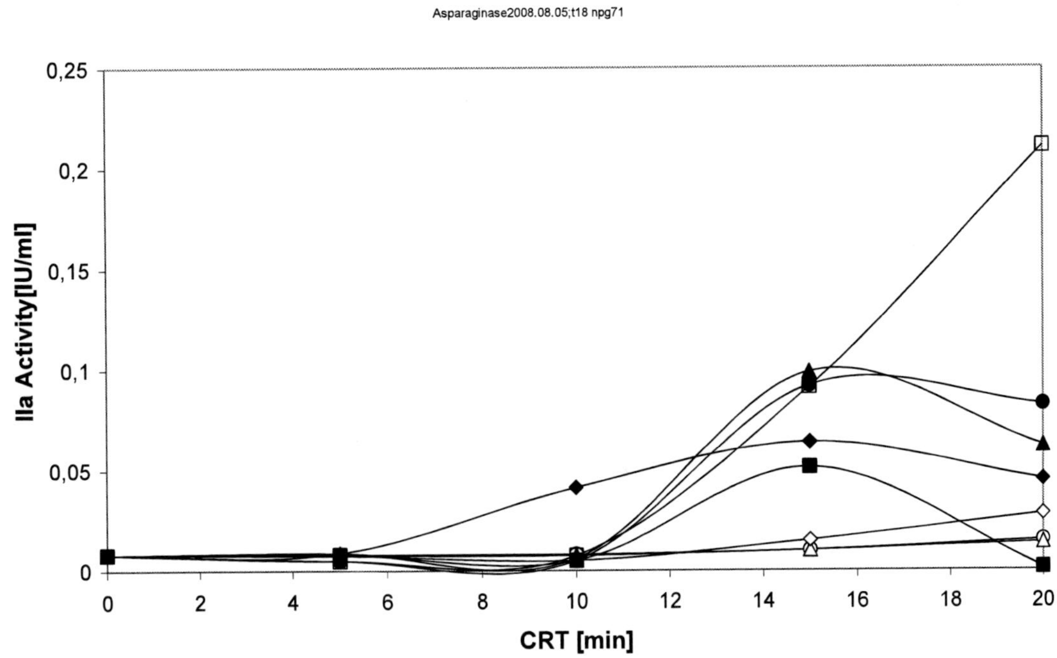

a

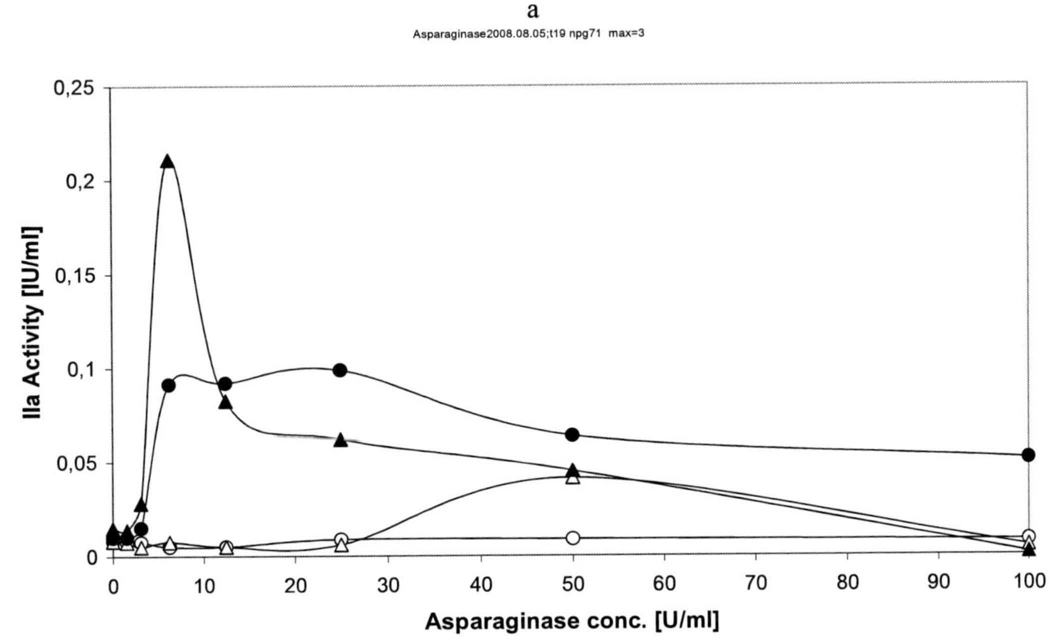

b

Figure 10. IIa generation in dependence of asparaginase concentration in sample 10. 50 µl unfrozen citrated normal plasma (sample 10) were supplemented in the U-microwells (Brand®701300) with 0-100 U/ml asparaginase by repetitive 1+1 dilution. The RECA was performed. Figure 10a: 0 (O), 1.6 (Δ), 3.1 (◊), 6.3 (□), 12.5 (●), 25 (▲), 50 (♦), or 100 (■) U/ml asparaginase. Figure 10b: coagulation reaction times (CRT) of 5 min (O), 10 min (Δ), 15 min (●), or 20 min (▲). Approx. SC200 = 3 U/ml asparaginase.

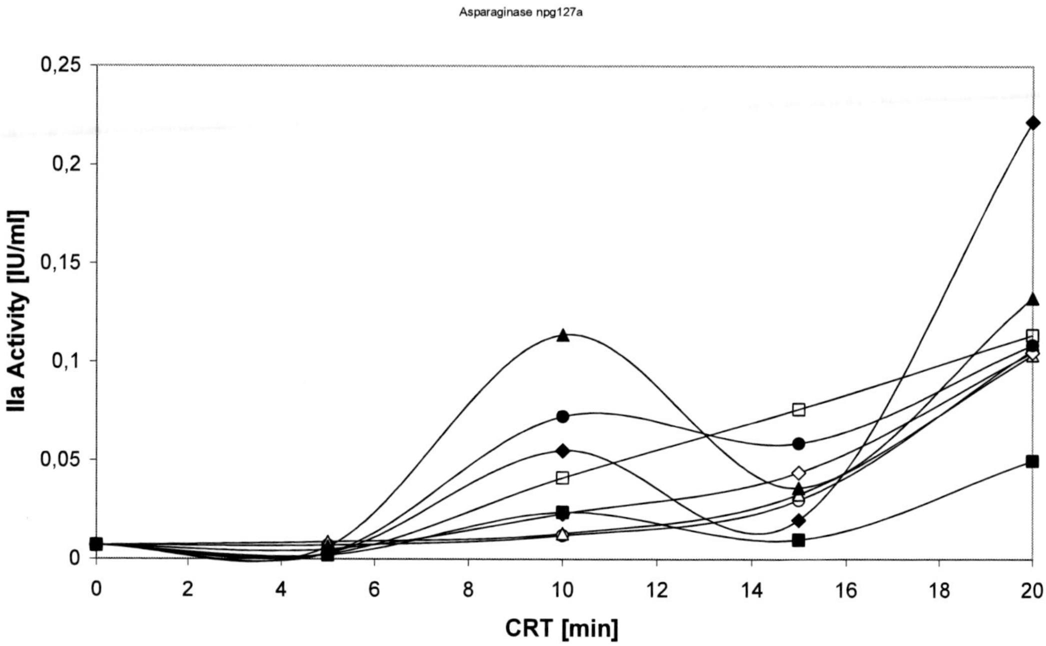

a

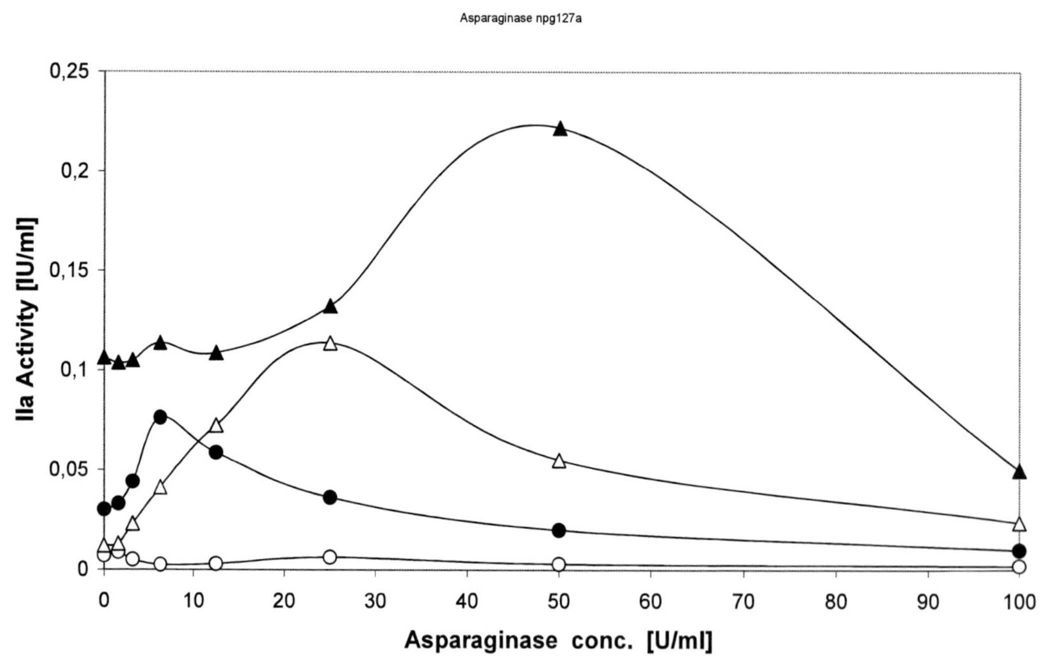

b

Figure 11. IIa generation in dependence of asparaginase concentration in sample 11. 50 μl unfrozen citrated normal plasma were supplemented in the U-microwells (Brand®701300) with 0-100 U/ml asparaginase by repetitive 1+1 dilution. The RECA was performed. Figure 11a: 0 (O), 1.6 (Δ), 3.1 (◊), 6.3 (□), 12.5 (●), 25 (▲), 50 (♦), or 100 (■) U/ml asparaginase. Figure 11b: coagulation reaction times (CRT) of 5 min (O), 10 min (Δ), 15 min (●), or 20 min (▲). Approx. SC200 = 3 U/ml asparaginase.

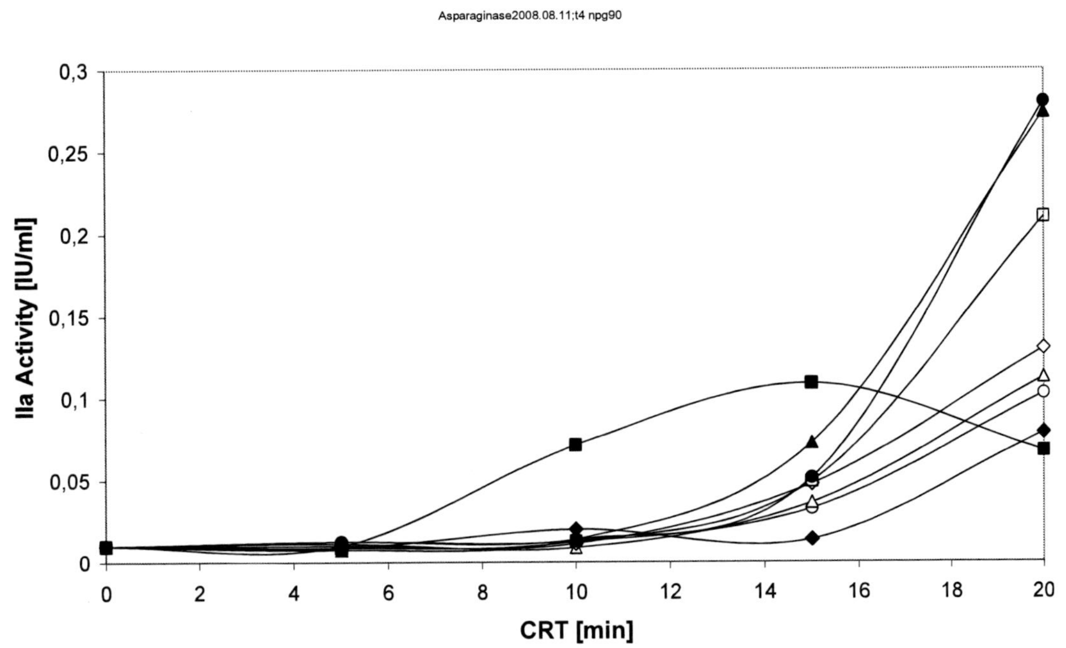

a

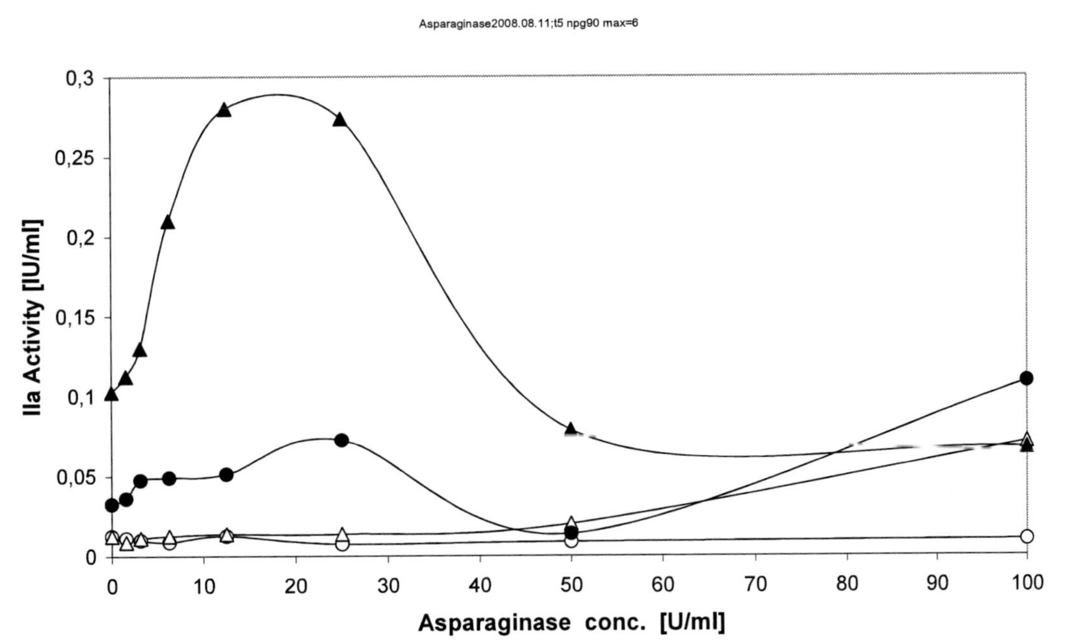

b

Figure 12. IIa generation in dependence of asparaginase concentration in sample 12. 50 µl unfrozen citrated normal plasma (sample 12) were supplemented in U-microwells (Brand®701300) with 0-100 U/ml asparaginase by repetitive 1+1 dilution. The RECA was performed. Figure 12a: 0 (O), 1.6 (Δ), 3.1 (◊), 6.3 (□), 12.5 (●), 25 (▲), 50 (♦), or 100 (■) U/ml asparaginase. Figure 12b: coagulation reaction times (CRT) of 5 min (O), 10 min (Δ), 15 min (●), or 20 min (▲). Approx. SC200 = 6 U/ml asparaginase.

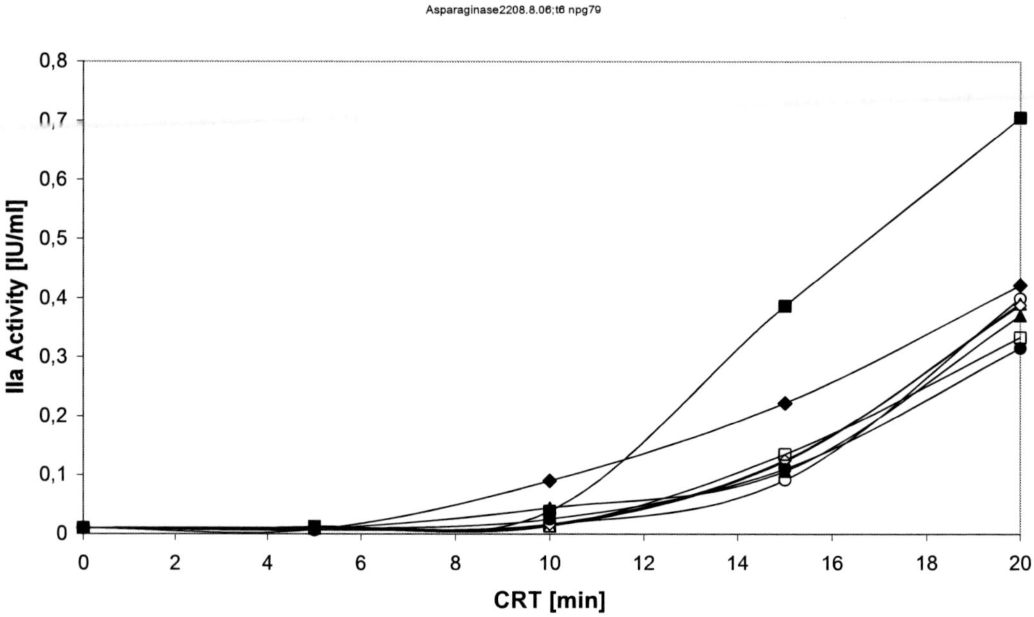

a

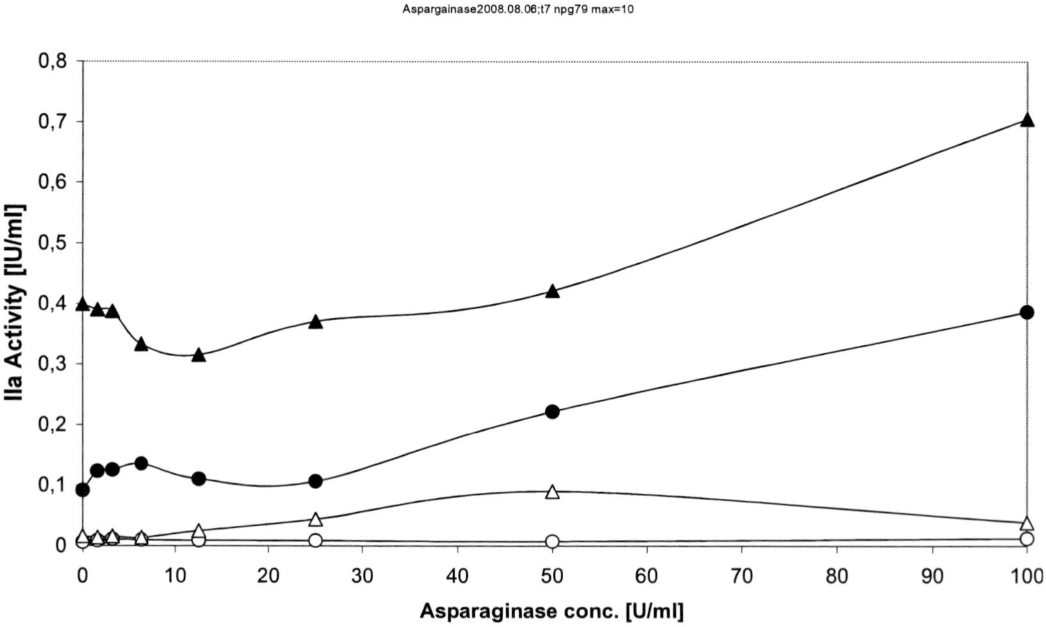

b

Figure 13. IIa generation in dependence of asparaginase concentration in sample 13. 50 µl unfrozen citrated normal plasma (sample 13) were supplemented in U-microwells (Brand®701300) with 0-100 U/ml asparaginase by repetitive 1+1 dilution. The RECA was performed. Figure 13a: 0 (O), 1.6 (Δ), 3.1 (◊), 6.3 (□), 12.5 (●), 25 (▲), 50 (♦), or 100 (■) U/ml asparaginase. Figure 13b: coagulation reaction times (CRT) of 5 min (O), 10 min (Δ), 15 min (●), or 20 min (▲). Approx. SC200= 10 U/ml asparaginase (analyzed at 10 min CRT).

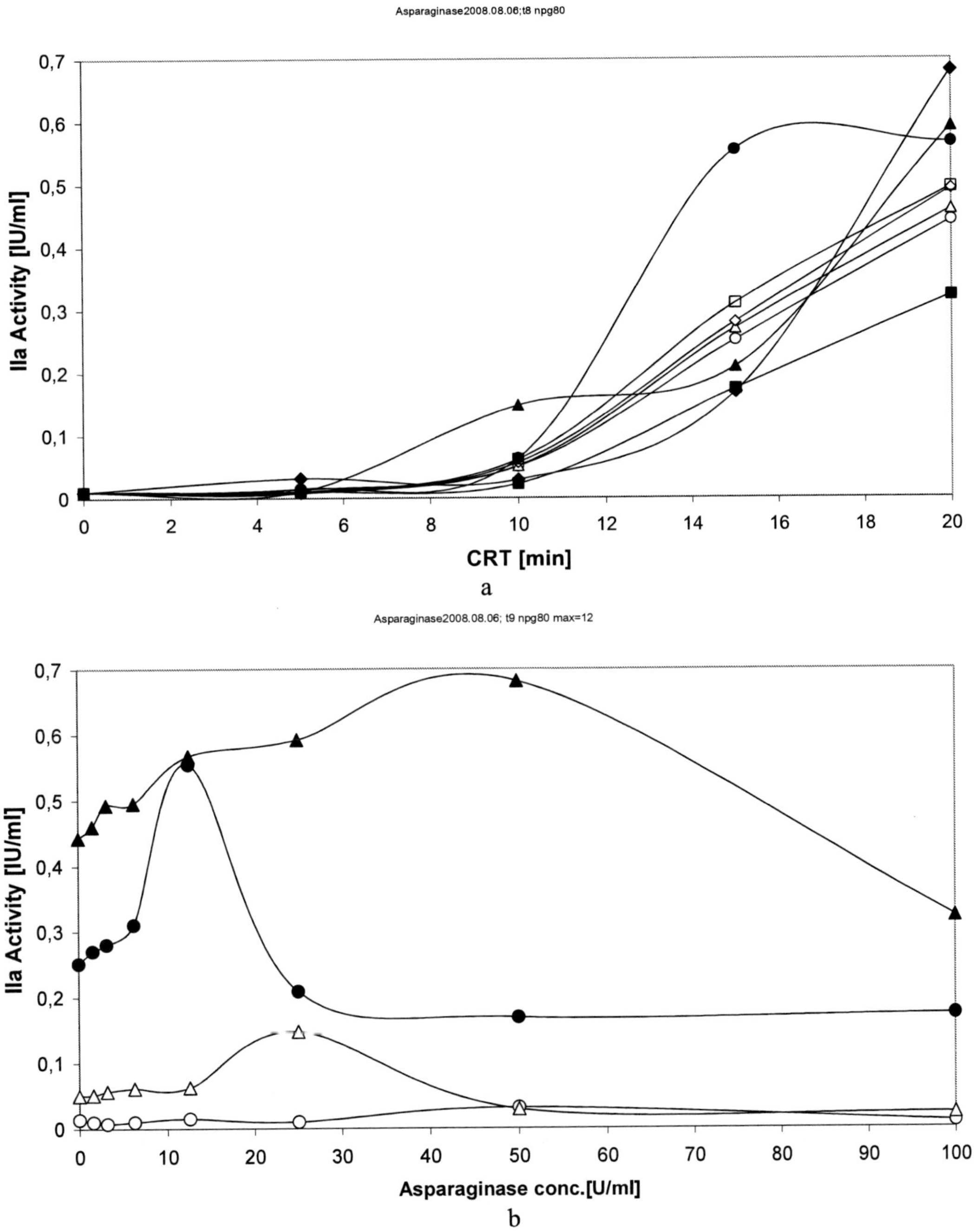

Figure 14. IIa generation in dependence of asparaginase concentration in sample 14. 50 µl unfrozen citrated normal plasma (sample 14) were supplemented in U-microwells (Brand®701300) with 0-100 U/ml asparaginase by repetitive 1+1 dilution. The RECA was performed. Figure 14a: 0 (O), 1.6 (Δ), 3.1 (◊), 6.3 (□), 12.5 (•), 25 (▲), 50 (♦), or 100 (■) U/ml asparaginase. Figure 14b: coagulation reaction times (CRT) of 5 min (O), 10 min (Δ), 15 min (•), or 20 min (▲). Approx. SC200= 12 U/ml asparaginase.

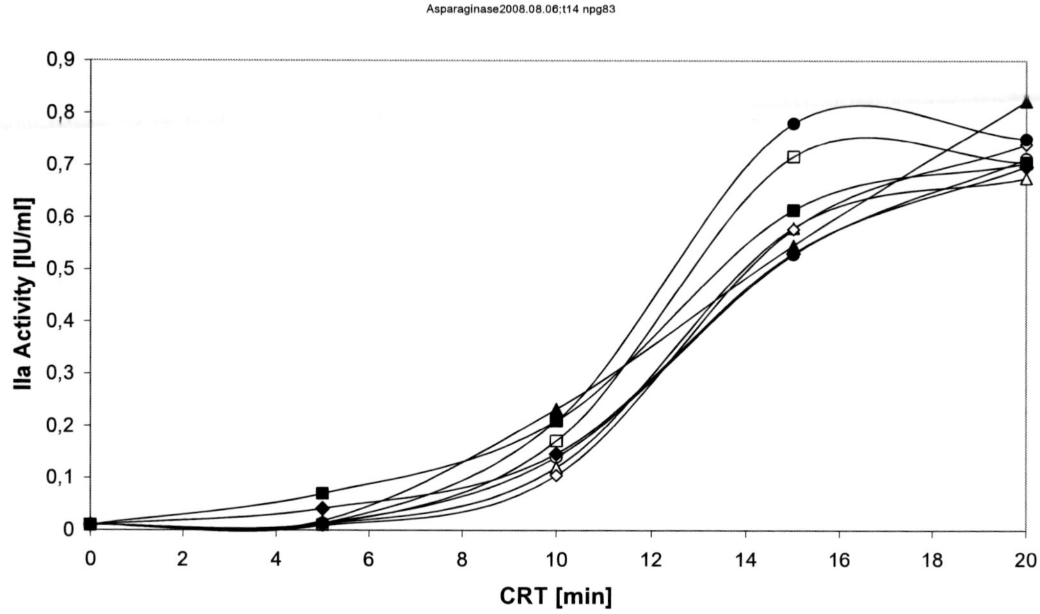

a

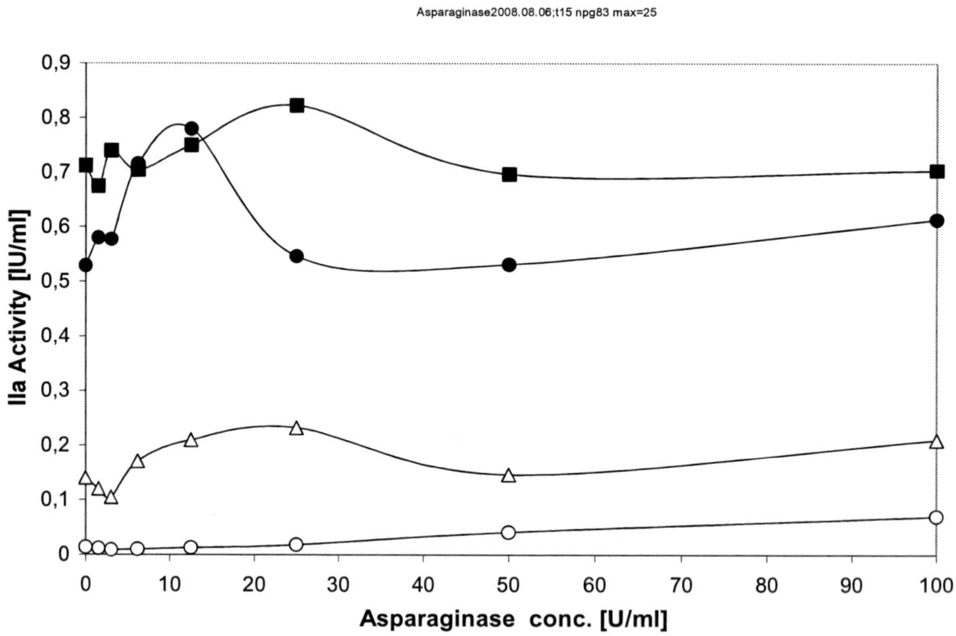

b

Figure 15. IIa generation in dependence of asparaginase concentration in sample 15. 50 µl unfrozen citrated normal plasma (sample 15) were supplemented in the U-microwells (Brand®701300) with 0-100 U/ml asparaginase by repetitive 1+1 dilution. The RECA was performed. Figure 15a: 0 (O) 1.6 (Δ), 3.1 (◊), 6.3 (□), 12.5 (●), 25 (▲), 50 (♦), or 100 (■) U/ml asparaginase.Figure 15b: coagulation reaction times (CRT) of 5 min (O), 10 min (Δ), 15 min (●), or 20 min (▲). Approx. SC200 = 25 U/ml asparaginase.

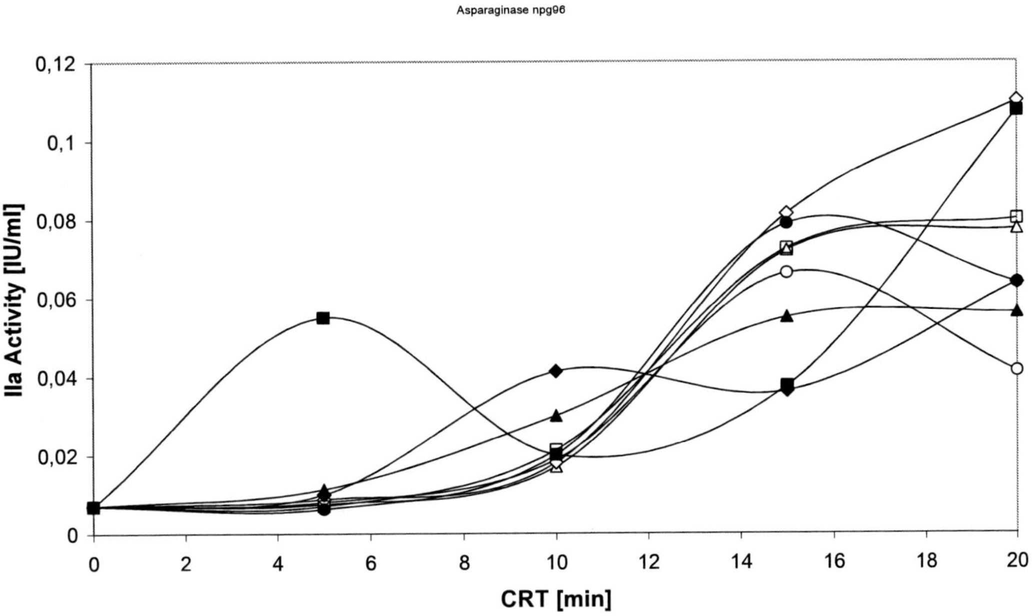

a

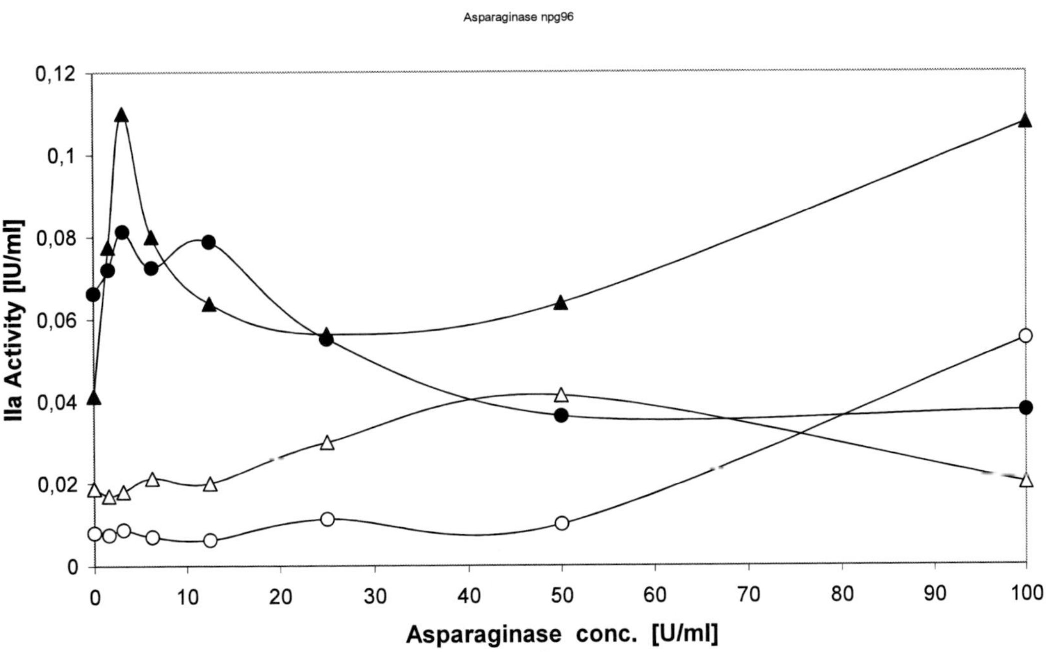

b

Figure 16. IIa generation in dependence of asparaginase concentration in sample 16. 50 µl unfrozen citrated normal plasma (sample 16) were supplemented in the U-microwells (Brand®701300) with 0-100 U/ml asparaginase by repetitive 1+1 dilution. The RECA was performed. Figure 16a: 0 (O), 1.6 (Δ), 3.1 (◊), 6.3 (□), 12.5 (●), 25 (▲), 50 (♦), or 100 (■) U/ml asparaginase. Figure 16b: coagulation reaction times (CRT) of 5 min (O), 10 min (Δ), 15 min (●), or 20 min (▲). Approx. SC200 = 25 U/ml asparaginase.

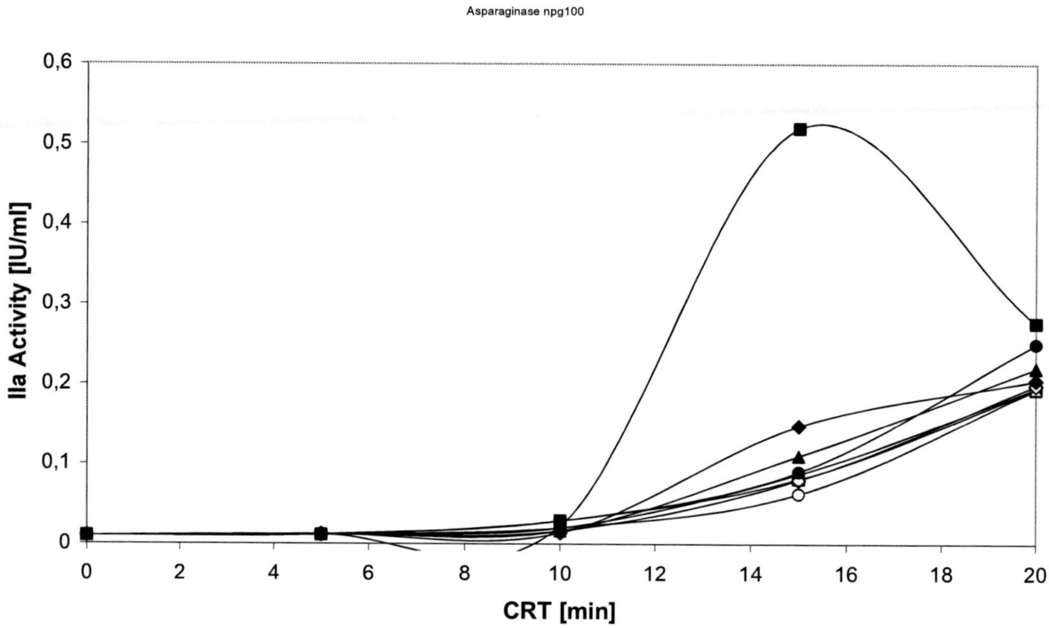

a

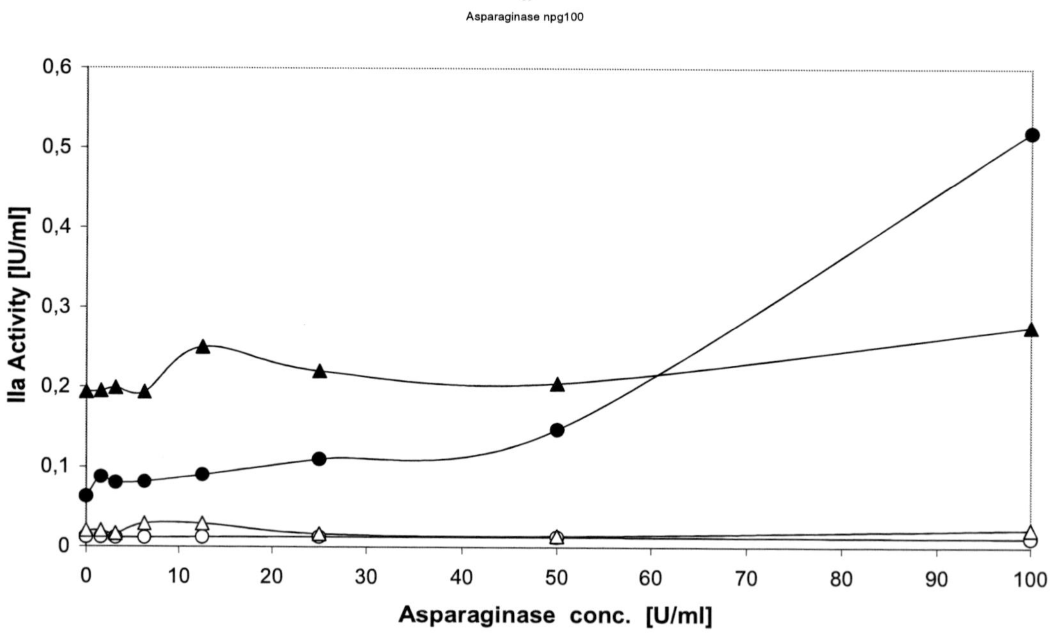

b

Figure 17. IIa generation in dependence of asparaginase concentration in sample 17. 50 µl unfrozen citrated normal plasma (sample 17) were supplemented in the U-microwells (Brand®701300) with 0-100 U/ml asparaginase by repetitive 1+1 dilution. The RECA was performed. Figure 17a: 0 (O), 1.6 (Δ), 3.1 (◊), 6.3 (□), 12.5 (●), 25 (▲), 50 (♦), or 100 (■) U/ml asparaginase. Figure 17b: coagulation reaction times (CRT) of 5 min (O), 10 min (Δ), 15 min (●), or 20 min (▲). Approx. SC200 = 25 U/ml asparaginase.

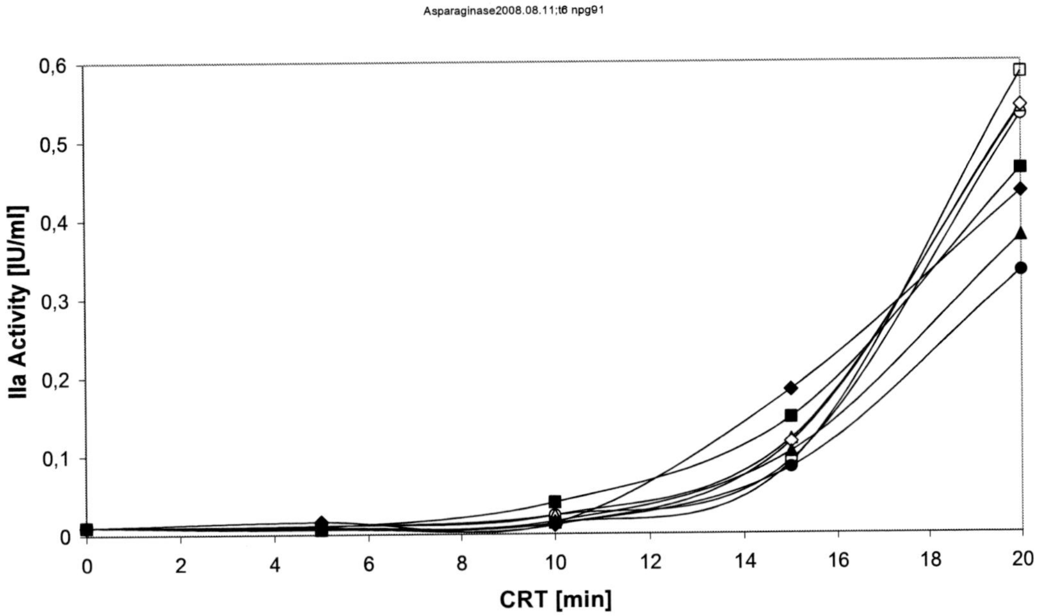

a

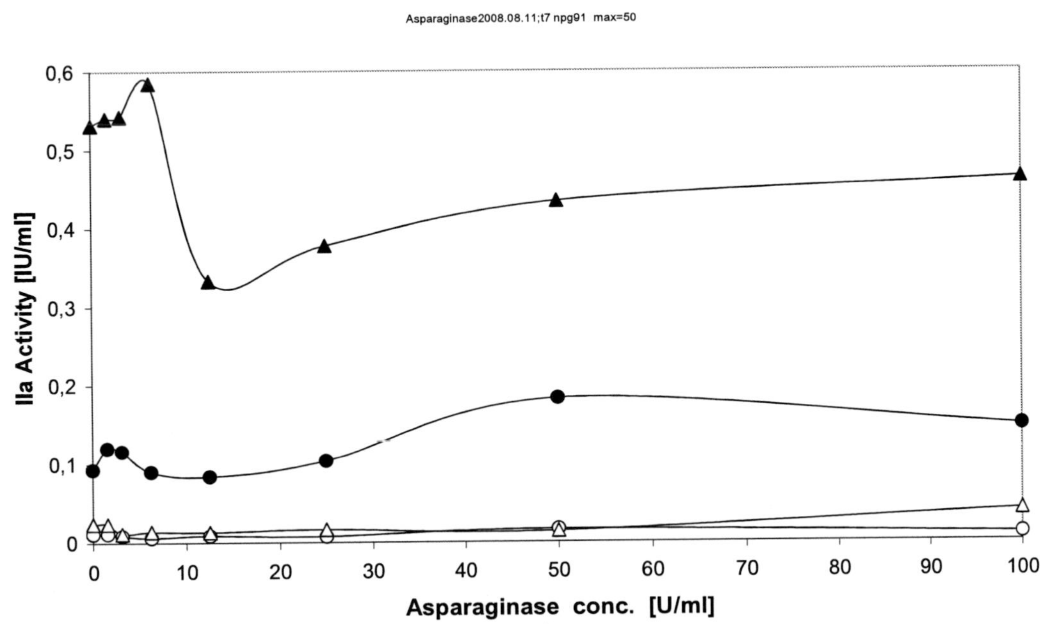

b

Figure 18. IIa generation in dependence of asparaginase concentration in sample 18. 50 µl unfrozen citrated normal plasma (sample 18) were supplemented in the U-microwells (Brand®701300) with 0-100 U/ml asparaginase by repetitive 1+1 dilution. The RECA was performed. Figure 18a: 0 (O), 1.6 (Δ), 3.1 (◊), 6.3 (□), 12.5 (●), 25 (▲), 50 (♦), or 100 (■) U/ml asparaginase. Figure 18b: coagulation reaction times (CRT) of 5 min (O), 10 min (Δ), 15 min (●), or 20 min (▲). Approx. SC200 = 50 U/ml asparaginase.

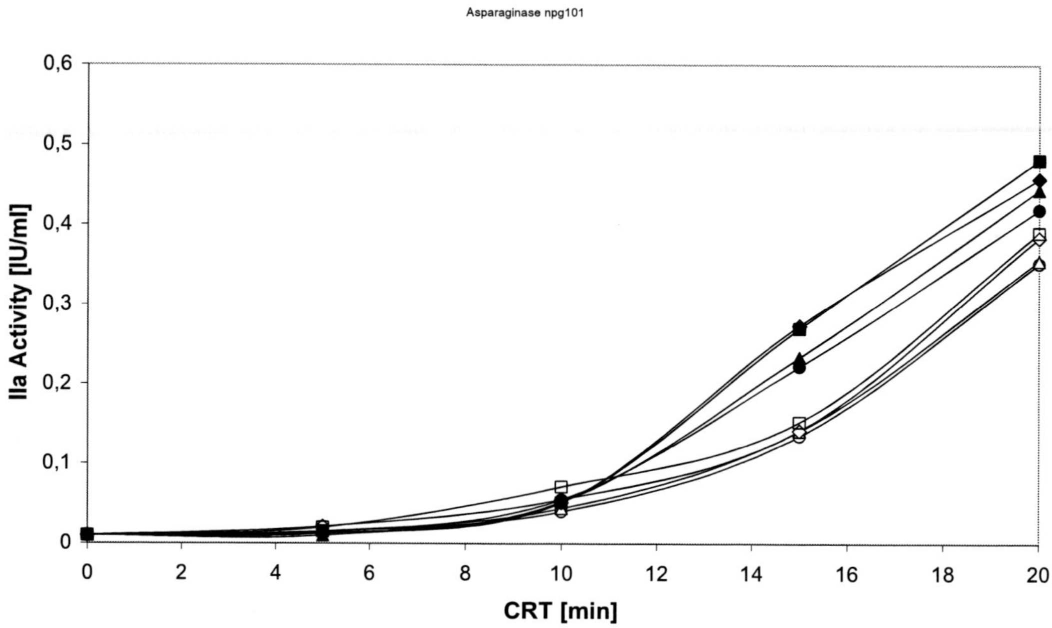

a

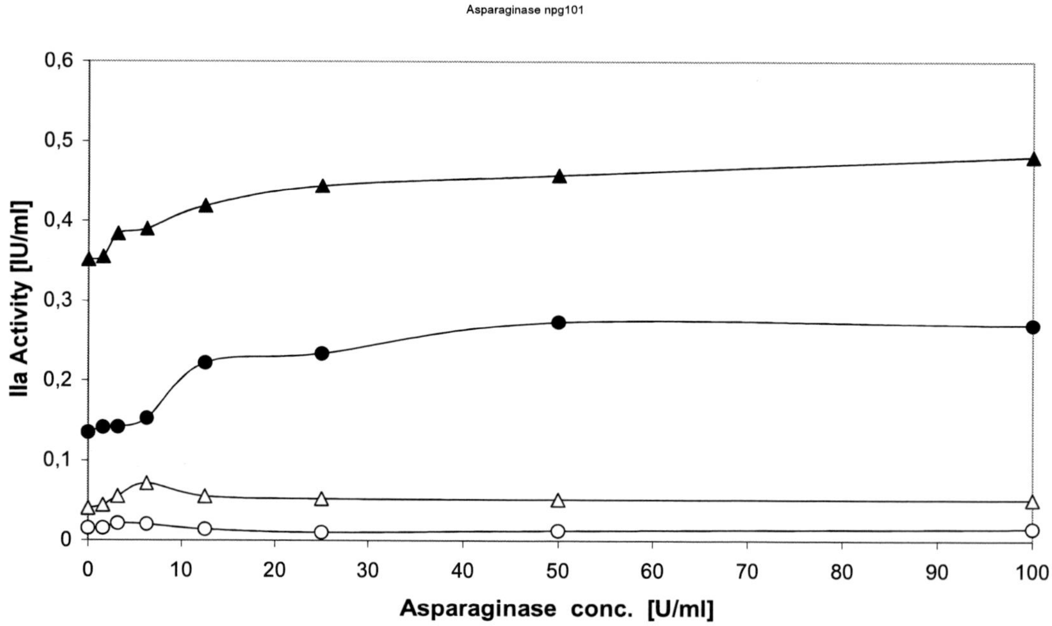

b

Figure 19. IIa generation in dependence of asparaginase concentration in sample 19. 50 µl unfrozen citrated normal plasma (sample 19) were supplemented in the U-microwells (Brand®701300) with 0-100 U/ml asparaginase by repetitive 1+1 dilution. The RECA was performed. Figure 19a: 0 (O), 1.6 (Δ), 3.1 (◊), 6.3 (□), 12.5 (●), 25 (▲), 50 (♦), or 100 (■) U/ml asparaginase. Figure 19b: coagulation reaction times (CRT) of 5 min (O), 10 min (Δ), 15 min (●), or 20 min (▲). Approx. SC200 = 50 U/ml asparaginase.

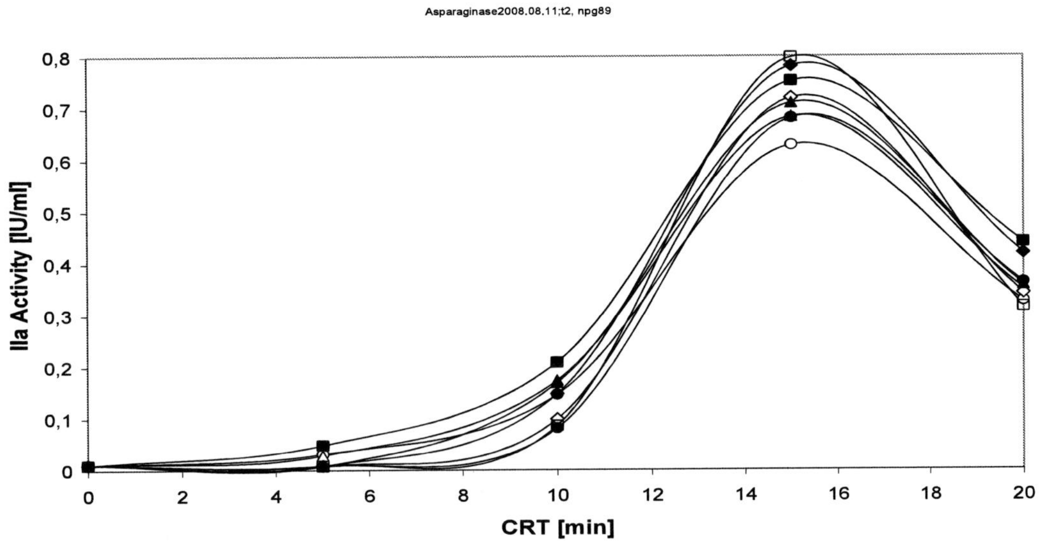

a

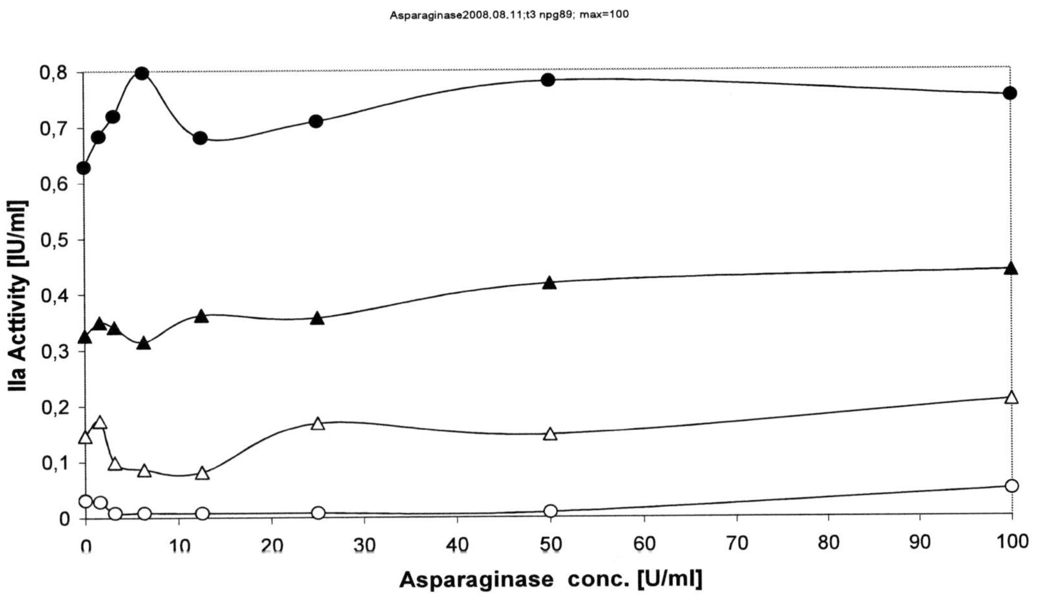

b

Figure 20. IIa generation in dependence of asparaginase concentration in sample 20. 50 µl unfrozen citrated normal plasma (sample 20) were supplemented in U-microwells (Brand®701300) with 0-100 U/ml asparaginase by repetitive 1+1 dilution. The RECA was performed. Figure 20a: 0 (O), 1.6 (Δ), 3.1 (◊), 6.3 (□), 12.5 (●), 25 (▲), 50 (♦), or 100 (■) U/ml asparaginase.Figure 20b: coagulation reaction times (CRT) of 5 min (O), 10 min (Δ), 15 min (●), or 20 min (▲). Approx. SC200 = 100 U/ml asparaginase.

Figures 21 and 22 show plasmas with an approximate SC200 of > 100 U/ml asparaginase. Plasma samples with an asparaginase-IC50 or with a combination of IC50 and SC200 are demonstrated in figures 23-46. The approximate IC50 values range from 1 to 40 U/ml asparaginase.

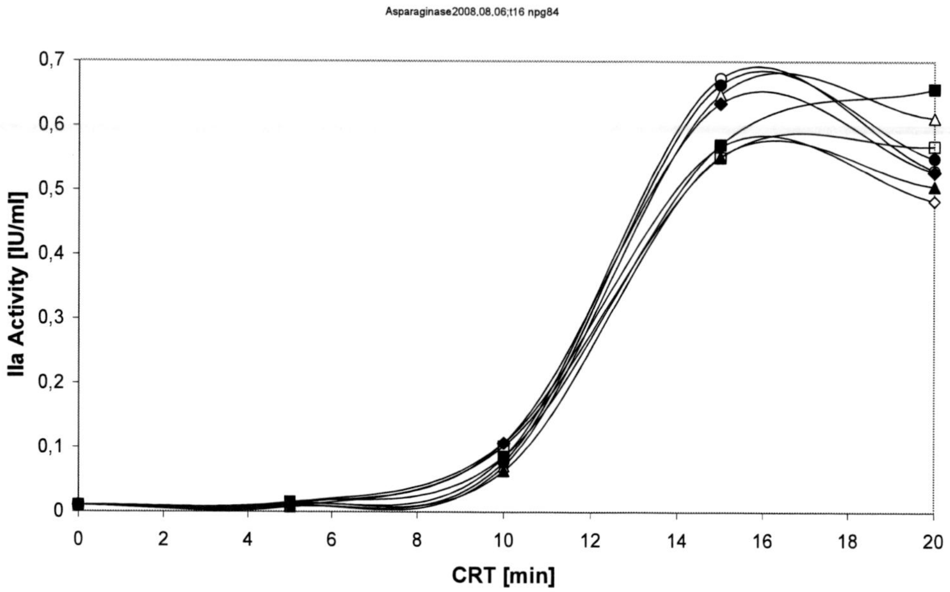

a

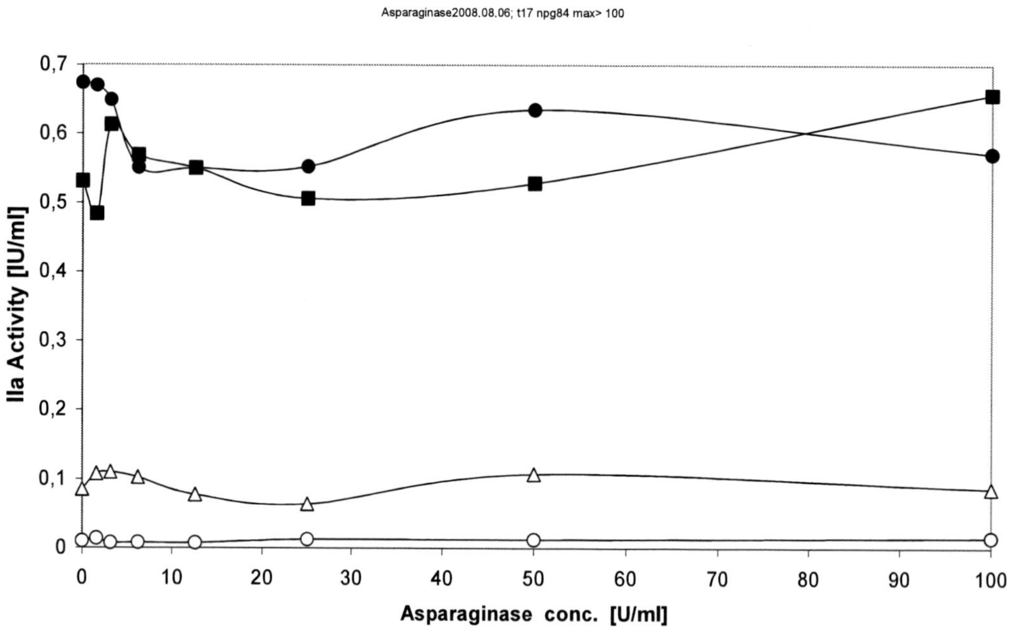

b

Figure 21. IIa generation in dependence of asparaginase concentration in sample 21. 50 µl unfrozen citrated normal plasma (sample 21) were supplemented in the U-microwells (Brand®701300) with 0-100 U/ml asparaginase by repetitive 1+1 dilution. The RECA was performed. Figure 21b: coagulation reaction times (CRT) of 5 min (O), 10 min (Δ), 15 min (●), or 20 min (▲). Figure 21a: (O), 1.6 (Δ), 3.1 (◊), 6.3 (□), 12.5 (●), 25 (▲), 50 (♦), or 100 (■) U/ml asparaginase. Approx. SC200 > 100 U/ml asparaginase.

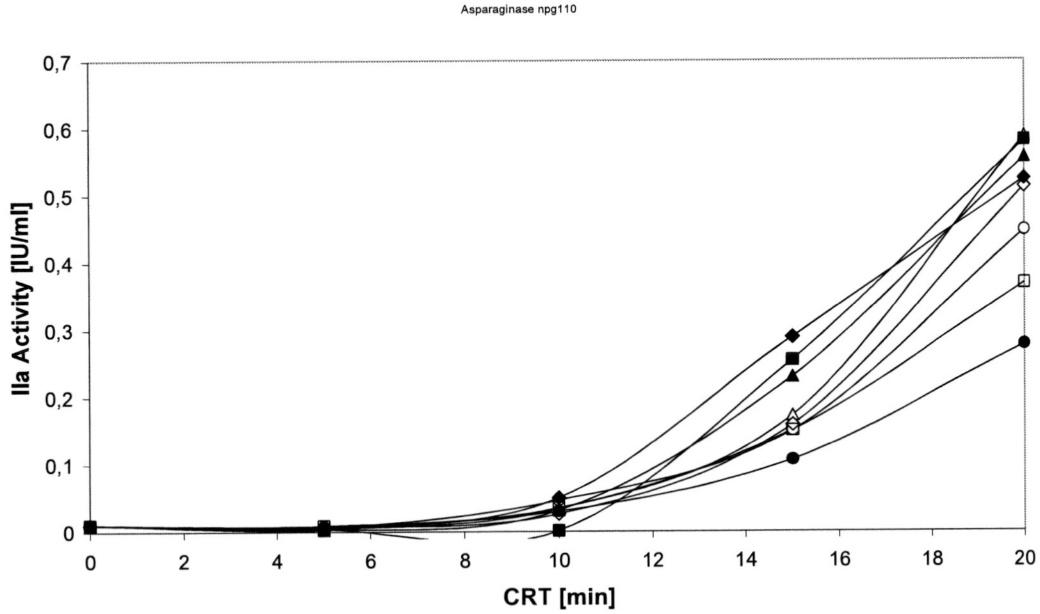

a

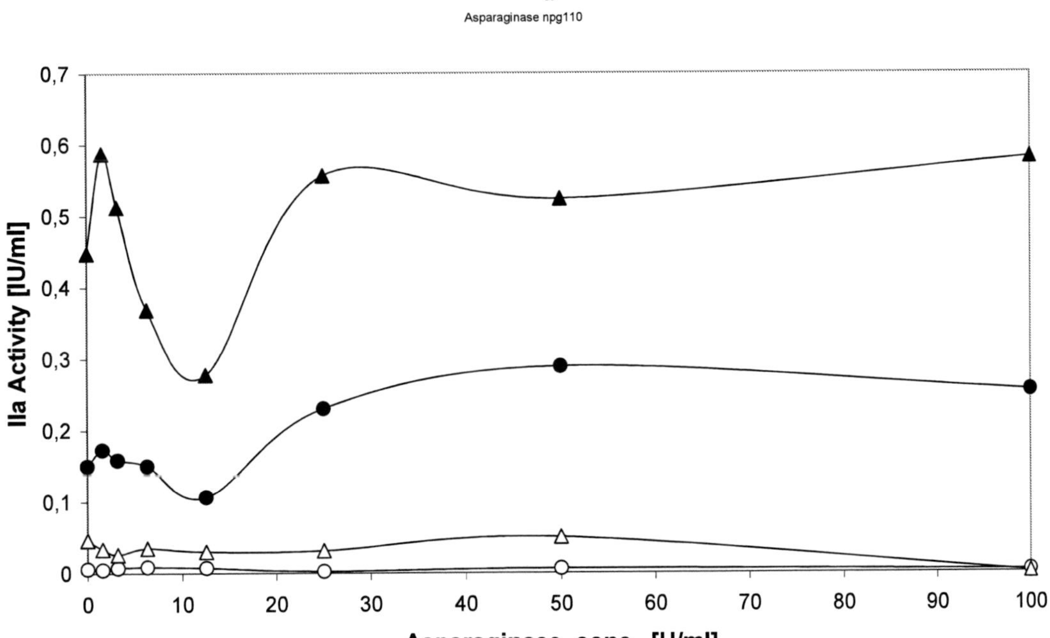

b

Figure 22. IIa generation in dependence of asparaginase concentration in sample 22. 50 µl unfrozen citrated normal plasma (sample 22) were supplemented in the U-microwells (Brand®701300) with 0-100 U/ml asparaginase by repetitive 1+1 dilution. The RECA was performed. Figure 22a: 0 (O), 1.6 (Δ), 3.1 (◊), 6.3 (□), 12.5 (•), 25 (▲), 50 (♦), or 100 (■) U/ml asparaginase. Figure 22b: coagulation reaction times (CRT) of 5 min (O), 10 min (Δ), 15 min (•), or 20 min (▲). Approx. SC200 > 100 U/ml asparaginase.

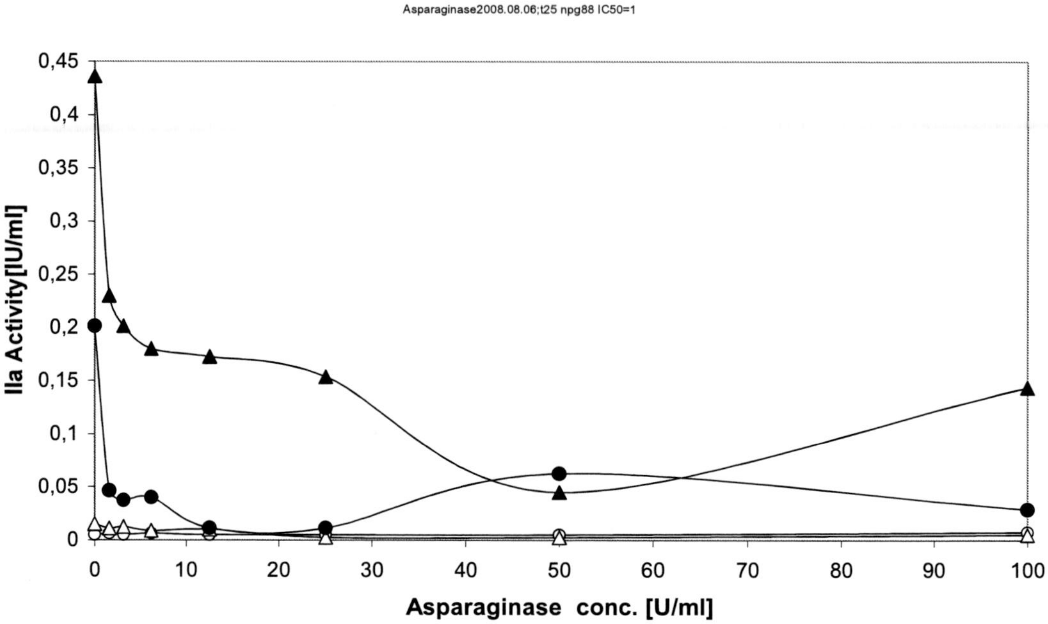

a

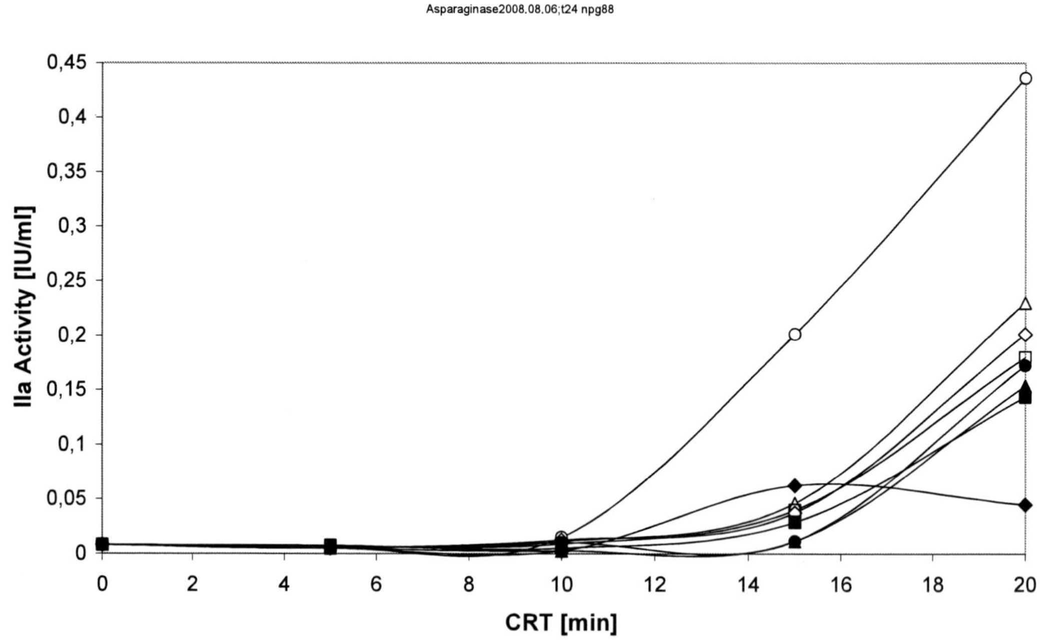

b

Figure 23. IIa generation in dependence of asparaginase concentration in sample 23. 50 µl unfrozen citrated normal plasma were supplemented in U-microwells (Brand®701300) with 0-100 U/ml asparaginase by repetitive 1+1 dilution. The RECA was performed. Figure 23a: 0 (O), 1.6 (Δ), 3.1 (◊), 6.3 (□), 12.5 (•), 25 (▲), 50 (♦), or 100 (■) U/ml asparaginase. Figure 23b: coagulation reaction times (CRT) of 5 min (O), 10 min (Δ), 15 min (•), or 20 min (▲). Approx. IC50 = 1 U/ml asparaginase.

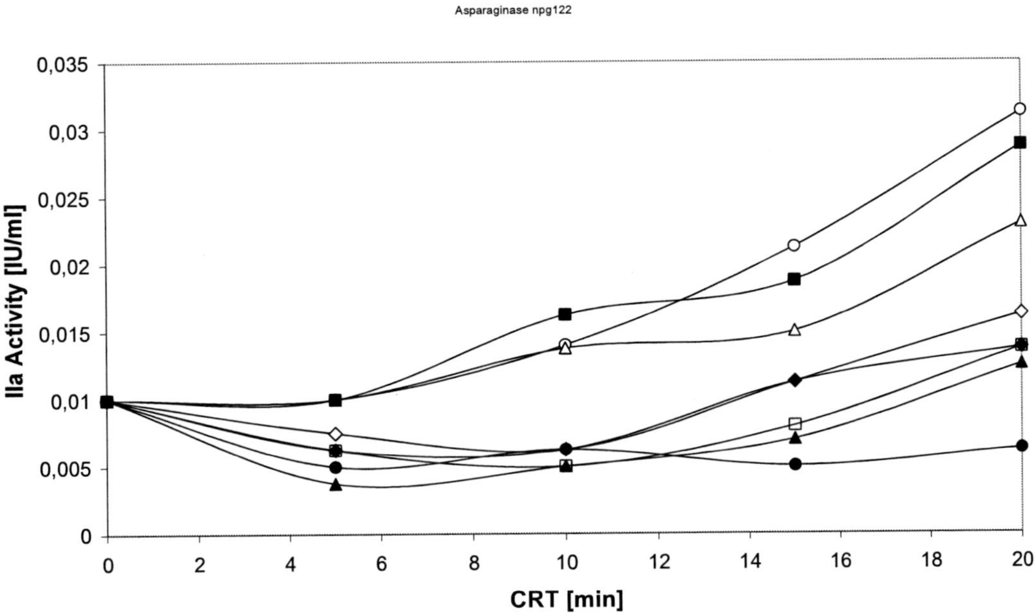

a

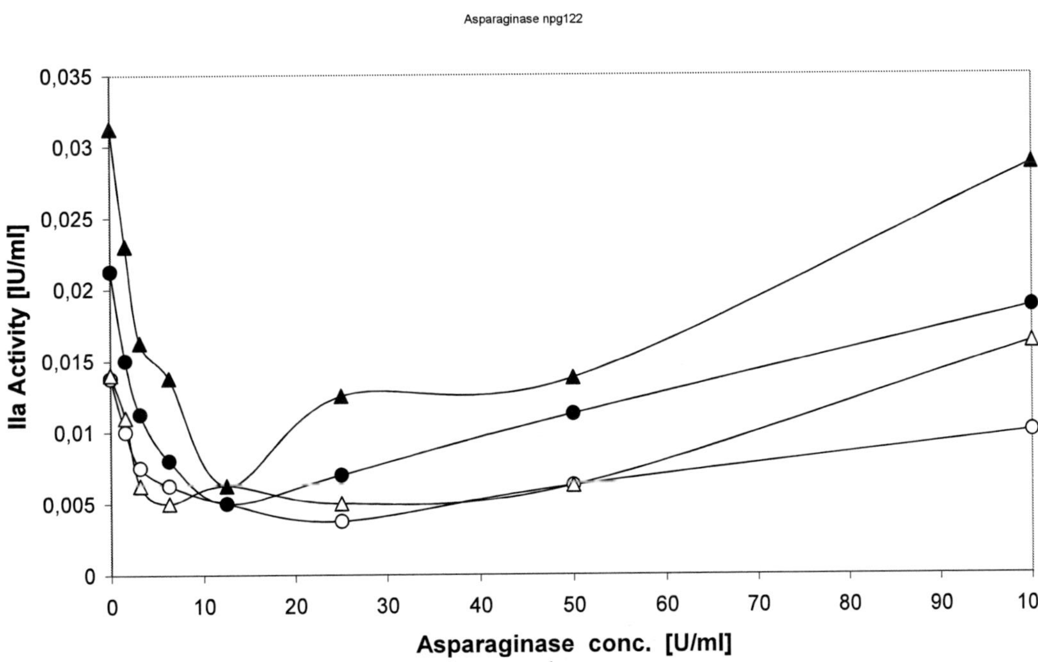

b

Figure 24. IIa generation in dependence of asparaginase concentration in sample 24. 50 µl unfrozen citrated normal plasma were supplemented in U-microwells (Brand®701300) with 0-100 U/ml asparaginase by repetitive 1+1 dilution. The RECA was performed. Figure 24a: 0 (O), 1.6 (Δ), 3.1 (◊), 6.3 (□), 12.5 (●), 25 (▲), 50 (♦), or 100 (■) U/ml asparaginase. Figure 24b: coagulation reaction times (CRT) of 5 min (O), 10 min (Δ), 15 min (●), or 20 min (▲). Approx. IC50 = 1 U/ml asparaginase.

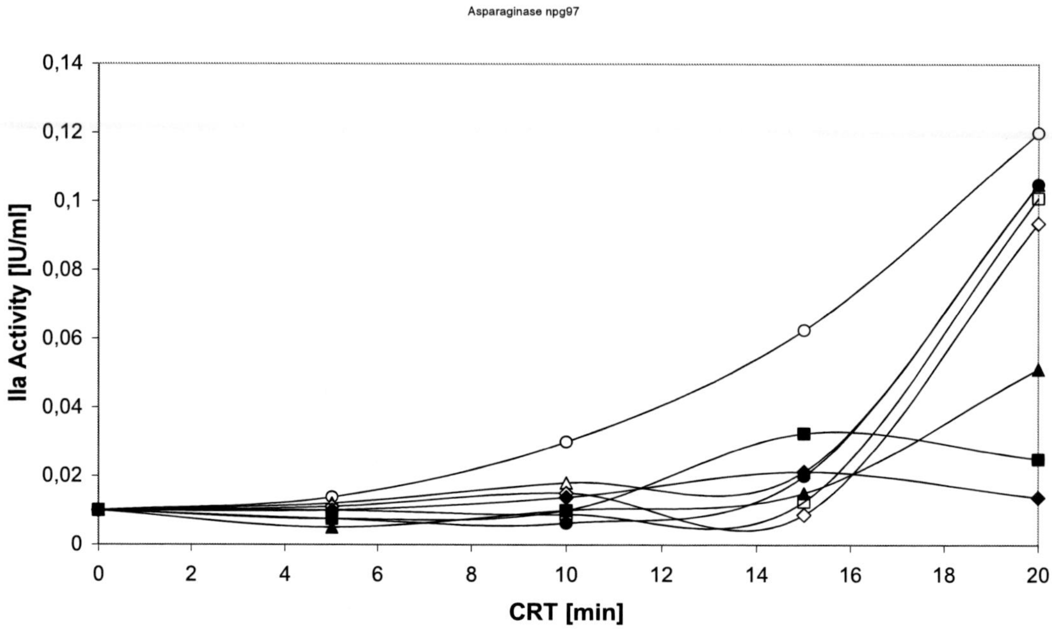

a

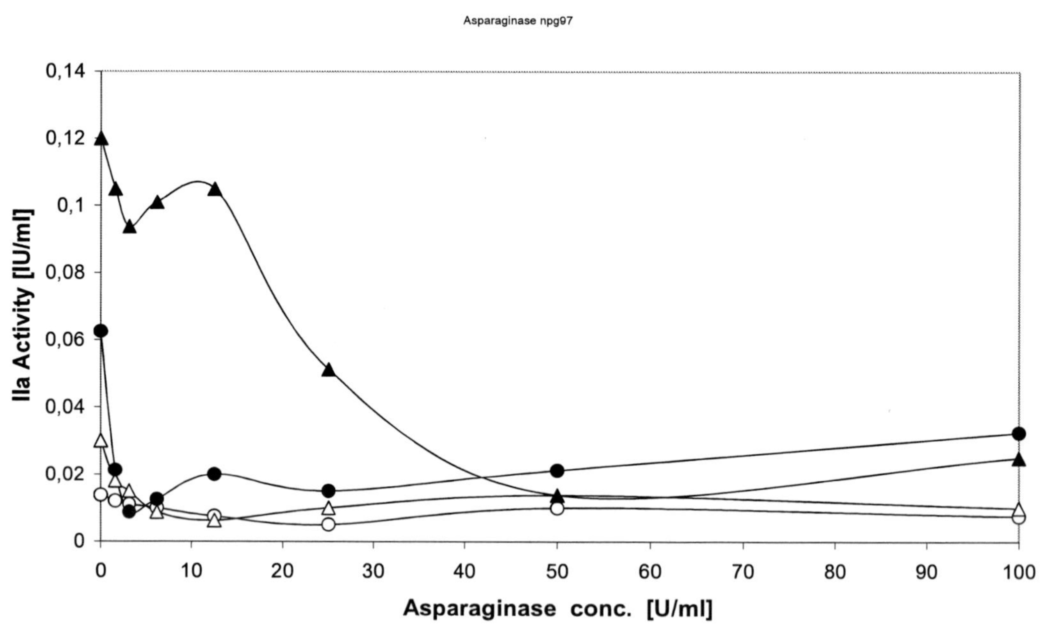

b

Figure 25. IIa generation in dependence of asparaginase concentration in sample 25. 50 µl unfrozen citrated normal plasma were supplemented in U-microwells (Brand®701300) with 0-100 U/ml asparaginase by repetitive 1+1 dilution. The RECA was performed. Figure 25a: 0 (O), 1.6 (Δ), 3.1 (◊), 6.3 (□), 12.5 (●), 25 (▲), 50 (♦), or 100 (■) U/ml asparaginase. Figure 25b: coagulation reaction times (CRT) of 5 min (O), 10 min (Δ), 15 min (●), or 20 min (▲). Approx. IC50 = 1 U/ml asparaginase.

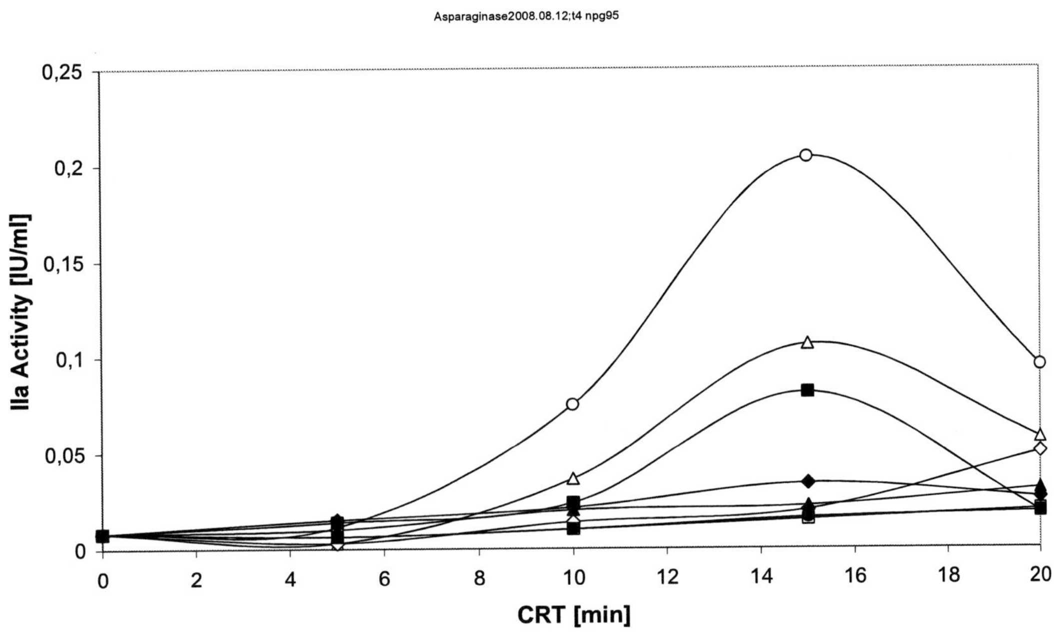

a

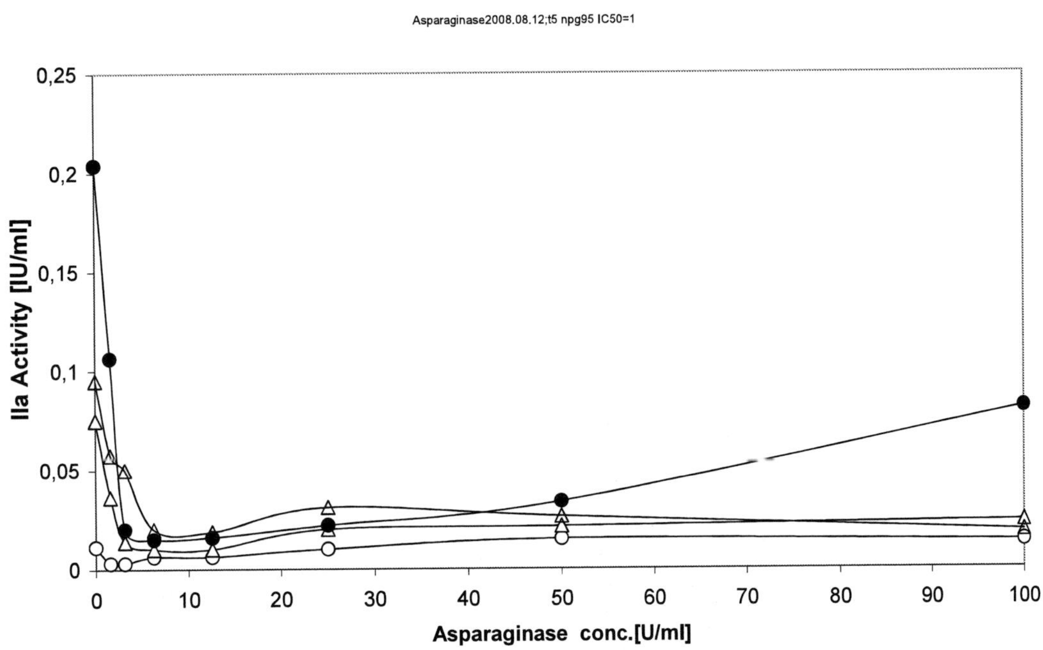

b

Figure 26. IIa generation in dependence of asparaginase concentration in sample 26. 50 µl unfrozen citrated normal plasma were supplemented in U-microwells (Brand®701300) with 0-100 U/ml asparaginase by repetitive 1+1 dilution. The RECA was performed. Figure 26a: 0 (O), 1.6 (Δ), 3.1 (◊), 6.3 (□), 12.5 (●), 25 (▲), 50 (♦), or 100 (■) U/ml asparaginase. Figure 26b: coagulation reaction times (CRT) of 5 min (O), 10 min (Δ), 15 min (●), or 20 min (▲). Approx. IC50 = 1 U/ml asparaginase.

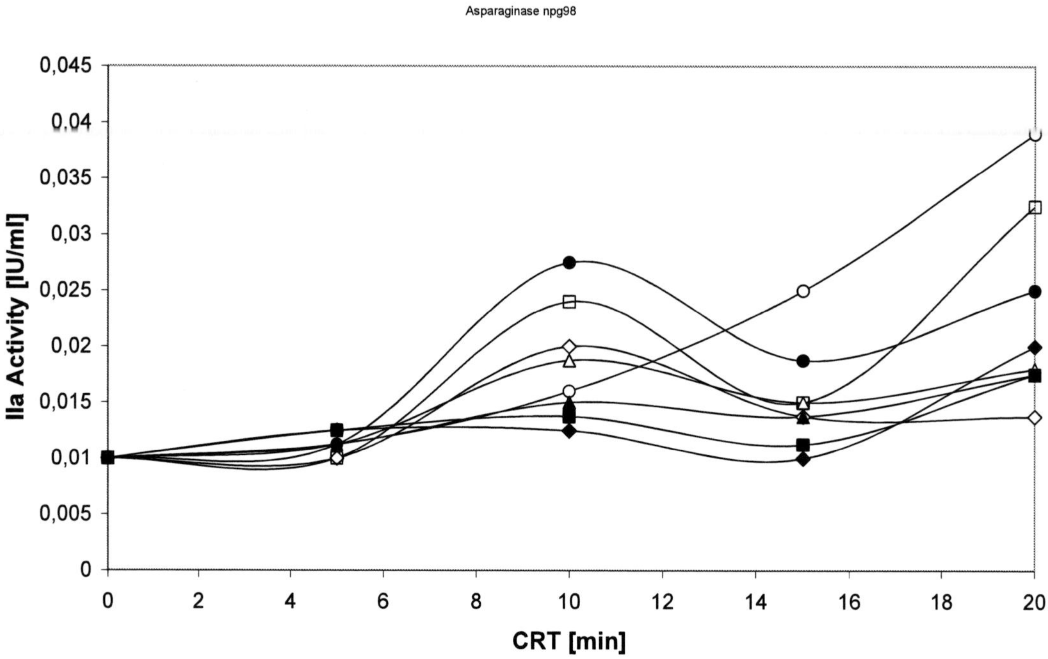

a

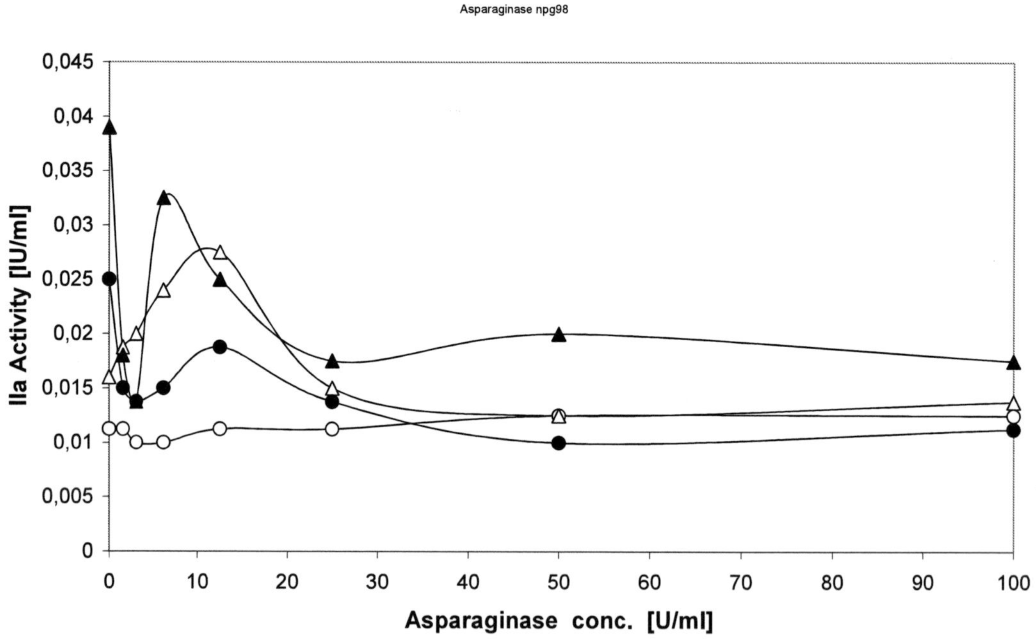

b

Figure 27. IIa generation in dependence of asparaginase concentration in sample 27. 50 µl unfrozen citrated normal plasma were supplemented in U-microwells (Brand®701300) with 0-100 U/ml asparaginase by repetitive 1+1 dilution. The RECA was performed. Figure 27a: 0 (O), 1.6 (Δ), 3.1 (◊), 6.3 (□), 12.5 (●), 25 (▲), 50 (♦), or 100 (■) U/ml asparaginase. Figure 27b: coagulation reaction times (CRT) of 5 min (O), 10 min (Δ), 15 min (●), or 20 min (▲). Approx. IC50 = 1 U/ml asparaginase.

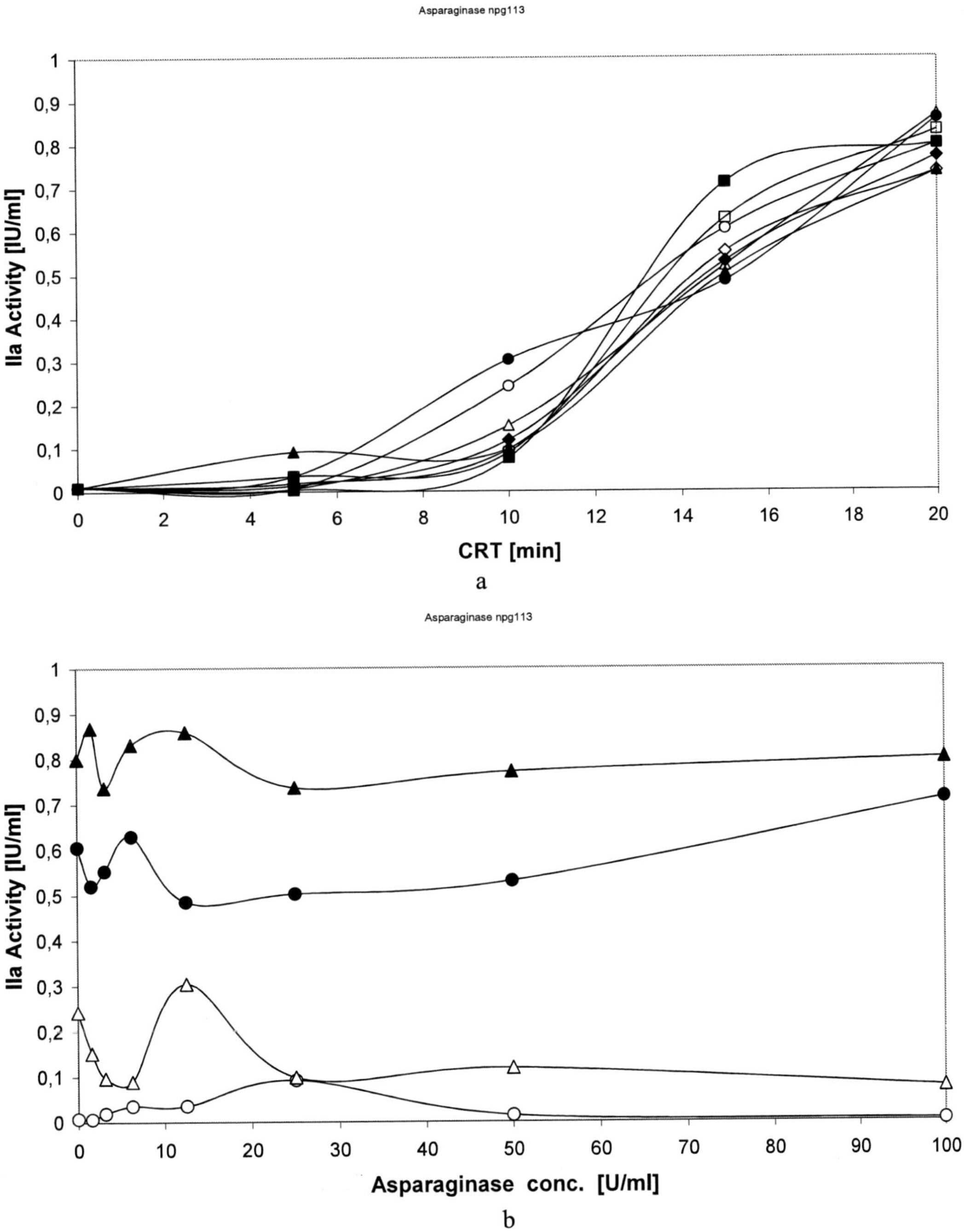

Figure 28. IIa generation in dependence of asparaginase concentration in sample 28. 50 µl unfrozen citrated normal plasma were supplemented in U-microwells (Brand®701300) with 0-100 U/ml asparaginase by repetitive 1+1 dilution. The RECA was performed. Figure 28a: 0 (O), 1.6 (Δ), 3.1 (◊), 6.3 (□), 12.5 (●), 25 (▲), 50 (♦), or 100 (■) U/ml asparaginase. Figure 28b: coagulation reaction times (CRT) of 5 min (O), 10 min (Δ), 15 min (●), or 20 min (▲). Approx. IC50 = 2 U/ml asparaginase.

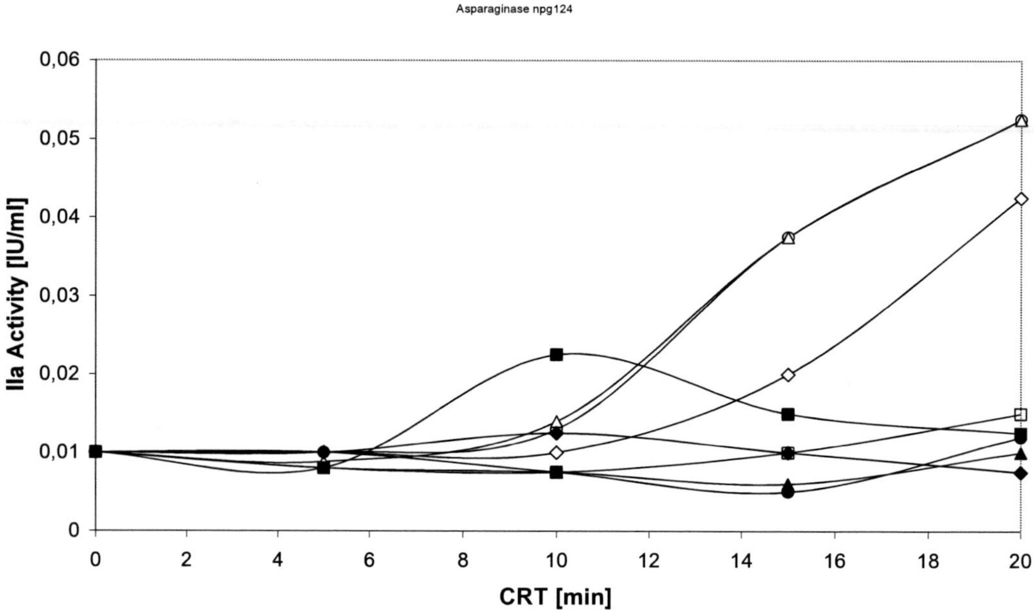

a

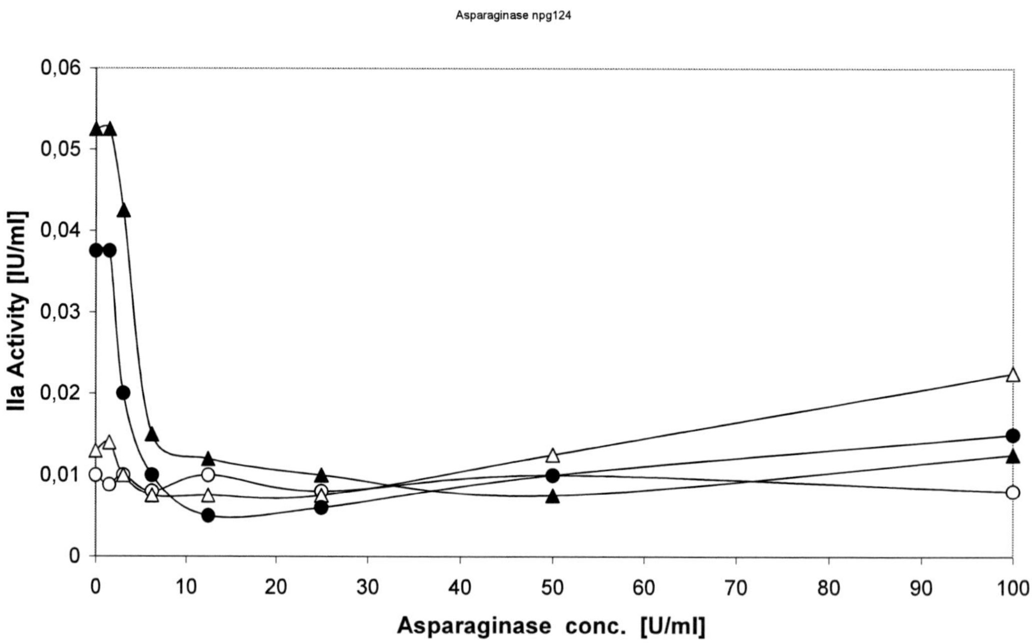

b

Figure 29. IIa generation in dependence of asparaginase concentration in sample 29. 50 µl unfrozen citrated normal plasma were supplemented in U-microwells (Brand®701300) with 0-100 U/ml asparaginase by repetitive 1+1 dilution. The RECA was performed. Figure 29a: 0 (O), 1.6 (Δ), 3.1 (◊), 6.3 (□), 12.5 (●), 25 (▲), 50 (♦), or 100 (■) U/ml asparaginase. Figure 29b: coagulation reaction times (CRT) of 5 min (O), 10 min (Δ), 15 min (●), or 20 min (▲). Approx. IC50 = 2 U/ml asparaginase.

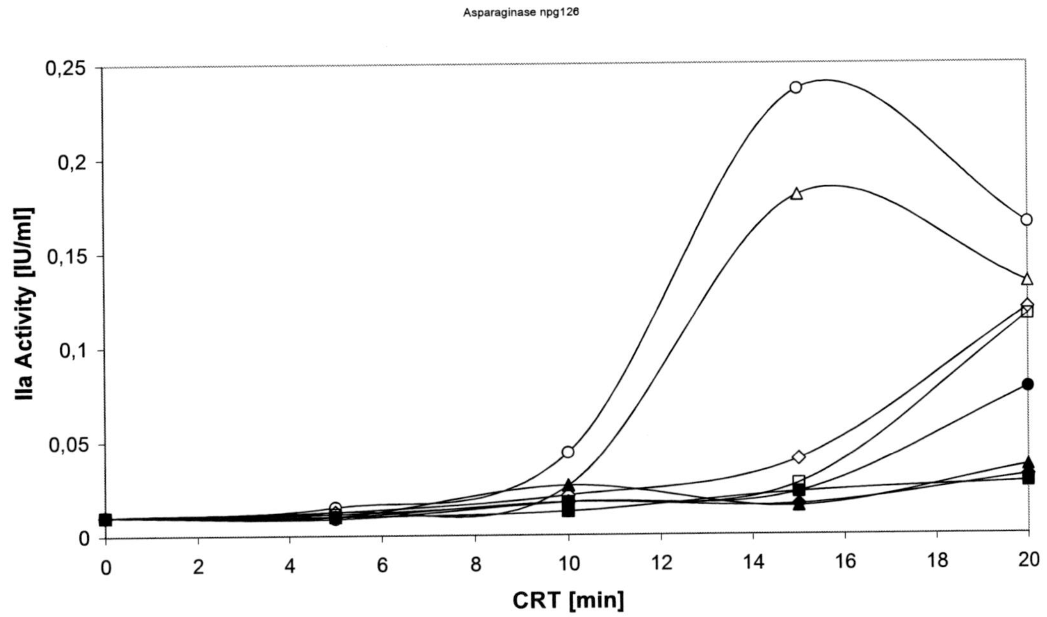

a

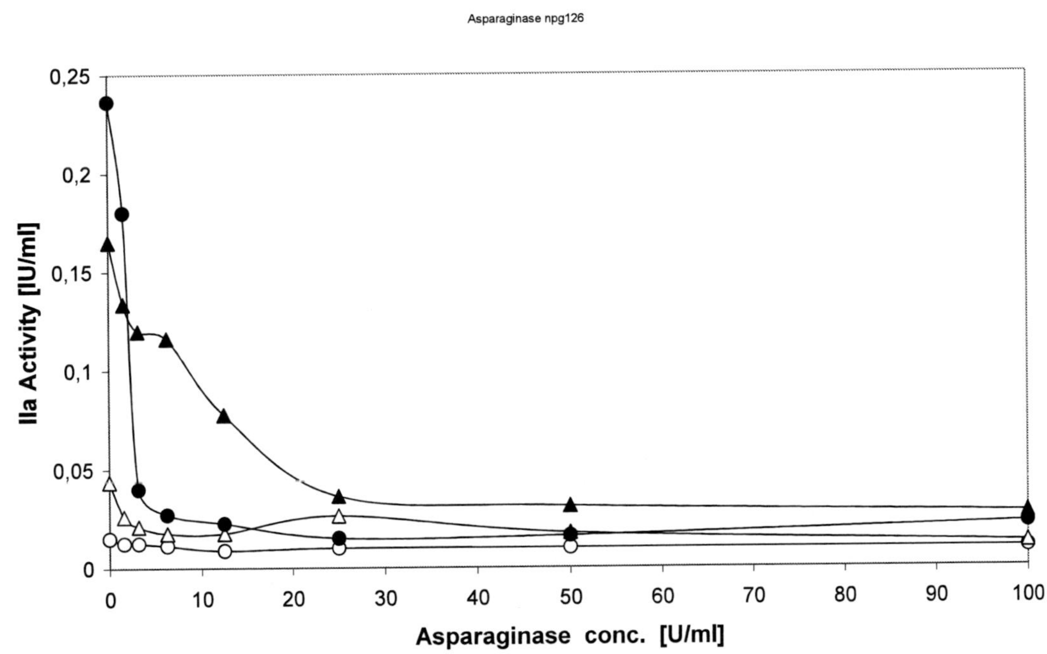

b

Figure 30. IIa generation in dependence of asparaginase concentration in sample 30. 50 µl unfrozen citrated normal plasma were supplemented in U-microwells (Brand®701300) with 0-100 U/ml asparaginase by repetitive 1+1 dilution. The RECA was performed. Figure 30a: 0 (O), 1.6 (Δ), 3.1 (◊), 6.3 (□), 12.5 (●), 25 (▲), 50 (♦), or 100 (■) U/ml asparaginase. Figure 30b: coagulation reaction times (CRT) of 5 min (O), 10 min (Δ), 15 min (●), or 20 min (▲). Approx. IC50 = 2 U/ml asparaginase.

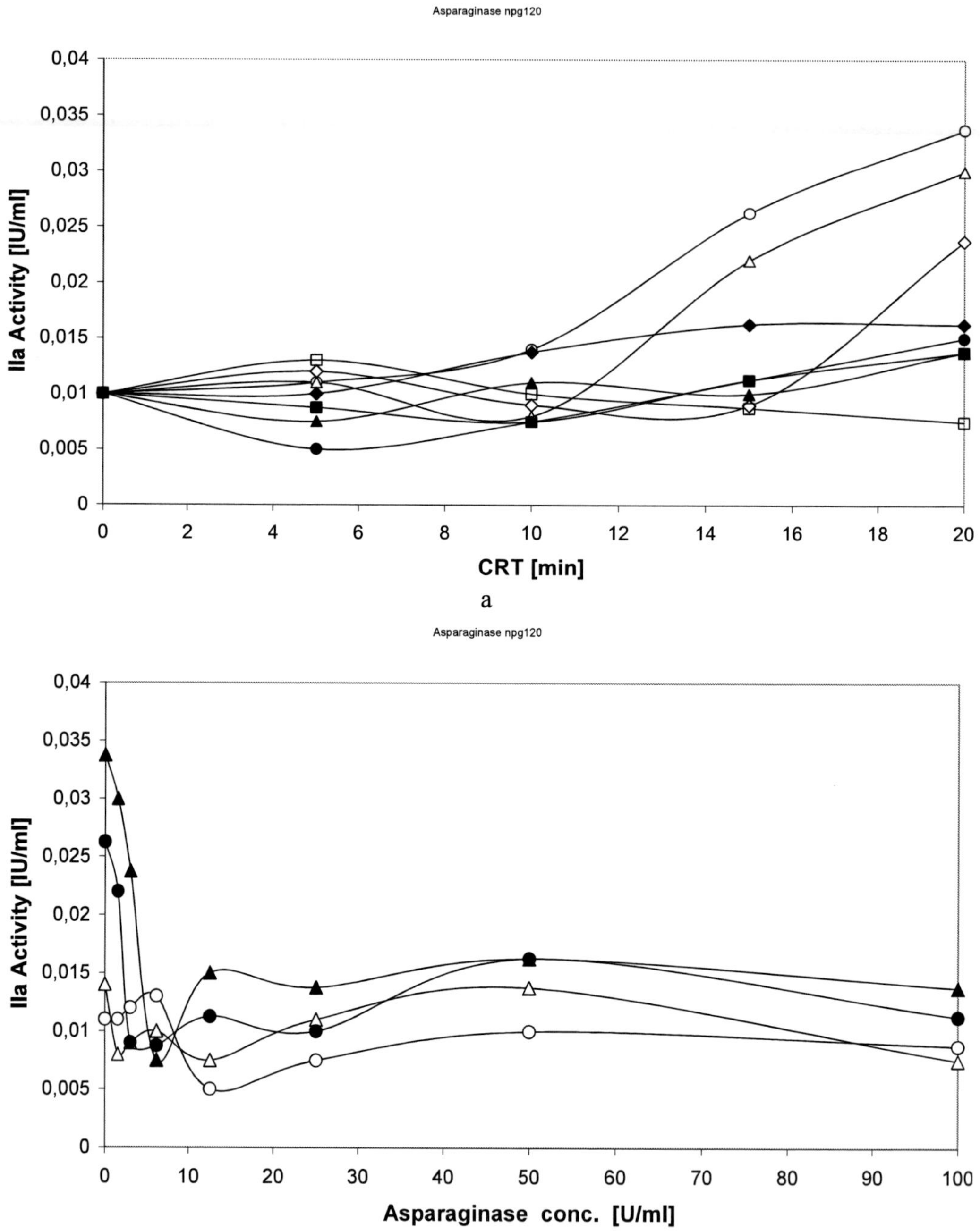

Figure 31. IIa generation in dependence of asparaginase concentration in sample 31. 50 µl unfrozen citrated normal plasma were supplemented in U-microwells (Brand®701300) with 0-100 U/ml asparaginase by repetitive 1+1 dilution. The RECA was performed. Figure 31a: 0 (O), 1.6 (Δ), 3.1 (◊), 6.3 (□), 12.5 (●), 25 (▲), 50 (♦), or 100 (■) U/ml asparaginase. Figure 31b: coagulation reaction times (CRT) of 5 min (O), 10 min (Δ), 15 min (●), or 20 min (▲). Approx. IC50 = 2 U/ml asparaginase.

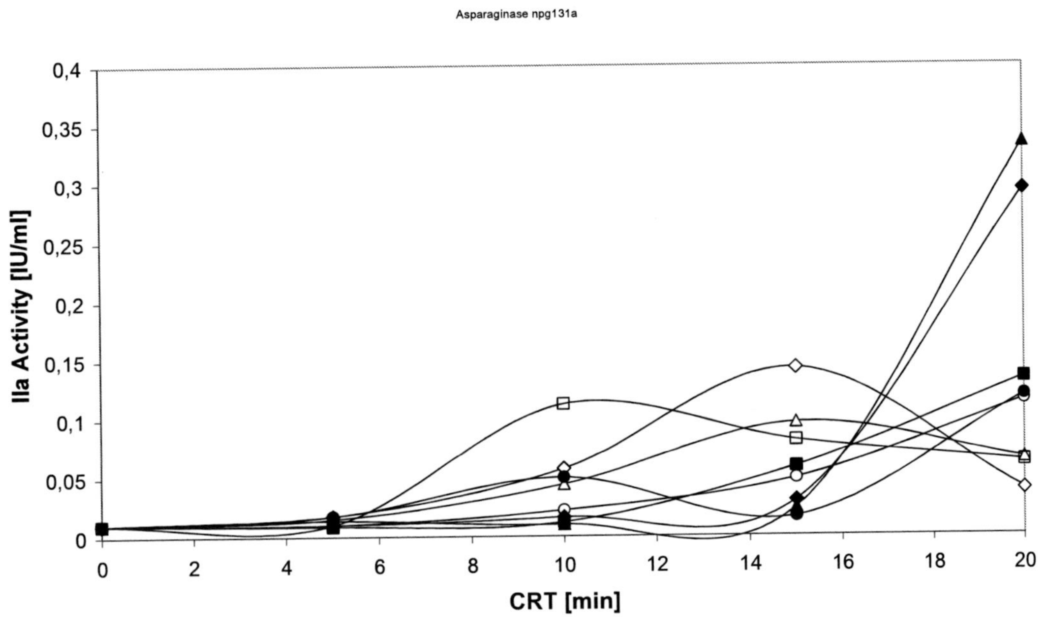

a

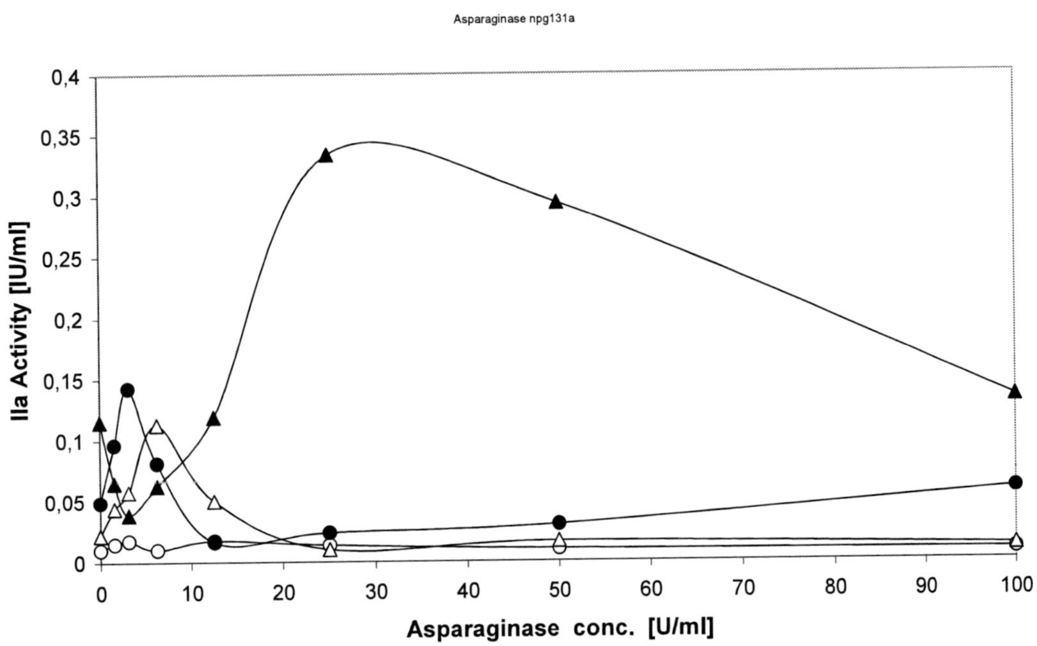

b

Figure 32. IIa generation in dependence of asparaginase concentration in sample 32. 50 µl unfrozen citrated normal plasma were supplemented in U-microwells (Brand®701300) with 0-100 U/ml asparaginase by repetitive 1+1 dilution. The RECA was performed. Figure 32a: 0 (O), 1.6 (Δ), 3.1 (◊), 6.3 (□), 12.5 (●), 25 (▲), 50 (♦), or 100 (■) U/ml asparaginase. Figure 32b: coagulation reaction times (CRT) of 5 min (O), 10 min (Δ), 15 min (●), or 20 min (▲). Approx. IC50 = 2 (RECA-20 with no plasmatic turbidity increase) or SC200 = 2 U/ml asparaginase (RECA-15).

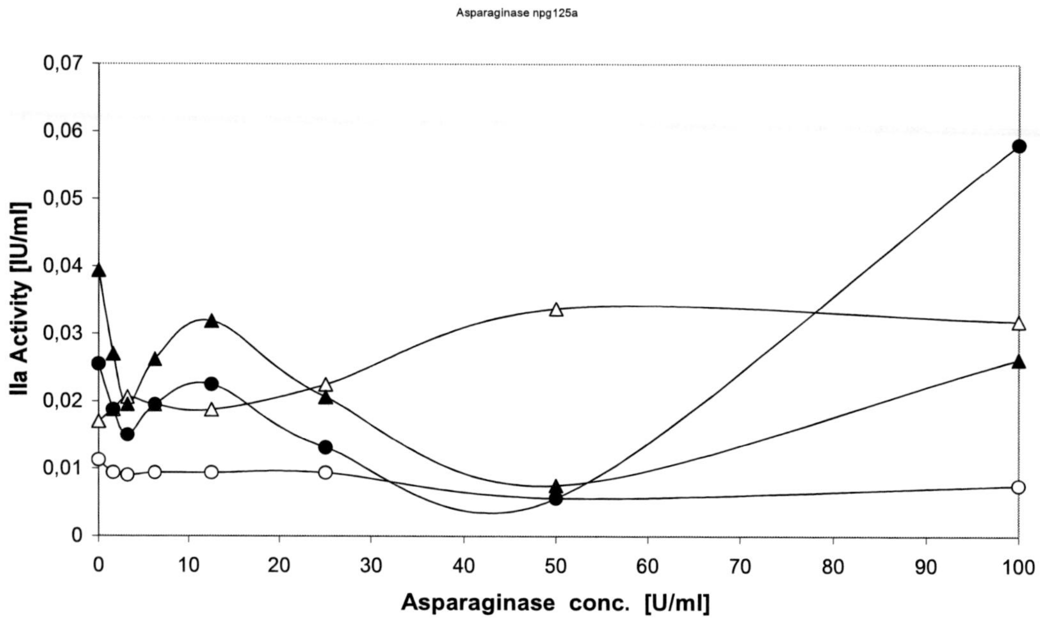

a

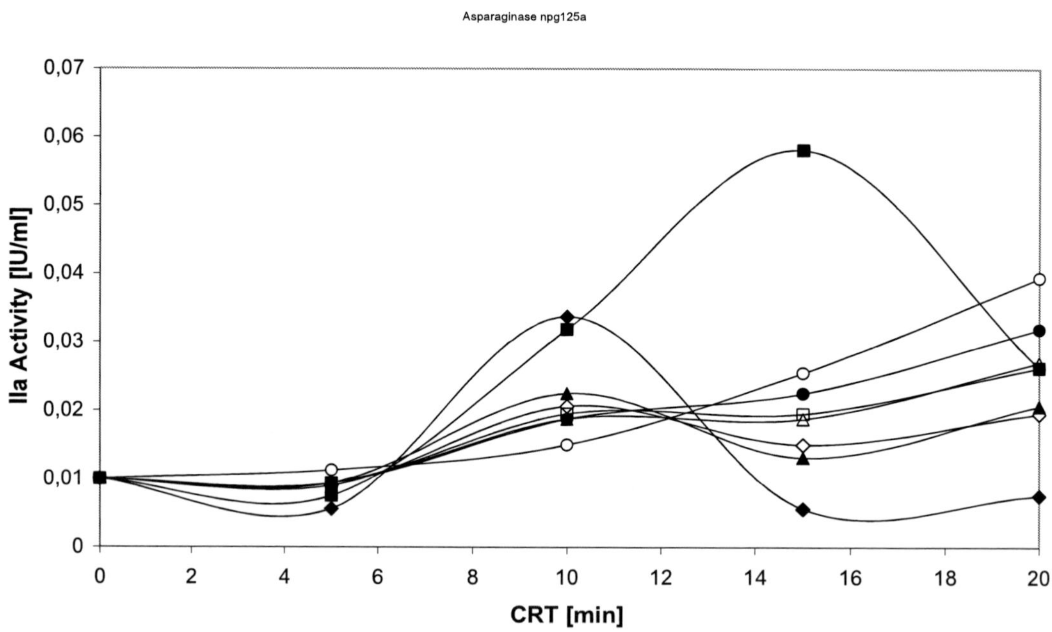

b

Figure 33. IIa generation in dependence of asparaginase concentration in sample 33. 50 μl unfrozen citrated normal plasma were supplemented in U-microwells (Brand®701300) with 0-100 U/ml asparaginase by repetitive 1+1 dilution. The RECA was performed. Figure 33a: 0 (O), 1.6 (Δ), 3.1 (◊), 6.3 (□), 12.5 (●), 25 (▲), 50 (♦), or 100 (■) U/ml asparaginase. Figure 33b: coagulation reaction times (CRT) of 5 min (O), 10 min (Δ), 15 min (●), or 20 min (▲).Approx. IC50 = 2 U/ml and approx. SC200 = 80 asparaginase.

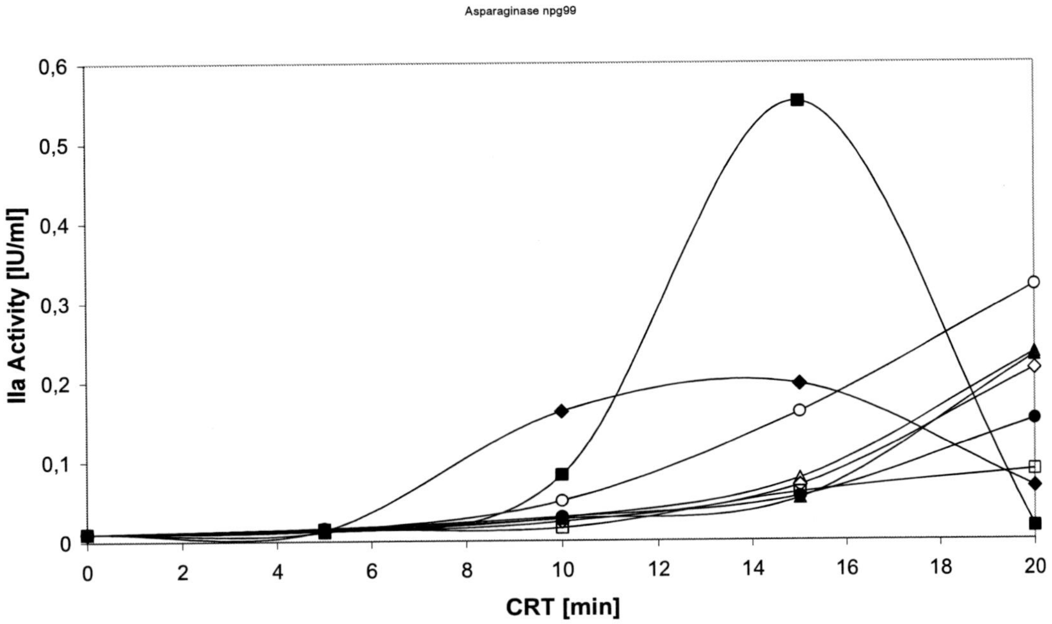

a

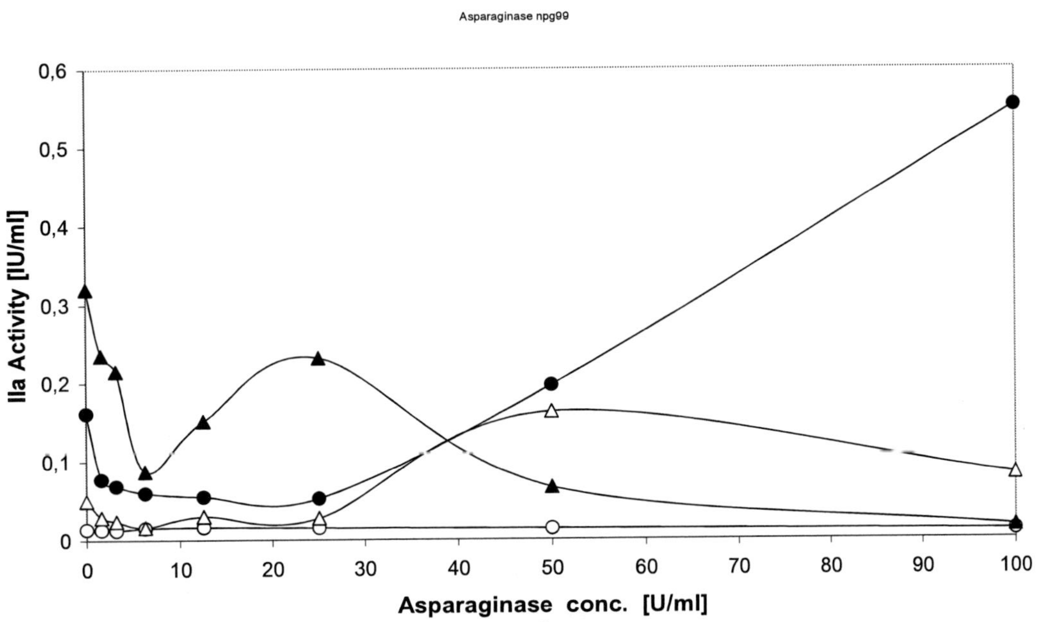

b

Figure 34. IIa generation in dependence of asparaginase concentration in sample 34. 50 µl unfrozen citrated normal plasma were supplemented in U-microwells (Brand®701300) with 0-100 U/ml asparaginase by repetitive 1+1 dilution. The RECA was performed. Figure 34a: 0 (O), 1.6 (Δ), 3.1 (◊), 6.3 (□), 12.5 (●), 25 (▲), 50 (♦), or 100 (■) U/ml asparaginase. Figure 34b: coagulation reaction times (CRT) of 5 min (O), 10 min (Δ), 15 min (●), or 20 min (▲).Approx. IC50 = 2 U/ml and approx. SC200 = 35 U/ml asparaginase.

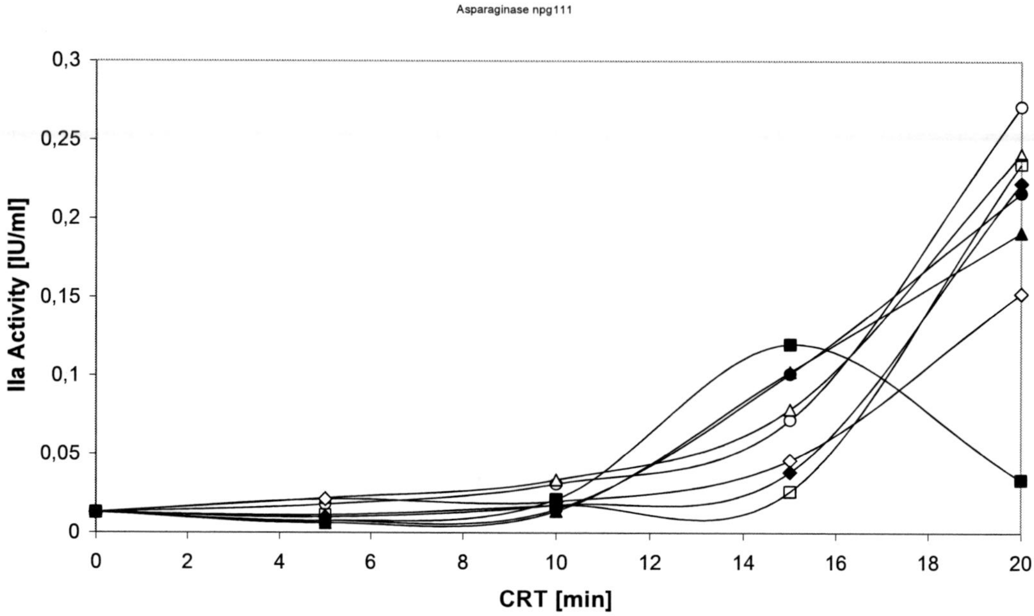

a

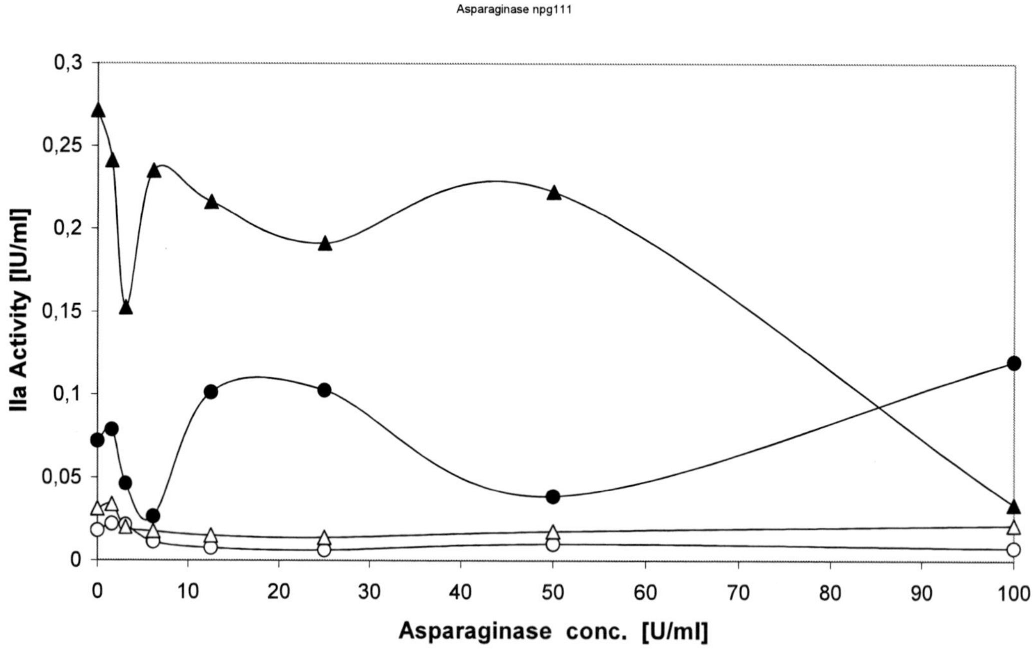

b

Figure 35. IIa generation in dependence of asparaginase concentration in sample 35. 50 µl unfrozen citrated normal plasma were supplemented in U-microwells (Brand®701300) with 0-100 U/ml asparaginase by repetitive 1+1 dilution. The RECA was performed. Figure 35a: 0 (O), 1.6 (Δ), 3.1 (◊), 6.3 (□), 12.5 (●), 25 (▲), 50 (♦), or 100 (■) U/ml asparaginase. Figure 35b: coagulation reaction times (CRT) of 5 min (O), 10 min (Δ), 15 min (●), or 20 min (▲). Approx. IC50 = 3 U/ml.

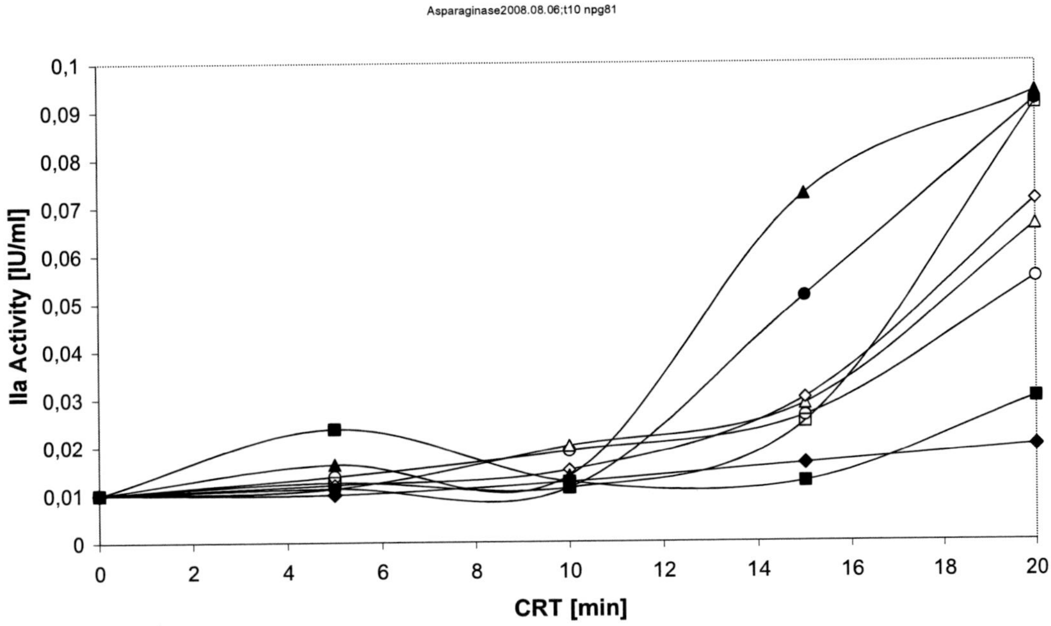

a

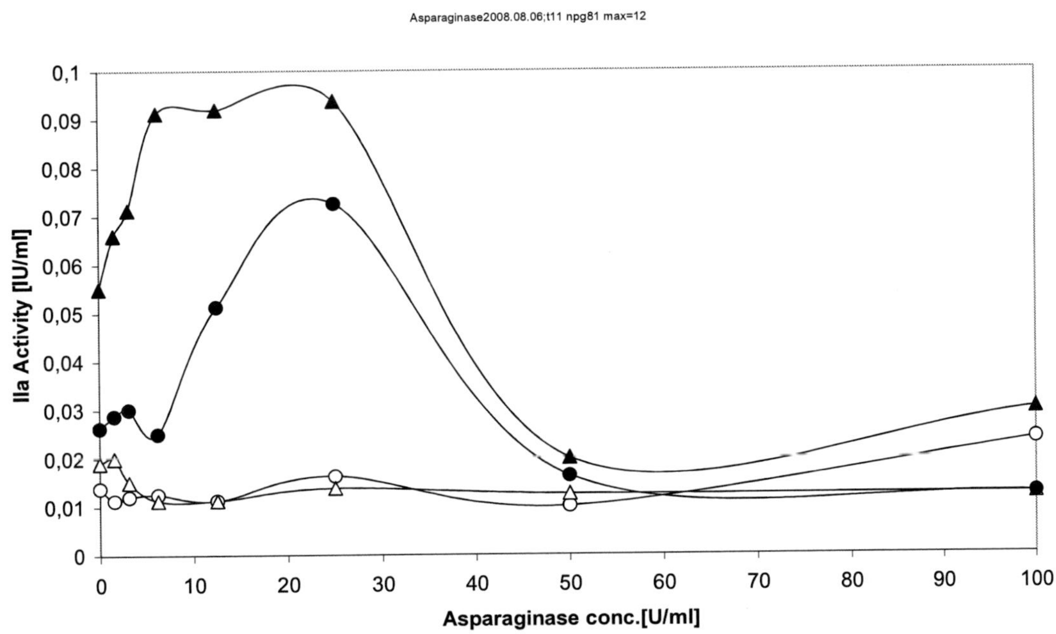

b

Figure 36. IIa generation in dependence of asparaginase concentration in sample 36. 50 μl unfrozen citrated normal plasma were supplemented in U-microwells (Brand®701300) with 0-100 U/ml asparaginase by repetitive 1+1 dilution. The RECA was performed. Figure 36a: 0 (O), 1.6 (Δ), 3.1 (◊), 6.3 (□), 12.5 (●), 25 (▲), 50 (♦), or 100 (■) U/ml asparaginase. Figure 36b: coagulation reaction times (CRT) of 5 min (O), 10 min (Δ), 15 min (●), or 20 min (▲).Approx. IC50 = 3 U/ml and approx. SC200 = 12 U/ml asparaginase.

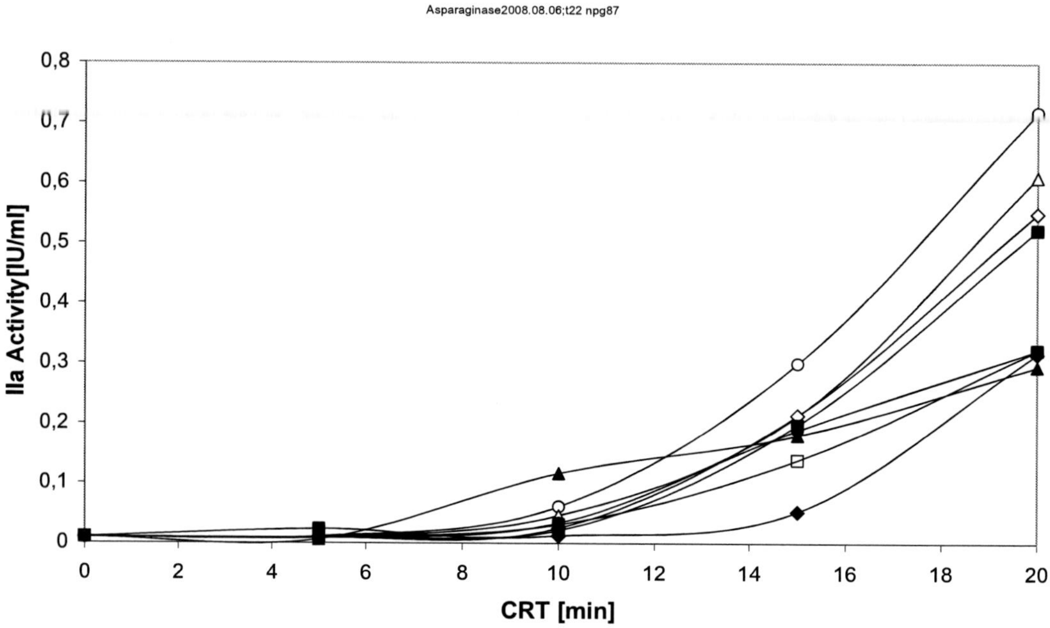

a

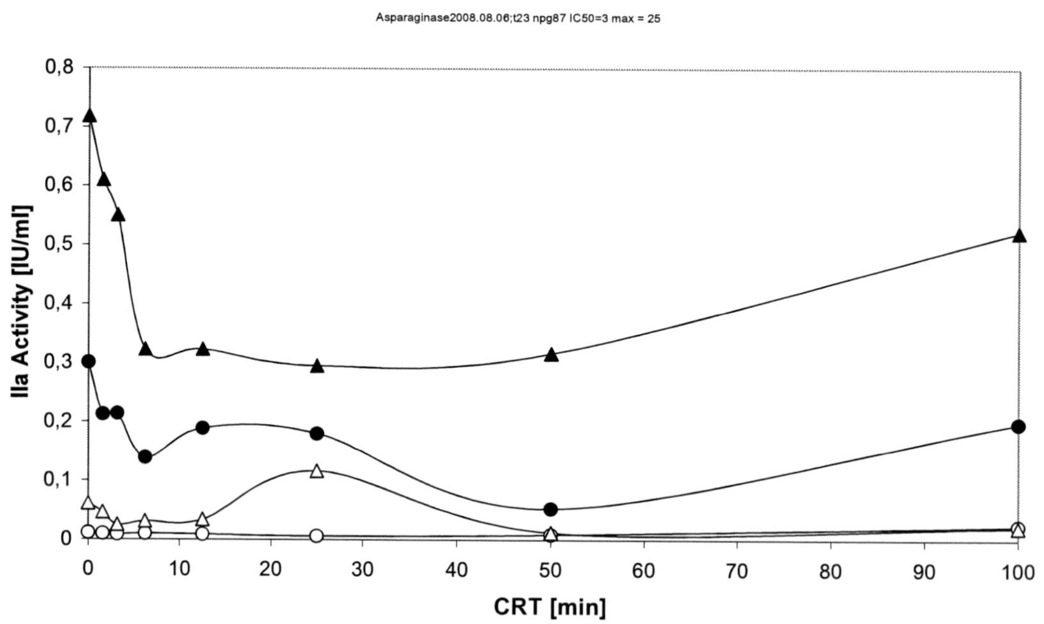

b

Figure 37. IIa generation in dependence of asparaginase concentration in sample 37. 50 µl unfrozen citrated normal plasma were supplemented in U-microwells (Brand®701300) with 0-100 U/ml asparaginase by repetitive 1+1 dilution. The RECA was performed. Figure 37a: 0 (O), 1.6 (Δ), 3.1 (◊), 6.3 (□), 12.5 (●), 25 (▲), 50 (♦), or 100 (■) U/ml asparaginase. Figure 37b: coagulation reaction times (CRT) of 5 min (O), 10 min (Δ), 15 min (●), or 20 min (▲).Approx. IC50 = 3 U/ml and approx. SC200 = 25 U/ml asparaginase.

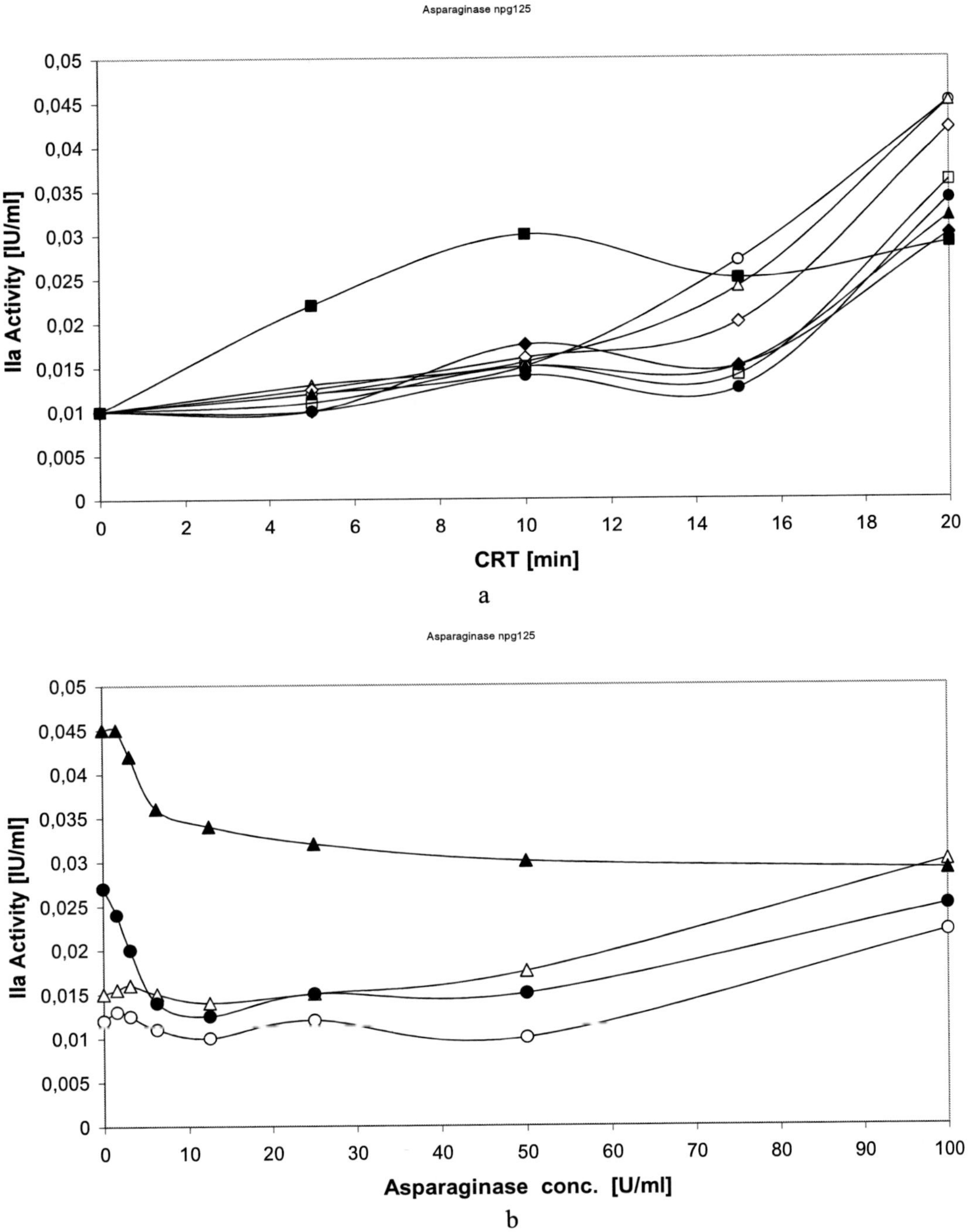

Figure 38. IIa generation in dependence of asparaginase concentration in sample 38. 50 µl unfrozen citrated normal plasma were supplemented in U-microwells (Brand®701300) with 0-100 U/ml asparaginase by repetitive 1+1 dilution. The RECA was performed. Figure 38a: 0 (O), 1.6 (Δ), 3.1 (◊), 6.3 (□), 12.5 (●), 25 (▲), 50 (♦), or 100 (■) U/ml asparaginase. Figure 38b: coagulation reaction times (CRT) of 5 min (O), 10 min (Δ), 15 min (●), or 20 min (▲).Approx. IC50 = 3 U/ml and approx. SC200 = 80 U/ml asparaginase.

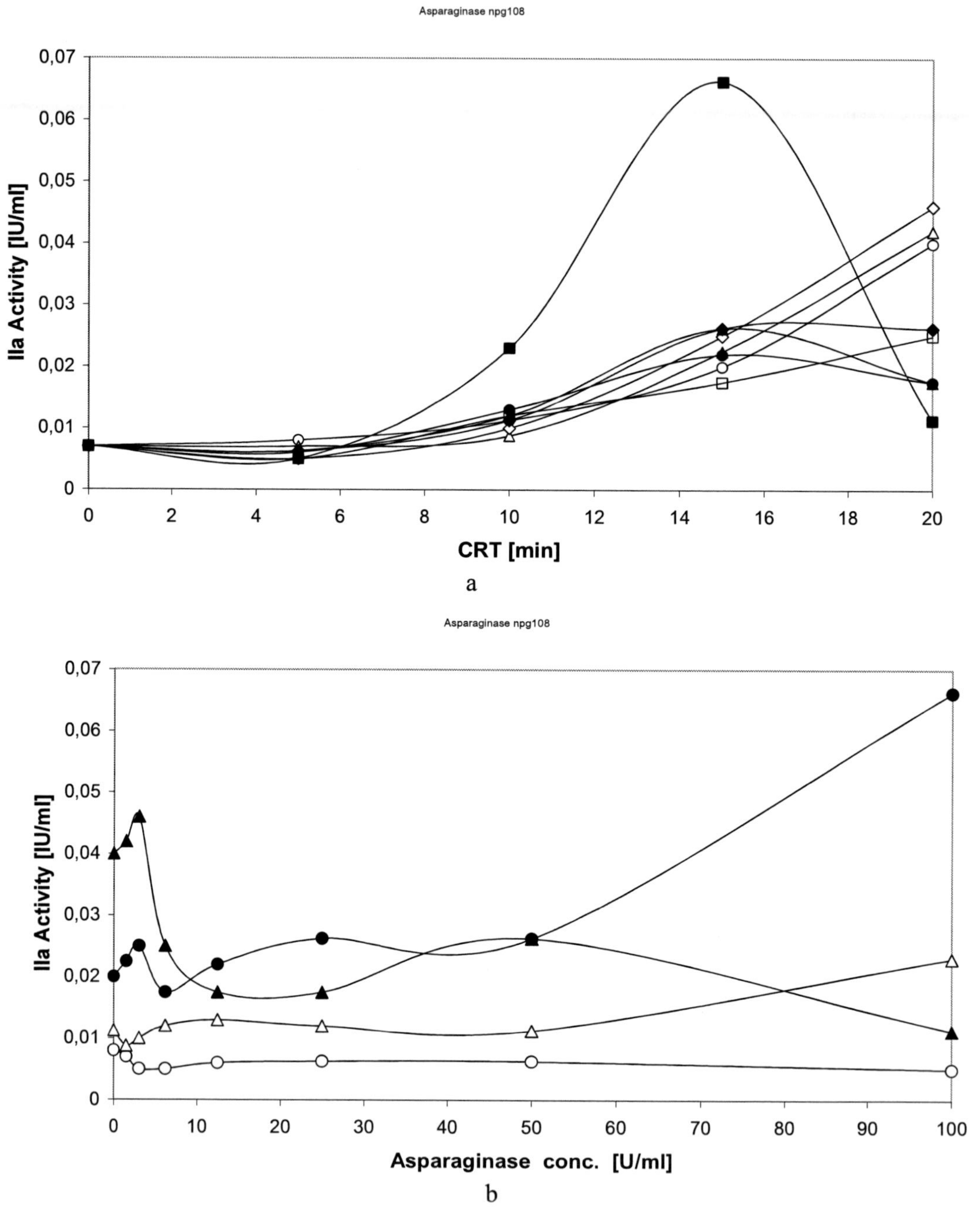

Figure 39. IIa generation in dependence of asparaginase concentration in sample 39. 50 µl unfrozen citrated normal plasma were supplemented in U-microwells (Brand®701300) with 0-100 U/ml asparaginase by repetitive 1+1 dilution. The RECA was performed. Figure 39a: 0 (O), 1.6 (Δ), 3.1 (◊), 6.3 (□), 12.5 (●), 25 (▲), 50 (♦), or 100 (■) U/ml asparaginase. Figure 39b: coagulation reaction times (CRT) of 5 min (O), 10 min (Δ), 15 min (●), or 20 min (▲). Approx. IC50 = 6 U/ml (analyzed at RECA-20, no significant basal increase of plasmatic turbidity) and approx. SC200 = 55 U/ml asparaginase.

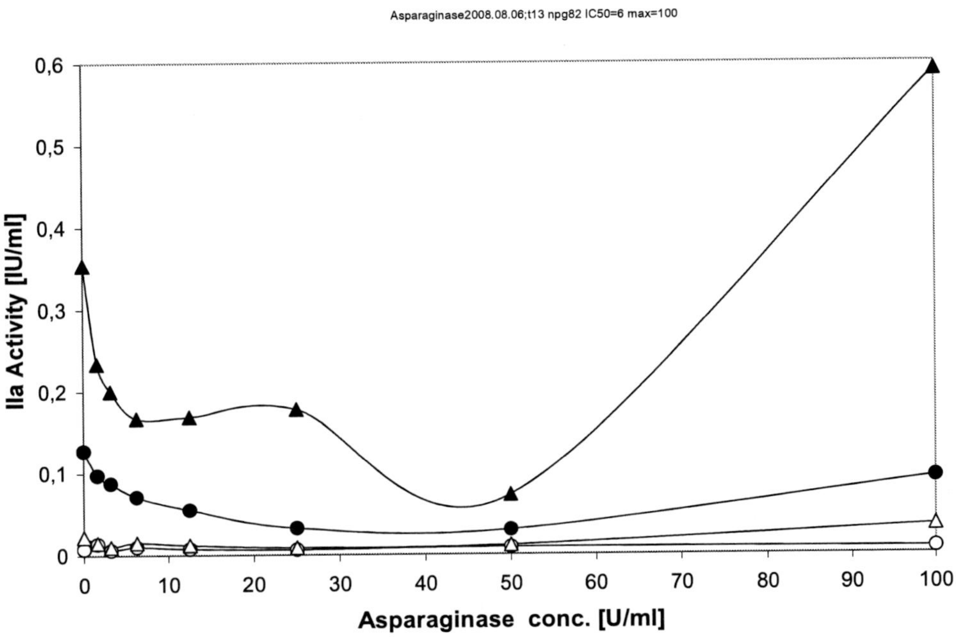

a

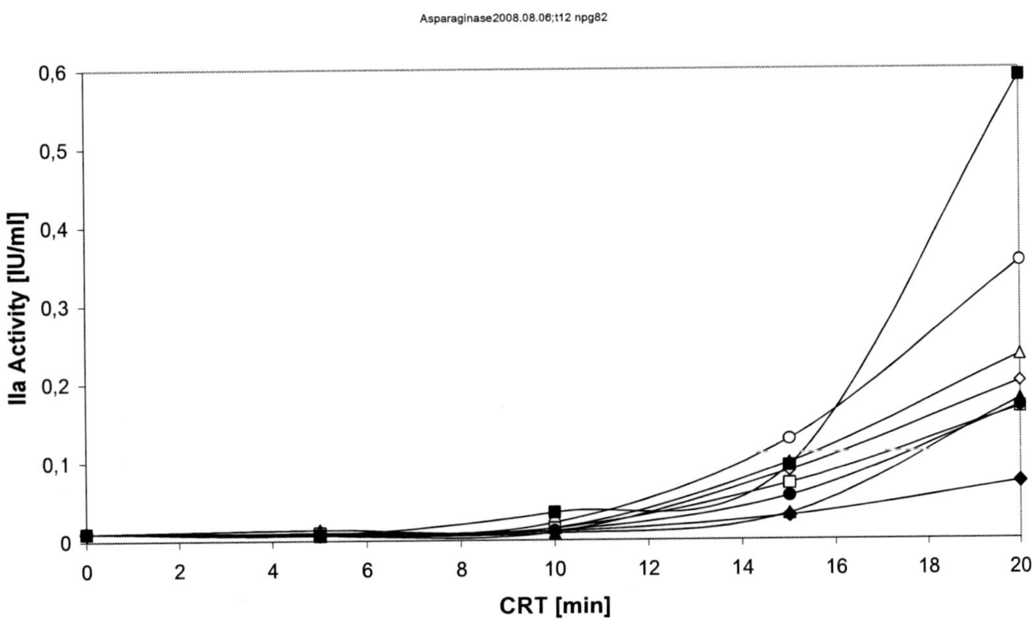

b

Figure 40. IIa generation in dependence of asparaginase concentration in sample 40. 50 µl unfrozen citrated normal plasma were supplemented in U-microwells (Brand®701300) with 0-100 U/ml asparaginase by repetitive 1+1 dilution. The RECA was performed. Figure 40a: 0 (O), 1.6 (Δ), 3.1 (◊), 6.3 (□), 12.5 (●), 25 (▲), 50 (♦), or 100 (■) U/ml asparaginase. Figure 40b: coagulation reaction times (CRT) of 5 min (O), 10 min (Δ), 15 min (●), or 20 min (▲).Approx. IC50 = 6 U/ml and approx. SC200 = 100 U/ml asparaginase.

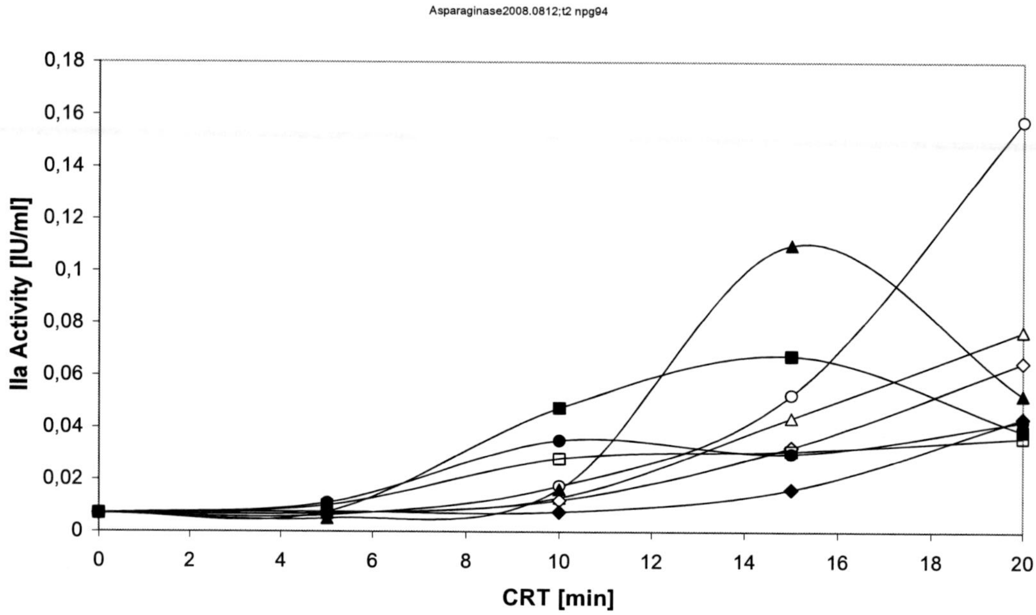

a

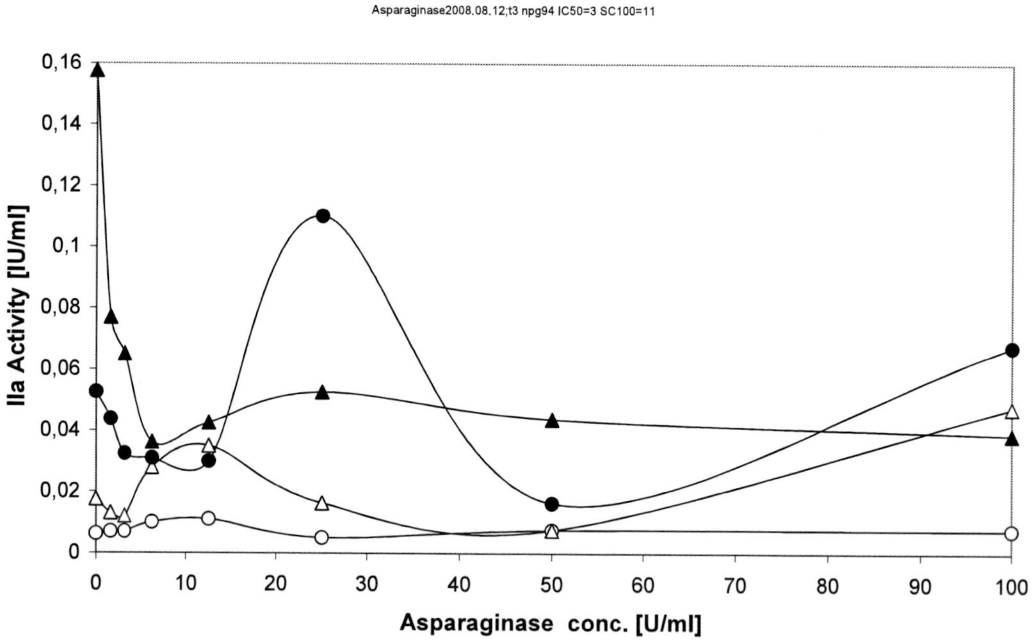

b

Figure 41. IIa generation in dependence of asparaginase concentration in sample 41. 50 µl unfrozen citrated normal plasma were supplemented in the U-microwells (Brand®701300) with 0-100 U/ml asparaginase by repetitive 1+1 dilution. The RECA was performed. Figure 41a: 0 (O), 1.6 (Δ), 3.1 (◊), 6.3 (□), 12.5 (•), 25 (▲), 50 (♦), or 100 (■) U/ml asparaginase. Figure 41b: coagulation reaction times (CRT) of 5 min (O), 10 min (Δ), 15 min (•), or 20 min (▲).Approx. IC50 = 3 U/ml and approx. SC200 = 11 U/ml asparaginase.

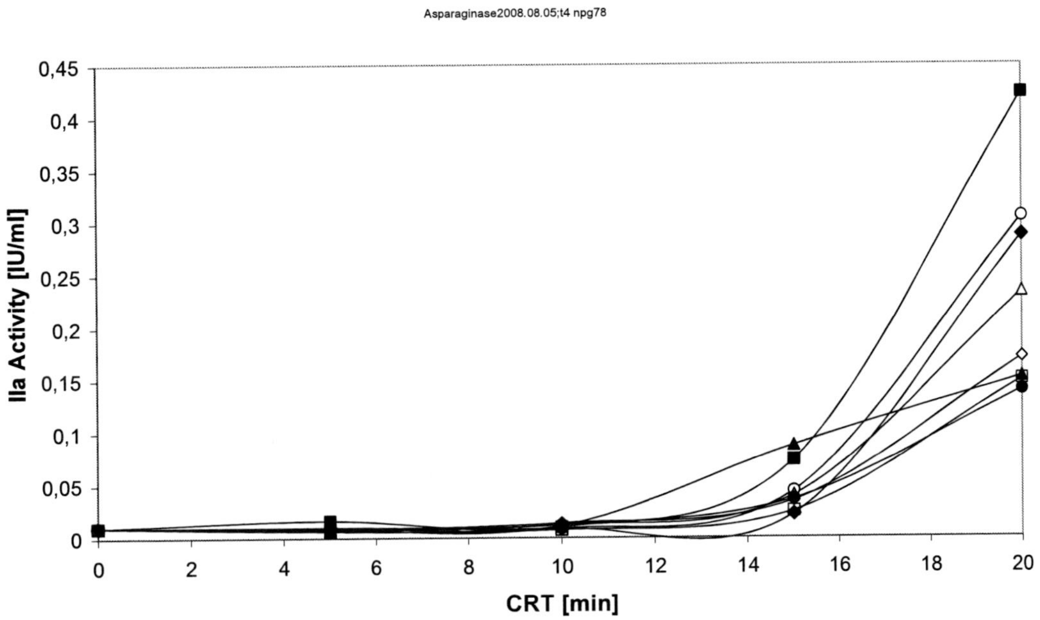

a

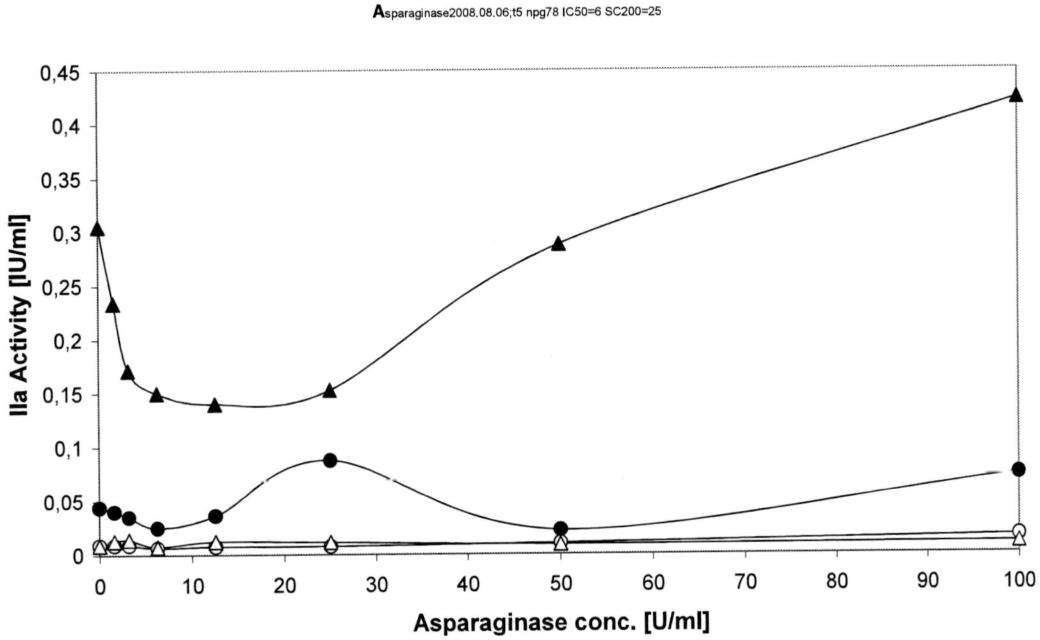

b

Figure 42. IIa generation in dependence of asparaginase concentration in sample 42. 50 µl unfrozen citrated normal plasma were supplemented in U-microwells (Brand®701300) with 0-100 U/ml asparaginase by repetitive 1+1 dilution. The RECA was performed. Figure 42a: 0 (O), 1.6 (Δ), 3.1 (◊), 6.3 (□), 12.5 (●), 25 (▲), 50 (♦), or 100 (■) U/ml asparaginase. Figure 42b: coagulation reaction times (CRT) of 5 min (O), 10 min (Δ), 15 min (●), or 20 min (▲). Approx. IC50 = 6 U/ml and approx. SC200=25 U/ml asparaginase.

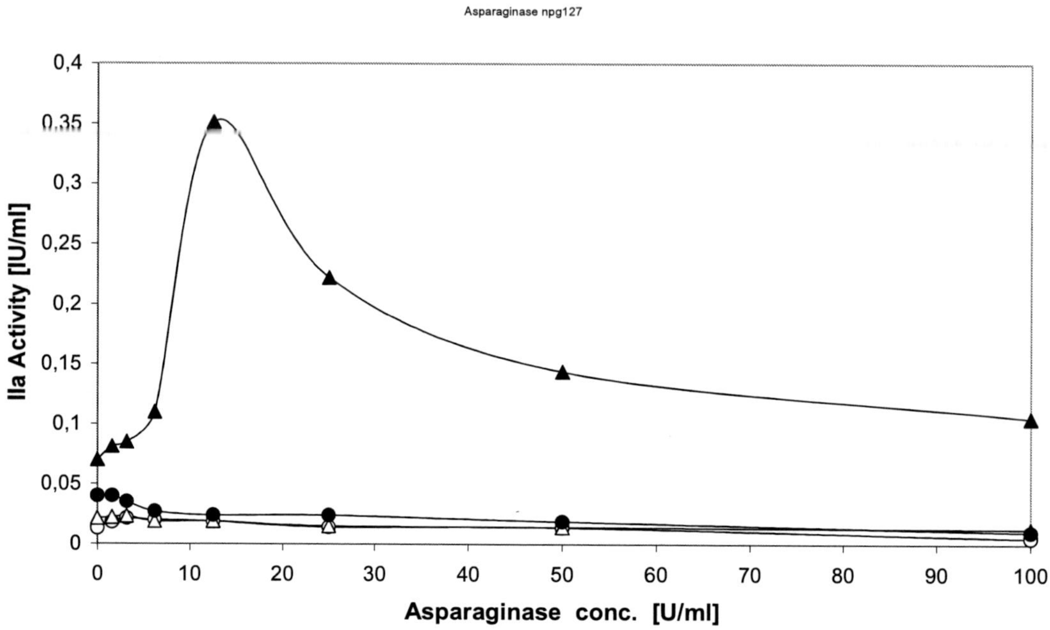

a

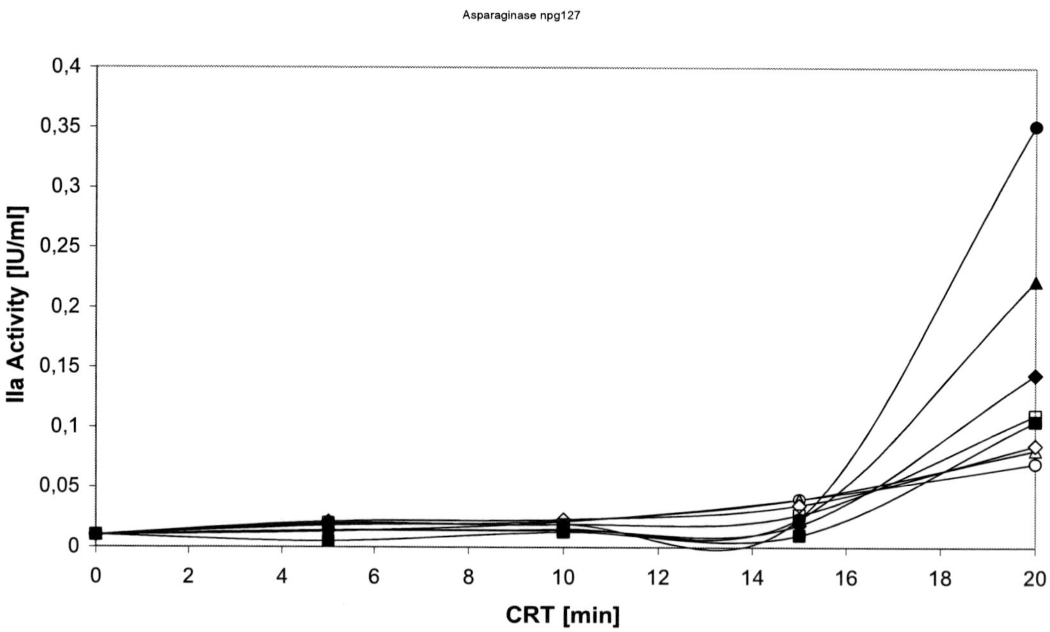

b

Figure 43. IIa generation in dependence of asparaginase concentration in sample 43. 50 μl unfrozen citrated normal plasma were supplemented in U-microwells (Brand®701300) with 0-100 U/ml asparaginase by repetitive 1+1 dilution. The RECA was performed. Figure 43a: 0 (O), 1.6 (Δ), 3.1 (◊), 6.3 (□), 12.5 (●), 25 (▲), 50 (♦), or 100 (■) U/ml asparaginase. Figure 43b: coagulation reaction times (CRT) of 5 min (O), 10 min (Δ), 15 min (●), or 20 min (▲). Approx. IC50 = 8 U/ml (analyzed at RECA-15) and approx. SC200= 8 U/ml asparaginase (analyzed at RECA-20).

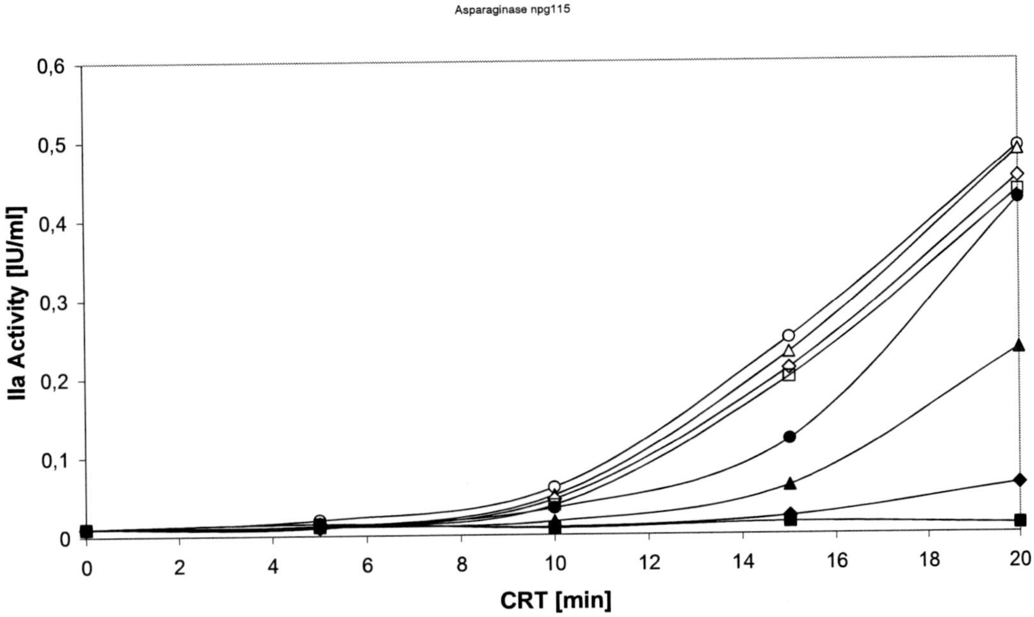

a

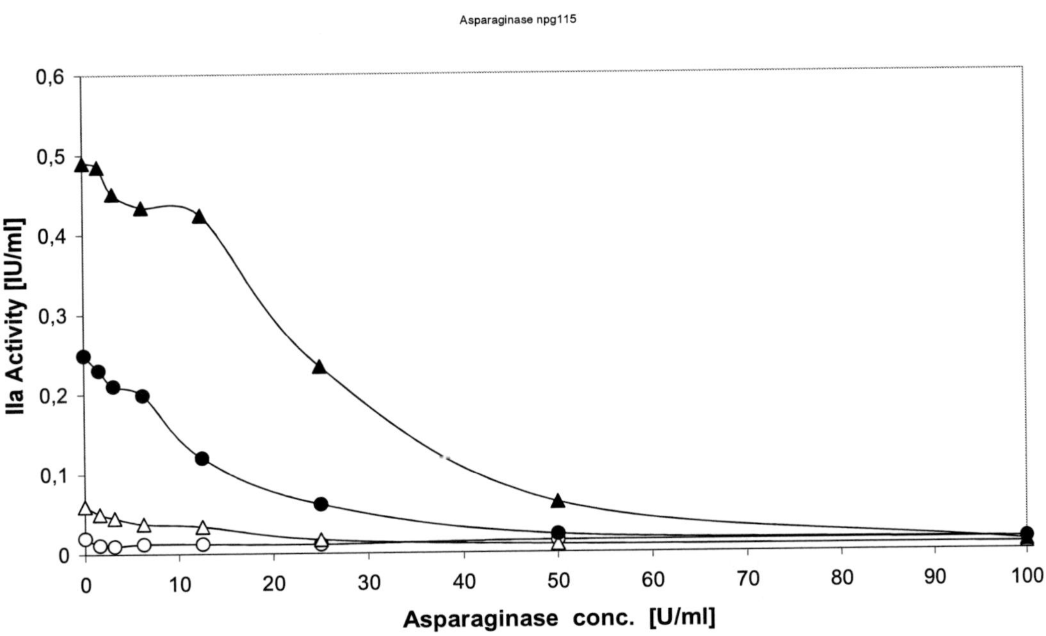

b

Figure 44. IIa generation in dependence of asparaginase concentration in sample 44. 50 µl unfrozen citrated normal plasma were supplemented in U-microwells (Brand®701300) with 0-100 U/ml asparaginase by repetitive 1+1 dilution. The RECA was performed. Figure 44a: 0 (O), 1.6 (Δ), 3.1 (◊), 6.3 (□), 12.5 (●), 25 (▲), 50 (♦), or 100 (■) U/ml asparaginase. Figure 44b: coagulation reaction times (CRT) of 5 min (O), 10 min (Δ), 15 min (●), or 20 min (▲). Approx. IC50 = 13 U/ml asparaginase.

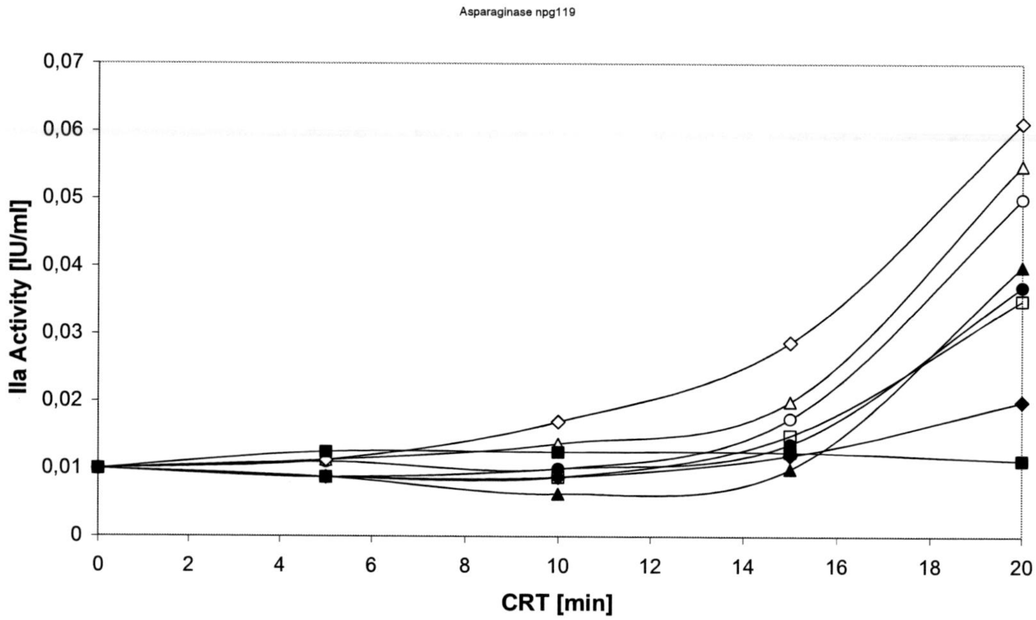

a

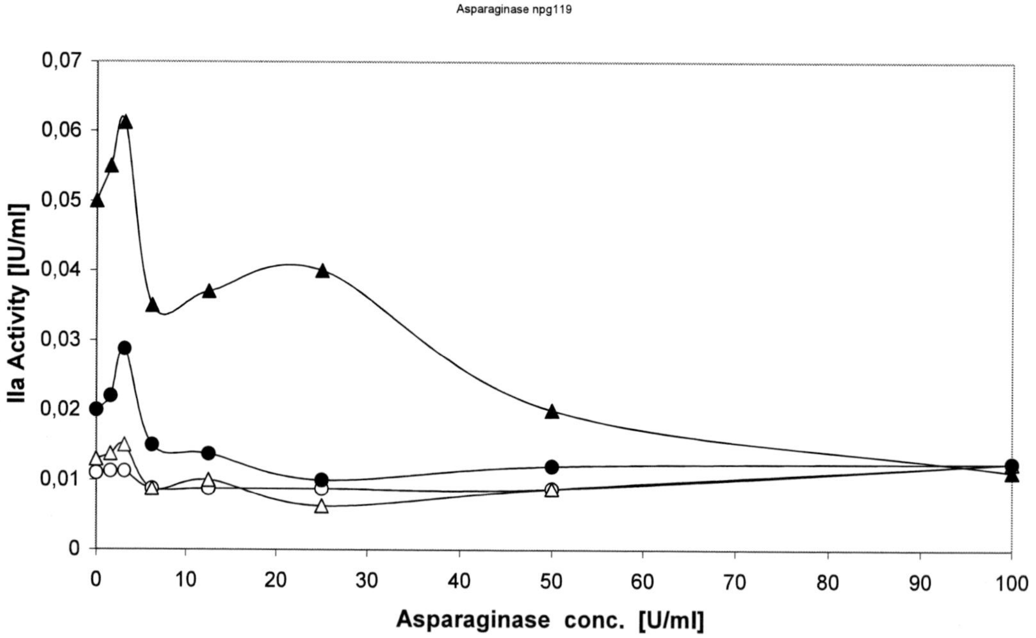

b

Figure 45. IIa generation in dependence of asparaginase concentration in sample 45. 50 µl unfrozen citrated normal plasma were supplemented in U-microwells (Brand®701300) with 0-100 U/ml asparaginase by repetitive 1+1 dilution. The RECA was performed. Figure 45a: 0 (O), 1.6 (Δ), 3.1 (◊), 6.3 (□), 12.5 (●), 25 (▲), 50 (♦), or 100 (■) U/ml asparaginase. Figure 45b: coagulation reaction times (CRT) of 5 min (O), 10 min (Δ), 15 min (●), or 20 min (▲). Approx. IC50 = 40 U/ml asparaginase.

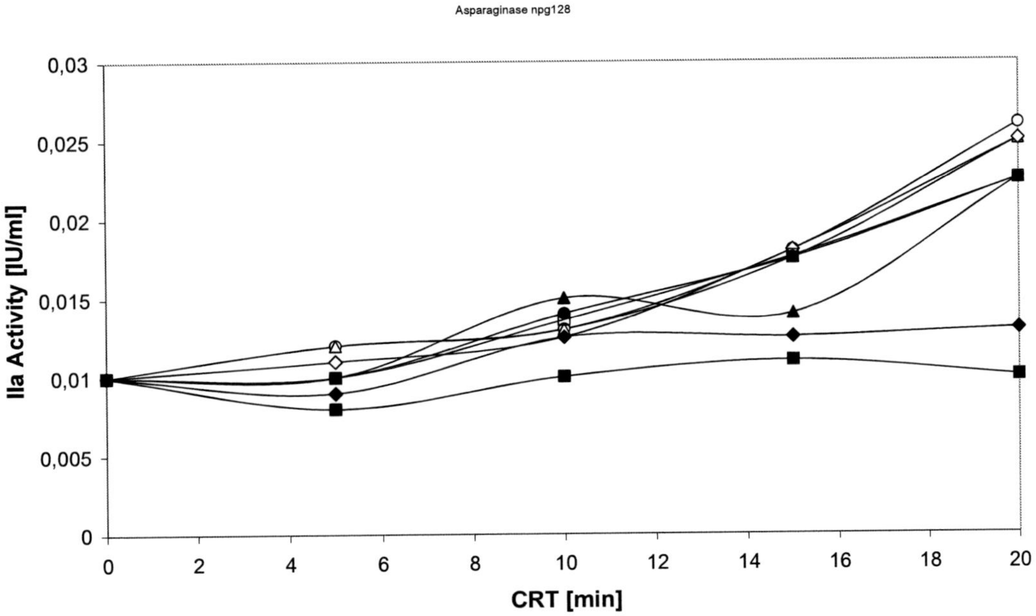

a

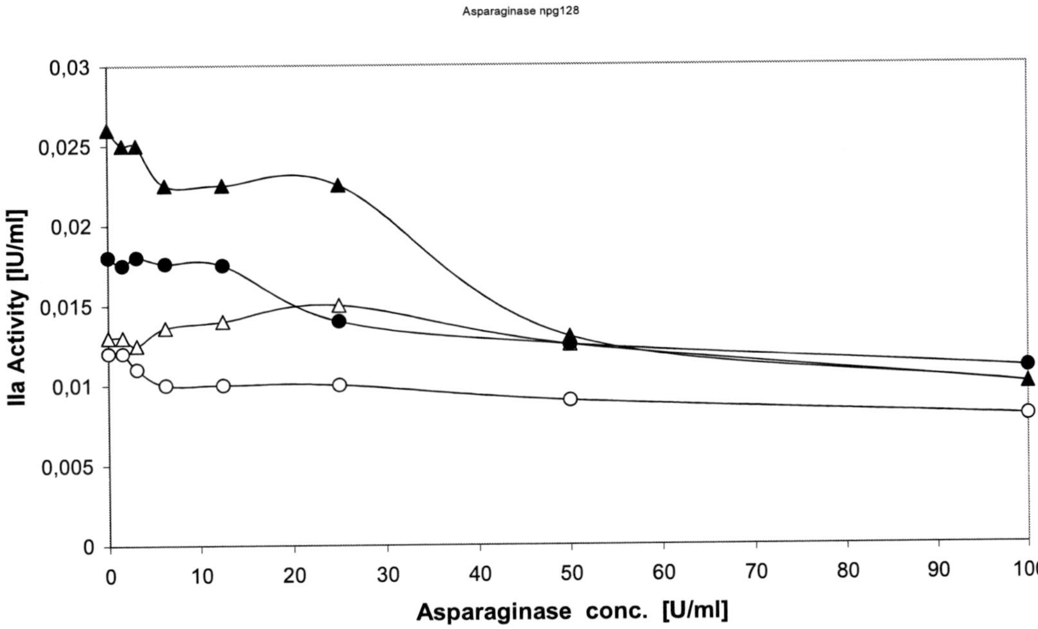

b

Figure 46. IIa generation in dependence of asparaginase concentration in sample 46. 50 μl unfrozen citrated normal plasma were supplemented in U-microwells (Brand®701300) with 0-100 U/ml asparaginase by repetitive 1+1 dilution. The RECA was performed. Figure 46a: 0 (O), 1.6 (Δ), 3.1 (◊), 6.3 (□), 12.5 (•), 25 (▲), 50 (♦), or 100 (■) U/ml asparaginase. Figure 46b: coagulation reaction times (CRT) of 5 min (O), 10 min (Δ), 15 min (•), or 20 min (▲). Approx. IC50 = 40 U/ml asparaginase.

The thrombin generation in pooled unfrozen normal plasma was analyzed in figures 47-52. Figure 53 demonstrates the mean values of thrombin activities in pools of unfrozen normal plasma. The approximate SC200 of the mean values was 6 U/ml asparaginase.

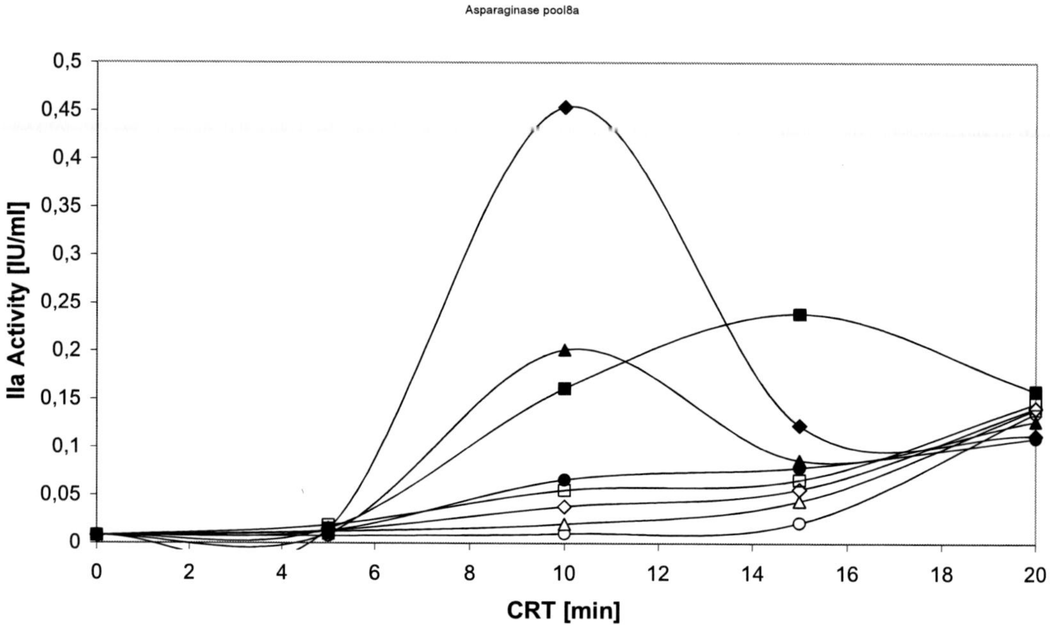

a

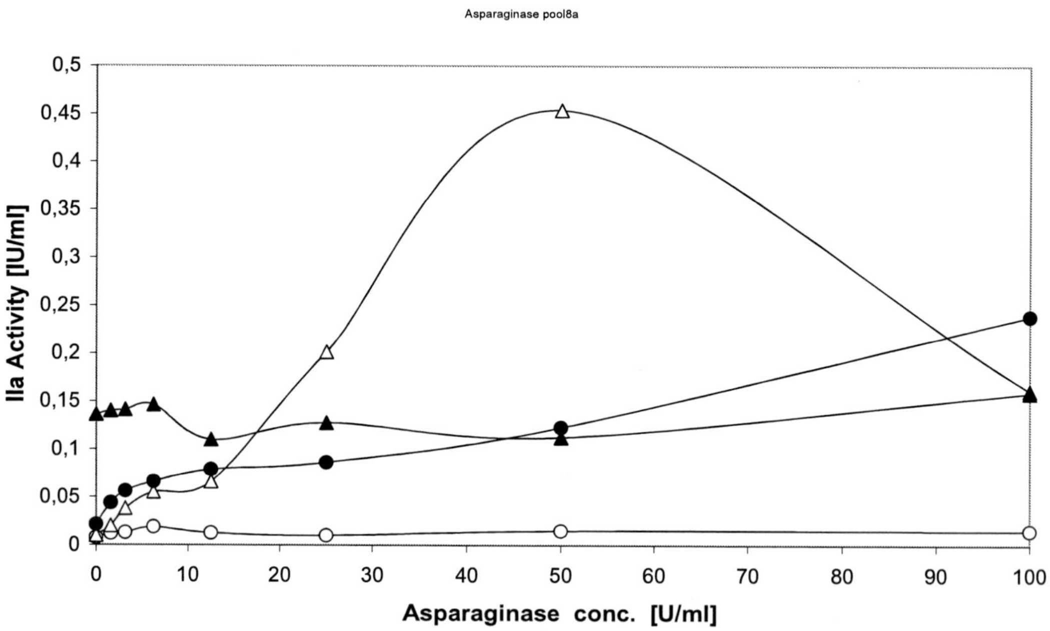

b

Figure 47. IIa generation in dependence of asparaginase concentration in pool 1. 50 µl pooled unfrozen citrated normal plasma were supplemented in U-microwells (Brand®701300) with 0-100 U/ml asparaginase by repetitive 1+1 dilution. The RECA was performed. Figure 47a: 0 (O), 1.6 (Δ), 3.1 (◊), 6.3 (□), 12.5 (●), 25 (▲), 50 (♦), or 100 (■) U/ml asparaginase. Figure 47b: coagulation reaction times (CRT) of 5 min (O), 10 min (Δ), 15 min (●), or 20 min (▲). Approx. SC200 = 1 U/ml asparaginase.

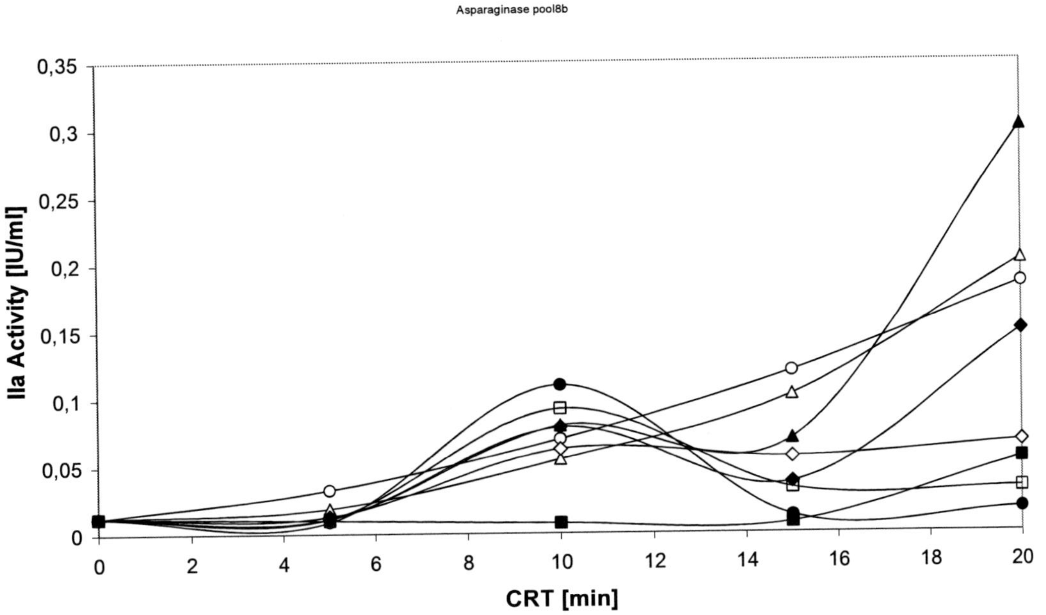

a

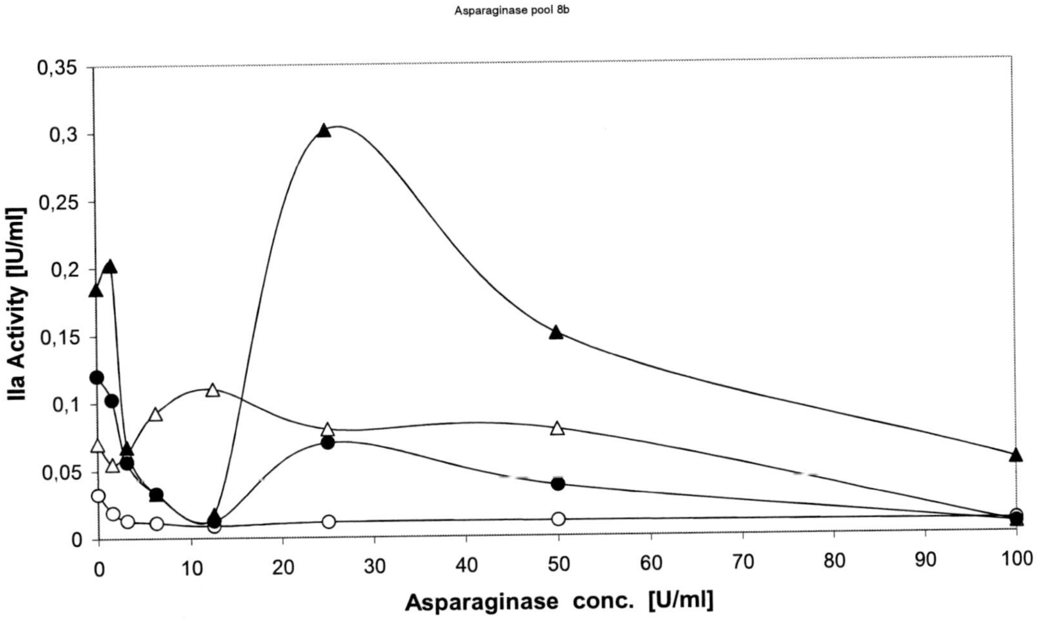

b

Figure 48. IIa generation in dependence of asparaginase concentration in pool 2. 50 µl pooled unfrozen citrated normal plasma were supplemented in U-microwells (Brand®701300) with 0-100 U/ml asparaginase by repetitive 1+1 dilution. The RECA was performed. Figure 48a: 0 (O), 1.6 (Δ), 3.1 (◊), 6.3 (□), 12.5 (●), 25 (▲), 50 (♦), or 100 (■) U/ml asparaginase. Figure 48b: coagulation reaction times (CRT) of 5 min (O), 10 min (Δ), 15 min (●), or 20 min (▲). Approx. IC50 = 3 U/ml asparaginase.

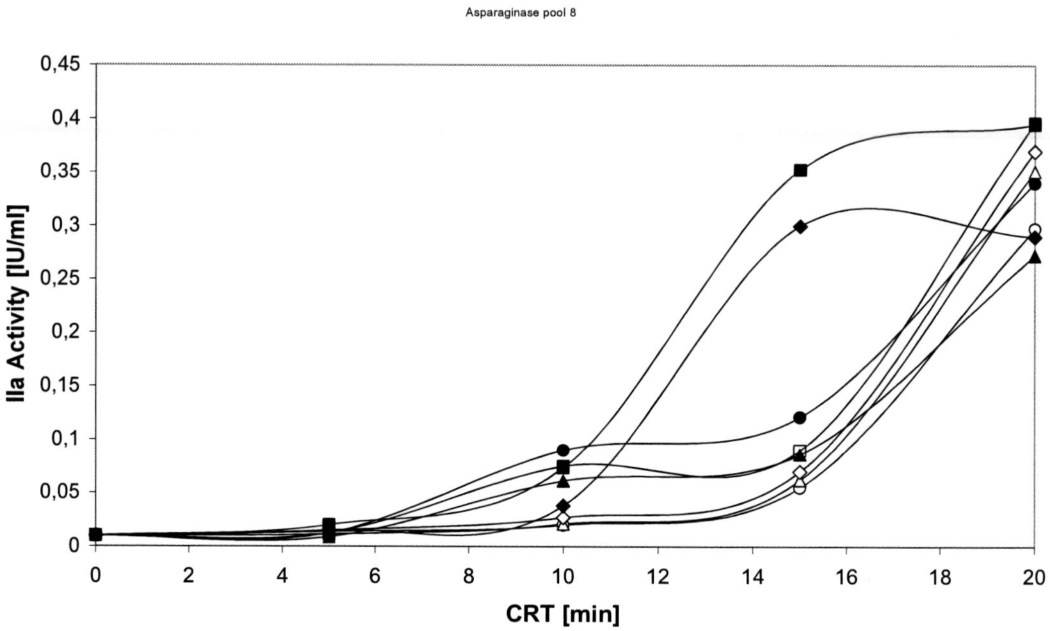

a

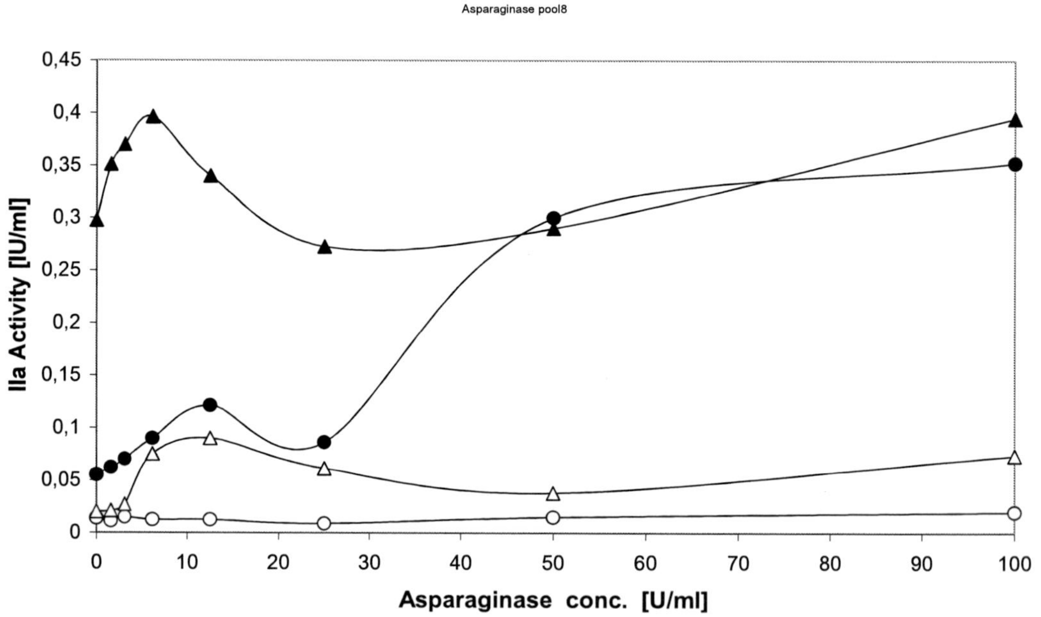

b

Figure 49. IIa generation in dependence of asparaginase concentration in pool 3. 50 µl pooled unfrozen citrated normal plasma were supplemented in U-microwells (Brand®701300) with 0-100 U/ml asparaginase by repetitive 1+1 dilution. The RECA was performed. Figure 49a: 0 (O), 1.6 (Δ), 3.1 (◊), 6.3 (□), 12.5 (●), 25 (▲), 50 (♦), or 100 (■) U/ml asparaginase. Figure 49b: coagulation reaction times (CRT) of 5 min (O), 10 min (Δ), 15 min (●), or 20 min (▲). Approx. SC200 = 8 U/ml asparaginase.

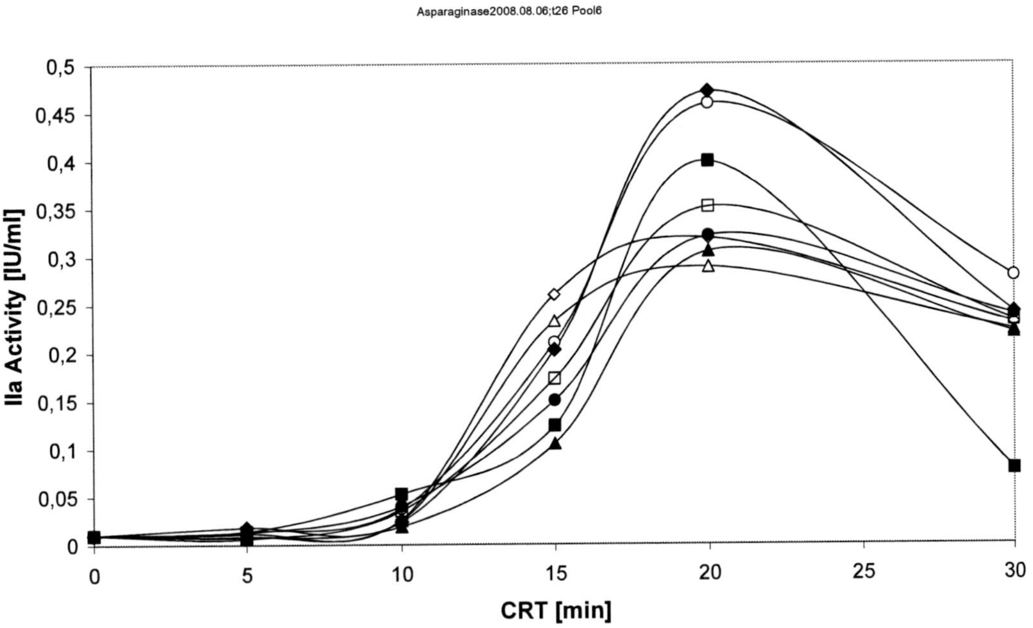

a

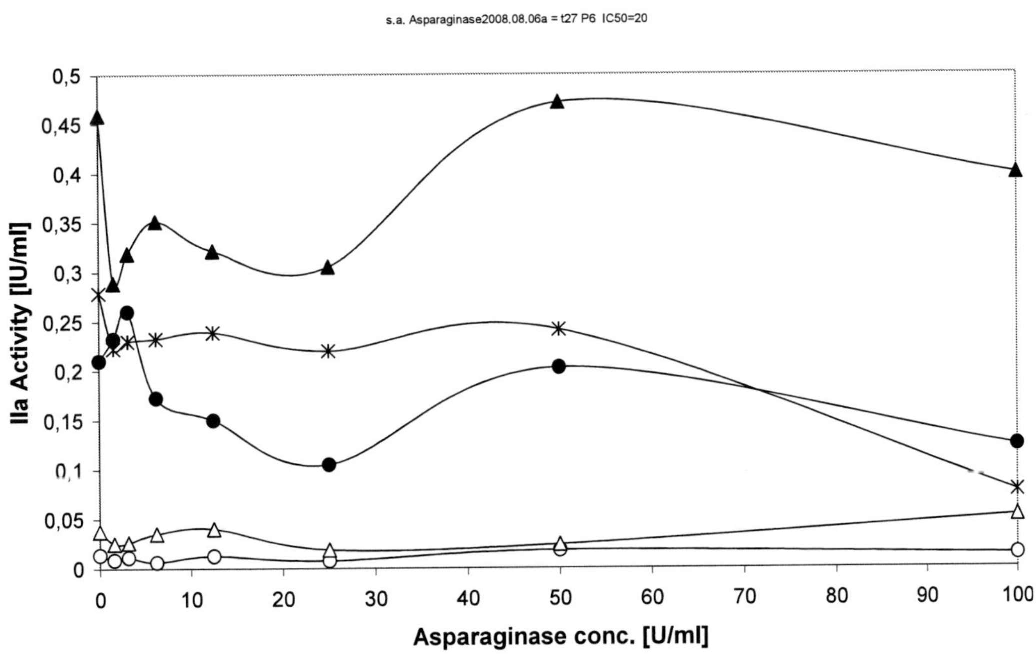

b

Figure 50. IIa generation in dependence of asparaginase concentration in pool 4. 50 µl pooled unfrozen citrated normal plasma were supplemented in U-microwells (Brand®701300) with 0-100 U/ml asparaginase by repetitive 1+1 dilution. The RECA was performed. Figure 50a: 0 (O), 1.6 (Δ), 3.1 (◊), 6.3 (□), 12.5 (●), 25 (▲), 50 (♦), or 100 (■) U/ml asparaginase. Figure 50b: coagulation reaction times (CRT) of 5 min (O), 10 min (Δ), 15 min (●), 20 min (▲), or 30 min (*). Approx. IC50 = 20 U/ml asparaginase.

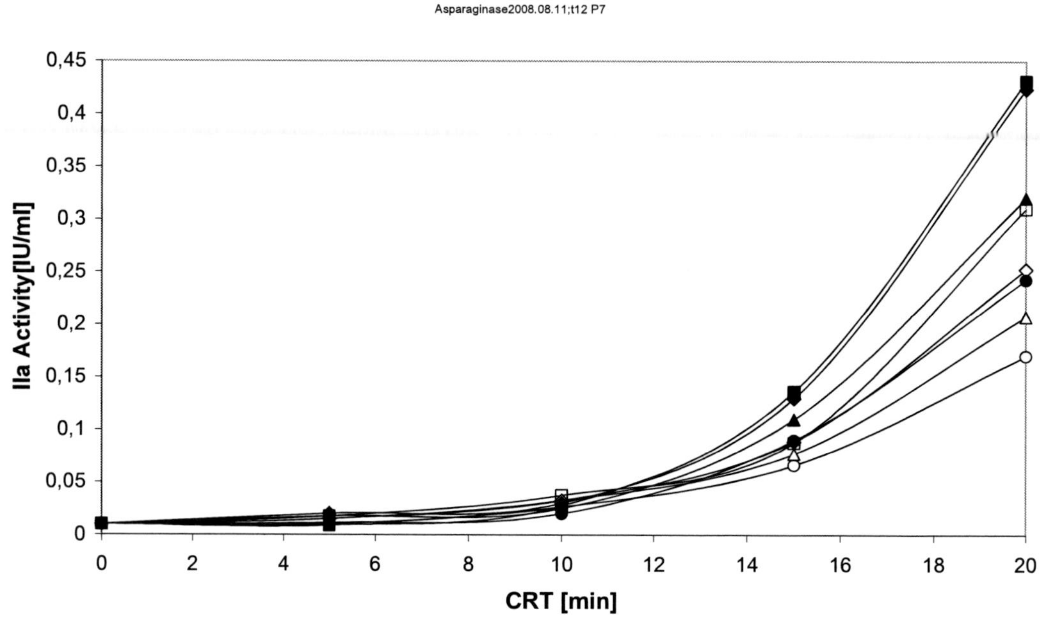

a

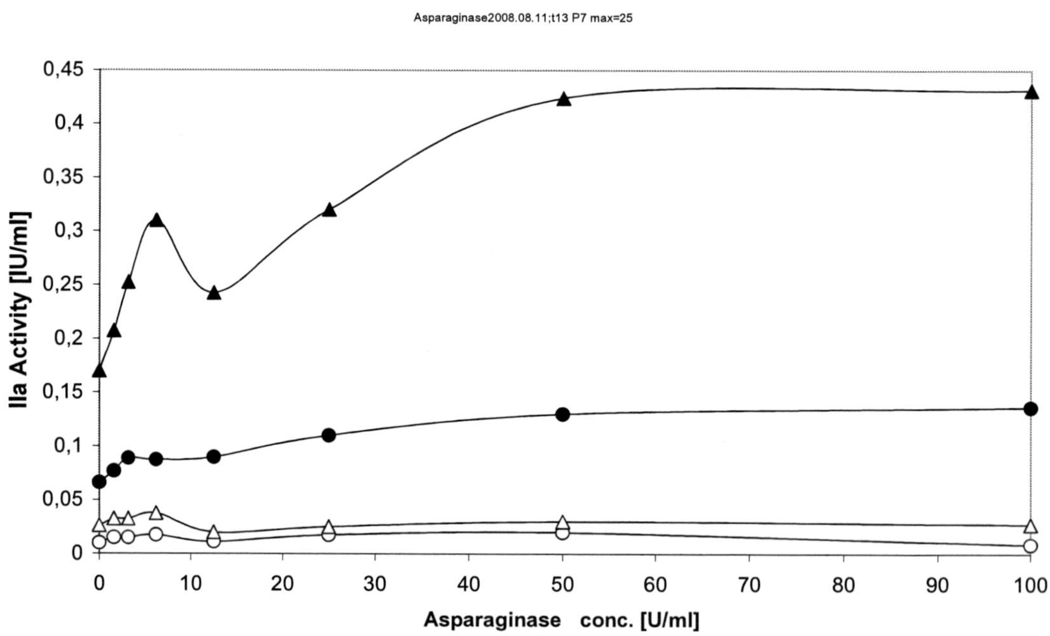

b

Figure 51. IIa generation in dependence of asparaginase concentration in pool 5. 50 µl pooled unfrozen citrated normal plasma were supplemented in U-microwells (Brand®701300) with 0-100 U/ml asparaginase by repetitive 1+1 dilution. The RECA was performed. Figure 51a: 0 (O), 1.6 (Δ), 3.1 (◊), 6.3 (□), 12.5 (●), 25 (▲), 50 (♦), or 100 (■) U/ml asparaginase. Figure 51b: coagulation reaction times (CRT) of 5 min (O), 10 min (Δ), 15 min (●), or 20 min (▲). Approx. IC50 = 25 U/ml asparaginase.

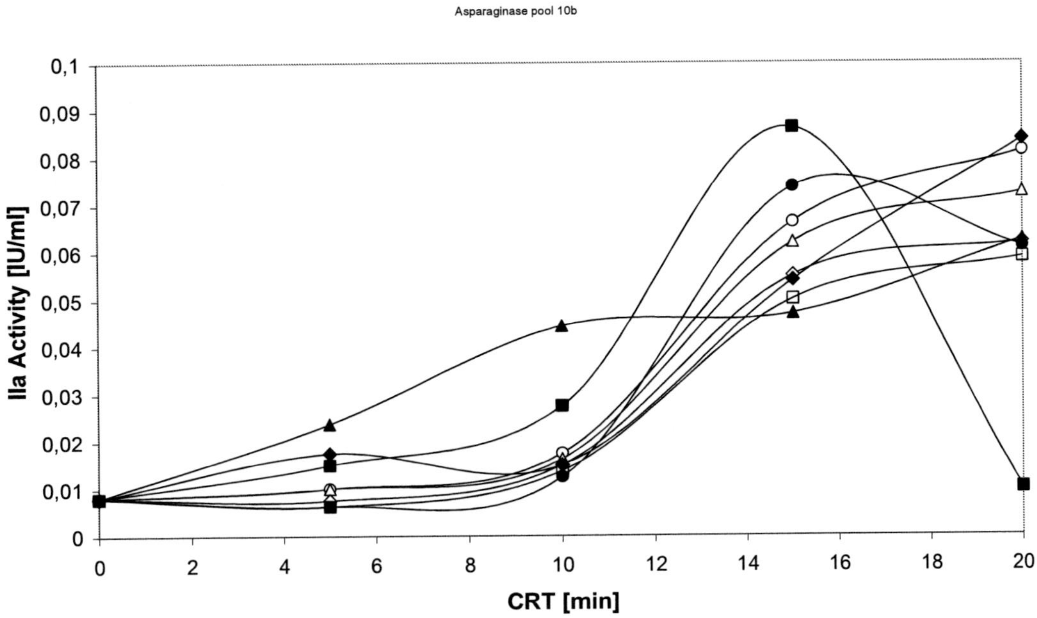

a

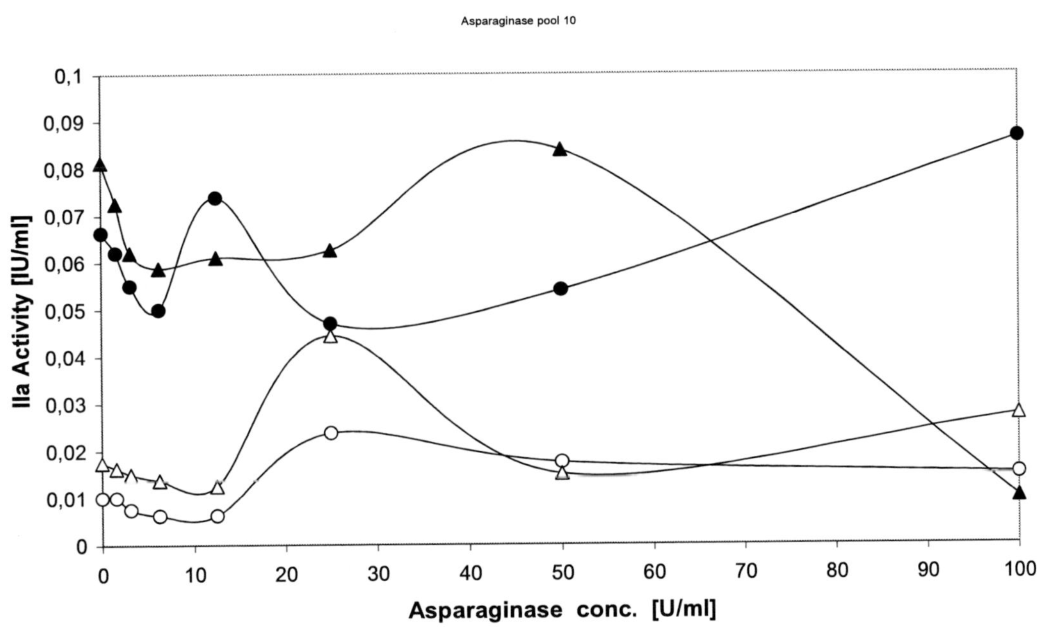

b

Figure 52. IIa generation in dependence of asparaginase concentration in pool 6. 50 µl pooled unfrozen citrated normal plasma were supplemented in U-microwells (Brand®701300) with 0-100 U/ml asparaginase by repetitive 1+1 dilution. The RECA was performed. Figure 52a: 0 (O), 1.6 (Δ), 3.1 (◊), 6.3 (□), 12.5 (●), 25 (▲), 50 (♦), or 100 (■) U/ml asparaginase. Figure 52b: coagulation reaction times (CRT) of 5 min (O), 10 min (Δ), 15 min (●), or 20 min (▲). The approx. IC 50 was 80 U/ml and the approx. SC200 was 15 U/ml asparaginase.

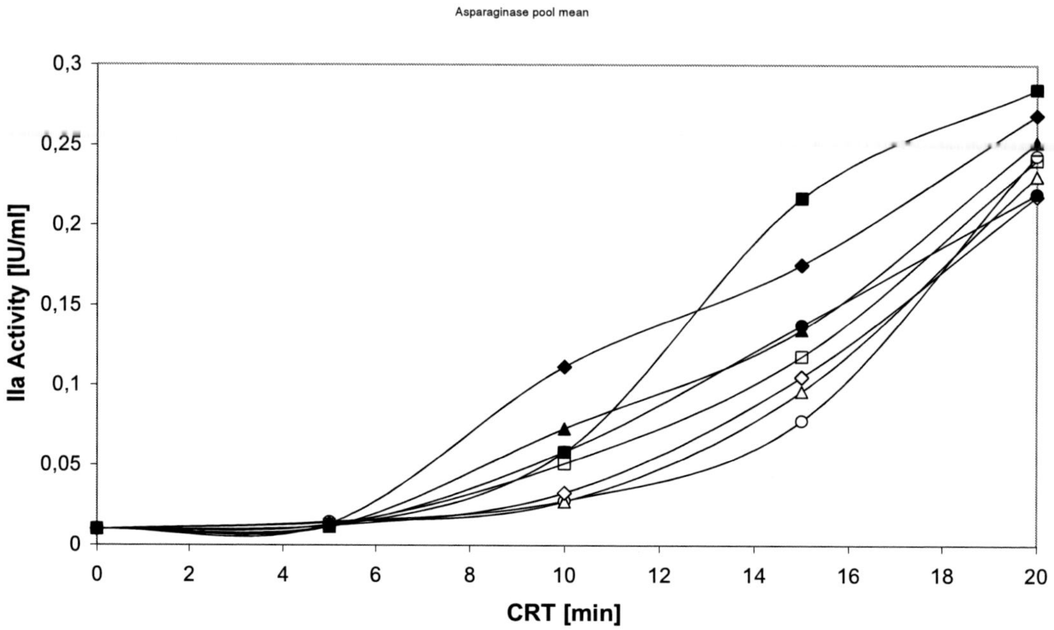

a

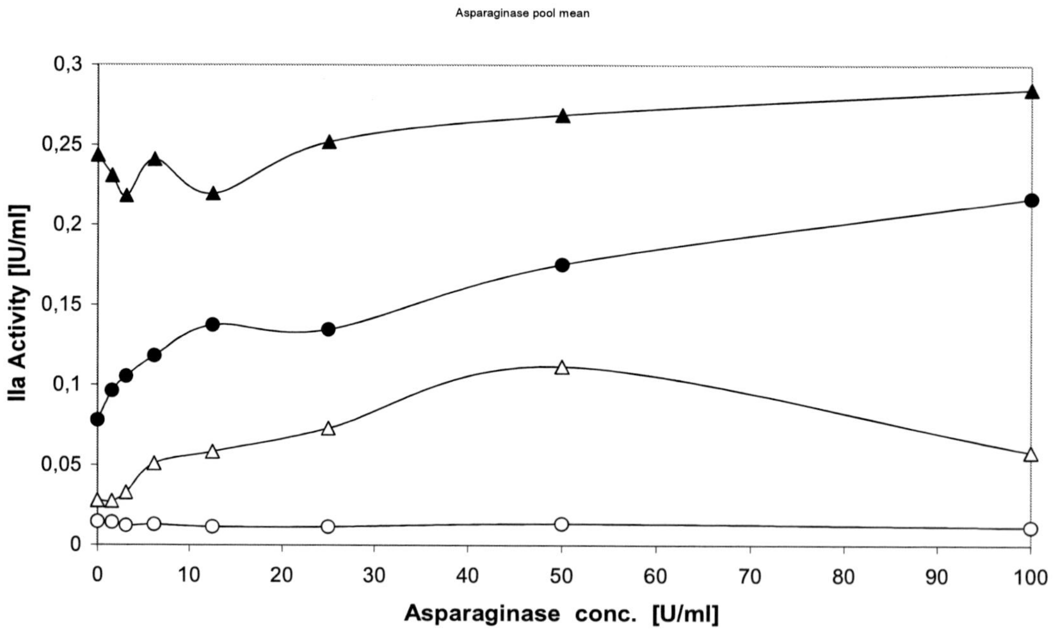

b

Figure 53. Mean value of IIa activities in pools in dependence of asparaginase concentration. The mean RECA-values of n=7 unfrozen plasma pools were calculated. Figure 53a: 0 (O), 1.6 (Δ), 3.1 (◊), 6.3 (□), 12.5 (●), 25 (▲), 50 (♦), or 100 (■) U/ml asparaginase. Figure 53b: coagulation reaction times (CRT) of 5 min (O), 10 min (Δ), 15 min (●), or 20 min (▲). The approx. SC200 was 6 U/ml asparaginase.

Figure 54 is the thrombin activity curve in a healthy donor. This plasma had with this lot of asparaginase an approximate IC50 of 4 U/ml (when analyzed at RECA-15) and an approximate SC200 of 5 U/ml (when analyzed at RECA-5) asparaginase, i.e. this individual might have a risk for both thrombosis and severe bleeding if therapied by this lot of asparaginase.

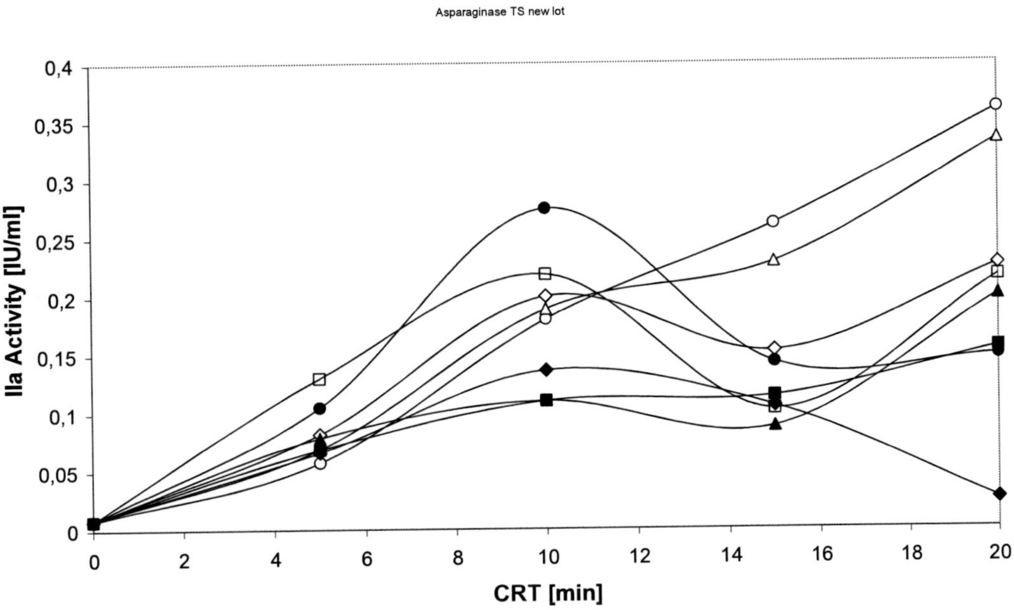

a

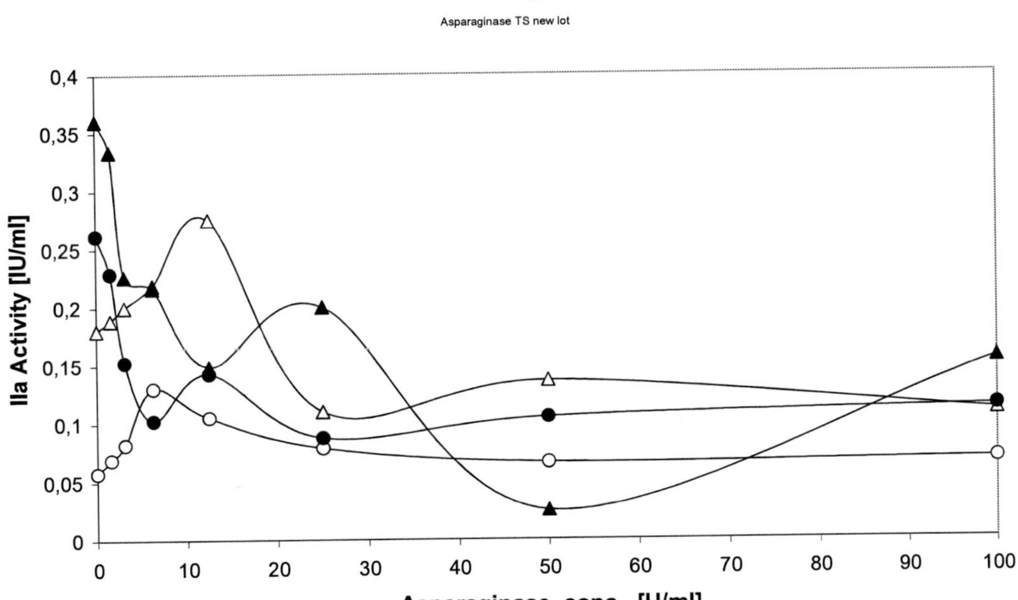

b

Figure 54. IIa generation in a healthy donor. 50 μl unfrozen citrated plasma of a healthy donor were supplemented in U-microwells (Brand®701300) with 0-100 U/ml asparaginase. The RECA was performed. Figure 54a: 0 (O), 1.6 (Δ), 3.1 (◊), 6.3 (□), 12.5 (●), 25 (▲), 50 (♦), or 100 (■) U/ml asparaginase. Figure 54b: coagulation reaction times (CRT) of 5 min (O), 10 min (Δ), 15 min (●), or 20 min (▲).The approx. IC50 was 4 U/ml and the approx. SC200 was 5 U/ml asparaginase.

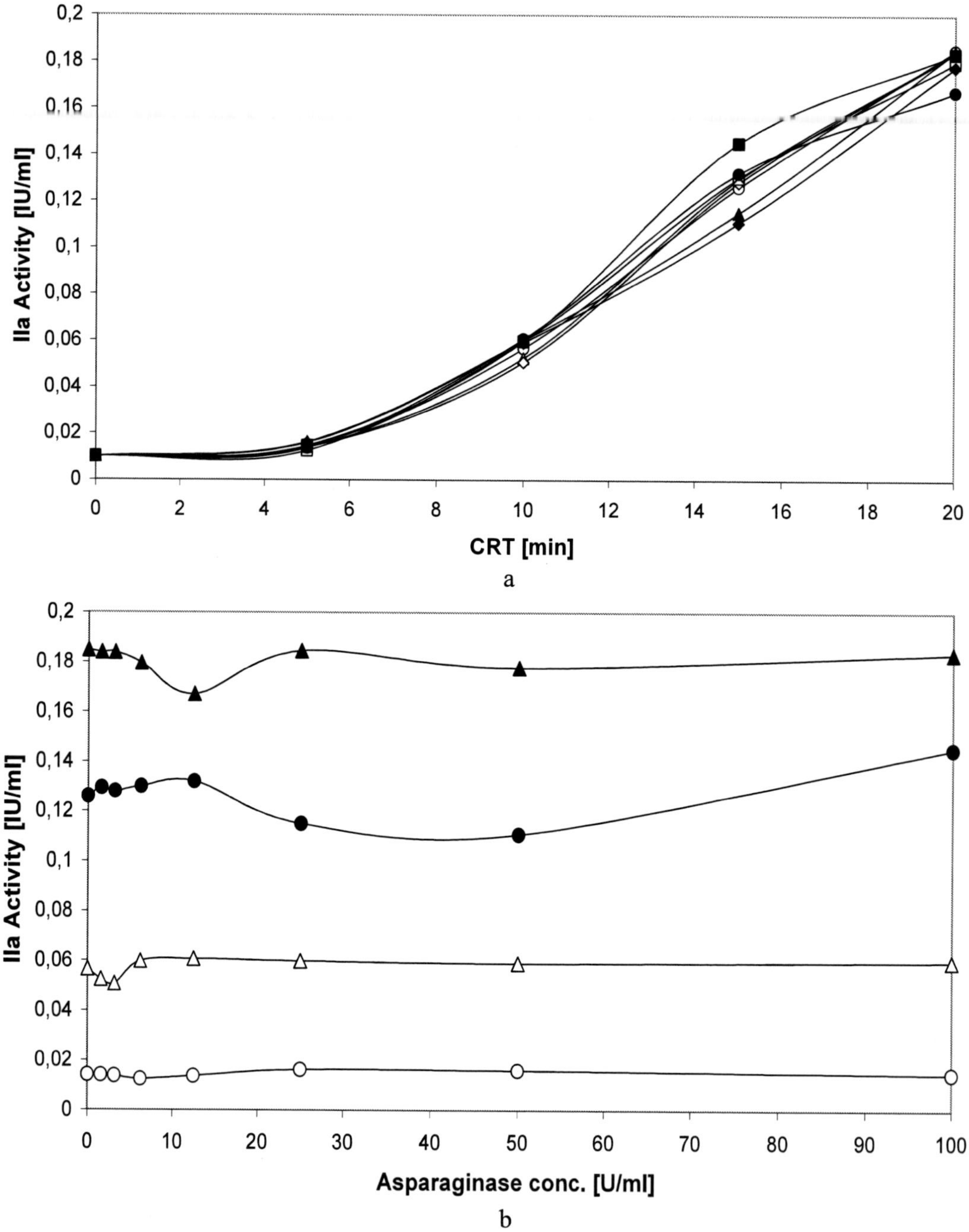

Figure 55. Mean values of IIa activities in dependence of asparaginase concentration. The mean RECA-values of n=58 patient samples were calculated. Figure 55a: 0 (O), 1.6 (Δ), 3.1 (◊), 6.3 (□), 12.5 (●), 25 (▲), 50 (♦), or 100 (■) U/ml asparaginase. Figure 55b: coagulation reaction times (CRT) of 5 min (O), 10 min (Δ), 15 min (●), or 20 min (▲). In the mean values there appeared neither an IC50 nor a SC200.

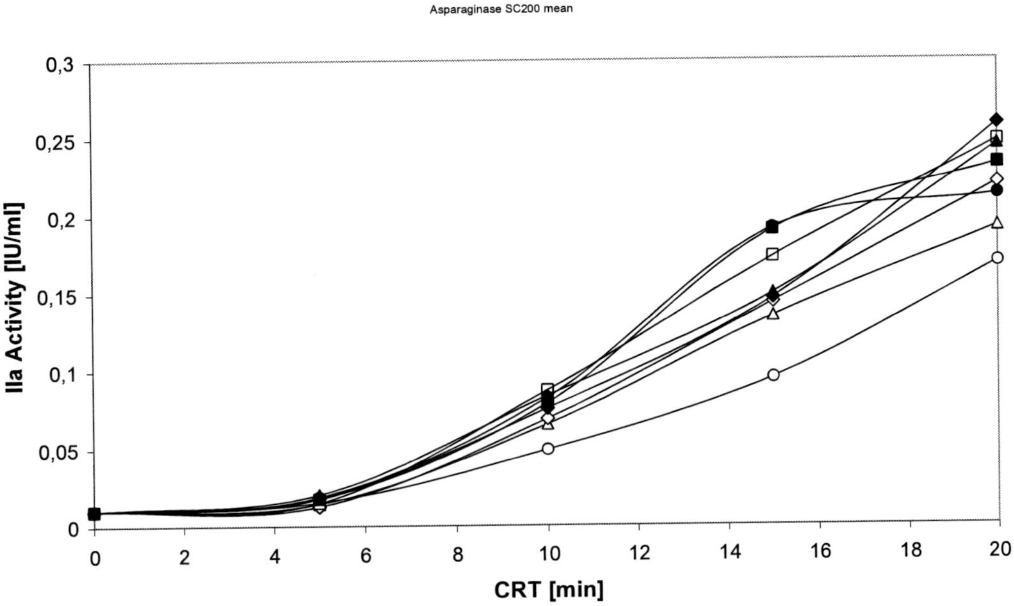

a

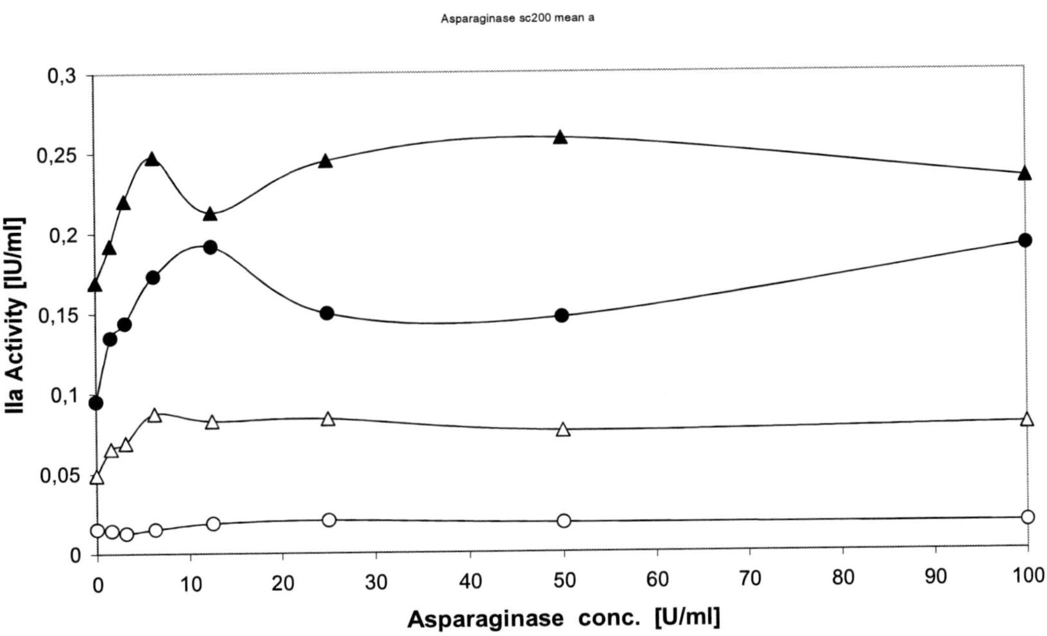

b

Figure 56. Mean IIa activities in samples with an asparaginase-SC200. The mean RECA values of n=29 samples with a SC200 of plasmatic asparaginase were calculated. Figure 56a: 0 (O), 1.6 (Δ), 3.1 (◊), 6.3 (□), 12.5 (●), 25 (▲), 50 (♦), or 100 (■) U/ml asparaginase. Figure 56b: coagulation reaction times (CRT) of 5 min (O), 10 min (Δ), 15 min (●), or 20 min (▲).The approx. SC200 was 10 U/ml asparaginase.

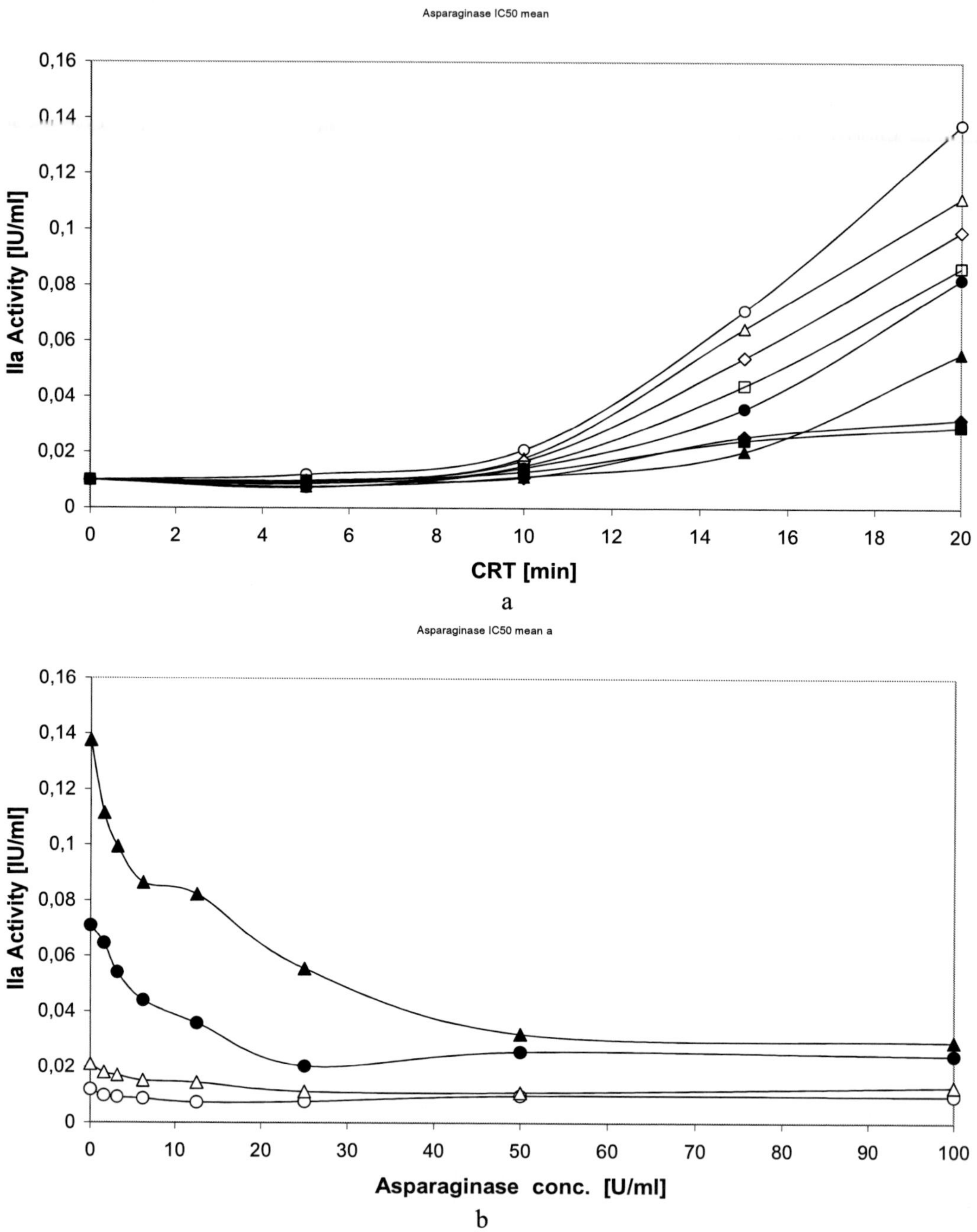

Figure 57. Mean IIa activities in samples with an asparaginase-IC50. The mean RECA values of n=12 samples with a SC200 of plasmatic asparaginase were calculated. Figure 57a: 0 (O), 1.6 (Δ), 3.1 (◊), 6.3 (□), 12.5 (●), 25 (▲), 50 (♦), or 100 (■) U/ml asparaginase. Figure 57b: coagulation reaction times (CRT) of 5 min (O), 10 min (Δ), 15 min (●), or 20 min (▲). The approx. IC50 was 10 U/ml asparaginase.

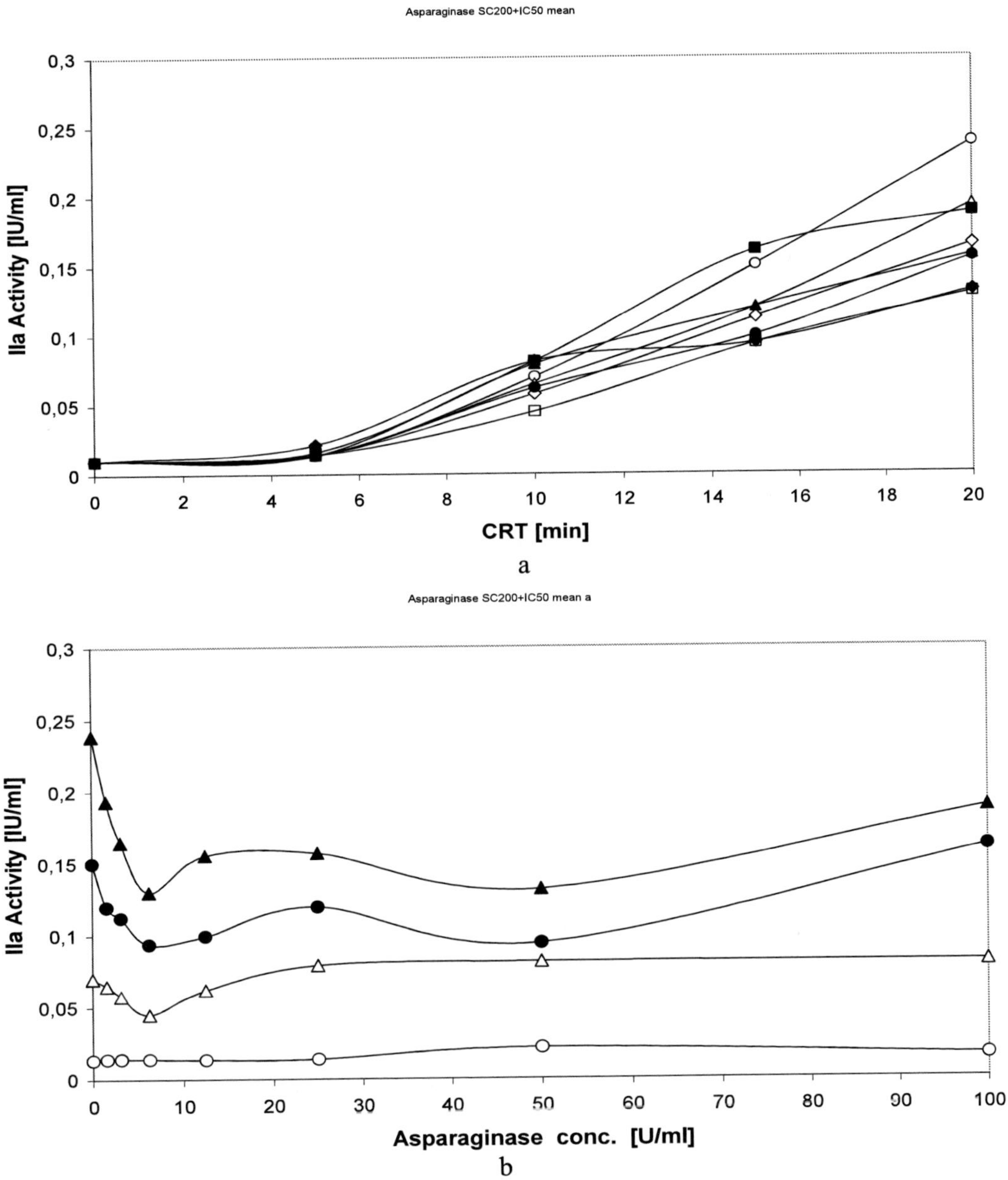

Figure 58. Mean IIa activities in samples with both an asparaginase - SC200 and an - IC50. The mean RECA values of n=15 samples with a SC200 of plasmatic asparaginase were calculated. Figure 58a: 0 (O), 1.6 (Δ), 3.1 (◊), 6.3 (□), 12.5 (•), 25 (▲), 50 (♦), or 100 (■) U/ml asparaginase. Figure 58b: coagulation reaction times (CRT) of 5 min (O), 10 min (Δ), 15 min (•), or 20 min (▲).The approx. SC200 was 40 U/ml asparaginase (analyzed at 5 min CRT = RECA-5), the approx. IC50 was 4 U/ml asparaginase (analyzed at 10 min CRT = RECA-10).

Figure 55 demonstrates the mean values of thrombin activities of n=57 normal samples. There appeared neither an IC50 nor a SC200. This means that the mean values of normal samples behaved as if the added asparaginase had no modulatory activity on plasmatic hemostasis, whereas asparaginase indeed modulates the hemostatic system of most individual plasmas (see figures 1-20, 23-46, 54).

Only 2 of the 57 individual plasma samples (3.5%) had neither an asparaginase - SC200 nor an asparaginase - IC50 up to asparaginase activities of 100 U/ml (Figure 21,22). 29 of 57 samples (51%) had only a SC200, 12 of 57 (21%) had only an IC50, and 14 of 57 (24.5%) had both a SC200 and an IC50. Of the n=29 individual plasma samples with only a SC200 for asparaginase about one third (10/29) of the samples had a SC200 < 3 U/ml, about one third (10/29) of the samples had a SC200 of 3-20 U/ml, and about one third (9/29) of the samples had a SC200 > 20 U/ml.

Figure 56 demonstrates the mean values of thrombin activities in plasmas with an asparaginase-SC200. The approximate SC200 of the mean values was 10 U/ml asparaginase. The mean values of thrombin activities in plasmas with an asparaginase-IC50 also gave an approximate IC50 of about 10 U/ml (Figure 57). The mean values of thrombin generation in plasmas with a combined SC200/IC50 resulted in an approximate SC200 of 40 U/ml (analyzed at RECA-5) and in an approximate IC50 of 4 U/ml asparaginase (analyzed at RECA-10).

Discussion

The clinical oncologist is often confronted with severe hemostasis problems that are induced in the blood of patients treated with agents that act against cancerous cells [3,11-16]. Asparaginase, e.g. attacks lymphoblasts, fragmented lymphoblasts together with the given asparaginase itself or cells that have been destroyed via NH_3-toxicity (via their phospholipid microparticles) can trigger the intrinsic phase of hemostasis. Asparaginase is used at doses of about 200 units/kg (about 6000 units/m^2) [15]. The dosage might be elevated to about 1000 units/kg, to about 1500 units/kg, or even more. The calculated corresponding plasma activities would be about 5 U/ml, about 25 U/ml, or > 25 U/ml.

The present study was undertaken to quantify the in-vitro hemostasis-altering action of asparaginase. Surprisingly, it was found that asparaginase not only might trigger intrinsic thrombin generation in many individual plasmas (here in about one half of the samples), it could also pathologically decrease thrombin generation (here in about one fourth of the samples), or it could both increase and decrease thrombin generation (here in about one fourth of the samples), depending on the reaction time of asparaginase on the recalcified contact system of hemostasis; i.e. the present preparation of asparaginase might activate or inactivate intrinsic factors of plasmatic coagulation. Some asparaginase-types might also attack critical diamino amino acids within susceptible proteins [17], especially within unglycosylated (immature) proteins glycosylated asparagine could be protected against the action of asparaginase.

Currently, there are 3 different asparaginases in clinical use: Escherichia coli – asparaginase, Erwinia chrysanthemi – asparaginase (both with half-lifes of about 1d), and pegylated asparaginase, i.e the Escherichia coli – asparaginase modified by covalent binding of polyethylene glycol (with a half-life of about 6d) [18-20]. Eschericia coli- asparaginase seems to activate coagulation more than Erwinia chrysanthemi–asparaginase, however at comparable doses the Escherichia coli-asparaginase depletes blood asparagines better than the Erwinia chrysanthemi-asparaginase, i.e. the Escherichia coli-asparaginase is more active [19,21]. The RECA is an interesting tool to predict the reactivity of the coagulation system of the individual patient towards any drug, e.g. all different types of asparaginase-preparations, allowing necessary individual adjustments of dosage [22].

In conclusion, the present work demonstrates that it is possible to establish the coagulation - altering capacity of asparaginase in individual plasma samples prior to administration of asparaginase against ALL or NHL. With such a test, the patient´s individual coagulation response to any drug could be pre-viewed, what currently is not possible [23]. Patients at risk for pathologically enhanced or for pathologically decreased plasmatic thrombin generation, which could result in thrombosis or in severe bleeding, respectively, could be identified prior to administration of a certain drug. Furthermore, the described RECA might determine the maximally tolerable dosage of plasmatic asparaginase for each individual patient. If there are different preparations of asparaginase available, the physician might prefer a preparation that slightly enhances thrombin generation to one that drastically decreases thrombin generation: patients at risk for asparaginase-induced thrombosis might be prophylactically given low molecular weight heparin [24].

ACKNOWLEDGMENTS

This work is part of the academic thesis (MD) of Danuta Chalkitis.

REFERENCES

[1] Panosyan EH, Grigoryan RS, Avramis IA, Seibel NL, Gaynon PS, Siegel SE, Fingert HJ, Avramis VI. Deamination of glutamine is a prerequisite for optimal asparagine deamination by asparaginases in vivo (CCG-1961).*Anticancer Res.* 2004; 24: 1121-5.

[2] Appel IM, Hop WC, van Kessel-Bakvis C, Stigter R, Pieters R. L-Asparaginase and the effect of age on coagulation and fibrinolysis in childhood acute lymphoblastic leukemia. *Thromb. Haemost.* 2008; 100: 330-7.

[3] Sutherland DE, Weitz IC, Liebman HA. Thromboembolic complications of cancer: epidemiology, pathogenesis, diagnosis, and treatment. *Am. J. Hematol.* 2003; 72: 43-52.

[4] Grigoryan RS, Panosyan EH, Seibel NL, Gaynon PS, Avramis IA, Avramis VI. *Changes of amino acid serum levels in pediatric patients with higher-risk acute lymphoblastic leukemia* (CCG-1961). In Vivo 2004; 18: 107-12.

[5] Mitchell L, Hoogendoorn H, Giles AR, Vegh P, Andrew M. Increased endogenous thrombin generation in children with acute lymphoblastic leukemia: risk of thrombotic complications in L-Asparaginase-induced antithrombin III deficiency. *Blood* 1994; 83: 386-91.

[6] Stief TW. Thrombin generation by exposure of blood to endotoxin: a simple model to study disseminated intravascular coagulation. *Clin. Appl. Thromb. Hemost.* 2006 ; 12: 137-61.

[7] Stief TW. Innovative tests of plasmatic hemostasis. *Laboratory Medicine* 2008; 39: 225-230.

[8] Stief TW. The Laboratory diagnosis of the pre-phase of pathologic disseminated intravascular coagulation. *Hemostasis Laboratory* 2008; 1: 2-20.

[9] Stief TW. Specific determination of plasmatic thrombin activity. *Clin. Appl. Thromb. Hemost.* 2006; 12: 324-9.

[10] Mosesson MW. Update on antithrombin I (fibrin). *Thromb. Haemost.* 2007; 98: 105-8.

[11] Payne JH, Vora AJ. Thrombosis and acute lymphoblastic leukaemia. *Br. J. Haematol.* 2007; 138: 430-45.

[12] Athale UH, Chan AK. Thromboembolic complications in pediatric hematologic malignancies. *Semin. Thromb. Hemost.* 2007; 33: 416-26.

[13] Appel IM, Hop WC, Pieters R. Changes in hypercoagulability by asparaginase: a randomized study between two asparaginases. *Blood Coagul. Fibrinolysis* 2006; 17: 139-46.

[14] Athale UH, Chan AK. Thrombosis in children with acute lymphoblastic leukemia. Part II. Pathogenesis of thrombosis in children with acute lymphoblastic leukemia: effects of the disease and therapy. *Thromb. Res.* 2003; 111: 199-212.

[15] Leone G, Gugliotta L, Mazzucconi MG, De Stefano V, Belmonte MM, Dragoni F, Specchia G, Centra A, Gamba G, Camera A, et al. Evidence of a hypercoagulable state in patients with acute lymphoblastic leukemia treated with low dose of E. coli L-asparaginase: a GIMEMA study. *Thromb. Haemost.* 1993; 69: 12-5.

[16] Barbui T, Rodeghiero F, Meli S, Dini E. Fatal pulmonary embolism and antithrombin III deficiency in adult lymphoblastic leukaemia during L-asparaginase therapy. *Acta Haematol.* 1983; 69: 188-91.

[17] Shapiro RS, Gerrard JM, Ramsay NK, Nesbit ME, Coccia PF, Stoddard SF, Plow EF, White JG, Krivit W. Selective deficiency in collagen-induced platelet aggregation during L-asparaginase therapy. *Am. J. Pediatr. Hematol. Oncol.* 1980; 2: 207-12.

[18] Asselin BL. The three asparaginases. Comparative pharmacology and optimal use in childhood leukemia. *Adv. Exp. Med. Biol.* 1999; 457: 621-9.

[19] Nowak-Göttl U, Ahlke E, Klösel K, Jürgens H, Boos J. Changes in coagulation and fibrinolysis in childhood acute lymphoblastic leukaemia re-induction therapy using three different asparaginase preparations. *Eur. J. Pediatr.* 1997; 156: 848-50.

[20] Graham ML, Asselin BL, Herndon JE 2nd, Casey JR, Chaffee S, Ciocci GH, Daeschner CW, Davis AR, Gold S, Halperin EC, Laughlin MJ, Martin PL, Olson JF, Kurtzberg J. Toxicity, pharmacology and feasibility of administration of PEG-L-asparaginase as consolidation therapy in patients undergoing bone marrow transplantation for acute lymphoblastic leukemia. *Bone Marrow Transplant* 1998 ; 21: 879-85.

[21] Castaman G, Rodeghiero F. Erwinia- and E. coli-derived L-asparaginase have similar effects on hemostasis. Pilot study in 10 patients with acute lymphoblastic leukemia. *Haematologica* 1993; 78 (6 Suppl 2): 57-60.

[22] Nowak-Göttl U, Ahlke E, Schulze-Westhoff P, Boos J. Changes in coagulation and fibrinolysis in childhood ALL: a two-step dose reduction of one E. coli asparaginase preparation. *Br. J. Haematol.* 1996; 95: 123-6.

[23] Payne JH, Vora AJ. Thrombosis and acute lymphoblastic leukaemia. *Br. J. Haematol.* 2007; 138: 430-45.

[24] Stief TW, Ajib S, Renz H. The sensibility of individual plasma to heparins. *Hemostasis Laboratory* 2008; 1: 143-157.

INDEX

A

D

E

H

I

K

L

M

N

O

P

Q

R

T

U